FOURTH EDITION

CASE FILES®
Family Medicine

Eugene C. Toy, MD
Assistant Dean for Educational Programs
Professor and Vice Chair of Medical Education
Department of Obstetrics and Gynecology
McGovern Medical School at The University
  of Texas Health Science Center at Houston
  (UTHealth)
Houston, Texas

Donald Briscoe, MD, FAAFP
Director, Family Medicine Residency Program
  and Chair
Department of Family Medicine, Houston
  Methodist Hospital
Family Medicine Clerkship Director
Texas A&M College of Medicine—Houston
  Campus
Chief Medical Officer, Vecino Health Centers
Associate Professor of Clinical Family Medicine
Houston Methodist Institute for Academic
  Medicine
Houston, Texas

Bruce Britton, MD
Professor of Family Medicine and Community
  Medicine
Family Medicine Director of Medical Student
  Education
Department of Family and Community
  Medicine
Eastern Virginia Medical School
Norfolk, Virginia

Joel J. Heidelbaugh, MD, FAAFP, FACG
Clinical Professor
Departments of Family Medicine and Urology
Clerkship Director
Department of Family Medicine
University of Michigan Medical School
Ann Arbor, Michigan

Mc
Graw
Hill
Education

New York   Chicago   San Francisco   Athens   London   Madrid
Mexico City   Milan   New Delhi   Singapore   Sydney   Toronto

Case Files®: Family Medicine, Fourth Edition

1 2 3 4 5 6 7 8 9 0   DOC/DOC   20 19 18 17 16

ISBN 978-1-259-58770-2
MHID 1-259-58770-3

Notice

Medicine is an ever-changing science. As new research and clinical experience broaden our knowledge, changes in treatment and drug therapy are required. The authors and the publisher of this work have checked with sources believed to be reliable in their efforts to provide information that is complete and generally in accord with the standard accepted at the time of publication. However, in view of the possibility of human error or changes in medical sciences, neither the editors nor the publisher nor any other party who has been involved in the preparation or publication of this work warrants that the information contained herein is in every respect accurate or complete, and they disclaim all responsibility for any errors or omissions or for the results obtained from use of the information contained in this work. Readers are encouraged to confirm the information contained herein with other sources. For example and in particular, readers are advised to check the product information sheet included in the package of each drug they plan to administer to be certain that the information contained in this work is accurate and that changes have not been made in the recommended dose or in the contraindications for administration. This recommendation is of particular importance in connection with new or infrequently used drugs.

This book was set in Adobe Jenson Pro by Cenveo® Publisher Services.
The editors were Catherine A. Johnson and Cindy Yoo.
The production supervisor was Catherine H. Saggese.
Project management was provided by Raghavi Khullar, Cenveo Publisher Services.
RR Donnelley was printer and binder.

This book is printed on acid-free paper.

Library of Congress Cataloging-in-Publication Data

Toy, Eugene C., author.
    Case files. Family medicine / Eugene C. Toy, Donald Briscoe, Bruce Britton, Joel J. Heidelbaugh. —Fourth edition.
        p. ; cm.
    Family medicine
    Includes bibliographical references and index.
    ISBN 978-1-259-58770-2 (pbk. : alk. paper)—ISBN 1-259-58770-3 (pbk. : alk. paper)
    I. Briscoe, Donald A., author.   II. Britton, Bruce, 1962- , author.   III. Heidelbaugh, Joel J., author.   IV. Title.   V. Title. Family medicine.
    [DNLM: 1. Family Practice—Case Reports.   2. Family Practice—Problems and Exercises.   WB 18.2]
    RC66
    610—dc23
                                                                    2015032679

International Edition ISBN 978-1-259-25120-7; MHID 1-25-925120-9. Copyright © 2016. Exclusive rights by McGraw-Hill Education Global Holdings, LLC for manufacture and export. This book cannot be re-exported from the country to which it is consigned by McGraw-Hill. The International Edition is not available in North America.

McGraw-Hill Education books are available at special quantity discounts to use as premiums and sales promotions or for use in corporate training programs. To contact a representative, please visit the Contact Us pages at www.mhprofessional.com.

To my incredible editor Catherine Johnson, whose imagination knows no bounds, whose compassion has no limits, and whose brilliance is a wonder to behold. I have been so fortunate to have you as my one and only editor for these Case Files books. You have been friend, encourager, and occasional bearer of the whip. Our successes are largely due to you and I will always be indebted to you.

– ECT

To my friends and colleagues at Hopital Saint Nicolas in St. Marc and Hopital Universitaire Justinien in Cap Haitien, Haiti.

– DB

To the students, residents, faculty, and patients of EVMS: the best teachers I could ever have.

And to May and Sean: for their infinite patience and love.

– BB

To my students and residents who teach me as much as I strive to teach them.

To my dedicated colleagues in academic family medicine who inspire me to become a greater teacher and clinician.

To Jacqui, Gwyneth, and Lilya for loving and supporting me.

– JJH

CONTENTS

Jessica K. Andrews, MD
Chief Resident, Portsmouth Family Medicine
Eastern Virginia Medical School
Portsmouth, Virginia
Congestive Heart Failure
Family Planning—Contraceptives
Major Depression
Postpartum Care

Sana I. Khan, DO
Resident, Family Medicine Residency Program
Houston Methodist Hospital
Houston, Texas
Chest Pain
Electrolyte Disorders
Geriatric Health Maintenance
Health Maintenance in Adult Female
Hematuria
Labor and Delivery
Musculoskeletal Injuries
Skin Lesions
Thyroid Disorders
Upper Respiratory Infections

Steven J. Lewis, MD, MPH
Chief Resident, Portsmouth Family Medicine
Eastern Virginia Medical School
Norfolk, Virginia
Family Violence
Hyperlipidemia
Migraine Headache
Obesity

William F. Mollenkopf, MD
Resident, Portsmouth Family Medicine
Eastern Virginia Medical School
Portsmouth, Virginia
Chronic Kidney Disease
Lower Gastrointestinal Bleeding
Pneumonia
Vaginitis

Dusty Marie Narducci, MD
Resident, Family Medicine Residency Program
Houston Methodist Hospital
Houston, Texas
Acute Diarrhea
Adult Male Health Maintenance
Allergic Disorders
Dyspnea (Chronic Obstructive Pulmonary Disease)
Geriatric Anemia
Joint Pain
Medical Ethics
Prenatal Care
Tobacco Use
Well-Child Care

Tuan D. Nguyen, MD, MPH, MBA
Resident, Family Medicine Residency Program
Houston Methodist Hospital
Houston, Texas
Electrolyte Disorders

Kartik Sidhar
Medical Student
Class of 2016
University of Michigan Medical School
Ann Arbor, Michigan
Cerebrovascular Accident/Transient Ischemic Attack
HIV, AIDS, and Other Sexually Transmitted Infections
Palpitations
Sting and Bite Injuries
Substance Abuse

Elizabeth R. Cochran Ward, MD, MappSci, MBBS (Hons)
Resident, Portsmouth Family Medicine
Eastern Virginia Medical School
Norfolk, Virginia
Abdominal Pain and Vomiting in a Child
Adolescent Health Maintenance
Dementia
Hypertension

Shea B. Wickland
Medical Student
Class of 2016
University of Michigan Medical School
Ann Arbor, Michigan
Chronic Pain Management
Lower Extremity Edema
Obstructive Sleep Apnea
Osteoporosis
Wheezing and Asthma

We appreciate all the kind remarks and suggestions from the many medical students over the past 3 years. Your positive reception has been an incredible encouragement, especially in light of the short life of the *Case Files®* series. In this fourth edition of *Case Files®: Family Medicine*, the basic format of the book has been retained. Improvements were made in updating many of the chapters. New cases include Substance Abuse, Asthma, Sleep Apnea, Osteoporosis, Chronic Pain Management, and Leg Swelling. We reviewed the clinical scenarios with the intent of improving them; however, their "real-life" presentations patterned after actual clinical experience were accurate and instructive. The multiple-choice questions (MCQs) have been carefully reviewed and rewritten to ensure that they comply with the National Board and USMLE format. Through this fourth edition, we hope that the reader will continue to enjoy learning diagnosis and management through the simulated clinical cases. It certainly is a privilege to be teachers for so many students, and it is with humility that we present this edition.

ACKNOWLEDGMENTS

The curriculum that evolved into the ideas for this series was inspired by two talented and forthright students, Philbert Yau and Chuck Rosipal, who have since graduated from medical school. It has been a pleasure to work with Dr. Don Briscoe, a brilliant, compassionate, and dedicated teacher and leader, Dr. Bruce Britton, who is an excellent teacher and communicator, and most recently Dr. Joel Heidelbaugh, who has a amazing breadth of knowledge and brings a fresh perspective. I am greatly indebted to my editor, Catherine Johnson, whose exuberance, experience, and vision helped to shape this series. I appreciate McGraw-Hill's believing in the concept of teaching through clinical cases; I am also grateful to Catherine Saggese for her excellent production expertise, and Cindy Yoo for her wonderful editing. I am thankful to Raghavi Khullar for the outstanding and precise project management. At the University of Texas Medical School at Houston, I appreciate Dr. Patricia Butler for her encouragement, Dr. Sean Blackwell for his example, role model and inspiration. Most of all, I appreciate my ever-loving wife Terri, and four wonderful children, Andy and his wife Anna, Michael, Allison, and Christina for their patience, encouragement, and understanding.

Eugene C. Toy, MD

Mastering the cognitive knowledge within a field such as family medicine is a formidable task. It is even more difficult to draw on that knowledge, procure, and filter through the clinical and laboratory data, develop a differential diagnosis, and, finally, to form a rational treatment plan. To gain these skills, the student often learns best at the bedside, guided and instructed by experienced teachers, and inspired toward self-directed, diligent reading. Clearly, there is no replacement for education at the bedside. Unfortunately, clinical situations usually do not encompass the breadth of the specialty. Perhaps the best alternative is a carefully crafted patient case designed to stimulate the clinical approach and decision making. In an attempt to achieve that goal, we have constructed a collection of clinical vignettes to teach diagnostic or therapeutic approaches that are relevant to family medicine. Most importantly, the explanations for the cases emphasize the mechanisms and underlying principles, rather than merely rote questions and answers.

This book is organized for versatility to allow the student "in a rush" to go quickly through the scenarios and check the corresponding answers, as well as enable the student who wants thought-provoking explanations to take a slower path. The answers are arranged from simple to complex: a summary of the pertinent points, the bare answers, an analysis of the case, an approach to the topic, a comprehension test at the end for reinforcement and emphasis, and a list of resources for further reading. The clinical vignettes are purposely placed in random order to simulate the way that real patients present to the practitioner. Section II includes a listing of cases to aid the student who desires to test his/her knowledge of a certain area, or to review a topic including basic definitions. Finally, we intentionally did not primarily use MCQ format because clues (or distractions) are not available in the real world. Nevertheless, several MCQs are included at the end of each scenario to reinforce concepts or introduce related topics.

HOW TO GET THE MOST OUT OF THIS BOOK

Each case is designed to simulate a patient encounter with open-ended questions. At times, the patient's complaint is different from the most concerning issue, and sometimes extraneous information is given. The answers are organized with four different parts.

PART I

1. The **Summary** identifies the salient aspects of the case, filtering out the extraneous information. The student should formulate his/her summary from the case before looking at the answers. A comparison to the summation in the answer will help to improve one's ability to focus on the important data, while appropriately discarding the irrelevant information, a fundamental skill in clinical problem solving.

2. A **Straightforward Answer** is given to each open-ended question.
3. The **Analysis of the Case**, which is comprised of two parts:
   a. **Objectives** of the Case: A listing of the two or three main principles that is crucial for a practitioner in managing the patient. Again, the student is challenged to make educated "guesses" about the objectives of the case upon initial review of the case scenario, which help to sharpen his/her clinical and analytical skills.
   b. **Considerations:** A discussion of the relevant points and a brief approach to the specific patient.

PART II

The Approach to the Disease Process, which has two distinct parts:
   a. **Definitions or Pathophysiology:** Terminology or basic science correlates that are pertinent to the disease process.
   b. **Clinical Approach:** A discussion of the approach to the clinical problem in general, including tables, figures, and algorithms.

PART III

The **Comprehension Questions** for each case is composed of several multiple-choice questions that either reinforce the material or introduce new and related concepts. Questions about material not found in the text have explanations in the answers.

PART IV

Clinical Pearls are a listing of several clinically important points that summarize the text, and allow for easy review of the material, such as before an examination.

How to Approach Clinical Problems

Part 1. Approach to the Patient

Applying "book learning" to a specific clinical situation is one the most challenging tasks in medicine. To do so, the clinician must not only retain information, organize facts, and recall large amounts of data but also apply all of this to the patient. The purpose of this text is to facilitate this process.

The first step involves gathering information, also known as establishing the database. This includes taking the history, performing the physical examination, and obtaining selective laboratory examinations, special studies, and/or imaging tests. Sensitivity and respect should always be exercised during the interview of patients. A good clinician also knows how to ask the same question in several different ways, using different terminology. For example, patients may deny having "congestive heart failure" but will answer affirmatively to being treated for "fluid on the lungs." Starting with open-ended questions for each section of the history often can help gather large amounts of information on the patient efficiently and allow the clinician's follow-up questions be targeted and more meaningful.

CLINICAL PEARL

▶ The history is usually the single most important tool in obtaining a diagnosis. The art of seeking this information in a nonjudgmental, sensitive, and thorough manner cannot be overemphasized.

HISTORY

1. **Basic information:**
   a. **Age:** Some conditions are more common at certain ages; for instance, chest pain in an elderly patient is more worrisome for coronary artery disease than the same complaint in a teenager.
   b. **Gender:** Some disorders are more common in men, such as abdominal aortic aneurysms. In contrast, women more commonly have autoimmune problems, such as chronic idiopathic thrombocytopenic purpura or systemic lupus erythematosus. Also, the possibility of pregnancy must be considered in any woman of childbearing age.
   c. **Ethnicity:** Some disease processes are more common in certain ethnic groups (such as type 2 diabetes mellitus in the Hispanic population).

CLINICAL PEARL

▶ *Family Medicine* illustrates the importance of longitudinal care, that is, seeing the patient in various phases and stages of life.

2. **Chief complaint:** What is it that brought the patient into the hospital? Has there been a change in a chronic or recurring condition or is this a completely new problem? The duration and character of the complaint, associated symptoms, and exacerbating/relieving factors should be recorded. The chief complaint engenders a differential diagnosis, and the possible etiologies should be explored by further inquiry.

> ### CLINICAL PEARL
>
> ▶ The first line of any presentation should include *age, ethnicity, gender, marital status, and chief complaint.* Example: A 32-year-old married white man complains of lower abdominal pain of 8-hour duration.

---

3. **Past medical history:**
   a. Major illnesses such as hypertension, diabetes, reactive airway disease, congestive heart failure, angina, or stroke should be detailed.
      i. Age of onset, severity, end-organ involvement.
      ii. Medications taken for the particular illness, including any recent changes to medications and reason for the change(s).
      iii. Last evaluation of the condition (eg, when was the last stress test or cardiac catheterization performed in the patient with angina).
      iv. Which physician or clinic is following the patient for the disorder?
   b. Minor illnesses such as recent upper respiratory infections.
   c. Hospitalizations, no matter how trivial, should be queried.

4. **Past surgical history:** Date and type of procedure performed, indication, and outcome. Laparoscopy versus laparotomy should be distinguished. Surgeon and hospital name/location should be listed. This information should be correlated with the surgical scars on the patient's body. Any complications should be delineated including anesthetic complications, difficult intubations, and so on.

5. **Allergies:** Reactions to medications should be recorded, including severity and temporal relationship to medication. Immediate hypersensitivity should be distinguished from an adverse reaction.

6. **Medications:** A list of medications, dosage, route of administration and frequency, and duration of use should be developed. Prescription, over-the-counter, supplements, and herbal remedies are all relevant. If the patient is currently taking antibiotics, it is important to note what type of infection is being treated.

7. **Immunization history:** Vaccination and prevention of disease is a principal goal of the family physician; hence, recording the immunizations received including dates, age, route, and adverse reactions, if any, is critical.

8. **Screening history:** Cost-effective surveillance for common diseases or malignancy is another cornerstone responsibility of the family physician. An organized record-keeping is important to a time-efficient approach to this area.

9. **Social history:** Occupation, marital status, family support, and tendencies toward depression or anxiety are important. Use or abuse of illicit drugs, tobacco, or alcohol should also be recorded. Social history, including marital stressors, sexual dysfunction, and sexual preference, is of importance. Patients, especially older patients or those with chronic illnesses, should be asked about medical power of attorney and advanced directives.

10. **Family history:** Many major medical problems are genetically transmitted (eg, hemophilia, sickle cell disease). In addition, a family history of conditions such as breast cancer and ischemic heart disease can be risk factors for the development of these diseases.

11. **Review of systems:** A systematic review should be performed but focused on the life-threatening and the more common diseases. For example, in a young man with a testicular mass, trauma to the area, weight loss, and infectious symptoms are important to note. In an elderly woman with generalized weakness, symptoms suggestive of cardiac disease should be elicited, such as chest pain, shortness of breath, fatigue, or palpitations.

PHYSICAL EXAMINATION

1. **General appearance:** Mental status, alert versus obtunded, anxious, in pain, in distress, interaction with other family members, and with examiner.

2. **Vital signs:** Record the temperature, blood pressure, heart rate, and respiratory rate. An oxygen saturation is useful in patients with respiratory symptoms. Height and weight are often placed here with a body mass index (BMI) calculated (weight in kg/height in meter squared = kg/m^2).

3. **Head and neck examination:** Evidence of trauma, tumors, facial edema, goiter and thyroid nodules, and carotid bruits should be sought. In patients with altered mental status or a head injury, pupillary size, symmetry, and reactivity are important. Mucous membranes should be inspected for pallor, jaundice, and evidence of dehydration. Cervical and supraclavicular nodes should be palpated.

4. **Breast examination:** Inspection for symmetry and skin or nipple retraction, as well as palpation for masses. The nipple should be assessed for discharge, and the axillary and supraclavicular regions should be examined.

5. **Cardiac examination:** The point of maximal impulse (PMI) should be ascertained, and the heart auscultated at the apex and base. It is important to note whether the auscultated rhythm is regular or irregular. Heart sounds (including S_3 and S_4), murmurs, clicks, and rubs should be characterized. Systolic flow murmurs are fairly common as a result of the increased cardiac output, but significant diastolic murmurs are unusual.

6. **Pulmonary examination:** The lung fields should be examined systematically and thoroughly. Stridor, wheezes, rales, and rhonchi should be recorded. The clinician should also search for evidence of consolidation (bronchial breath sounds, egophony) and increased work of breathing (retractions, abdominal breathing, accessory muscle use).

7. **Abdominal examination:** The abdomen should be inspected for scars, distension, masses, and discoloration. For instance, the Grey-Turner sign of bruising at the flank areas may indicate intra-abdominal or retroperitoneal hemorrhage. Auscultation should identify normal versus high-pitched and hyperactive versus hypoactive bowel sounds. The abdomen should be percussed for the presence of shifting dullness (indicating ascites). Then careful palpation should begin away from the area of pain and progress to include the whole abdomen to assess for tenderness, masses, organomegaly (ie, spleen or liver), and peritoneal signs. Guarding and whether it is voluntary or involuntary should be noted.

8. **Back and spine examination:** The back should be assessed for symmetry, tenderness, and masses. The flank regions particularly are important to assess for pain on percussion that may indicate renal disease.

9. **Genital examination:**
   a. **Female:** The external genitalia should be inspected, then the speculum used to visualize the cervix and vagina. A bimanual examination should attempt to elicit cervical motion tenderness, uterine size, and ovarian masses or tenderness.
   b. **Male:** The penis should be examined for hypospadias, lesions, and discharge. The scrotum should be palpated for tenderness and masses. If a mass is present, it can be transilluminated to distinguish between solid and cystic masses. The groin region should be carefully palpated for bulging (hernias) upon rest and provocation (coughing, standing).
   c. **Rectal examination:** A rectal examination will reveal masses in the posterior pelvis and may identify gross or occult blood in the stool. In females, nodularity and tenderness in the uterosacral ligament may be signs of endometriosis. The posterior uterus and palpable masses in the cul-de-sac may be identified by rectal examination. In the male, the prostate gland should be palpated for tenderness, nodularity, and enlargement.

10. **Extremities and skin:** The presence of joint effusions, tenderness, rashes, edema, and cyanosis should be recorded. It is also important to note capillary refill and peripheral pulses.

11. **Neurologic examination:** Patients who present with neurologic complaints require a thorough assessment, including mental status, cranial nerves, strength, sensation, reflexes, and cerebellar function.

CLINICAL PEARL

▶ A thorough understanding of functional anatomy is important to optimally interpret the physical examination findings.

12. **Laboratory assessment depends on the circumstances**

    a. CBC, or complete blood count, can assess for anemia, leukocytosis (infection), and thrombocytopenia.

    b. Basic metabolic panel: electrolytes, glucose, blood urea nitrogen (BUN), and creatinine (renal function).

    c. Urinalysis and/or urine culture to assess for hematuria, pyuria, or bacteriuria. A pregnancy test is important in women of childbearing age.

    d. Aspartate aminotransferase (AST), alanine aminotransferase (ALT), bilirubin, alkaline phosphatase for liver function; amylase and lipase to evaluate the pancreas.

    e. Cardiac markers (creatine kinase myocardial band [CK-MB], troponin, myoglobin) if coronary artery disease or other cardiac dysfunction is suspected.

    f. Drug levels such as acetaminophen level **in possible overdoses.**

    g. Arterial blood gas measurements give information about oxygenation, carbon dioxide, and pH readings.

13. **Diagnostic adjuncts**

    a. Electrocardiogram if cardiac ischemia, dysrhythmia, or other cardiac dysfunction is suspected.

    b. Ultrasound examination is useful in evaluating pelvic processes in female patients (eg, pelvic inflammatory disease, tuboovarian abscess) and in diagnosing gall stones and other gallbladder disease. With the addition of color-flow Doppler, deep venous thrombosis and ovarian or testicular torsion can be detected.

    c. Computed tomography (CT) is useful in assessing the brain for masses, bleeding, strokes, and skull fractures. CTs of the chest can evaluate for masses, fluid collections, aortic dissections, and pulmonary emboli. Abdominal CTs can detect infection (abscess, appendicitis, diverticulitis), masses, aortic aneurysms, and ureteral stones.

    d. Magnetic resonance imaging (MRI) helps to identify soft-tissue planes very well. In the emergency department setting, this is most commonly used to rule out spinal cord compression, cauda equina syndrome, and epidural abscess or hematoma.

    e. **Screening tests:** Fasting lipid panel can demonstrate the cholesterol level, including the low-density lipoprotein (LDL) levels, which have prognostic significance in coronary heart disease; fasting glucose and thyroid tests may be important; in many centers, dual-energy x-ray absorptiometry (DEXA) is the test of choice to monitor bone mineral density; the mammogram is the examination of choice to assess for subclinical breast cancer; fecal occult blood testing, flexible sigmoidoscopy, double-contrast barium enema, and colonoscopy are used to screen for colon cancer.

Part 2. Approach to Clinical Problem Solving

CLASSIC CLINICAL PROBLEM SOLVING

There are typically four distinct steps that the family physician undertakes to systematically solve most clinical problems:

1. Making the diagnosis

2. Assessing the severity of the disease

3. Treating based on the stage of the disease

4. Following the patient's response to the treatment

Making the Diagnosis

This is achieved by carefully evaluating the patient, analyzing the information, assessing risk factors, and developing a list of possible diagnoses (the differential). Usually a long list of possible diagnoses can be pared down to a few of the most likely or most serious ones, based on the clinician's knowledge, experience, assessment of the likelihood of having a condition (pretest probability), and selective testing. For example, a patient who complains of upper abdominal pain and has a history of nonsteroidal anti-inflammatory drug (NSAID) use may have peptic ulcer disease; another patient who has abdominal pain, fatty food intolerance, and abdominal bloating may have cholelithiasis. Yet another individual with a 1-day history of periumbilical pain that now localizes to the right lower quadrant may have acute appendicitis.

> ## CLINICAL PEARL
>
> ▶ The first step in clinical problem solving is making the diagnosis.

Assessing the Severity of the Disease

After establishing the diagnosis, the next step is to characterize the severity of the disease process; in other words, to describe "how bad" the disease is. This may be as simple as determining whether a patient is "sick" or "not sick." Is the patient with a urinary tract infection septic or stable for outpatient therapy? In other cases, a more formal staging may be used. For example, cancer staging is used for the strict assessment of extent of malignancy.

> ## CLINICAL PEARL
>
> ▶ The second step in clinical problem solving is to establish the severity or stage of disease. This usually impacts the treatment and/or prognosis.

Treating Based on Stage

Many illnesses are characterized by stage or severity because this affects prognosis and treatment. As an example, a formerly healthy young man with pneumonia and no respiratory distress may be treated with oral antibiotics at home. An older person with emphysema and pneumonia would probably be admitted to the hospital for IV antibiotics. A patient with pneumonia and respiratory failure would likely be intubated and admitted to the intensive care unit for further treatment.

> ### CLINICAL PEARL
>
> ▶ The third step in clinical problem solving is tailoring the treatment to fit the severity or "stage" of the disease.

Following the Response to Treatment

The final step in the approach to disease is to follow the patient's response to the therapy. Some responses are clinical, such as improvement (or lack of improvement) in a patient's pain. Other responses may be followed by testing (eg, monitoring the anion gap in a patient with diabetic ketoacidosis). The clinician must be prepared to know what to do if the patient does not respond as expected. Is the next step to treat again, to reassess the diagnosis, or to follow up with another more specific test?

> ### CLINICAL PEARL
>
> ▶ The fourth step in clinical problem solving is to monitor treatment response or efficacy. This may be measured in different ways—symptomatically or based on physical examination or other testing. For the emergency physician, the vital signs, oxygenation, urine output, and mental status are the key parameters.

Part 3. Approach to Reading

The clinical problem-oriented approach to reading is different from the classic "systematic" research of a disease. Patients rarely present with a clear diagnosis; hence, the student must become skilled in applying textbook information to the clinical scenario. Because reading with a purpose improves the retention of information, the student should read with the goal of answering specific questions. There are several fundamental questions that facilitate clinical thinking. These are:

1. What is the most likely diagnosis?

2. How would you confirm the diagnosis?

3. What should be your next step?

4. What is the best screening strategy in this situation?

5. What are the risk factors for this condition?

6. What are the complications associated with the disease process?

7. What is the best therapy?

CLINICAL PEARL

▶ Reading with the purpose of answering the seven fundamental clinical questions improves retention of information and facilitates the application of "book knowledge" to "clinical knowledge."

What Is the Most Likely Diagnosis?

The method of establishing the diagnosis was discussed in the previous section. One way of determining the most likely diagnosis is to develop standard "approaches" to common clinical problems. It is helpful to understand the most common causes of various presentations, such as "the worst headache of the patient's life is worrisome for a subarachnoid hemorrhage" (see the Clinical Pearls at end of each case).

The clinical scenario would be something such as:

A 38-year-old woman is noted to have a 2-day history of unilateral, throbbing headache with photophobia. What is the most likely diagnosis?

With no other information to go on, the student would note that this woman has a unilateral headache with photophobia. Using the "most common cause" information, the student would make an educated guess that the patient has a migraine headache. If instead the patient is noted to have "the worst headache of her life," the student would use the Clinical Pearl:

The worst headache of the patient's life is worrisome for a subarachnoid hemorrhage.

CLINICAL PEARL

▶ The more common cause of a unilateral, throbbing headache with photophobia is a migraine, but the main concern is subarachnoid hemorrhage. If the patient describes this as "the worst headache of her life," the concern for a subarachnoid bleed is increased.

How Would You Confirm the Diagnosis

In the scenario above, the woman with "the worst headache" is suspected of having a subarachnoid hemorrhage. This diagnosis could be confirmed by a CT scan of the head and/or lumbar puncture (LP). The student should learn the limitations of various diagnostic tests, especially when used early in a disease process. The LP **showing xanthochromia (red blood cells) is the "gold standard" test for diagnosing subarachnoid hemorrhage, but it may be negative early in the disease course.**

What should be your next step? This question is difficult because the next step has many possibilities; the answer may be to obtain more diagnostic information, stage the illness, or introduce therapy. It is often a more challenging question than "What is the most likely diagnosis?" because there may be insufficient information to make a diagnosis and the next step may be to pursue more diagnostic information. Another possibility is that there is enough information for a probable diagnosis, and the next step is to stage the disease. Finally, the most appropriate answer may be to treat. Hence, from clinical data, a judgment needs to be rendered regarding how far along one is on the road of:

1. **Make the diagnosis** → 2. **Stage the disease** →
3. **Treat based on stage** → 4. **Follow response**

Frequently, the student is taught "to regurgitate" the same information that someone has written about a particular disease, but is not skilled at identifying the next step. This talent is learned optimally at the bedside, in a supportive environment, with freedom to make educated guesses, and with constructive feedback. A sample scenario might describe a student's thought process as follows:

1. **Make the diagnosis:** "Based on the information I have, I believe that the patient has a small bowel obstruction from adhesive disease *because* he presents with nausea and vomiting, abdominal distension, and high-pitched hyperactive bowel sounds, and has dilated loops of small bowel on x-ray."

2. **Stage the disease:** "I don't believe that this is severe disease as he does not have fever, evidence of sepsis, intractable pain, peritoneal signs, or leukocytosis."

3. **Treat based on stage:** "Therefore, my next step is to treat with nothing per mouth, nasogastric (NG) tube drainage, IV fluids, and observation."

4. **Follow response:** "I want to follow the treatment by assessing his pain (I will ask him to rate the pain on a scale of 1 to 10 every day), his bowel function (I will ask whether he has had nausea, vomiting, or passed flatus), his temperature, abdominal examination, serum bicarbonate (for metabolic acidemia), white blood cell count, and then reassess him in 48 hours."

In a similar patient, when the clinical presentation is unclear, perhaps the best "next step" may be diagnostic such as an oral contrast radiologic study to assess for bowel obstruction.

CLINICAL PEARL

▶ Usually, the vague query, "What is your next step?" is the most difficult question because the answer may be diagnostic, staging, or therapeutic.

What Is the Best Screening Strategy in This Situation?

A major role of the family physician is screening for common and/or dangerous conditions where there may be interventions to alleviate disease. Cost-effectiveness, ease of the screening modality, wide availability, and presence of intervention are some of the important issues. The age, gender, and risk factors for the disease process in question play roles. In general, age is one of the most important risk factors for cancer. For instance, with breast cancer, an annual or biannual mammogram is recommended in women older than age 50. This imaging technique is widely available, inexpensive, safe, has been shown to decrease mortality. In the United States, screening examinations with strong evidence for effectiveness are fully covered by insurance.

What Are the Risk Factors for This Process?

Understanding the risk factors helps the practitioner to establish a diagnosis and to determine how to interpret tests. For example, understanding risk-factor analysis may help in the management of a 55-year-old woman with anemia. If the patient has risk factors for endometrial cancer (such as diabetes, hypertension, anovulation) and complains of postmenopausal bleeding, she likely has endometrial carcinoma and should have an endometrial biopsy. Otherwise, occult colonic bleeding is a common etiology. If she takes NSAIDs or aspirin, then peptic ulcer disease is the most likely cause.

CLINICAL PEARL

▶ Being able to assess risk factors helps to guide testing and develop the differential diagnosis.

What Are the Complications to This Process?

Clinicians must be cognizant of the complications of a disease, so that they will understand how to follow and monitor the patient. Sometimes the student has to make the diagnosis from clinical clues and then apply his/her knowledge of the consequences of the pathologic process. For example, "A 26-year-old man complains of right lower-extremity swelling and pain after a trans-Atlantic flight" and his Doppler ultrasound reveals a deep vein thrombosis. Complications of this process include pulmonary embolism (PE). Understanding the types of consequences also helps the clinician to be aware of the dangers to a patient. If the patient has any symptoms consistent with a PE, a ventilation-perfusion scan or CT scan with angiographic imaging of the chest may be necessary.

What Is the Best Therapy?

To answer this question, not only does the clinician need to reach the correct diagnosis and assess the severity of the condition, but (s)he must also weigh the situation to determine the appropriate intervention. For the student, knowing exact dosages is not as important as understanding the best medication, route of delivery, mechanism of action, and possible complications. It is important for the student to be able to verbalize the diagnosis and the rationale for the therapy. It is also important that the therapy choice takes into consideration patient beliefs and desires. Evidence-based medicine combines the best available evidence, the clinicians' experience and the patient's beliefs and values.

CLINICAL PEARL

▶ Therapy should be logical and based on the severity of disease and the specific diagnosis. An exception to this rule is in an emergent situation, such as respiratory failure or shock, when the patient needs treatment even as the etiology is being investigated.

Summary

1. There is no replacement for a meticulous history and physical examination.

2. There are four steps in the clinical approach to the family medicine patient: making the diagnosis, assessing severity, treating based on severity, and following response.

3. There are seven questions that help to bridge the gap between the textbook and the clinical arena.

REFERENCES

South-Paul J, Matheny S. *Current Diagnosis and Treatment in Family Medicine*. 4th ed. New York, NY: McGraw-Hill Education; 2015.

Taylor RB, David AK, Fields SA, Phillips DM, Scherger JE. *Family Medicine: Principle and Practice*. 7th ed. New York, NY: Springer-Verlag; 2007.

Listing of Cases

Listing by Case Number

Listing by Disorder (Alphabetical)

Listing by Case Number

Listing by Disorder (Alphabetical)

Clinical Cases

CASE 1

A 52-year-old man comes to your office for a routine physical examination. He is a new patient to your practice. He has no significant medical history and takes no medications regularly. His father died at the age of 74 of a heart attack. His mother is alive at the age of 80. She has hypertension. He has two younger siblings with no known chronic medical conditions. He does not smoke cigarettes, drink alcohol, or use any recreational drugs. He does not exercise. On examination, his blood pressure is 127/82 mm Hg, pulse is 80 beats/min, respiratory rate is 18 breaths/min, height is 67 in, and weight is 190 lb. On careful physical examination, no abnormalities are noted.

▶ What screening test(s) for cardiovascular disease should be recommended for this patient?
▶ What screening test(s) for cancer should be recommended?
▶ What immunization(s) should be recommended?

ANSWERS TO CASE 1:
Adult Male Health Maintenance

Summary: A 52-year-old man with no active medical problems is being evaluated during an "annual physical." He has no complaints on history and has a normal physical examination.

- **Recommended screening tests for cardiovascular conditions:** Blood pressure measurement (screening for hypertension) and lipid measurement (screening for dyslipidemia)

- **Recommended screening tests for cancer:** Fecal occult blood testing, flexible sigmoidoscopy (with or without occult blood testing), colonoscopy or double-contrast barium enema to screen for colorectal cancer; there is insufficient evidence to recommend for or against universal prostate cancer screening by prostate-specific antigen (PSA) testing

- **Recommended immunizations:** Tetanus toxoid, reduced diphtheria toxoid, and acellular pertussis vaccine (Tdap) if he has not had one before and if it has been 10 years or more since he has had a tetanus-diphtheria (Td) vaccine, or if he requires booster protection against pertussis; influenza vaccine annually, in the fall or winter months

ANALYSIS

Objectives

1. Know the components of an adult health-maintenance visit.

2. Learn the screening tests and immunizations that are routinely recommended for adult men.

Considerations

The patient described is a healthy 52-year-old man. Health maintenance should be employed to prevent future disease. In general, the approach is immunizations, cancer screening, and screening for common diseases. Generally, colon cancer screening should be initiated at age 50 and beyond. The influenza vaccine should be recommended annually, and the tetanus vaccine every 10 years. The acellular pertussis vaccine is also recommended as many adults have had waning immunity to pertussis and occasional outbreaks of whooping cough have been noted. Other vaccinations, including pneumococcal, meningococcal, hepatitis A and B, are recommended in those who have certain risk factors but are otherwise not routinely used for someone of his age and overall health. Since cardiovascular disease is the most common cause of mortality in his age group, screening for cardiovascular disease or risk factors is appropriate.

APPROACH TO:
Health Maintenance

DEFINITIONS

SCREENING TEST: Assessment device or test that should be cost-effective with high sensitivity and can be used on a large population to identify persons with disease

HEALTH MAINTENANCE: Systematic program or procedure planned to prevent illness, maintain maximum function, and promote health

CLINICAL APPROACH

For years, one of the cornerstones of primary care was the "annual physical," which often consisted of a complete physical examination, blood tests, including complete blood counts (CBCs) and multichemistry panels, and, frequently, annual chest x-rays and electrocardiograms (ECGs). The concept of the "annual physical," or "health-maintenance examination" is still important; however, the components of the examination have changed over time.

The purposes of the health-maintenance visit are to identify the individual patient's health concerns, manage the patient's current medical conditions, identify the patient's risks for future health problems, perform rational and cost-effective health screening tests, and promote a healthy lifestyle. Prevention is divided into primary, secondary and tertiary approaches. **Primary prevention** is an intervention designed to prevent a disease before it occurs. It usually involves the identification and management of risk factors for a disease. Examples of this would be immunization against communicable disease, public health education about good nutrition, exercise and stress management, or removal of colon polyps to prevent the development of colon cancer. **Secondary prevention** is an intervention intended to promote early detection of a disease or condition, so prompt treatment can be initiated. Examples of secondary prevention are the use of mammography for the detection of breast cancer or eye examinations for the detection of glaucoma. **Tertiary prevention** involves both therapeutic and rehabilitative measures once a disease has been diagnosed. Examples of tertiary prevention include core measure medications for congestive heart failure, rehabilitation programs for stroke patients to improve functioning, and chronic pain management programs.

Effective screening for diseases or health conditions should meet several established criteria. First, the disease should be of **high enough prevalence** in the population to make the screening effort worthwhile. There should be a time frame during which the person is asymptomatic, but during which the disease or risk factor can be identified. There needs to be a test available for the disease that has **sufficient sensitivity and specificity, is cost-effective**, and is **acceptable** to patients. Finally, there must be an intervention that can be made during the asymptomatic period that will prevent the development of the disease or reduce the morbidity/mortality of the disease process.

The United States Preventive Services Task Force (USPSTF) is an independent panel of experts in primary care and preventive medicine that reviews evidence and makes recommendations on the effectiveness of clinical preventive services, specifically in the areas of screening, immunization, preventive medications, and counseling. USPSTF recommendations are "gold standards" for clinical preventive medicine. The recommendations of the USPSTF are available online for free at uspreventiveservicetaskforce.org. USPSTF grades its recommendations in five categories to reflect evidence strength and overall benefit of an intervention.

Recommendation Grade	Definition	Suggestion for Practice
A	There is high certainty that the net benefit of the intervention is substantial.	Offer or provide this service.
B	There is high certainty that the net benefit of the intervention is moderate or moderate certainty that it is moderate to substantial.	Offer or provide this service.
C	There may be considerations that support providing the service in an individual patient. There is moderate or high certainty that there is no net benefit or harm.	Offer or provide the service only if there are other considerations that support offering or providing for the individual.
D	There is moderate or high certainty that there is no net benefit or that the harms outweigh the benefits.	Discourage use of this service.
I	There is insufficient evidence, or the available evidence is of such poor quality, that the balance of benefits and harms cannot be weighed and recommendations for or against the service cannot be made.	If service is offered, patients should understand the uncertainty about the balance of benefits and harms.

SCREENING TESTS

Cardiovascular Diseases

Diseases of the cardiovascular system are the leading cause of death in adult men and the management of risk factors for these diseases reduces both morbidity and mortality from these diseases. The USPSTF strongly recommends (Level A) screening of adults (age 18 and older) for **hypertension** by measurement of blood pressure, as screening causes little harm and management of hypertension is effective at reducing the risk of cardiovascular diseases. USPSTF also strongly recommends (Level A) screening men aged 35 or more and women aged 45 or more for **lipid disorders** and recommends (Level B) screening adults older than 20 years who are at increased risk for cardiovascular diseases. The screening can take the form of nonfasting total cholesterol and high-density lipoprotein (HDL)-cholesterol levels or fasting lipid panels that include the low-density lipoprotein (LDL)-cholesterol. Men aged 45 to 79 are recommended (Level A) to take aspirin daily to reduce the risk of a myocardial infarction (MI) as long as the benefit outweighs their risk of a gastrointestinal hemorrhage. Ultrasonography to assess for **abdominal aortic aneurysm** (AAA) is recommended (Level B) for men aged 65 to 75 who have ever smoked. There is no recommendation (Level C) for AAA screening for men who have never smoked and it is recommended against (Level D) for women who have never smoked. For women aged 65 to 75 who have smoked, there is insufficient evidence (Level I) whether screening for AAA would be beneficial.

The routine use of ECG, exercise stress testing, or computed tomography (CT) scanning for coronary calcium is not recommended (Level D) for screening for **coronary artery disease** in adults at low risk for coronary events. There is insufficient evidence to recommend for or against these modalities (Level I) in adults at higher risk of coronary events. There is insufficient evidence (Level I) for screening peripheral artery disease and coronary artery disease with ankle-brachial index (ABI). There is evidence to suggest against screening asymptomatic individuals among the general adult population for carotid artery stenosis.

Cancer

Adults (men and women) older than 50 years are strongly advised (Level A) to have screening for **colorectal cancer**. This screening can take the form of fecal occult blood testing (FOBT) using guaiac cards on three consecutive bowel movements collected at home, flexible sigmoidoscopy with or without occult blood testing, or colonoscopy. The optimal intervals for testing are not clear, but FOBT is generally recommended annually, sigmoidoscopy every 3 to 5 years, and colonoscopy every 10 years. An abnormal test result of FOBT or sigmoidoscopy leads to the performance of a colonoscopy.

The USPSTF currently recommends against (Level D) routine screening for **prostate cancer** using digital examination or PSA. Men and women aged 50 to 80 with a 30 or more pack-year history who continue to smoke or who quit less than 15 years ago should undergo annual low-dose CT of chest to screen for **lung cancer** (Level B), but screening for lung cancer with routine chest x-ray is not recommended.

Screening for **testicular and pancreatic** cancer in asymptomatic adults is not recommended (Level D). There is insufficient evidence to recommend screening for bladder cancer in asymptomatic individuals (Level I).

Other Health Conditions

All adults (Level B) should be screened for obesity by calculating their body mass index (BMI). Individuals with a BMI greater than 30 kg/m^2 should be offered or referred for intensive multicomponent behavioral intervention. There is insufficient evidence to recommend screening of asymptomatic adults for **type 2 diabetes mellitus** (Level I), although screening is recommended (Level B) for adults with hypertension (135/89 or more sustained or untreated) or hyperlipidemia. **Depression** screening is recommended (Level B) if there are mechanisms in place for ensuring accurate diagnosis, treatment, and follow-up. Screening and counseling to identify and promote cessation of **tobacco use** is strongly recommended (Level A). Screening and counseling to identify and prevent the **misuse of alcohol** is also recommended (Level B). The USPSTF states there is insufficient evidence (Level I) for or against routine screening of thyroid disease in asymptomatic individuals.

IMMUNIZATIONS

As is the case for well-child care, the provision of age- and condition-appropriate immunizations is an important component of well-adult care. Recommendations for immunizations change from time to time and the most up-to-date source of vaccine recommendations is the Advisory Committee on Immunization Practices. Its immunization schedules are widely published and are available at the Centers for Disease Control and Prevention (CDC) Website (among other places), www.cdc.gov.

The CDC has recently recommended that all adults between 19 and 65 years of age should receive a booster of Tdap in place of a scheduled dose of Td due to waning immunity against pertussis and the presence of an increasing number of cases of pertussis nationwide. Adults who have not had a Td booster in 10 years or more and who have never had a dose of Tdap as an adult should receive a booster vaccination with Tdap. Persons who may need an increase in protection against pertussis, including health-care workers, childcare providers, or those who anticipate having close contact with infants younger than 1 year, should also receive a Tdap booster.

In a 2010 update, the CDC recommended routine vaccination against **influenza** for everyone 6 months of age and older. This replaced a recommendation of vaccination based upon risk factors.

Pneumococcal polysaccharide (PPSV-23) and pneumococcal conjugate (PCV-13) vaccination are recommended for all adults aged 65 or older. PPSV-23 and/or PCV-13 may also be recommended for previously unvaccinated adults younger than 65 in the presence of immunocompromising or certain chronic medical conditions.

Other vaccinations may be recommended for specific populations, although not for all adults. **Hepatitis B** vaccination should be recommended for those at high risk of exposure, including health-care workers, those exposed to blood or blood products, dialysis patients, intravenous drug users, persons with multiple sexual partners or recent sexually transmitted diseases, and men who engage in sexual relations with other men. A new recommendation also suggests routine vaccination against hepatitis B for all patients with diabetes who have not previously been immunized. **Hepatitis A** vaccine is recommended for persons with chronic liver disease, who use clotting factors, who have occupational exposure to the hepatitis A virus, who use IV drugs, men who have sex with men, or who travel to countries where hepatitis A is endemic. **Varicella** vaccination is recommended for those with no reliable history of immunization or disease, who are seronegative on testing for varicella immunity, and who are at risk for exposure to varicella virus. **Meningococcal** vaccine is recommended for persons in high-risk groups, college dormitory residents and military recruits, with certain complement deficiencies, functional or anatomic asplenia, or who travel to countries where the disease is endemic.

HEALTHY LIFESTYLE

Along with the discussion of screening and promotion of tobacco cessation and prevention of alcohol misuse, other aspects of healthy living should be promoted by physicians. **Exercise** has been consistently shown to reduce the risk of cardiovascular disease, diabetes, obesity, and overall mortality. Even exercise of moderate amounts, such as walking for 30 minutes on most days of the week, has a positive effect on health. The benefits increase with increasing the amount of exercise performed. Studies performed on counseling physically inactive persons to exercise have shown inconsistent results. However, the benefits of exercise are clear and should be promoted. Counseling to promote a healthy **diet** in persons with hyperlipidemia, other risk factors for cardiovascular disease, or other conditions related to diet is beneficial. Intensive counseling by physicians or, when appropriate, referral to dietary counselors or nutritionists, can improve health outcomes. In selected patients, recommendations regarding **safer sexual practices**, including the use of condoms, may be appropriate to reduce the risk or recurrence of sexually transmitted diseases. Finally, all patients should be encouraged to use **seat belts** and avoid driving while under the influence of alcohol or drugs, as motor vehicle accidents remain a leading cause of morbidity and mortality in adults.

COMPREHENSION QUESTIONS

1.1 A 52-year-old man comes into the outpatient clinic for an annual "checkup." He is in good health, and has a relatively unremarkable family history. He has never smoked cigarettes. For which of the following disorders should a screening test be performed?

    A. Prostate cancer

    B. Lung cancer

    C. Abdominal aortic aneurysm

    D. Colon cancer

1.2 A 62-year-old man with recently diagnosed emphysema presents to your office in November for a routine examination. He has not had any immunizations in more than 10 years. Which of the following immunizations would be most appropriate for this individual?

    A. Tetanus-diphtheria (Td) only

    B. Tdap, pneumococcal, and influenza

    C. Pneumococcal and influenza

    D. Tdap, pneumococcal, influenza, and meningococcal

1.3 A 49-year-old sedentary man has made an appointment because his best friend died of an MI at age 50. He asks about an exercise and weight loss program. In counseling him, which of the following statements regarding exercise is most accurate?

    A. To be beneficial, exercise must be performed every day.

    B. Walking for exercise has not been shown to improve meaningful clinical outcomes.

    C. Counseling patients to exercise has not been shown consistently to increase the number of patients who exercise.

    D. Intense exercise offers no health benefit over mild to moderate amounts of exercise.

ANSWERS

1.1 **D.** Colon cancer screening is given a Level A recommendation by the USPSTF and is routinely offered or provided to all adults older than 50 years. There is insufficient evidence to recommend for or against routine lung or prostate cancer screening. Abdominal aortic aneurysm screening is recommended in men aged 65 to 75 years who have smoked.

1.2 **B.** In an adult with a chronic lung disease, one-time vaccination with pneumococcal vaccine and annual vaccination with influenza vaccine are recommended. A Tdap booster should be recommended to all adults who have not had a Td booster within 10 years and have never had a Tdap vaccine as an adult.

1.3 **C.** The benefits of exercise are clear. Exercise decreases cardiovascular risk factors, increases insulin sensitivity, decreases the incidence of the metabolic syndrome, and decreases cardiovascular mortality regardless of obesity. The benefits of counseling patients regarding exercise are not so clear and counseling does not seem to increase the number of patients who exercise.

CLINICAL PEARLS

▶ There is no such thing as a "routine blood test" or a "routine chest x-ray." All tests that are ordered should have evidence to support their benefit.

▶ High-quality, evidence-based recommendations for preventive health services are available at www.uspreventiveservicestaskforce.org.

REFERENCES

Blaha, MJ, Bansal S, Rouf R, Golden SH, Blumenthal RS, Defilippis AP. A practical "ABCDE" approach to the metabolic syndrome. *Mayo Clin Proc.* 2008 Aug;83(8):932-941.

Centers for Disease Control and Prevention. Vaccines and immunizations. Available at: http://www. cdc.gov/vaccines/. Accessed May 24, 2015.

Mosby's Marie T. O'Toole, editor Medical Dictionary. 8th ed. St Louis, MO: Mosby Elsevier; 2008.

United States Preventive Services Task Force. Recommendations for primary care practice. Available at: http://www.uspreventiveservicestaskforce.org/Page/Name/recommendations. Accessed May 24, 2015.

A 52-year-old man presents to your office for an acute visit because of coughing and shortness of breath. He is well known to you because of multiple office visits in the past few years for similar reasons. He has a chronic "smoker's cough," but reports that in the past 2 days his cough has increased, his sputum has changed from white to green in color, and he has had to increase the frequency with which he uses his albuterol inhaler. He denies having a fever, chest pain, peripheral edema, or other symptoms. His medical history is significant for hypertension, peripheral vascular disease, and two hospitalizations for pneumonia in the past 5 years. He has a 60-pack-year history of smoking and continues to smoke two packs of cigarettes a day.

On examination, he is in moderate respiratory distress. His temperature is 98.4°F, his blood pressure is 152/95 mm Hg, his pulse is 98 beats/min, his respiratory rate is 24 breaths/min, and he has an oxygen saturation of 94% on room air. His lung examination is significant for diffuse expiratory wheezing and a prolonged expiratory phase of respiration. There are no signs of cyanosis. The remainder of his examination is normal. A chest x-ray done in your office shows an increased anteroposterior (AP) diameter and a flattened diaphragm, but otherwise he has clear lung fields.

▶ What is the most likely cause of this patient's dyspnea?
▶ What acute treatment(s) are most appropriate at this time?
▶ What interventions would be most helpful to reduce the risk of future exacerbations of this condition?

ANSWERS TO CASE 2:

Dyspnea (Chronic Obstructive Pulmonary Disease)

Summary: A 52-year-old man with a long history of smoking presents with dyspnea, increased sputum production, change in sputum character, coughing, and wheezing.

- **Most likely cause of current symptoms:** Acute exacerbation of chronic obstructive pulmonary disease (COPD)

- **Appropriate treatment of exacerbation:** Antibiotic, bronchodilators, systemic corticosteroids

- **Interventions to reduce exacerbations:** Smoking cessation, long-acting bronchodilator, inhaled corticosteroid, influenza and pneumococcal polysaccharide vaccination

ANALYSIS

Objectives

1. Be able to diagnose and determine the stage of COPD in adults.

2. Know the management of stable COPD and COPD exacerbations.

Considerations

Two of the most common causes of dyspnea and wheezing in adults are asthma and COPD. There can be substantial overlap between the two diseases, as patients with chronic asthma can develop chronic obstructive disease over time. As in most medical situations, the patient's history will usually provide the key information to the appropriate diagnosis. Asthma often presents earlier in life, may or may not be associated with cigarette smoking, and is characterized by episodic exacerbations with return to relatively normal baseline lung functioning. COPD, on the other hand, tends to present in midlife or later, is usually the result of a long history of smoking, and is a slowly progressive disorder in which measured pulmonary functioning never returns to normal.

In the setting of an acute exacerbation, the differentiation between an exacerbation of asthma and an exacerbation of COPD is not necessary for determination of the immediate management. The assessment of the patient presenting with dyspnea should always start with the ABCs—Airway, Breathing, and Circulation. Intubation with mechanical ventilation should be performed when the patient is unable to protect his own airway (eg, when he has a reduced level of consciousness), when he is tiring because of the amount of work required to overcome his airway obstruction, or when adequate oxygenation cannot be maintained.

For both asthma and COPD exacerbations, the mainstays of medical therapy are oxygen, bronchodilators, and steroids. All dyspneic patients should have an assessment of their level of oxygenation. Clinical signs of hypoxemia, such as cyanosis of the perioral region or digits, should be noted on examination. Objective levels of oxygenation using pulse oximetry or arterial blood gas measurements should also be performed. Hypoxemia must be addressed by providing supplemental oxygen. Inhaled β_2-agonists, most commonly albuterol, can rapidly result in bronchodilation and reduction in airway obstruction. The addition of an inhaled anticholinergic agent, such as ipratropium, may work synergistically with the β-agonist. Corticosteroids, given systemically (orally, intramuscularly, or intravenously), act to reduce the airway inflammation that underlies the acute exacerbation. Clinically significant effects of steroids take hours to occur; consequently, steroids should be used with bronchodilators because bronchodilators act rapidly. Steroids used in combination with bronchodilators significantly improve short-term outcomes in the management of acute exacerbations of asthma and COPD.

APPROACH TO:
Chronic Obstructive Pulmonary Disease

DEFINITIONS

CHRONIC BRONCHITIS: Cough and sputum production on most days for at least 3 months during at least 2 consecutive years

EMPHYSEMA: Shortness of breath caused by the enlargement of respiratory bronchioles and alveoli caused by destruction of lung tissue

CLINICAL APPROACH

Evaluation

COPD is the third leading cause of death in the United States, affecting more than 5% of the adult population. COPD is defined as airway obstruction that is not fully reversible, is usually progressive, and is associated with chronic bronchitis, emphysema, or both. The most common etiology is **cigarette smoking**, which is **associated with approximately 90% of cases of COPD**. Other etiologies of COPD include passive exposure to cigarette smoke ("second-hand smoke") and occupational exposures to dusts (including mining, cotton, silica, plastics), chemicals, and fumes (welding, heavy metals). Patients with symptoms of COPD, who do not smoke and work in high-risk occupations, warrant further evaluation. A rare cause of COPD is a genetic deficiency in α_1-**antitrypsin**, which is more common in Caucasians and should be considered when emphysema develops at younger ages (<45 years), especially in nonsmokers. COPD is a disease of inflammation of the airways, lung tissue, and vasculature. Pathologic changes include mucous gland hypertrophy with hypersecretion, ciliary dysfunction, destruction of lung parenchyma, and airway remodeling. The results of these changes are narrowing of the airways, causing a fixed airway obstruction, poor mucous clearance, cough, wheezing, and dyspnea.

The most common initial symptom of COPD is cough, which is at first intermittent and then frequently becomes a daily occurrence. The cough is often productive of white, thick mucus. Patients will present with intermittent episodes of worsening cough, with change in mucus from clear to yellow/green, and often with wheezing. These exacerbations are usually caused by viral or bacterial infections.

As COPD progresses, lung function continues to deteriorate and dyspnea develops. Dyspnea is the primary presenting symptom of COPD. Dyspnea also tends to worsen over time—initially the dyspnea will occur only with significant effort, then with any exertion, and finally at rest. **By the time dyspnea develops, lung function (as measured by forced expiratory volume in the first second of expiration [FEV_1]) has been reduced by about half and the COPD has been present for years.** When evaluating the patient with dyspnea, it is important to consider other diagnoses. Eighty-five percent of dyspnea causes are due to one of the following conditions: congestive heart failure, COPD, asthma, interstitial lung disease, pneumonia, and psychogenic disturbances (including anxiety).

Examination of a patient with mild or moderate COPD, who is not having an exacerbation, is usually normal. As the disease progresses, patients are often noted to have "barrel chests" (increased anteroposterior chest diameter) and distant heart sounds, as a result of hyperinflation of the lungs. Breath sounds may also be distant and expiratory wheezes with a prolonged expiratory phase of respiration may be noted. During an acute exacerbation, patients often appear anxious and tachypneic; they may be using accessory muscles of respiration, usually have wheezes or rales, and may have signs of cyanosis.

Chest x-rays in patients with COPD are typically normal until the disease is advanced. In more severe cases, hyperinflation of the lungs with an increased posteroanterior (PA) diameter and flattening of diaphragms may be seen. Bullae—areas of pulmonary parenchymal destruction—can also be seen in x-rays in more severe disease.

The primary diagnostic test of lung function is spirometry. In normal aging, both the forced vital capacity (FVC) (a measure of the total amount of air that can be expired after a maximal inspiration) and FEV_1 reduce gradually over time. In normal-functioning lungs, the ratio of the FEV_1 to FVC is greater than 0.7. **In COPD, both the FVC and FEV_1 are reduced and the ratio of FEV_1 to FVC is less than 0.7**, indicating an airway obstruction. **Reversibility is defined as an increase in FEV_1 of greater than 12% or 200 mL.** Using a bronchodilator may result in some improvement of both FVC and FEV_1, but neither will return to normal, making the diagnosis of a fixed obstruction. The severity of COPD, which can help to determine treatment, can be assessed using these measurements (Table 2–1).

Management of Stable COPD

The goals of COPD management are to relieve symptoms, prevent/slow disease progression, reduce/prevent/treat exacerbations, and reduce/prevent/treat complications. Several components of treatment are common to all stages of COPD, whereas pharmacologic treatment is guided by the stage of disease.

All patients with COPD should be encouraged to quit smoking. The pulmonary function of smokers declines more rapidly than that of nonsmokers. **Although smoking cessation does not result in significant improvement in pulmonary function, smoking cessation does reduce the rate of further deterioration to that of a nonsmoker.** Cessation also reduces the risks of other comorbidities, including cardiovascular diseases and cancers. Case 7 more thoroughly discusses smoking cessation. All patients with COPD should be appropriately vaccinated. Those with chronic pulmonary diseases and all smokers should receive a pneumococcal vaccination and

Table 2-1 • CLASSIFICATION OF COPD SEVERITY

Stage	Classification	Findings	Treatment
0	At risk	Cough, sputum production Normal spirometry	Vaccines and address risk factors (exposure to tobacco smoke, occupational dust/chemicals, or smoke from home cooking/heating fuel)
I	Mild COPD	FEV_1/FVC <0.7 FEV_1 ≥80% predicted With or without symptoms	Short-acting bronchodilators
II	Moderate COPD	FEV_1/FVC <0.7 FEV_1 50%-80% predicted With or without symptoms	Long-acting bronchodilators
III	Severe COPD	FEV_1/FVC <0.7 FEV_1 30%-50% predicted With or without symptoms	Inhaled steroids
IV	Very severe COPD	FEV_1/FVC <0.7 FEV_1 <30% predicted FEV_1 <50% predicted with chronic hypoxemia	Long-term oxygen therapy and consider surgical interventions

Adapted from National Heart, Lung and Blood Institute/World Health Organization. Global initiative for chronic obstructive lung disease. Executive summary. Updated 2009. Available at: http://www.goldcopd.com/Guidelineitem.asp?l1 = 2&l2 = 1&intld = 2205. Accessed October 20, 2010.

annual influenza vaccination. Regular exercise and efforts to maintain normal body weight should be encouraged. Avoidance of second-hand smoke, aggravating occupational exposures, and indoor and outdoor pollution is recommended.

Although pharmacologic treatment cannot reverse lung changes or modify long-term decline in lung function, it does reduce the severity of symptoms, decrease the frequency of exacerbations, and improve exercise tolerance and overall health. **Short-acting bronchodilators used as needed are the recommended treatment in stage I COPD.** These include β_2-agonists (albuterol) and anticholinergics (ipratropium). **Inhaled medications are preferred over oral,** as they tend to have fewer side effects. The choice of specific agent is based on availability, individual response to therapy, and side effects.

In stage II COPD, a long-acting bronchodilator should be added. Commonly used agents in the United States are salmeterol (an inhaled β_2-agonist) and tiotropium (an inhaled anticholinergic). Oral methylxanthines (aminophylline, theophylline) are also options, but have narrow therapeutic windows (high toxicity) and multiple drug-drug interactions, making their use less common. The use of long-acting bronchodilators is more convenient and more effective than using short-acting agents, but is much more expensive and does not replace the need for short-acting agents for rescue therapy in exacerbations.

Inhaled steroids (fluticasone, triamcinolone, mometasone, etc) do not affect the rate of decline of lung function in COPD but do reduce the frequency of exacerbations. For that reason, **inhaled steroids are recommended for stages III and IV COPD with frequent exacerbations.** Long-term treatment with oral steroids is not recommended, as there is no evidence of benefit, and there can be multiple complications (myopathy, osteoporosis, glucose intolerance, etc). Although continuous prophylactic antibiotic use decreases the number of COPD exacerbations for a few years, there is no decrease in mortality and the risk of antibiotic resistance makes this a controversial issue.

Oxygen therapy is recommended in stage IV COPD if there is evidence of hypoxemia (PaO_2 ≤55 mm Hg or SaO_2 ≤88% at rest) or where the PaO_2 is less than or equal to 60 mm Hg and there is polycythemia, pulmonary hypertension, or peripheral edema suggesting heart failure. **Oxygen therapy is the only intervention that has been shown to decrease mortality and must be worn for at least 15 h/d.**

As COPD is a chronic condition that is expected to worsen over time, routine follow-up is imperative. Spirometry is the best method to monitor lung function. The COPD Assessment Test (CAT) is a questionnaire given to patients every 3 months. The CAT is an objective tool to assess changes overtime and the impact that COPD is having on a patient's life. Depending on the stage of the patients, COPD, pulmonary rehabilitation, and possibly lung resection surgery should be considered with the appropriate specialists.

Management of Exacerbations of COPD

An acute COPD exacerbation is defined as a change in respiratory function causing worsening of symptoms which leads to a change in medication. Acute exacerbations of COPD are common and typically present with change in sputum color or amount, cough, wheezing, and increased dyspnea. Although respiratory tract infections (viral and bacterial) are the most common precipitant, air pollutants are another common cause of acute COPD exacerbations. Diagnoses that can cause similar symptoms (eg, pulmonary embolism, congestive heart failure, myocardial infarction, pneumonia, pneumothorax, pleural effusion) must be excluded so that appropriate therapy can occur.

The severity of the exacerbation should be evaluated by history, examination, assessment of oxygenation using a pulse oximetry, and focused testing. The following questions from the medical history may help to assist in assessing the exacerbation: number of previous episodes and hospitalizations, other chronic conditions, current treatment regimen, history of intubation/mechanical ventilation, and duration and new symptoms. Physical examination signs of severity include the use of respiratory muscles, worsening or new cyanosis, unstable blood pressure and heart rate, altered mental status, and peripheral edema. Oxygen should be given with a target saturation of 88% to 92% or PaO_2 levels at about 60 mm Hg.

Patients with more severe symptoms, comorbidities, altered mental status, an inability to care for themselves at home, or whose symptoms fail to respond promptly to office or emergency room treatments should be hospitalized. If hospitalized, a baseline arterial blood gas should be ordered to evaluate for hypercapnia, hypoxemia, and respiratory acidosis. Ventilatory support with either noninvasive (nasal or face mask) or invasive ventilation (intubation) should be considered in deteriorating or critical patients.

All acute exacerbations should be treated with short-acting bronchodilators. Combinations of short-acting agents with different mechanisms of action (ie, β-agonist and anticholinergic) can be used until symptoms improve. **Systemic** steroids shorten the course of the exacerbation and may reduce the risk of relapse. A steroid dose of 40 mg prednisolone (or equivalent) for 10 to 14 days is recommended.

Exacerbations associated with increased amounts of sputum or with purulent sputum should be treated with antibiotics. A sputum culture should be performed. *Pneumococcus, Haemophilus influenzae, and Moraxella catarrhalis* are the most common bacteria implicated. In milder exacerbations, treatment with oral agents directed against these pathogens is appropriate. In severe exacerbations, gram-negative bacteria (*Klebsiella, Pseudomonas*) can also play a role, so antibiotic coverage needs to be broader.

Measures taken to prevent COPD exacerbation should be discussed and reviewed at each patient encounter. The number of annual exacerbations can be reduced by receiving appropriate vaccinations (influenza and pneumococcal), smoking cessation counseling, education about current medications and their proper use. Patients should be encouraged to discuss social concerns, psychiatric problems (such as anxiety), and proper nutrition and exercise with their physician.

COMPREHENSION QUESTIONS

2.1 A 38-year-old woman presents with progressively worsening dyspnea and cough. She has never smoked cigarettes, has no known passive smoke exposure, and does not have any occupational exposure to chemicals. Pulmonary function testing shows obstructive lung disease that does not respond to bronchodilators. Which of the following is the most likely etiology?

   A.   Radon exposure at home

   B.   COPD

   C. α_1-Antitrypsin deficiency

   D.   Asthma

2.2 A 60-year-old man is diagnosed with moderately severe (stage II) COPD. He admits to a long history of cigarette smoking and is still currently smoking. In counseling him about the benefits of smoking cessation, which of the following statements is most accurate?

   A.   By quitting, his pulmonary function will significantly improve.

   B.   By quitting, his current pulmonary function will be unchanged, but the rate of pulmonary function decline will slow.

   C.   By quitting, his current pulmonary function and the rate of decline are unchanged, but there are cardiovascular benefits.

   D.   By quitting, his pulmonary function will approach that of a nonsmoker of the same age.

2.3 A 68-year-old patient of your practice with known COPD has pulmonary function testing showing an FEV_1 of 40% predicted has been having frequent exacerbations of his COPD. His SaO_2 by pulse oximetry is 91%. Which of the following medication regimens is the most appropriate?

A. Inhaled salmeterol BID and albuterol as needed

B. Oral albuterol daily and inhaled fluticasone BID

C. Inhaled fluticasone BID, inhaled tiotropium BID, and inhaled albuterol as needed

D. Inhaled fluticasone BID, inhaled tiotropium BID, inhaled albuterol as needed, and home oxygen therapy

2.4 A 59-year-old man with a known history of COPD presents with worsening dyspnea. On examination, he is afebrile. His breath sounds are decreased bilaterally. He is noted to have jugular venous distension (JVD) and 2+ pitting edema of the lower extremities. Which of the following is the most likely cause of his increasing dyspnea?

A. COPD exacerbation

B. Pneumonia

C. Cor pulmonale

D. Pneumothorax

ANSWERS

2.1 **C.** This patient has a fixed airway obstruction consistent with COPD. The airway obstruction of asthma would be at least partially reversible on testing with a bronchodilator. α_1-Antitrypsin deficiency should be considered in a patient who develops COPD at a young age, especially if there is no other identifiable risk factor.

2.2 **B.** Smoking cessation will not result in reversal of the lung damage that has already occurred, but can result in a slowing in the rate of decline of pulmonary function. In fact, smoking cessation can result in the rate of decline returning to that of a nonsmoker.

2.3 **C.** This patient has stage III COPD with frequent exacerbations. He is best treated by a long-acting bronchodilator (eg, tiotropium) and an inhaled steroid (eg, fluticasone) used regularly, along with an inhaled, short-acting bronchodilator on an as-needed basis.

2.4 **C.** JVD and lower extremity edema are suggestive of cor pulmonale, which is right heart failure due to chronically elevated pressures in the pulmonary circulation. Right heart failure causes increased right atrial pressures and right ventricular end-diastolic pressures, which then lead to liver congestion, jugular venous distension, and lower extremity edema.

CLINICAL PEARLS

▶ All smokers should be counseled on the benefits of smoking cessation before they develop symptomatic COPD; by the time symptoms develop, the patient's FEV$_1$ will have reduced by approximately 50%.

▶ Always remember to evaluate the ABCs—**A**irway, **B**reathing, **C**irculation— when evaluating a dyspneic patient.

REFERENCES

Armstrong C. ACP updated guidelines on diagnosis and management of stable COPD. *Am Fam Physician*. 2012 Jan 15;85(2):204-205.

Herath SC, Pooler P. Prophylactic antibiotic therapy for chronic obstructive pulmonary disease (COPD). *Cochrane Database Syst Rev*. 2013 Nov 28;11:CD009764.

National Heart, Lung and Blood Institute/World Health Organization. Global initiative for chronic obstructive lung disease. Executive summary. Updated 2011. Available at: http://www.goldcopd.com/Guidelineitem.asp?l1=2&l2=1&intId=2205. Accessed January 28, 2015.

Reilly JJ Jr., Silverman EK, Shapiro SD. Chronic obstructive pulmonary disease. In: Kasper D, Fauci A, Hauser S, Longo D, Jameson J, Loscalzo J, eds. *Harrison's Principles of Internal Medicine*. 19th ed. New York, NY: McGraw-Hill Education; 2015. Available at: http://accessmedicine.mhmedical.com. Accessed May 25, 2015.

A 45-year-old white man presents to your office complaining of left knee pain that started last night. He says that the pain started suddenly after dinner and was severe within a span of 3 hours. He denies any trauma, fever, systemic symptoms, or prior similar episodes. He has a history of hypertension for which he takes hydrochlorothiazide (HCTZ). He admits to consuming a great amount of wine last night with dinner.

On examination, his temperature is 98°F, his pulse is 90 beats/min, his respirations are 22 breaths/min, and his blood pressure is 129/88 mm Hg. Heart and lung examinations are unremarkable. The patient is reluctant to flex the left knee, wincing in pain at touch, and has passive range of motion. The knee is edematous, hot to touch, and has erythema of the overlying skin. No crepitation or deformity is apparent. No other joints are involved. Inguinal lymph nodes are not enlarged. Complete blood count (CBC) reveals a white blood cell count of 10,900 cells/mm^3 and is otherwise normal.

▶ What is the next diagnostic step?
▶ What is the most likely diagnosis?
▶ What is the next step in therapy?

ANSWERS TO CASE 3:
Joint Pain

Summary: This is a 45-year-old man who presents with the sudden onset of monoarticular, nontraumatic joint pain. Evolution from onset to severe pain was rapid. The patient denies any trauma, systemic signs of illness, or any prior episodes. The history that he took HCTZ and drank a lot of alcohol the night that his symptoms started is important. His vital signs are stable, and he does not appear to be systemically ill. There is pain to movement and touch of the left knee, with evident edema, erythema, and warmth of the joint. No other joints are involved. His white blood cell count is not indicative of an acute infectious process.

- **Next diagnostic step:** Joint aspiration for examination of joint fluid to identify crystals and exclude infection

- **Most likely diagnosis:** Crystal-induced gout of the left knee

- **Next step in therapy:** Nonsteroidal anti-inflammatory drug (NSAID) and provide analgesia; may consider using colchicine

ANALYSIS

Objectives

1. Have a differential diagnosis for nontraumatic joint pain, based on clinical presentation.

2. Be familiar with the most common diagnostic tests for the above conditions, and have a rationale when ordering these tests.

3. Know the most common treatment options in the acute onset of gout and infectious arthritis, as well as the chronic management of rheumatoid arthritis (RA) and osteoarthritis (OA).

Considerations

This 45-year-old man presents with the sudden onset of monoarticular joint pain. **The first diagnosis that needs to be excluded is an infected joint.** A joint becomes septic by blood inoculation, by contiguous infection (such as from bone or soft tissue), or from direct inoculation from trauma or surgery. Exclusion of an infectious etiology is paramount as cartilage can be destroyed within the first 24 hours of infection. In this case, the patient's history and clinical scenario do not favor an infectious cause, although it cannot be excluded by history and physical examination alone.

There are several additional pieces of information that guide the diagnosis in this case. Most gout attacks occur between the ages of 30 and 50 in men and in postmenopausal women (50-70 years of age). Premenopausal women are less likely to suffer from gout due to the increased level of female sex hormones, which aid in the urinary excretion of uric acid. Genetic mutations associated with the overproduction or underexcretion of uric acid can be the contributing factor for gout attacks. African Americans have a higher risk of having a gout attack. Other factors that may also increase the risk of a gout attack include trauma, surgery, or a large meal (especially one high in purines such as red meat, liver, nuts, or seafood) that induces hyperuricemia. The patient's recent increase in alcohol consumption can be considered an exacerbating factor. Finally, the patient's history of taking a **thiazide diuretic** is also important, as these drugs **may induce hyperuricemia** by increasing urinary urate reabsorption. Other medications that increase the risk of a gout attack include loop diuretics and chemotherapeutic agents. Weight loss has been proven to lower the risk of gout.

The examination of a joint aspirate is essential for the diagnosis. The **gross appearance of fluid is not very specific**, as both a septic aspirate and a heavily condensed crystal-induced arthritis may have a thick, yellowish/chalky appearance. To diagnose crystal-induced arthritis, polarizing microscopy must reveal monosodium urate (MSU) crystals, which will look like needles and have a strong negative bire-fringence. Other crystals that may be seen are **calcium pyrophosphate dehydrate (CPPD), calcium hydroxyapatite, and calcium oxalate.**

- **CPPD:** Rod-shaped, rhomboid, weakly positive birefringence

- **Calcium hydroxyapatite:** Seen by electron microscopy, cytoplasmic inclusions those are nonbirefringent

- **Calcium oxalate:** Bipyramidal appearance, strongly positive birefringence; seen mostly in end-stage renal disease patients

In crystal-induced arthritis, the white blood cell count of the joint aspirate is on average 2000 to 60,000/μL, with less than 90% neutrophils, while a septic joint will have an average of 100,000 WBC/μL (25,000-250,000 cells) with more than 90% neutrophils. Aspirate that has been determined to be crystal-induced must also be cultured so as to rule out a coexisting infection.

APPROACH TO:
Nontraumatic Joint Pain/Swelling

DEFINITIONS

GOUTY ARTHRITIS: Condition of excess uric acid leading to deposition of MSU crystals in joints

PSEUDOGOUT: Condition of joint pain and inflammation due to **calcium pyrophosphate dehydrate crystals in the joints**, which can be diagnosed by noting rod-shaped, rhomboid, weakly positive birefringence by crystal analysis

CLINICAL APPROACH

Depending on the etiology, pain may be present in one, two, or more joints. Considering the patient's age, medical history, and medication profile are important.

The patient's lifestyle and social history should also be considered, as certain activities may predispose a patient to specific infections. Among **the major diagnoses that have to be considered in a nontraumatic swollen joint are gout (or any crystal-induced arthritis), infectious arthritis, osteoarthritis, and rheumatoid arthritis.** For acute monoarticular arthritis in adults, the most common causes include trauma, crystals, and infection.

Clinical Presentation

Gout can be divided into four stages: (1) asymptotic tissue deposition of crystals, (2) acute gout flares, (3) intercritical segments (occurring after an acute flare, but before the next flare), and (4) chronic gout (symptoms of chronic arthritis and/or tophi). Gout's first episode can often be confused with cellulitis. It presents with swelling and pain, usually of one joint, accompanied by erythema and warmth. **Classically, a gout attack involves the metatarsophalangeal joint of the first toe, called podagra,** but it may involve any joint in the body. Some cases, left untreated, resolve spontaneously within 3 to 10 days, with no residual signs or symptoms. **During an acute attack, the serum uric acid level may be normal or even low,** likely as a result of the existing deposition of the urate crystals. Uric acid levels are, however, useful in monitoring hypouricemic therapy between attacks. Radiographs may show cystic changes in the joint surface, with punched-out lesions and soft-tissue calcifications. These findings are nonspecific and are also seen in osteoarthritis and rheumatoid arthritis. In patients suspected to have gout, it is important to ask about recent trauma or injury. Following a traumatic event, an increase in the concentration of urate can be seen within the synovial fluid. Although imaging studies are not often necessary for the diagnosis of gout, a history of trauma may warrant such testing to rule out a fracture.

An infection usually involves only one joint if it is of bacterial origin (>90% of cases). Most cases of infectious arthritis occur in large joints including the knee, hip, and shoulder. A *chronic* monoarticular arthritis or involvement of two to three joints may be caused by fungi or mycobacteria. In the case of acute polyarticular (more than three joints) arthritis, the etiology may be from endocarditis or a disseminated gonococcal infection. The three ways that microorgranisms can infect joints include (1) direct penetration (surgery, bite, and trauma), (2) hematogenous spread from a distant infection, (3) extension from a nearby infected joint. Along with arthrocentesis with examination of synovial fluid, a blood culture, Gram stain and culture, CBC and erythrocyte sedimentation rate (ESR) should be obtained.

Risk factors for infectious arthritis include alcoholism, malignancy, diabetes, hemodialysis, immunodeficiency (HIV), immunosuppressive drugs (corticosteroids), chronic medical conditions (endocrine, pulmonary or hepatic disease), hemophilia, and the use of intravenous drugs. Bacterial infections of a joint occur most commonly in persons with rheumatoid arthritis. The chronic inflammation of joints coupled with the use of steroids predisposes this group to *Staphylococcus aureus* infections. HIV-positive patients may develop pneumococcal, *Salmonella*, or even *Haemophilus influenzae* joint infections. Intravenous drug users are most likely to get a streptococcal, staphylococcal, gram-negative, or *Pseudomonas* infection.

Range of motion (ROM) of the joint is an important maneuver of the physical examination. **A septic joint will have a very limited ROM due to pain** coupled with a joint effusion and fever. However, a nearby cellulitis, bursitis, or osteomyelitis will usually maintain the ROM of a joint. The aspirate of a septic joint will have a positive culture in more than 90% of cases.

Osteoarthritis (OA) is most commonly found in people older than 65 years (68% of patients) and is associated with trauma, history of repetitive joint use, and obesity (specifically for knee OA). It primarily affects the cartilage, but ends up damaging the bone surface, synovium, meniscus, and ligaments. The clinical presentation is usually that of a dull, deep, ache-type pain. The onset is usually gradual, with activity exacerbating the pain, and rest decreasing it. In the latter stages, pain is usually constant. On physical examination, a bony crepitus may be felt on passive ROM. There may be a small joint effusion and periarticular muscle atrophy. In the advanced stage, joint deformity with decreased ROM will be seen. **X-rays are usually normal at first**, with the gradual development of bone sclerosis, subchondral cysts, and osteophytes.

Rheumatoid arthritis (RA) is another common disorder that may affect people from any age group, but will usually present initially in those 30 to 55 years old. The presentation of RA can be varied, ranging from a monoarticular arthritis that is intermittent, to a polyarthritis that progresses gradually in intensity, leading to disability. It affects more women than men (3:1), and the treatment will usually depend on the stage at which the disease is diagnosed. It is thought that the increase in proinflammatory cytokines (such as tumor necrosis factor [TNF] and interleukin-6) within the synovial cells of joints is responsible for the destruction of cartilage and bony erosions seen in RA. Among the laboratory tests that may be abnormal in patients with RA are a positive rheumatoid factor (RF) and anti-citrullinated protein antibody (anti-CCP), an elevated ESR, an elevated C-reactive protein (CRP), anemia, thrombocytosis, and low albumin. The level of hypoalbuminemia usually correlates with the severity of the disease. The anti-CCP autoantibody is more specific than RF; additionally, a positive anti-CCP may precede the clinical manifestation of disease by many years.

In 2010, the American College of Rheumatology/European League Against Rheumatism (ACR/EULAR) developed a new approach to diagnose RA that focuses on features found in the earlier stages of disease. According to this new classification, RA is diagnosed if a person presents with synovitis (swelling) in at least one joint, all other diagnoses for the synovitis are excluded, and has a calculated individual score of 6 points or more (maximum of 10 points). This individual score is based upon both clinical and laboratory factors, including the number and site of involved joints, serologic abnormalities (RF and anti-CCP), elevated acute-phase response markers (CRP and ESR), and symptom duration (Table 3–1).

Treatment

Analgesia is a common factor to consider in therapy for all the conditions described earlier. In the case of an acute gout attack, colchicines, nonsteroidal anti-inflammatory drugs (NSAIDs), and glucocorticoids are the drugs mainly used. Rapid and complete resolution of symptoms from acute gout treatment should begin within 24 hours of symptom onset. NSAIDs should be used with caution or avoided entirely in elderly patients (possibility of gastrointestinal [GI] complications), heart failure patients, those with peptic ulcer disease, and individuals with liver or renal disease.

Table 3–1 • ACR/EULAR CRITERIA FOR DIAGNOSIS OF RHEUMATOID ARTHRITIS
1. Synovitis (swelling) is present in at least 1 joint
2. All other diagnoses for clinical synovitis are excluded

3. Individual score ≥6 points is reached based on the following criteria:
   a. Joint involvement: 1 large[a] joint (no points), 2-10 large joints (1 point), 1-3 small[b] joints +/– large joint (2 points), 4-10 small joints +/– large joints (3 points), >10 joints (5 points)
   b. Serology: Negative RF **and** anti-CCP (no points), low positive RF **or** anti-CCP (2 points), high positive RF **or** anti-CCP (3 points)
   c. Acute-phase reactants: normal CRP **and** normal ESR (no points), abnormal CRP **or** abnormal ESR (1 point)
   d. Duration of symptoms: <6 weeks (no point), >6 weeks (1 point)

[a]*Large joints include shoulders, elbows, hips, knees, and ankles.*
[b]*Small joints include wrists, MCP, PIP, 2nd to 5th MTPs, and thumb interphalangeal joints.*
Data from Aletaha D, Neogi T, Silman AJ, et al. Rheumatoid arthritis classification criteria. Arthritis Rheum. 2010;62(9);2569-2581.

To reduce these risks, intra-articular steroids, ice packs, and low-dose colchicine are more often used. In patients with recurrent gout attacks, chronic medication therapy can be used to maintain serum uric acid levels below 5 mg/dL. The maintenance therapy is usually with either probenecid, which increases the urinary excretion of uric acid, or allopurinol, which reduces the production of uric acid. **Maintenance therapy should not be used during an acute gout attack.** Consider short-term corticosteroids once septic arthritis is ruled out. Use immunosuppressive therapy with caution, especially in patients with diabetes mellitus.

    The preferred treatment for septic arthritis includes IV antimicrobials and surgery for drainage of the infected joint. Methicillin-resistant *S aureus* (MRSA) will usually require vancomycin, but coverage with antibiotics is dependent on the specific organisms isolated.

    Degenerative joint disease treatment involves mobility exercises, maintenance of adequate ROM, and weight loss, if appropriate. Intra-articular corticosteroid injections may provide relief for varying amounts of time, but should only be done every 4 to 6 months so as to avoid cartilage destruction. Surgery, such as joint replacement, is usually reserved for people with severe disease that affects their daily functions.

    Therapy for RA involves multiple modalities. Education and counseling of the patient regarding disease progression, treatment options, and implications to lifestyle is essential. Exercises, such as those that maintain joint mobility and muscle strength, are very important, as the natural course of RA is to develop a stiff joint that becomes disabling. Physical therapy and occupational therapy are important to address specific areas in which the patient may need additional devices to perform activities of daily living.

    Many different categories of medications are used in RA. **Disease-modifying antirheumatic drugs (DMARDs)**, are the first-line agent for the treatment of RA. Among the DMARDs are sulfasalazine and methotrexate. NSAIDs, glucocorticoids, anticytokines, and topical analgesics can be used with DMARDs as adjuvant medication during the first month of treatment. Infliximab and etanercept are examples of anticytokine agents. Treatment regimens are individualized, and will often include a combination of two or three of these agents. Although effective, monitoring for hepatotoxicity must be performed.

COMPREHENSION QUESTIONS

3.1 A 26-year-old man presents with fever, dysuria, and left knee pain. He reports being sexually active with a new partner as recently as 2 weeks ago. On physical examination, he is febrile and his left knee is erythematous, swollen, and tender. He denies a previous history of arthritis. Which of the following is the next best step?

A. CBC with differential

B. X-ray of the knee

C. Aspiration of synovial fluid

D. Serum uric acid level

3.2 A 44-year-old woman has a 5-month history of malaise and stiff hands in the morning that improve as the day goes by. She notes that both hands are involved at the wrists. Initial laboratory tests show an elevated ESR and high positive anti-CCP. Which of the following treatments is most likely to lead to the best long-term disease outcome for this patient?

A. Allopurinol

B. Ibuprofen

C. Naproxen

D. Methotrexate

E. Intravenous ceftriaxone

3.3 A 52-year-old man complains of bilateral knee pain for about 1 year. He is noted to have a body mass index (BMI) of 40 kg/m². Which of the following is the best therapy?

A. Allopurinol

B. Ibuprofen

C. Methotrexate

D. Intravenous ceftriaxone

E. Oral glucocorticoids

3.4 A 35-year-old man with hypertension presents with the sudden onset of right big toe pain. Which of the following is the best treatment?

A. Ibuprofen

B. Methotrexate

C. Colchicine

D. Intravenous antibiotics

ANSWERS

3.1 **C.** Infectious arthritis would need to be high on the differential diagnosis because of the danger of gonococcal arthritis. The history supports this diagnosis. This patient needs a joint aspiration to look for gram-negative diplococci, crystals, and to obtain a sample for culture. He will likely require surgical drainage of the swollen joint and IV antibiotic therapy.

3.2 **D.** Morning stiffness, involvement of the hands, and symmetric arthritis are common features of RA. According to the ACR/EULAR, this patient meets the criteria for the diagnosis of newly presenting RA in that she has joint involvement, positive serology, elevated acute-phase reactants, and duration of symptoms more than 6 weeks. DMARD therapy, such as the use of methotrexate, would be indicated. Methotrexate as a disease-modifying agent would alter the natural history of the disease rather than just treat the symptoms.

3.3 **B.** Obesity is a risk factor for osteoarthritis, which is common in the knees and typically presents with a gradual onset and worsening of symptoms. Along with exercise and efforts to lose weight, an NSAID medication, such as ibuprofen, may provide symptomatic relief.

3.4 **C.** Gouty arthritis often initially presents in the big toe ("podagra") and the use of HCTZ, a common treatment for hypertension, also can increase the risk. Colchicine can provide effective acute treatment.

CLINICAL PEARLS

▶ A red, swollen joint **must** be aspirated to rule out a joint infection.

▶ Trauma, infection, and crystals are the most common causes of acute monoarthritis in adults.

REFERENCES

Aletaha D, Neogi T, Silman AJ, et al. Rheumatoid arthritis classification criteria. *Arthritis Rheum.* 2010;62(9):2569-2581.

Bieber JD, Terkeltaub RA. Gout. On the brink of novel therapeutic options for an ancient disease. *Arthritis Rheum.* 2004;50:2400-2414.

Cush J. Approach to articular and musculoskeletal disorders. In: Kasper D, Fauci A, Hauser S, et al, eds. *Harrison's Principles of Internal Medicine.* 19th ed. New York, NY: McGraw-Hill Education, 2015. Available at: http://accessmedicine.mhmedical.com. Accessed May 25, 2014.

Hainer BL, Matheson E, Wilkes RT. Diagnosis, treatment and prevention of gout. *Am Fam Physician.* 2014;90(12):831-836.

Mochan E, Ebell MH. Predicting rheumatoid arthritis risk in adults with undifferentiated arthritis. *Am Fam Physician.* 2008;77:1451-1453.

Shah A, St. Clair EW. Rheumatoid arthritis. In: Kasper D, Fauci A, Hauser S, et al, eds. *Harrison's Principles of Internal Medicine*. 19th ed. New York, NY: McGraw-Hill Education, 2015. Available at: http://accessmedicine.mhmedical.com. Accessed May 24, 2015.

The Merk Manual. *Acute Infectious Arthritis*. Whitehouse Station, NJ: Merck Sharp & Dohme Corp.; 2015.

Wasserman AM. Diagnosis and management of rheumatoid arthritis. *Am Fam Physician*. 2011:84(11): 1245-1252.

A 22-year-old woman who has never been pregnant before presents to you after having a positive home pregnancy test. She has no significant medical history. Upon further questioning, she states that she is unsure of the date of her last menstrual period. She denies any symptoms and is worried as she has not felt the baby move thus far. She is also concerned as she recently had dental x-rays taken prior to discovering that she was pregnant. Patient denies the use of any drugs, alcohol, or tobacco. She inquires about when she can get an ultrasound and a genetic test to rule out Down syndrome.

▶ When is an ultrasound indicated in prenatal care?
▶ What laboratory studies are routinely indicated at an initial prenatal visit?
▶ What is the risk to the pregnancy based on the radiation exposure that the patient has encountered?
▶ When is the optimal time for screening with a trisomy screen test?

ANSWERS TO CASE 4:
Prenatal Care

Summary: A 22-year-old primigravida woman with no significant past medical history presents for initial prenatal care visit. She has numerous questions regarding her care and recently has had dental x-rays taken.

- **Indications for an ultrasound in pregnancy:** According to the American College of Obstetricians and Gynecologists (ACOG), an ultrasound is not mandatory in routine, low-risk prenatal care. An ultrasound is indicated for the evaluation of uncertain gestational age, size/date discrepancies, vaginal bleeding, multiple gestations, or other high-risk situations.

- **Laboratory studies recommended at the initial prenatal visit:** Complete blood count (CBC), hepatitis B surface antigen (HBsAg), HIV testing, syphilis screening with a rapid plasma reagin (RPR), urinalysis and urine culture, rubella antibody, blood type and Rh status with antibody screen, Papanicolaou (Pap) smear, and cervical swab for gonorrhea and *Chlamydia*.

- **Risk to the pregnancy based on the radiation exposure from dental x-rays:** Risk for the baby is increased once the radiation exposure is greater than 5 rad; the radiation exposure from routine dental x-rays is 0.00017 rad.

- **The optimal time for the trisomy screen:** The options for trisomy screening include first trimester testing for nuchal translucency (NT) via ultrasound or a combined test of NT and serum markers human chorionic gonadotropin (hCG) and pregnancy-associated plasma protein A (PAPP-A) testing between 10 and 13 weeks and second trimester triple (AFP, hCG, estriol) or quadruple (triple screen and inhibin-A) screen between 16- and 18-week gestation; however, it may be performed between 15- and 20-week gestation, if necessary. Emerging evidence shows that combining results of first- and second-trimester screening tests improves trisomy detection rate; consequently, the optimal time for screening should be discussed at initial prenatal visit. Concerning results from the above tests may warrant more invasive testing to confirm chromosomal abnormalities. These tests include chronic villous sampling at 10 to 13 weeks or amniocentesis at 16 to 18 weeks.

ANALYSIS

Objectives

1. Learn the components of the preconception counseling and the initial prenatal visit.

2. Know the recommended screening tests and visit intervals in routine prenatal care.

3. Learn the relevant psychosocial aspects of providing prenatal care, including important counseling issues.

Considerations

Prenatal, or antenatal, care affords the opportunity to both perform appropriate medical testing and provide counseling and anticipatory guidance. Pregnancy can be a time of anxiety and patients frequently have many questions. One of the goals of prenatal care is to provide appropriate education in order to help reduce anxiety and help women to be active participants in their own care.

APPROACH TO:
Prenatal Care

DEFINITIONS

ADVANCED MATERNAL AGE: Pregnant woman who will be 35 years or beyond at the estimated date of delivery (EDD).

ISOIMMUNIZATION: The development of specific antibodies as a result of antigenic stimulation by material from the red blood cells of another individual. For example, Rh isoimmunization means a Rh-negative woman who develops anti-D (Rh factor) antibodies in response to exposure to Rh (D) antigen.

ASYMPTOMATIC BACTERIURIA (ASB): 100,000 cfu/mL or more of a pure pathogen of a mid-stream voided specimen without clinical symptoms. ASB in pregnant women increase risk of acute pyelonephritis, preterm delivery, and low birth weight; therefore, early detection is paramount and treatment is mandated.

GENETIC COUNSELING: An educational process provided by a health-care professional for individuals and families who have a genetic disease or who are at risk for such a disease. It is designed to provide patients and their families with information about their condition or potential condition and help them make informed decisions.

VERTICAL TRANSMISSION: Infectious passage of infection from mother to fetus, whether in utero, during labor and delivery, or postpartum.

ANTENATAL TESTING: A procedure that attempts to identify whether the fetus is at risk for uteroplacental insufficiency and perinatal death. Some of these tests include nonstress test and biophysical profile.

CLINICAL APPROACH

Preconception

In the United States, the first visit for prenatal care frequently is at 8 weeks of gestation or later, and yet it is the time preceding this that poses the greatest risk to fetal development. **A preconception visit is an ideal opportunity for the patient to discuss with her physician any issue related to possible pregnancy or contraception occurring within 1 year of pregnancy.** The preconception visit can be included during visits for many reasons, including fertility problems, contraception, periodic health assessment, recent amenorrhea, or specifically for preconception counseling. Roughly one-half of patients with a negative pregnancy test may have some risk that could adversely affect a future pregnancy. Because roughly 50% of pregnancies are unplanned or unintended, physicians should consider the potential of pregnancy when writing each prescription. The primary care physician should ask women of reproductive age about their intention to become pregnant. Contraceptive counseling should be given based on the patient's intentions.

Women who intend to become pregnant should be advised to avoid, whenever possible, potentially harmful agents such as radiation, drugs, alcohol, tobacco, over-the-counter (OTC) medications, herbs, and other environmental agents. **Radiation exposure greater than 5 rad is associated with fetal harm. Most commonly performed x-ray procedures, including dental, chest, and extremity x-rays, expose a fetus to only very small fractions of this amount of radiation.** Fetuses are particularly sensitive to radiation during the early stages of development, between 2 and 15 weeks after conception. Whenever possible, the abdomen and pelvis should be shielded and x-rays performed only when the benefit outweighs the potential risk. Imaging procedures not associated with ionizing radiation, including ultrasound or magnetic resonance imaging, should be considered as alternatives to x-ray during pregnancy when appropriate.

Women should refrain from OTC medicines, herbs, vitamins, minerals, and nutritional products until cleared by their obstetric provider. The US Public Health Service and CDC recommend that all women of childbearing take folic acid daily and women considering conception should start a folic acid supplement at least 1 month prior to attempting to conceive. **For low-risk women, 400 to 800 μg of folic acid daily is recommended to reduce the risk of neural tube defects.** Higher doses are recommended in the presence of certain risk factors. For women with diabetes mellitus or epilepsy, 1 mg of folic acid a day is recommended. **A woman who has had a child with a neural tube defect should take 4 mg of folic acid daily.**

Women from certain ethnic backgrounds may be offered specific genetic screening. African and African-American women may be offered sickle cell trait screening. A French-Canadian or Ashkenazi Jewish background is an indication to consider screening for a Tay-Sachs carrier state. Southeast Asian and Middle Eastern women may be offered screening for thalassemia. Ashkenazi Jews and Caucasian women may be offered screening for cystic fibrosis.

Women who will be 35 years old or older at the anticipated time of delivery should be educated about age-related risk, particularly the increased risk of Down syndrome. They should be counseled about the available screening and diagnostic testing available, along with the appropriate time frame in which each test may be performed.

Women with medical conditions such as diabetes, asthma, thyroid disease, hypertension, lupus, thromboembolism, and seizures should be referred to providers with experience in managing high-risk pregnancies. Women with psychiatric disorders should be comanaged with a psychiatrist and counselor/therapist so that the patient can benefit from pharmacologic and behavioral therapy. These patients may require more frequent visits.

Pregnant women and those looking to become pregnant should be screened for tobacco use. Patients who have drug, tobacco, or alcohol dependence should be educated about the risks and referred to rehab/treatment centers to quit the drug prior to conception. Women should also be educated about proper nutrition and exercise during pregnancy. Preconception counseling may also address issues such as financial readiness, social support during pregnancy and the postpartum period, and issues of domestic violence.

Initial Prenatal Visit

The initial visit should address all the concepts in the preconception visit, if no preconception counseling was done. Ideally, the initial visit should be in the first trimester. A detailed history and physical examination, initial obstetric laboratory tests, and counseling regarding the logistics for prenatal care should be done at this visit. The history should begin with an assessment of the last menstrual period (LMP) and its reliability. **One of the most crucial pieces of information is the accuracy of the dating.** The first day of the LMP is used to obtain the EDD using Naegele's rule (from the first day of the LMP subtract 3 months and add 7 days). The LMP is considered reliable if the following criteria are met: the date is certain, the last menstrual period was normal, there has been no contraceptive use in the past 1 year, the patient has had no bleeding since the LMP, and her menses are regular. If these criteria are not met, an ultrasound should be performed. ACOG has established further criteria that can be used to ensure that a fetus is mature at the time of delivery, which include criteria such as early sonography and the timing of the positive pregnancy test.

History should also be obtained with particular attention to medical history, prior pregnancies, delivery outcomes, pregnancy complications, neonatal complications, and birth weights. Gynecologic history should focus on the menstrual history, contraceptive use, and history of sexually transmitted diseases (STDs). Allergies, current medications—both prescription and OTC—and substance use should also be investigated. Social history should consider whether the pregnancy was planned, unplanned, or unintentional. A discussion of social supports for the patient during the prenatal and postpartum period is also warranted. Genetic history should be obtained for the patient and partner's family, if known.

The initial examination should be thorough and should assess height, weight, blood pressure, thyroid, breast, and general physical and pelvic examinations. Pregnancy-specific examinations, including an estimation of gestational age by uterine size or fundal height measurement and an attempt to hear fetal heart tones by Doppler fetoscope should be performed. Heart tones should be obtainable by 10-week gestation using a handheld Doppler fetoscope. Pelvimetry has been removed as a recommended required intervention, but it may be useful to have a subjective assessment for risks of problems during delivery.

The initial laboratory screen (Table 4–1) should include blood type and Rh status antibody screen, rubella status, HIV, HBsAg, RPR, urinalysis, urine culture, Pap smear, cervical swab for gonorrhea and *Chlamydia*, and a CBC. The inactivated influenza vaccination should be offered to all pregnant women during flu season.

The logistics of the prenatal visits should be addressed. A typical protocol includes follow-up visits every 4 weeks until 28-week gestation, every 2 weeks from 28- to 36-week gestation, and every week from 36-week gestation until delivery.

Table 4–1 • SUMMARY OF PRENATAL LABORATORIES, RAMIFICATIONS, AND EVALUATION

Lab Test	Finding	Ramifications	Next Step	Comments
Hemoglobin	<10.5 g/dL	Preterm delivery Low fetal iron stores Identify thalassemia	Mild: therapeutic trial of iron Moderate: ferritin and Hb electrophoresis	
Rubella	Negative	Nonimmune to rubella	Stay away from sick individuals, vaccinate postpartum	Live attenuated vaccine in the post-partum period
Blood type	Any type	May help pediatricians identify ABO incompatibility		
Rh factor	Negative	May be sus-ceptible to Rh disease	If antibody screen negative, give RhoGAM at 28 weeks, after any trauma, obstetrical complication, or invasive procedure, and if baby is Rh+, then also after delivery	RhoGAM (D immu-noglobulin) 300 μg IM × 1 dose at 28-wk gestation or within 72 h of trauma, complication, procedure, or delivery
Antibody screen	Positive	May indicate isoimmunization	Need to identify the antibody, and then titer	Lewis lives, Kell kills, Duffy dies
HIV ELISA	Positive	May indicate infection with HIV	Western blot or PCR, if positive then place pt on anti-HIV meds, offer elective cesarean, or IV ZDV (zidovudine) in labor	Intervention reduces vertical transmission from 25% to 2% Antiretroviral therapy is started in 2nd trimester
RPR or VDRL	Positive	May indicate syphilis	Specific antibody such as MHA-TP, and if positive, then stage disease	Less than 1 y, penicillin IM × 1; >1 y or unknown, penicillin IM each week × 3
Gonorrhea	Positive	May cause preterm labor, blindness	Ceftriaxone 125 mg IM × 1 dose	
Chlamydia	Positive	May cause neo-natal blindness, pneumonia	Azithromycin 1 g PO × 1 or amoxicillin 500 mg PO TID × 7 days	

(Continued)

Table 4–1 • SUMMARY OF PRENATAL LABORATORIES, RAMIFICATIONS, AND EVALUATION (CONTINUED)

Lab Test	Finding	Ramifications	Next Step	Comments
Hepatitis B surface antigen	Positive	Patient is infectious	Check LFTs and hepatitis serology to determine if chronic carrier vs active hepatitis	Baby needs HBIG and hepatitis B vaccine
Urine culture	Positive	Asymptomatic bacteriuria may lead to pyelonephritis 25%	Treat with antibiotic and recheck urine culture	If GBS is organism, then give penicillin in labor
Pap smear	Positive	Only invasive cancer would alter management	ASC–US = repap postpartum; LGSIL, HSIL = colposcopy	Reflexive HPV not recommended with ASC–US
Nuchal translucency (NT) (10-13 wk) or combined test (NT, hCG, and PAPP-A)	Positive	May indicate trisomy	Offer karyotype, follow-up ultrasounds, chorionic villas sampling (CVS) or second-trimester screening	Increased NT means increased risk, not definitive diagnosis
Trisomy screen (15-20 wk)	Positive	At risk for trisomy or NTD	Basic ultrasound for dates; if dates confirmed, offer genetic amniocentesis	Most common reason for abnormal serum screening: wrong dates
1-h diabetic screen (26-28 wk)	Positive (elevated >140)	May indicate gestational diabetes	Go to 3-h GTT	About 15% of those screened will be positive
3-h glucose tolerance test	Two abnormal values	Gestational diabetes	Try ADA diet, monitor blood sugars, if elevated may need meds or insulin	About 15% of abnormal 1-h GCT will have gestational diabetes
GBS culture (35-37 wk)	Positive	GBS colonizing genital tract	Penicillin during labor	Helps to prevent early GBS sepsis, pneumonia, or meningitis of newborn

Abbreviations: ELISA, enzyme-linked immunosorbent assay; PCR, polymerase chain reaction; ASC-US, atypical squamous cell of uncertain significance; LGSIL, low-grade squamous intraepithelial lesion; HSIL, high-grade squamous intraepithelial lesion.
Reproduced, with permission, from Toy EC, Baker B, Ross P, Jennings J. Case Files: Obstetrics and Gynecology. 3rd ed. New York, NY: McGraw-Hill; 2009.

More frequent visits should be performed if any problems arise or if all issues are not addressed in the scheduled visits.

The **ACOG does not stipulate routine ultrasonography in patients without complications.** Ultrasound is considered accurate for establishing gestational age, fetal number, viability, and placental location. Therefore, ultrasonography should be performed in patients without reliable dating criteria, with a discrepancy between the measured and expected uterine growth, and in case of a postdated pregnancy, suspicion for twin gestation, suspicion for placental issues, chromosomal abnormalities, or other problems. For gestational-age estimations, ultrasonography is accurate to within 1 week if performed in the first trimester, 2 weeks in the second trimester, and 3 weeks in the third trimester. If the ultrasound dates and LMP are off by more than the aforementioned intervals, the due date should be recalculated based on the ultrasound findings.

The visit should end with an adequate explanation of all patient/partner concerns. Women should be counseled that sexual activity is not associated with any harm during an uncomplicated pregnancy, although there may be conditions that arise during the course of a pregnancy that would make sexual activity inadvisable. A follow-up visit should be scheduled prior to her leaving the office. She should also be educated about preterm labor precautions, signs of ectopic pregnancy, and situations in which to call the physician or go to the obstetrics triage unit for evaluation.

Subsequent Visits

At follow-up prenatal visits, concerns or questions brought up by the patient should be addressed. The examiner should ask questions specifically targeted at symptoms suggestive of complications that include gestational hypertension, preeclampsia, infections (urinary tract, vaginal, etc), fetal compromise, placenta previa/abruption, and preterm labor or premature rupture of membranes. At each visit, the patient should be asked about vaginal bleeding, loss of fluid, headaches, visual changes, abdominal pain, dysuria, facial or upper-extremity edema, vaginal discharge, and subjective sensation of fetal movements.

The examination on each subsequent visit should include weight, blood pressure, fundal height measurement, and fetal heart tones by handheld Doppler. In addition, a urinalysis should be performed at every visit to assess for protein, glucose, or infection.

Subsequent Testing and Laboratory Studies

At 15 to 20 weeks' gestation (preferably between 16 and 18 weeks' gestation), a multiple marker test, which screens for trisomy 21, trisomy 18, and neural tube defects, should be offered to patients. The two most common modalities of screening the fetus for these anomalies are the triple screen and the quad screen. The triple screen tests for serum hCG, unconjugated estriol, and α-fetoprotein; the quad screen tests for those three-plus inhibin-A. **The triple screen has a sensitivity of approximately 65% to 69% and specificity of 95% for detecting aneuploidy.** The quad screen increases sensitivity to approximately 80% without reducing specificity. The most common cause for a false-positive serum screen is incorrect gestational age dating. During the first trimester, fetal nuchal translucency can be measured by ultrasonography combined with maternal serum analyte levels (ie, free hCG and PAPP-A). This testing can be performed at 10 to 14 weeks' gestation. Sensitivity and specificity of these tests are determined by the risk cutoff used (eg, for trisomy 21, sensitivity is 85.2% when specificity is 90.6%; at 95% specificity, the sensitivity is 78.7%). Women should be counseled about the limited sensitivity and specificity of the tests, the psychological implications of a positive test, the potential impact of delivering a child with Down syndrome, the risks associated with pre-natal diagnosis and second-trimester abortion, and delays inherent in the process.

Women at increased risk of aneuploidy should be offered prenatal diagnosis by amniocentesis or chorionic villus sampling (CVS). Persons at increased risk include women who will be older than 35 years at delivery and who have a single-ton pregnancy (older than 32 years at delivery for women pregnant with twins); women carrying a fetus with a major structural anomaly identified by ultrasonog-raphy; women with ultrasound markers of aneuploidy (including increased nuchal thickness); women with a previously affected pregnancy; couples with a known translocation, chromosome inversion, or aneuploidy; and women with a positive maternal serum screen. Amniocentesis may be performed after 15-week gestation and is associated with a 0.5% risk of spontaneous abortion. CVS is performed at 10- to 12-week gestation and has a 1% to 1.5% risk of spontaneous abortion. CVS may be associated with transverse limb defects (1 per 3000 to 1 per 1000 fetuses). Women undergoing CVS also should be offered maternal serum α-fetoprotein testing for neural tube defects. Women older than 35 years at time of delivery may opt for serum screening and ultrasonography before deciding whether to proceed with amniocentesis. **Although the risk for trisomy 21 increases with maternal age, an estimated 75% of affected fetuses are born to mothers younger than 35 years at time of delivery.**

The United States Preventive Services Task Force recommends screening for gestational diabetes in asymptomatic pregnant women after 24 weeks of gestation (Level B). At 24 to 28 weeks' gestation, patients should be screened for gestational diabetes with a 1-hour 50-g glucose challenge test. When the screening test is posi-tive, a 3-hour glucose tolerance test (GTT) should be performed (after an over-night fast) by giving the patient a 100-g glucose load and obtaining fasting, 1-hour, 2-hour, and 3-hour postload serum glucose samples; two out of four positive values generally establish the diagnosis of gestational diabetes. A diagnosis of gestational diabetes impacts the pregnancy, but also increases the risk of type 2 diabetes in the patient throughout her life. Women diagnosed with gestational diabetes should be screened for type 2 diabetes at 12 weeks' postpartum.

At 28 weeks' gestation, a repeat RPR and hemoglobin/hematocrit should be obtained in those at risk for syphilis and anemia, respectively. In addition, a patient who is Rh-negative should receive Rho(D) immune globulin (RhoGAM) at this time. An Rh-negative patient should also receive Rho(D) immune globulin at deliv-ery and in any instance of trauma. Nonsensitized, Rh-negative women also should be offered a dose of Rho(D) immune globulin after spontaneous or induced abor-tion, ectopic pregnancy termination, CVS, amniocentesis, cordocentesis, exter-nal cephalic version, abdominal trauma, and second- or third-trimester bleeding. Administration of Rho(D) immune globulin can be considered before 12-week gestation in women with a threatened abortion and live embryo, but Rh alloim-munization is rare.

The Centers for Disease Control and Prevention and ACOG recommend that **all women be offered group B *Streptococcus* (GBS) screening by vaginorectal culture at 35 to 37 weeks' gestation** and that colonized women be treated with intravenous antibiotics at the time of labor or rupture of membranes in order to reduce the risk of neonatal

GBS infection. The **proper method of collection is to swab the lower vagina, perineal area, and rectum.** Of tested women, 10% to 30% will test positive for GBS colonization. Because GBS bacteriuria indicates heavy maternal colonization, women with GBS bacteriuria at any time during their pregnancy should be offered intrapartum antibiotics and do not require a vaginorectal culture. Similarly, women with a previous infant who was diagnosed with a GBS infection should be offered intrapartum antibiotics.

Late-term pregnancy is from 41 weeks, 0 days to 41 weeks, 6 days. Postterm pregnancy is defined as a pregnancy that has extended beyond 42 weeks or 294 days. Several studies found that induction of labor at 41 weeks reduced the need for cesarean delivery and reduced neonatal mortality and morbidity. Women who deliver postterm are at greater risk for maternal complications such as postpartum hemorrhage, dystocia, and maternal infection.

Birth before 37 weeks' gestation is considered preterm. To decrease the risk of neonatal morbidity and mortality, it is important to distinguish women with a history of preterm delivery and premature rupture of membranes. Women with these known risk factors should be given progesterone injections weekly from 16 to 37 weeks' gestation. Women diagnosed with a short cervix have an increased risk of preterm labor. Placing a cervical cerclage may reduce this risk, but current evidence is not definitive.

Vaccinations During Pregnancy

All pregnant women should receive the influenza vaccination at their initial prenatal visit. Influenza vaccine is safe in any stage of pregnancy provided there is no allergy to any of its components. Tetanus toxoid, diphtheria and acellular pertussis vaccination (Tdap) should be administered between 27 and 36 weeks' gestation of each pregnancy, regardless of prior vaccination status. Varicella, rubella, and the live attenuated intranasal influenza vaccinations are not advised during pregnancy. For pregnant mothers with a rubella nonimmune status, a rubella vaccination should be given after delivery of the infant. During the first prenatal visit, the mother's history of varicella should be documented. Women with a negative varicella history should undergo serologic testing, to confirm immunoglobulin G. Those not immunized to varicella should be advised to avoid exposure during pregnancy and should be offered the vaccine postpartum.

COMPREHENSION QUESTIONS

4.1 A 24-year-old woman presents for an initial prenatal visit. She is at 9 weeks' gestation based on her LMP but, on further questioning, she is not certain of the first day of her LMP. Which of the following would be the most accurate estimate of her gestational age?

A. Using her LMP if her uterine size is consistent

B. A first-trimester ultrasound

C. A second-trimester ultrasound

D. A quantitative serum hCG level

4.2 A 38-year-old pregnant woman presents for initial visit at 12 weeks' gestation. She requests a "genetic screen" because she is concerned about her advanced maternal age. She does not want any invasive testing that may cause a potential miscarriage. Which of the following is most appropriate to offer this patient?

A. If no prior personal or family history of genetic defects, no screen is needed.

B. Draw and send blood for the triple or quad screen, as patient has advanced maternal age.

C. Nuchal translucency screening and hCG and PAPP-A testing.

D. Offer the patient chorionic villus sampling.

4.3 A 28-year-old woman with a history of epilepsy presents for a preconception consultation visit. Which of the following is the most important advice to give to this patient?

A. Diabetes screening prior to pregnancy.

B. EEG reading that is normal prior to conception.

C. Preconception folate supplementation.

D. Stop epilepsy medication prior to pregnancy and through the first trimester.

4.4 A 28-year-old G1P0 woman at 16 weeks' gestation is noted to be Rh negative. Which of the following is the most appropriate next step for this patient?

A. Administer RhoGAM at this time.

B. Check the patient's antibody screen (indirect Coombs).

C. Schedule the patient for amniocentesis to assess for isoimmunization.

D. Counsel the patient to terminate the pregnancy.

ANSWERS

4.1 **B.** A first-trimester ultrasound is accurate to within ±1 week for gestational dating and would be the most accurate assessment of gestational age of the options listed.

4.2 **C.** In the 10 to 13 weeks' gestational age, first-trimester trisomy screening may be performed by ultrasound looking at an echolucent area behind the fetal neck called the nuchal translucency. That measurement together with serum hCG and PAPP-A can give a risk for trisomy.

4.3 **C.** Women with a history of epilepsy should receive 1 mg of folic acid supplementation daily to help prevent neural tube defects. In general, epilepsy medications should be continued, although the type of medication may be changed. For instance, valproic acid has a relatively high rate of neural tube defects associated with its use, and if possible, another medication should be used.

4.4 **B.** For women who are Rh negative, the next step is to assess the antibody screen or indirect Coombs test. If the antibody screen is negative, there is no isoimmunization, and RhoGAM is given at 28 weeks' gestation and again at delivery if the baby is confirmed as Rh positive. The RhoGAM is given to prevent isoimmunization. If the antibody screen is positive and the identity of the antibody is confirmed as Rh (anti-D), then assessment of its titer will assist in knowing the probability of fetal effect. A low titer can be observed, whereas a high titer should initiate further testing such as ultrasound and possibly amniocentesis.

CLINICAL PEARLS

▶ The initial prenatal visit often is scheduled after fetal organogenesis has occurred. For this reason, a preconception visit can be very beneficial. Furthermore, when prescribing medications, physicians must consider the possibility that any woman of reproductive age may become pregnant.

▶ Genetic counseling should be offered to any woman who *will be* 35 years old or older at her estimated date of confinement (EDC).

▶ Folic acid supplementation is important for every woman, and the recommended daily dose is based on individual risk factors such as anticonvulsant therapy or a previous pregnancy with a neural tube defect.

▶ If all criteria are met, Naegele's rule can be used to determine the EDC (subtract 3 months, add 7 days). If there is any uncertainty, the dating should be confirmed by ultrasound, preferably in the first trimester.

REFERENCES

Centers for Disease Control and Prevention. Immunization schedules. Available at: http://www.cdc.gov/vaccines/schedules. Accessed April 5, 2015.

Institute for Clinical Systems Improvement (ICSI). *Health Care Guideline: Routine Prenatal Care.* Bloomington, MN: Institute for Clinical Systems Improvement (ICSI); July 2010.

Kirkham C, Harris S, Grzybowski S. Evidence-based prenatal care: part I. General prenatal care and counseling issues. *Am Fam Physician.* 2005;71(7):1307-1316.

Kirkham C, Harris S, Grzybowski S. Evidence-based prenatal care: part II. Third-trimester care and prevention of infectious diseases. *Am Fam Physician.* 2005;71(8):1555-1560.

National Collaborating Centre for Women's and Children's Health. *Antenatal Care: Routine Care for the Healthy Pregnant Woman.* London, UK: RCOG Press; June 2008.

U.S. Preventive Services Task Force. Gestational diabetes mellitus, screening. Available at: http://www.uspreventiveservicestaskforce.org. Accessed April 5, 2015.

Veterans Health Administration, Department of Defense. DoD/VA *Clinical Practice Guidelines for the Management of Uncomplicated Pregnancy, version 2.0.* Washington, DC: Department of Veteran Affairs; 2009.

Wang M. Common questions about late-term postterm pregnancy. *Am Fam Physician.* 2014;90(3):160-165.

Wapner R, Thom E, Simpson JL, et al. First-trimester screening for trisomies 21 and 18. *N Engl J Med.* 2003;349:1405-1413.

Zolotor A, Carlough MC. Update on prenatal care. *Am Fam Physician.* 2014 Feb 1;89(3):199-208.

A 6-month-old male infant is brought to your office by his mother for a routine well-child visit. His mother is concerned that he is not yet saying "mama," because her best friend's baby said "mama" by age 6 months. Your patient was born via an uncomplicated pregnancy to a 23-year-old G1P1 mother. He was delivered by a spontaneous vaginal delivery at full term and there were no complications in the neonatal period. You have been following him since his birth. He has had appropriate growth and development up to this age and is up-to-date on his routine immunizations. He had one upper respiratory infection at age 5 months that was treated symptomatically. There is no family history of any developmental, hearing, or speech disorders. He has been fed since birth with an iron-fortified infant formula. Cereals and other baby foods were added starting at age 4 months. He lives with both parents, neither of whom smokes cigarettes.

On examination, he is a vigorous infant who is at the 50th percentile for length and weight and 75th percentile for head circumference. His physical examination is normal. On developmental examination, he is seen to sit for a short period of time without support, reach out with one hand for your examining light, pick up a Cheerio with a raking grasp and put it in his mouth, and he is noted to babble frequently.

▶ What immunizations would be recommended at this visit?
▶ By what age should an infant say "mama" and "dada"?
▶ The child's mother asks when she can place him in front-facing car seat. What is your recommendation?

ANSWERS TO CASE 5:
Well-Child Care

Summary: A 6-month-old healthy infant is brought in for a routine well-child examination.

- **Recommended immunizations for a 6-month well-child visit (in a child who is up-to-date on routine immunizations):** *Diphtheria, tetanus,* and acellular *pertussis* (DTaP) no. 3, hepatitis B no. 3, *Haemophilus influenzae* type b (Hib) no. 3, pneumococcal conjugate vaccine (PCV 13) no. 3, and rotavirus no. 3; inactivated polio vaccine (IPV) no. 3 can be given between 6 and 18 months. If the encounter is during "flu season," annual influenza vaccination is recommended beginning at 6 months.

- **Age by which a child should say "mama" and "dada":** Most children will start to say "dada" or "mama" nonspecifically between 6 and 9 months. It usually becomes specific between 8 and 15 months.

- **Recommendations for continuing in a rear-facing car seat:** A child should stay in a rear-facing car seat until the age of 2 or until the child reaches the maximum height and weight limit for the car seat.

ANALYSIS

Objectives

1. Learn the basic components of a well-child examination.
2. Know the routine immunization schedule for children.
3. Know common developmental milestones for young children.

Considerations

The pediatric well-child examination serves many valuable purposes. It provides an opportunity for parents, especially first-time parents, to ask questions about, and for the physician to address specific concerns regarding, their child. It allows the physician to assess the child's growth and development in a systematic fashion and to perform an appropriate physical examination. It also allows for a review of both acute and chronic medical conditions. When performed at recommended time intervals, it gives the opportunity to provide age-appropriate immunizations, screening tests, and anticipatory guidance. Finally, it supports the development of a good doctor-patient-family relationship, which can promote health and serve as an effective tool in the management of illness.

APPROACH TO:
Well-Child Examination

DEFINITIONS

AMBLYOPIA: Monocular childhood vision reduction caused by abnormal vision development. Strabismus is the most common cause of amblyopia.

STRABISMUS: Ocular misalignment.

CLINICAL APPROACH

Pediatric History

For the purposes of routine well-child visits, a comprehensive history should be obtained at the initial visit with more focused, interval histories obtained at subsequent encounters. The initial history should include an opportunity for the parent to raise any questions or concerns that the parent may have. New parents, especially first-time parents and young parents, often have many questions or anxieties about their child. The ability to discuss them with the physician will help to engender a positive physician-patient-family relationship and improve the parent's satisfaction with their child's care.

A complete past medical history should be obtained. This should start with a detailed prenatal and pregnancy history, including the duration of the pregnancy, any complications of pregnancy, any medications taken, the type of delivery performed, the child's birth weight, and any neonatal problems. Any significant chronic or acute illnesses should be recorded. The use of any medications, both prescription and over-the-counter, should be reviewed.

A detailed family history, including information (when available) on both maternal and paternal relatives should be obtained. A thorough social history is critical in pediatric care. Information, including the parents' education levels, relationships, religious beliefs, use of substances (tobacco, alcohol, drugs), and socioeconomic factors, can provide significant insight into the health and development of the child.

Efforts should be made to obtain old medical records, if any are available. Growth charts, immunization records, results of screening tests, and other valuable information that can assist with the child's assessment can often be found and reduce the unnecessary duplication of previously performed interventions.

Growth

At each well-child visit, the child's height and weight should be recorded and plotted on a standard growth chart. Head circumference is measured and plotted in children of 3 years and younger. Children older than 3 years should have their blood pressure recorded using an appropriate-size pediatric cuff. Significant variances from accepted, age-adjusted, population norms, or growth that deviates from predicted growth curves, may warrant further evaluation. The CDC and the American Academy of Pediatrics (AAP) recommend measuring body mass index (BMI) to screen for overweight and obesity in children of 2 years and older. The measurement of BMI in children is calculated the same way as it is for adults, but it is compared to typical values for other children of the same age. Weight classifications based on BMI in children are as follows:

Definition	BMI
• Obese	>95 percentile
• Overweight	85-95 percentile
• Healthy bodyweight	5-85 percentile
• Underweight	<5 percentile

Failure to thrive is defined by some as weight below the third or fifth percentile for age, and by others as decelerations of growth that have crossed two major growth percentiles in a short period of time. Either significant loss or gain of weight may prompt an in-depth discussion of nutrition and caloric intake.

Development

An assessment of the child's development in the areas of **gross motor, fine motor/ adaptive, language, and social/personal** skills is an important aspect of each well-child visit. Numerous screening tools, such as the Denver II developmental screening test, the Parents' Evaluations of Developmental Status (PEDS), and others, are available to assist with these assessments. These assessments typically involve both responses from the parents regarding the child's behavior at home and observations of the child in the office setting. Persistent delays in development, either globally or in individual skill areas, should prompt a more in-depth developmental assessment, as early intervention may effectively aid in the management of some developmental abnormalities. Children who are raised in a bilingual environment may have some language and development delay. Proficiency in both languages is often reached by age 5. The threshold for referral to a specialist should be the same for bilingual children as monolingual children. Table 5−1 summarizes many of the important motor, language, and social developmental milestones of early childhood.

Screening Tests

There are a variety of screening tests used to prevent disease and promote proper developmental and physical growth. These include tests for congenital diseases, lead screening, evaluating children for anemia, and hearing and vision screens.

Each state requires screening of all newborns for specified congenital diseases; however, the specific diseases for which screening is done vary from state to state. **All states require testing for phenylketonuria (PKU) and congenital hypothyroidism,** as early treatment can prevent the development of profound mental retardation. Diseases for which testing commonly occurs include hemoglobinopathies (including sickle cell disease), galactosemia, and other inborn errors of metabolism. This screening is done by collecting blood from newborns prior to discharge from the hospital. In some states, newborn screening is repeated at the first routine well visit, usually at about 2 weeks of age.

TABLE 5-1 · DEVELOPMENTAL MILESTONES

Age	Motor	Language	Social	Other
1 mo	Reacts to pain	Responds to noise	Regards human face Establishes eye contact	
2 mo	Eyes follow object to midline Head up prone	Vocalizes	Social smile Recognizes parent	
4 mo	Eyes follow object past midline Rolls over	Laughs and squeals	Regards hand	
6 mo	Sits well unsupported Transfers objects hand to hand (switches hands) Rolls prone to supine	Babbles	Recognizes strangers	Mnemonic: Six strangers switch sitting at 6 mo
9 mo	Pincer grasp (10 mo) Crawls Cruises (walks holding furniture)	Says "mama," "dada," and "bye-bye"	Starts to explore	Can crawl, therefore can explore It takes 9 mo to be a "mama" Grabs furniture to walk
12 mo	Walks Throws object	1-3 words Follows 1-step commands	Stranger and separation anxiety	Walking away from mom causes anxiety Knows 1 word at 1 y
2 y	Walks up and down stairs Copies a line Runs Kicks ball	2-3-word phrases 1/2 of speech is understood by strangers Refers to self by name Pronouns	Parallel play	Puts 2 words together at 2 At age 2, 2/4 (1/2) of speech understood by strangers
3 y	Copies a circle Pedals a tricycle Can build a bridge of 3 cubes Repeats 3 numbers	Speaks in sentences 3/4 of speech is understood by strangers Recognizes 3 colors	Group play Plays simple games Knows gender Knows first and last name	Tricycle, 3 cubes, 3 numbers, 3 colors, 3 kids make a group At age 3, 3/4 of speech understood by strangers

(Continued)

TABLE 5–1 • DEVELOPMENTAL MILESTONES (CONTINUED)				
Age	Motor	Language	Social	Other
4 y	Identifies body parts Copies a cross Copies a square (4 1/2 y) Hops on one foot Throws overhand	Speech is completely understood by strangers Uses past tense to speak of things that happened before Tells a story	Plays with kids, social interaction	Song "head, shoulder, knees, and toes," 4 parts reminds you that at age 4 can identify body parts At age 4, 4/4 of speech is understood by strangers A 4-year-old can copy 2 lines to draw a cross and a square, which has 4 sides
5 y	Copies a triangle Catches a ball Partially dresses self	Writes name Counts 10 objects		
6 y	Draws a person with 6 parts Ties shoes Skips with alternating feet	Identifies left and right		Mnemonic: At 6 y: skips, shoes, person with parts

Modified, with permission, from Hay WW, Hayword AR, Levin MJ, Sondheimer JM. Current Pediatric Diagnosis and Treatment. *17th ed. New York, NY: McGraw-Hill; 2005.*

Nationwide, the prevalence of childhood lead poisoning has declined, primarily because of the use of unleaded gasoline and lead-free paints. However, in some communities, the risk of lead exposure is higher. The Advisory Committee on Childhood Lead Poisoning Prevention recommends that all children not previously enrolled in Medicaid be screened for elevated blood levels between 12 and 24 months or at 36 and 72 months. All children at risk of lead exposure should be screened at 1 year. All children born outside of the United States should have a blood level measured on arrival to the United States. In other communities, screening should be targeted to high-risk children (Table 5–2).

Iron deficiency is the most common cause of anemia in children. Iron-containing formula and cereals have helped to reduce the occurrence of iron deficiency. Children who drink more than 24 oz of cow's milk, have iron-restricted diets, were low birth weight or preterm, or whose mother was iron deficient are at higher risk. In 2010, the AAP recommended universal screening for anemia in all children at 1 year. Additional laboratory screening for iron deficiency is recommended at later ages in those children at high risk for iron deficiency anemia. The American Academy of Family Physicians (AAFP) and the United States Preventive Services Task Force (USPSTF) found insufficient evidence to recommend for or against screening asymptomatic children for anemia. An anemic child can empirically be given a trial of an iron supplement and dietary modification. Failure to respond to iron therapy should warrant further evaluation of other causes of anemia.

TABLE 5-2 • ELEMENTS OF A LEAD RISK QUESTIONNAIRE
Recommended questions
• Does your child live in or regularly visit a house built before 1950? This could include a day care center, preschool, the home of a babysitter or relative, and so on.
• Does your child live in or regularly visit a house built before 1978 with recent, ongoing, or planned renovation or remodeling?
• Does your child have a sister or brother, housemate, or playmate who is being followed for lead poisoning?
Questions that may be considered by region or locality
• Does your child live with an adult whose job (eg, at a brass/copper foundry, firing range, automotive or boat repair shop, or furniture refinishing shop) or hobby (eg, electronics, fishing, stained-glass making, pottery making) involves exposure to lead?
• Does your child live near a work or industrial site (eg, smelter, battery recycling plant) that involves the use of lead?
• Does your child use pottery or ingest medications that are suspected of having a high lead content?
• Does your child have exposure to burning lead-painted wood?

Reproduced, with permission, from Stead LG, Stead SM, Kaufman MS. First Aid for the Pediatrics Clerkship. New York, NY: McGraw-Hill Education; 2004:39-40.

Most states now mandate newborn hearing screening by auditory brainstem response or evoked otoacoustic emission. All high-risk infants, regardless of requirement, should be screened. High-risk infants include those with a family history of childhood hearing loss, craniofacial abnormalities, syndromes associated with hearing loss (such as neurofibromatosis), or infections associated with hearing loss (such as bacterial meningitis). Older infants and toddlers can be assessed for hearing problems by questioning the parents or performing office testing by snapping fingers, or by using rattles or other noisemakers. Office-based audiometry should be performed in children aged 4 and older. Any hearing loss should be promptly evaluated and referred for early intervention, if necessary.

Vision screening can also start in the newborn nursery. Evaluation of the neonate for red reflexes on ophthalmoscopy should be a standard part of the newborn examination. The presence of red reflexes helps to rule out the possibility of congenital cataracts and retinoblastoma. The evaluation of an older infant should include a subjective evaluation of the child's vision by the parent. Infants should be able to focus on a face by 1 month and should move their eyes consistently and symmetrically by 6 months. An examining light should reflect symmetrically off of both corneas; asymmetric light reflex may be a sign of strabismus. The cover-uncover test also is a screening examination for strabismus. The child focuses on an object with both eyes and the examiner covers one eye. Strabismus is suggested when the uncovered eye deviates to focus on the object. **Strabismus should be referred to a pediatric ophthalmologist as soon as it is detected**, as early intervention results in a lower incidence of amblyopia. After the age of 3, most children can be tested for visual acuity using a Snellen chart, modified with a "tumbling E" or pictures, instead of letters.

Other screening tests may be recommended for high-risk children. Tuberculosis (TB) screening is recommended for children who were born or live in a region of high TB prevalence or who have close contact with someone known to have TB.

TABLE 5-3 • FIRST-TIME LIPID SCREENING RECOMMENDATIONS
Perform first-time lipid screening in children and adolescents if:
• Family history of dyslipidemia
• Family history of premature (men <55 years or women <65 years) cardiovascular disease or dyslipidemia
• Unknown family history
• Other cardiovascular risk factors:
Overweight (BMI >85th percentile and <95th percentile)
Obese (BMI >95th percentile)
Hypertension (blood pressure >95th percentile)
Cigarette smoking
Diabetes mellitus

Data from Daniels SR, Greer FR. Lipid screening and cardiovascular health in childhood. Pediatrics. 2008;122(1):198-202.

The Mantoux test (an intradermal injection of PPD tuberculin) is the screening test of choice. In accordance with the National Heart, Lung and Blood Institute (NHLBI), the American Heart Association (AHA), and AAP recommend universal screening of high cholesterol for all children at least one time between the ages of 9 and 11 and again between 17 and 21. Screening for hyperlipidemia should begin at age 2 in children with a family history of hyperlipidemia, premature cardiovascular disease, or other risk factors (Table 5–3).

With early childhood caries being one of the most prevalent chronic conditions during childhood, it is important to discuss good oral hygiene and the establishment of a dental home during well-child visits. At the 4-month visit, sources of systemic fluoride should be assessed. One of the most effective tools to prevent teeth decay is systemic fluoride. If there are concerns with the amount of fluoride in drinking water supplies, especially well water, appropriate testing should be performed. At 6 months, infants should begin to receive appropriate topical (fluoride toothpaste) and systemic fluoride. By the 12-month visit, each appointment should include a complete dental screening during the physical examination and reassurance that the child has a regular source of dental care. The American Academy of Pediatric Dentistry recommends that all children see a dentist by 12 months.

Anticipatory Guidance

A primary feature of the well-child visit should be education of the patient and family on issues that promote health and prevent illness, injury, or death. This anticipatory guidance should be focused and age appropriate. The use of preprinted handouts can reinforce issues discussed in the office, address issues that could not be discussed because of time limitations, and allow for the parent to review the information as needed at home. Subjects that should routinely be addressed include injury prevention, nutrition, development, discipline, exercise, mental health issues, and the need for ongoing care (eg, immunization schedules, future well-child visits, dental care). During the well-child examination, it is important to evaluate how much time is spent watching television, using the computer, and playing video games. Screen time should be limited to 1 to 2 hours or less daily. The number and quality of sleep should be asked at each visit. Abnormalities in sleep should be further investigated and managed appropriately.

Accidents and injuries are the leading cause of death in children older th Accidents involving motor vehicles, both traffic and pedestrian accidents, leading cause of these accidental deaths. All states now require the use of car s seats for children, although the regulations vary from state to state. The gener recommendation is that a child should be in the back seat of the vehicle whenever possible. If there is no back seat, the child should only ride in the front seat if there is no air bag or if the air bag can be disabled. **A child should sit in a rear-facing car seat until the child is 2 years old or has reached the maximum height or weight limit of the rear-facing seat.** When the child weighs more than 40 lb, the child may use a booster-type seat along with the lap and shoulder seatbelts. The child can stop using the booster when he or she can sit with his or her back squarely against the back of the seat with the legs bent at the knees over the front of the seat. The child usually will need to be at least 4 ft 9 in in height and 8 to 12 years of age to meet these requirements. No child should ride in the front seat unless they are 13 years or older and meet height and weight requirements.

According to the CDC, the top three causes of death in infants younger than 1 year are congenital abnormalities, short gestation, and **sudden infant death syndrome** (SIDS). The Back-to-Sleep campaign advises parents to place their infant on the infant's back—not abdomen or side—when the infant is put down to sleep, as this reduces the risk of dying of SIDS. In addition, the infant should be placed on a firm mattress with nothing else in the crib—this includes pillows, positioning devices, and toys. Heavy coverings and soft mattresses have been associated with an increased risk of SIDS.

As children get older, anticipatory guidance on other safety issues become important. As children learn to crawl and walk, stairwells should be blocked to reduce the risk of injuries from falling. Cleaning supplies, medications, and other potential poisons need to be stored safely out of reach of children, preferably in locked cabinets. Similarly, firearms should be stored safely, preferably unloaded and in locked cabinets or safes. Parents should be counseled on keeping matches and lighters in a safe place out of the reach of children. Older children should be advised regarding the importance of wearing a helmet while riding a bicycle, skateboard, scooter, or other similar vehicle. The National Highway Traffic Safety Administration recommends that in addition to helmets, bicyclists should wear clothing that is right and reflective, ride with the flow of traffic and obey all traffic laws. All families should be advised to have smoke detectors throughout the home, especially in rooms where people sleep, and to keep the hot water heater set at or below 120°F to reduce the risk of scald injuries. The AAFP recommends that all caregivers be trained in cardiopulmonary resuscitation. When a pool or hot tub is accessible to children, a nearby telephone with emergency contacts should be at poolside. All children under the age of 4 should have supervision within arm's length at all times.

Nutrition is another important area of anticipatory guidance. Infants younger than 1 year should be breast-fed or receive an iron-containing formula. Cereals, other baby foods, and water can be introduced between 4 and 6 months. Whole cow's milk is introduced at 12 months and continued until at least the age of 2, before considering changing to reduced fat milk.

Figure 1. Recommended immunization schedule for persons aged 0 through 18 years – United States, 2015.
(FOR THOSE WHO FALL BEHIND OR START LATE, SEE THE CATCH-UP SCHEDULE [FIGURE 2]).
These recommendations must be read with the footnotes that follow. For those who fall behind or start late, provide catch-up vaccination at the earliest opportunity as indicated by the green bars in Fi
To determine minimum intervals between doses, see the catch-up schedule (Figure 2). School entry and adolescent vaccine age groups are shaded.

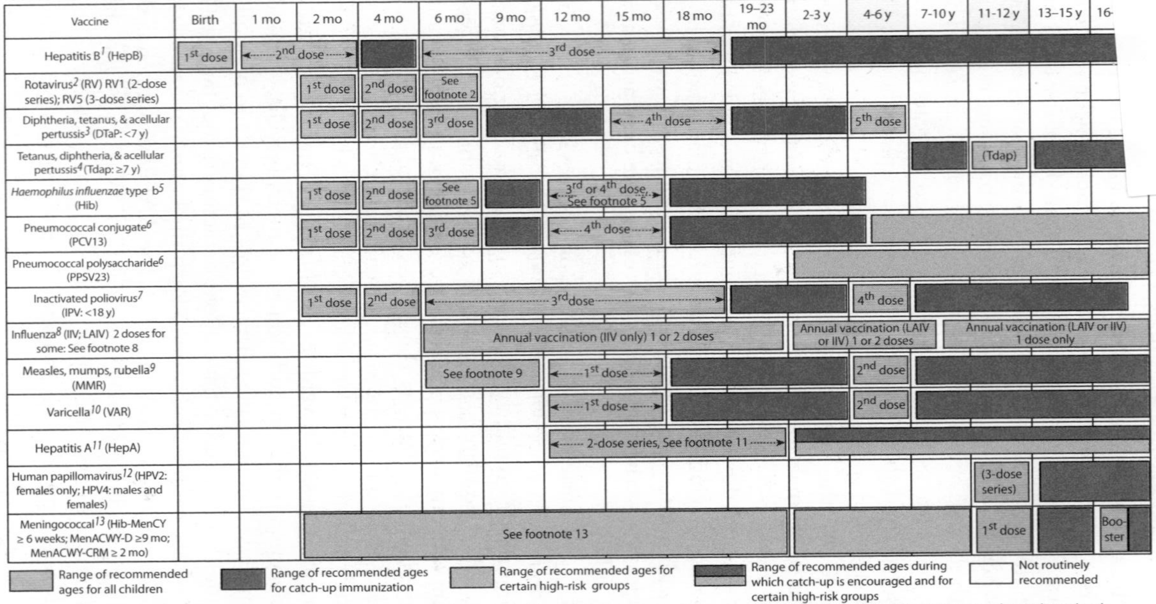

This schedule includes recommendations in effect as of January 1, 2015. Any dose not administered at the recommended age should be administered at a subsequent visit, when indicated and feasible. The use of a combination vaccine generally is preferred over separate injections of its equivalent component vaccines. Vaccination providers should consult the relevant Advisory Committee on Immunization Practices (ACIP) statement for detailed recommendations, available online at http://www.cdc.gov/vaccines/hcp/acip-recs/index.html. Clinically significant adverse events that follow vaccination should be reported to the Vaccine Adverse Event Reporting System (VAERS) online (http://www.vaers.hhs.gov) or by telephone (800-822-7967). Suspected cases of vaccine-preventable diseases should be reported to the state or local health department. Additional information, including precautions and contraindications for vaccination, is available from CDC online (http://www.cdc.gov/vaccines/recs/vac-admin/contraindications.htm) or by telephone (800-CDC-INFO [800-232-4636]).

This schedule is approved by the Advisory Committee on Immunization Practices (http//www.cdc.gov/vaccines/acip), the American Academy of Pediatrics (http://www.aap.org), the American Academy of Family Physicians (http://www.aafp.org), and the American College of Obstetricians and Gynecologists (http://www.acog.org).

NOTE: The above recommendations must be read along with the footnotes of this schedule.

Figure 5–1. Recommended immunization schedule for persons aged 0 through 18—United States, 2015. Available at: http://www.cdc.gov/vaccines/schedules/downloads/child/0-18yrs-child-combined-schedule.pdf. (Accessed April 11, 2015.)

Immunizations

Ensuring that each child has received the child's age-appropriate immunizations is a key component of each well-child visit. The child's immunization status also should be reviewed at acute care visits. Minor illnesses, even those causing low-grade fevers, are not contraindications to vaccinating children, allowing an acute care visit to be an excellent opportunity to provide this service. **True contraindications to providing a vaccination include a history of an anaphylactic reaction to a specific vaccine or vaccine component or a severe illness,** with or without a fever. The recommended childhood vaccination schedule (Figure 5–1) and catch-up schedules for children who are either completely unimmunized or who have missed doses of the recommended vaccines are published by the CDC.

COMPREHENSION QUESTIONS

5.1 A 7-month-old male infant is brought into the office for a possible ear infection. In assessing the infant's posture, you note that he is not able to sit very well without support. You also observe other fine motor skills and speech. Which of the following is the most accurate statement?

A. By 3 months, a child should be able to sit up without support.

B. By 6 months, a child should be able to transfer objects from one hand to another.

C. By 9 months, a child should be able to walk.

D. By 12 months, a child should be able to put two words together.

5.2 A 5-year-old child presents to your clinic for a school physical. The child weighs 42 lb and is up-to-date on his immunizations. Which of the following anticipatory guidances is most appropriate for a child at this age?

A. He should ride in a rear-facing car seat in the back seat of the vehicle.

B. He should ride in a forward-facing car seat in the back seat of the vehicle.

C. He should ride in a forward-facing car seat in the front seat of the vehicle.

D. He should ride in a booster seat in the back seat of the vehicle.

5.3 A 4-month-old infant is brought into the family physician's office for routine checkup and immunizations. Which of the following vaccines is routinely recommended at this time?

A. Diphtheria, tetanus, and acellular pertussis (DTaP)

B. Oral polio vaccine (OPV)

C. Measles, mumps, rubella (MMR)

D. Varicella

5.4 A 5-year-old child is brought into the pediatrician's office for immunization and physical examination. The mother is concerned that her child is a little "under the weather". Which of the following is a contraindication to vaccinating the child?

A. Acute otitis media with a temperature of 100°F requiring antibiotic therapy

B. Previous vaccination reaction that consisted of fever and fussiness that lasted for 2 days

C. History of an allergic reaction to penicillin

D. Previous vaccination reaction that consisted of wheezing and hypotension

ANSWERS

5.1 **B.** It is critical to understand the normal milestones for gross motor, fine motor, speech, and social categories. Delay in one or more areas can indicate problems which if addressed can alleviate long-term issues. Most 6-month-old infants would be expected to sit without support. They would also be expected to transfer objects from one hand to the other, roll from a prone to supine position, babble, and recognize strangers.

5.2 **D.** A child who is older than 2 years may sit in a forward-facing car seat in the back seat of the car. A child who weighs more than 40 lb is usually big enough to use a booster seat, also in the back seat of the car.

5.3 **A.** DTaP is routinely recommended at 2, 4, 6, 12 to 18 months, and 4 to 6 years. Oral polio vaccination is no longer routinely recommended in children; the inactivated, injectable polio vaccine is recommended in its place and is recommended at 2, 4, 6 to 18 months, and 4 to 6 years. MMR and varicella vaccination are recommended at 12 to 15 months and 4 to 6 years.

5.4 **D.** A previous anaphylactic reaction is a true contraindication to vaccination. Minor illnesses or vaccination reactions, even with fever, are not contraindications. Penicillin is not a component of vaccines and history of allergy to this medication is not a contraindication.

CLINICAL PEARLS

▶ True contraindications to providing vaccinations are rare; acute care visits are an excellent opportunity to provide childhood vaccinations.

▶ SIDS is the leading cause of death in infants younger than 1 year. Parents should place their children on their "Back-to-Sleep".

REFERENCES

Bright Futures/American Academy of Pediatrics. Recommendations for Preventive Pediatric Health Care, 2014. Available at: https://www.aap.org/en-us/professional-resources/practice-support/Periodicity/Periodicity%20Schedule_FINAL.pdf. Accessed May 24, 2015.

Centers for Disease Control and Prevention. Vaccines and Immunizations. Available at: http://www.cdc.gov/vaccines/. Accessed May 24, 2015.

Douglass JM, Douglass AB, Silk HJ. A practical guide to infant oral health. *Am Fam Physician*. 2004 Dec 1;70(11):2113-2120.

Durbin DR for the AAP Committee on Injury, Violence and Poison Prevention. American Academy of Pediatrics Policy Statement: Child passenger safety. *Pediatrics*. 2011 April 1;127(4):788-793.

Warniment C, Tsang K, Galazka SS. Lead poisoning in children. *Am Fam Physician*. 2010 Mar 15;81(6):751-757.

A 35-year-old woman with a history of asthma presents to your office with symptoms of nasal itching, sneezing, and rhinorrhea. She states she feels this way most days but her symptoms are worse in the spring and fall. She has had difficulty sleeping because she is always congested. She states she has taken diphenhydramine (Benadryl) with no relief. She does not smoke cigarettes and does not have exposure to passive smoke but she does have two cats at home. On examination, she appears tired but is in no respiratory distress. Her vital signs are temperature, 98.8°F; blood pressure, 128/84 mm Hg; pulse, 88 beats/min; and respiratory rate, 18 breaths/min. The mucosa of her nasal turbinates appears swollen (boggy) and has a pale, bluish-gray color. Thin and watery secretions are seen. No abnormalities are seen on ear examination. There is no cervical lymphadenopathy noted and her lungs are clear.

▶ What is the most likely diagnosis?
▶ What is your next step?
▶ What are important considerations and potential complications of management?

ANSWERS TO CASE 6:
Allergic Disorders

Summary: A 35-year-old asthmatic woman complains of chronic nasal congestion that is worse in the spring and the fall.

- **Most likely diagnosis:** Allergic rhinitis.

- **Next step in management of this patient:** Treatment with antihistamines, decongestants, or intranasal steroids. These treatments can also be used in combination with each other. First-line treatment is intranasal corticosteroids for mild to moderate disease. With moderate to severe allergic rhinitis, antihistamines and decongestants should be added.

- **Considerations and possible complications of therapy:** Recognition and reduction of potential allergen exposure will yield more success in management than pharmacotherapy alone. Excessive use of topical decongestants can cause rebound congestion.

ANALYSIS

Objectives

1. Understand the inflammatory nature of allergic rhinitis.

2. Recognize physical examination findings consistent with allergic rhinitis.

3. Develop an approach to the management of allergic rhinitis, including the roles of pharmacotherapy and reduction of allergen exposure.

4. Recognition and management of asthma.

5. Identification of essential features and treatment of anaphylaxis.

Considerations

This patient presents with a classic history of allergic rhinitis. Her history of itchy eyes, nasal congestion and discharge, and seasonal in nature (worse in spring and fall) are all consistent with allergic rhinitis. Her examinations are also consistent with the diagnosis. The mucosa of her nasal turbinates appears swollen (boggy) and has a pale, bluish-gray color. Thin and watery secretions are seen. The best therapy for this condition is avoidance of allergens, but due to the probable allergy to pollen, this can be very difficult. Nasal corticosteroids offer the most consistent symptomatic relief.

APPROACH TO:
Allergic Disorders

DEFINITIONS

ALLERGIC RHINITIS: Inflammation of the nasal passages caused by immuno-globulin E (IgE)–mediated response to airborne substances.

ANAPHYLAXIS: Rapidly progressing, life-threatening allergic reaction, mediated by IgE immediate hypersensitivity reaction.

CLINICAL APPROACH

Background

Rhinitis is inflammation of the nasal membranes and is characterized by any combination of the following: sneezing, nasal congestion, nasal itching, obstruction, pruritus, and rhinorrhea. The eyes, ears, sinuses, and throat can also be involved. Allergic rhinitis is the most common cause of rhinitis, occurring in up to 30% of adults and 40% of children.

Pathophysiology

Allergic rhinitis involves inflammation of the mucous membranes of the nose, eyes, eustachian tubes, middle ear, sinuses, and pharynx. Inflammation of the mucous membranes is characterized by a complex interaction of inflammatory mediators but, ultimately, is triggered by an IgE-mediated response to an extrinsic protein.

In susceptible individuals, exposure to certain foreign proteins leads to allergic sensitization, which is characterized by the production of specific IgE directed against these proteins. This specific IgE coats the surface of mast cells, which are present in the nasal mucosa. When the specific allergen is inhaled into the nose, it can bind to the IgE in the mast cells, leading to the delayed release of a number of mediators.

Mediators that are immediately released include histamine, tryptase, chymase, and kinase. Mast cells quickly synthesize other mediators, including leukotrienes and prostaglandin D_2. Symptoms can occur quickly after exposure. Mucous glands are stimulated, leading to increased secretions. Vasodilation occurs, causing congestion. Stimulation of sensory nerves leads to sneezing and itching. Other symptoms include the redness and tearing of eyes, postnasal drip, and ear pressure.

Over the next 4 to 8 hours, these mediators, through a complex interplay of events, recruit neutrophils, eosinophils, lymphocytes, and macrophages to the mucosa. These inflammatory cells cause more congestion and mucus production that may persist for hours or days. Systemic effects, including fatigue, sleepiness, and malaise, can result from the inflammatory response as well.

History

Obtaining a detailed history is important in the evaluation of allergic rhinitis, as specific triggers may be identified. Evaluation should include the nature, duration, and time course of symptoms. The recent use of medications is another important consideration as is a family history of allergic diseases, environmental exposures, and comorbid conditions.

Part of the history should include the time pattern of symptoms and whether symptoms occur at a consistent level throughout the year (**perennial rhinitis**), only occur in specific seasons (**seasonal rhinitis**), a combination of the two, or in relation to a workplace (**occupational rhinitis**). Trigger factors such as exposure to pollens, mold spores, specific animals, or cleaning of the house can sometimes be identified. Irritant triggers such as smoke, pollution, and strong smells can aggravate symptoms of allergic rhinitis. Response to treatment with antihistamines supports the diagnosis of allergic rhinitis.

Symptoms

Symptoms that can be associated with allergic rhinitis include sneezing, itching (of nose, eyes, or ears), rhinorrhea, postnasal drip, congestion, anosmia, headache, earache, tearing, red eyes, and drowsiness.

Physical Examination

Common findings on examination include "allergic shiners," which are dark circles around the eyes related to vasodilation or nasal congestion. The "nasal crease" can be seen in some cases. It is a horizontal crease across the lower half of the bridge of the nose caused by repeated upward rubbing of the tip of the nose by the palm of the hand ("allergic salute").

Examination of the nose may reveal mucosa of the nasal turbinates to be swollen (boggy) and have a pale, bluish-gray color. Assessment of the character and quantity of nasal mucus may be helpful in ascertaining a diagnosis. Thin and watery secretions are frequently associated with allergic rhinitis, whereas thick and purulent secretions are usually associated with sinusitis. The characteristic of the mucous is not always diagnostic, as thick, purulent, colored mucus can also occur with allergic rhinitis.

The nasal cavity should be inspected for growths such as polyps or tumors. Polyps are firm, gray masses that are often attached by a stalk, which may not be visible. After spraying a topical decongestant, polyps do not shrink, whereas the surrounding nasal mucosa does shrink. Examine the nasal septum to look for any deviation or septal perforation that may be present as a consequence of chronic rhinitis, granulomatous disease, cocaine abuse, prior surgery, topical decongestant abuse, or, rarely, topical steroid overuse.

Otoscopy should be performed to look for tympanic membrane retraction, air-fluid levels, or bubbles. Performing pneumatic otoscopy can be considered to look for abnormal tympanic membrane mobility. These findings can be associated with allergic rhinitis, particularly if eustachian tube dysfunction or secondary otitis media is present. Ocular examination may reveal findings of injection and swelling of the palpebral conjunctivae, with excess tear production. Dennie-Morgan lines (prominent creases below the inferior eyelid) are associated with allergic rhinitis.

"Cobblestoning" of the posterior pharynx is often observed. This is caused by the presence of streaks of lymphoid tissue on the posterior pharynx. Tonsillar hypertrophy can also be seen. The neck should be examined for the presence of lymphadenopathy. The respiratory system must be examined for findings consistent with asthma. These include wheezing, tachypnea, and a prolonged expiratory phase of respiration.

CAUSES OF ALLERGIC RHINITIS

The causes of allergic rhinitis can differ depending on whether the symptoms are seasonal, perennial, or sporadic/episodic. Some patients are sensitive to multiple allergens and can have perennial allergic rhinitis with seasonal exacerbations. Although food allergy can cause rhinitis, particularly in children, it is rarely a cause of allergic rhinitis in the absence of gastrointestinal or skin symptoms. Seasonal allergic rhinitis is commonly caused by allergy to seasonal pollens and outdoor molds.

Pollens (Tree, Grass, and Weed)

Tree pollens, which vary by geographic location, are typically present in high counts during the spring, although some species produce their pollens in the fall. Grass pollens also vary by geographic location. Most of the common grass species are associated with allergic rhinitis. A number of these grasses is cross-reactive, meaning that they have similar antigenic structures (ie, proteins recognized by specific IgE in allergic sensitization). Consequently, a person who is allergic to one species is also likely to be sensitive to a number of other species. The grass pollens are most prominent from the late spring through the fall, but can be present year-round in warmer climates.

Weed pollens also vary geographically. Many weeds, such as short ragweed, a common cause of allergic rhinitis in much of the United States, are most prominent in the late summer and fall. Other weed pollens are present year-round, particularly in warmer climates.

Perennial allergic rhinitis is typically caused by allergens within the home, but can also be caused by outdoor allergens that are present year-round. In warmer climates, grass pollens can be present throughout the year. In some climates, individuals may be symptomatic because of trees and grasses in the warmer months and molds and weeds in the winter.

House Dust Mites

In the United States, two major house dust mite species are associated with allergic rhinitis. These mites feed on organic material in households, particularly the skin that is shed from humans and pets. They can be found in carpets, upholstered furniture, pillows, mattresses, comforters, and stuffed toys. Exposure can be reduced by methods such as carpet removal; however, current studies have not found any benefit to using mite-proof mattresses or pillow covers.

Animals

Allergy to indoor pets is a common cause of perennial allergic rhinitis. Cat and dog allergies are encountered most commonly in clinical practice. However, allergies have been reported to occur with most of the furry animals and birds that are kept as indoor pets. Although cockroach allergy is most frequently considered to be a cause of asthma, particularly in the inner city, it can also cause perennial allergic rhinitis in infested households. Rodent infestation may also be associated with allergic sensitization.

TREATMENT

The management of allergic rhinitis consists of four major categories of treatment: patient education, allergen avoidance, pharmacologic management, and immunotherapy. All aspects of treatment are more successful when exposure to allergens is decreased. Recommendations for treatment are primarily based on symptoms and patient's age. Pharmacotherapy can involve the use of **antihistamines, decongestants, intranasal corticosteroids, and, in severe cases, systemic corticosteroids.**

Antihistamines competitively antagonize the receptors for histamine, which is released from mast cells. This reduces the production of symptoms mediated by the release of histamine. "First-generation" antihistamines including diphenhydramine, chlorpheniramine, and hydroxyzine are inexpensive and available over the counter. Side effects include sedation and the anticholinergic effects of dry mouth, dry eyes, blurred vision, and urinary retention; therefore, their use should be monitored in sensitive populations, such as the elderly. "Second-generation" antihistamines, including loratadine, desloratadine, fexofenadine, azelastine, and cetirizine, have a lower incidence of sedation and anticholinergic side effects, therefore are preferred over first-generation antihistamines. Caution should be used with cetirizine because sedative side effects can occur at recommended doses. Oral antihistamines begin to take effect within 15 to 30 minutes after ingestion and are best used in persons with mild and intermittent symptoms.

Corticosteroid nasal sprays are the most effective treatment and first-line therapy for the long-term management of mild to moderate persistent symptoms of allergic rhinitis. They reduce the production of inflammatory mediators and the recruitment of inflammatory cells. Systemic absorption of the steroid is relatively low, reducing the risk of complications associated with the chronic use of systemic corticosteroids. Side effects include nosebleeds, nasal irritation, and rarely nasal septum perforation. Maximal effectiveness is achieved after 2 to 4 weeks of use.

Decongestants, either given orally or intranasally, can be used to provide symptomatic relief of nasal congestion. These α-adrenergic agonist agents constrict blood vessels in the nasal mucosa and reduce the overall volume of the mucosa. Common decongestants include pseudoephedrine and phenylephrine. Oral decongestants can cause tachycardia, tremors, and insomnia. Rebound hyperemia and worsening of symptoms can occur with chronic use or upon discontinuation of nasal decongestants. Caution should be used in the elderly, young children, during the first trimester of pregnancy and individuals with cardiac arrhythmias, glaucoma, or hyperthyroidism.

Leukotriene inhibitors (zafirlukast, montelukast, zileuton) are indicated both for allergic rhinitis and for maintenance therapy for persistent asthma. They are particularly useful in patients with both asthma and allergies or in those whose asthma may be triggered by allergens. These medications can be taken alone or in combination with antihistamines.

Oral corticosteroids are potent inhibitors of cell-mediated immunity. The use of systemic steroids is limited by adverse effects, including suppression of the hypothalamic-pituitary-adrenal axis and hyperglycemia. Long-term use can lead to peptic ulcer formation, increased susceptibility to infection, poor wound healing, and the reduction of bone density. Because of these significant risks, systemic steroids are used only for severe allergies unresponsive to other pharmacologic modalities or a diagnosis of nasal polyposis. Oral steroids should be used in the lowest effective dose for the shortest possible time.

Desensitization therapy is frequently attempted in patients who remain symptomatic despite maximal medical therapy. Skin allergy testing is used to detect reactivity against specific antigens. The next step is to inject the patient with highly diluted concentrations of this antigen. The concentration of the antigen(s) in the injection is gradually increased, in an effort to reduce the patient's inflammatory response to the antigen(s). Injections are typically given weekly or biweekly. This process is expensive, time-consuming, and requires numerous injections. Patients and physicians must be prepared to address severe, even anaphylactic, reactions that may occur during the process.

ANAPHYLAXIS, URTICARIA, AND ANGIOEDEMA

Urticaria is characterized by large, irregularly shaped, pruritic, erythematous wheals. **Angioedema** is painless, deep, subcutaneous swelling that often involves the periorbital, circumoral, and facial regions. **Anaphylaxis** is a systemic reaction with cutaneous symptoms that is associated with dyspnea, visceral edema, and hypotension. Insect bites or stings, foods, and medications are the most common culprits of anaphylactic reactions. The manifestations of anaphylaxis include hypotension or shock from widespread vasodilation, respiratory distress from bronchospasm or laryngeal edema, gastrointestinal and uterine muscle contraction, and urticaria and angioedema.

At the first suspicion of anaphylaxis, aqueous epinephrine 1:1000, in a dose of 0.2 to 0.5 mg, is injected subcutaneously or intramuscularly. Repeated injections can be given every 5 to 15 minutes when necessary. Epinephrine administration increases peripheral resistance by causing immediate vasoconstriction. Airway obstruction and vascular collapse improve due to the inotropic properties of epinephrine on the heart and bronchodilator effects on the lungs. Rapid intravenous infusion of large volumes of fluids (saline, lactated Ringer solution, plasma or plasma expanders) is essential to replace loss of intravascular plasma into tissues. Airway obstruction may be caused by edema of the larynx or by bronchospasm. In addition to securing the airway, oxygen therapy should be provided. Endotracheal intubation may be required. Antihistamines may be useful as adjuvant therapy for alleviating cutaneous manifestations of urticaria or angioedema and pruritus. Caution is recommended with antihistamine use given the sedative effects, which could be problematic in compromised patients. Systemic corticosteroids can be beneficial, but should not be used as first line due to its delayed onset of action. All patients with anaphylaxis should be monitored for a period of time, for example, 24 hours.

CONJUNCTIVITIS

Conjunctivitis is an infection of the palpebral and/or bulbar conjunctiva. It is the most common eye disease seen in community medicine. Most cases are caused by bacterial or viral infection. Other causes include allergy and chemical irritants. The mode of transmission of infectious conjunctivitis is usually direct contact to the opposite eye or to other persons via fingers, towels, or handkerchiefs.

The organisms isolated most commonly in bacterial conjunctivitis are *Staphylococcus*, *Streptococcus*, *Haemophilus*, *Moraxella*, and *Pseudomonas*. There is no blurring of vision and only mild discomfort. In severe cases, immunocompromised patients, contact lens wearers, and those who failed initial treatment, examination of stained conjunctival scrapings and cultures are recommended. The disease is usually self-limited, lasting about 10 to 14 days if untreated. A sulfonamide instilled locally three times daily will usually clear the infection in 2 to 3 days.

Epidemic keratoconjunctivitis (pink eye) is highly contagious and spread by person-to-person contact or fomites. The most common cause is adenovirus. It is usually associated with pharyngitis, fever, malaise, and preauricular lymphadenopathy. Locally, the palpebral conjunctiva is red with a copious watery discharge and scanty exudates. Symptomatic treatment includes ocular decongestants, artificial tears, and cool or warm compresses to reduce the discomfort of the associated lid edema. Weak topical steroids may be necessary to treat the corneal infiltrates. The disease usually lasts at least 2 weeks.

Noninfectious causes of conjunctivitis include allergic and chemical irritants. Symptoms of allergic conjunctivitis include itching, tearing, redness, stringy discharge, and sometimes photophobia. In addition to avoiding the irritant, treatment can include the use of oral antihistamines or topical antihistamine or anti-inflammatory eye drops.

COMPREHENSION QUESTIONS

6.1 A 30-year-old man has both mild persistent asthma and chronic environmental allergies. Which of the following medications is indicated for the management of this patient's conditions?

A. Inhaled albuterol (short-acting β-adrenergic agonist)

B. Intranasal fluticasone (corticosteroid)

C. Oral montelukast (leukotriene modifier)

D. Oral cetirizine (second-generation antihistamine)

6.2 A 12-year-old boy presents with eye itching and redness. He has clear drainage from his eyes but no crusting. Examination today is normal except for mildly injected conjunctiva bilaterally. Which of the following is the most appropriate treatment?

A. Antibiotic eye drops

B. Ophthalmology consultation

C. Anti-inflammatory eye drops

D. Oral leukotriene inhibitor

6.3 A 56-year-old man presents to his physician with symptoms consistent with allergic rhinitis. His past medical history is positive for benign prostatic hyperplasia. He continues to work in a warehouse as a forklift operator. Which of the following medications should be used to treat this patient?

A. Diphenhydramine

B. Hydroxyzine

C. Chlorpheniramine

D. Fexofenadine

ANSWERS

6.1 **C.** Montelukast is indicated for both the management of persistent asthma and chronic allergies. Nasal steroids and oral antihistamines are indicated only for allergies.

6.2 **C.** This patient has allergic conjunctivitis. Topical anti-inflammatory drops are appropriate therapy. Other options would include topical or oral antihistamines. The other therapies listed are not appropriate in this condition.

6.3 **D.** The second-generation antihistamines, such as fexofenadine, are less sedating and have fewer anticholinergic side effects than the first-generation antihistamines. They would be a better choice for someone who operates heavy machinery and has benign prostatic hyperplasia. However, they are no more effective at symptom relief than the first-generation antihistamines listed earlier.

CLINICAL PEARLS

▶ The management of allergic rhinitis consists of four major categories of treatment: patient education, allergen avoidance, pharmacologic management, and immunotherapy.

▶ At the first suspicion of anaphylaxis, aqueous epinephrine 1:1000 in a dose of 0.2 to 0.5 mL (0.2-0.5 mg) is injected subcutaneously or intramuscularly. The airway should always be assessed and patient intubated if necessary to secure breathing.

REFERENCES

American Academy of Allergy Asthma & Immunology. Allergy testing: tips to remember. Available at: http://www.aaaai.org/conditions-and-treatments/library/at-a-glance/allergy-testing.aspx. Accessed May 24, 2015.

Arnold JJ, Williams PM. Anaphylaxis: recognition and management. *Am Fam Physician*. 2011 Nov 15;84(10):1111-1118.

Barnes PJ. Asthma. In: Kasper D, Fauci A, Hauser S, et al, eds. *Harrison's Principles of Internal Medicine*. 19th ed. New York, NY: McGraw-Hill Education; 2015. Available at: http://accessmedicine. mhmedical.com/. Accessed May 24, 2015.

Boyce AJ, Austen KF. Allergies, anaphylaxis and systemic mastocytosis. In: Kasper D, Fauci A, Hauser S, et al, eds. *Harrison's Principles of Internal Medicine*. 19th ed. New York, NY: McGraw-Hill Education; 2015. Available at: http://accessmedicine.mhmedical.com. Accessed May 24, 2015.

Cronau H, Kankanala RR, Mauger T. Diagnosis and management of red eye in primary care. *Am Fam Physician*. 2010 Jan 15;81(2):1137-1441.

Lambert M. Practice parameters for for allergic rhinitis. *Am Fam Physician*. 2009 Jul 1;80(1):79-85.

Quillen DM, Feller DB. Diagnosing rhinitis: allergic vs. non-allergic. *Am Fam Physician*. 2006;73(9):1583-1590.

Scow DT, Luttermoser GK, Dickerson KS. Leukotriene inhibitor in the treatment of allergy and asthma. *Am Fam Physician*. 2007;75(1):65-70.

Sur DK, Scandale S. Treatment of allergic rhinitis. *Am Fam Physician*. 2010;81(12):1440-1446.

A 55-year-old man comes into your office for follow-up of a chronic cough. He also complains of shortness of breath with activity. He reports that this has been getting worse over time. As you are interviewing the patient, you note that he smells of cigarette smoke. Upon further questioning, he reports smoking 1 pack of cigarettes per day for the past 35 years and denies ever being advised to quit. On examination, he is in no respiratory distress at rest, his vital signs are normal, and he has no obvious signs of cyanosis. His pulmonary examination is notable for reduced air movement and faint expiratory wheezing on auscultation.

▶ What would you recommend to this patient?
▶ What interventions are available to aid with smoking cessation?

ANSWERS TO CASE 7:

Tobacco Use

Summary: A 55-year-old man with a 35-pack-year history of smoking presents with a chronic cough and progressively worsening dyspnea.

- **Recommendations to this patient:** This patient should be advised to quit smoking; one strategy, using the 5 A's, is discussed below.

- **Interventions available to help with smoking cessation:** Counseling to quit smoking along with pharmacologic assistance with bupropion, varenicline, or nicotine replacement.

ANALYSIS

Objectives

1. Know the many medical conditions and complications related to tobacco use.

2. Develop a framework for the discussion of tobacco use and promotion of smoking cessation.

3. Know the currently available pharmacologic agents that are used to aid in smoking cessation.

Considerations

This is a 55-year-old man with a long history of smoking who presents with a chronic cough and worsening dyspnea. The most important first steps are to address the airway and breathing, and ensure that there is no respiratory emergency. Assessment of the patient's air movement, oxygenation, and degree of respiratory distress are important. After evaluating his condition and ascertaining whether it is chronic lung disease or an exacerbation such as bronchitis superimposed on chronic obstructive pulmonary disease (COPD), therapy may be enacted. Bronchodilator therapy, antibiotic therapy depending on the character of the sputum, and the chest radiograph findings are typically used. One critical component to therapy includes smoking cessation. Physician intervention is paramount, and the use of adjuvant therapies helps to increase the success.

APPROACH TO:

Tobacco Cessation

DEFINITIONS

PREGNANCY CATEGORY B: *Food and Drug Administration* (FDA) category for use of a medication in pregnancy in which animal studies have shown no harm to a fetus but human studies are not available *or* animal studies have shown harm to a fetus but studies in pregnant women have not shown harm.

PREGNANCY CATEGORY C: Animal studies have shown adverse fetal effects and there are no adequate studies in humans *or* no animal studies have been conducted and there are no adequate studies in humans.

PREGNANCY CATEGORY D: Human studies have shown potential adverse fetal effects; however, the benefits of therapy may outweigh the potential risks.

CLINICAL APPROACH

Tobacco use is the single greatest cause of preventable death. It is responsible for increased death rates from cancer, cardiac, cerebrovascular, and chronic pulmonary disease. Approximately, 18% of the adult population reported smoking in 2012 and over 480,000 deaths per year are a result of tobacco use. Smoking also affects the health of those in close contact with people who smoke. Each year, 41,000 deaths from cancer and heart disease in nonsmokers are attributable to secondhand smoke. Secondhand smoke increases a nonsmoker's risk of lung cancer up to 30%. Data pooled in 2010 by the CDC showed nearly 11% of pregnant women reported tobacco use. Smoking in pregnancy is associated with prematurity, intrauterine growth restriction, stillbirth, spontaneous abortion, and infant death. Smoking cessation reduces all of these risks. However, despite this evidence, it is difficult for smokers to quit. Health-care providers are important in the effort to reduce tobacco use and its related disease burden.

Research indicates that physician intervention, even in brief encounters, increases tobacco cessation rate. Furthermore, cessation rates increase with increased physician time and frequency of encounters to address tobacco use, but the optimal duration and frequency has not been defined. **The process of discussing tobacco use and cessation involves several steps; one useful framework is the "five A's":**

- **Ask** about tobacco use: Ask the patient at each visit about current tobacco use.

- **Advise** to quit through clear personalized messages: Let the patient know of his/her specific risks of tobacco use; in the sample case, talk to the patient about how the persistent cough and dyspnea can be related to the tobacco use and how cessation might be helpful.

- **Assess** willingness to quit: Find out the patient's thoughts about quitting and if the patient is ready to proceed.

- **Assist** to quit: Including individual, group, or telephone counseling and pharmacologic treatment. For the patient that does not desire to quit, provide interventions that increase future quit attempts (motivational interviewing or the five R's enhancing motivation strategy).

- **Arrange** follow-up and support.

Individuals who fail to quit smoking or those who relapse should be reassessed using the five A framework. Once a new plan of cessation is in place, patients should determine a new quit date.

Multiple factors may be part of a patient's unwillingness to quit. **A strategy to enhance motivation (five R's strategy)** includes discussing the specific **relevance** to the patient of smoking cessation, **risks** of ongoing tobacco use, **rewards** of quitting (financial, health, social), **roadblocks** to quitting (withdrawal, discouragement because of failed past attempts, enjoyment of smoking), and **repetition** (readdressing the problem at each visit and reminding patients most people attempt to quit several times before being successful).

In pregnancy, it has been found to be helpful to discuss specific risks to the mother and fetus of continued tobacco use. While cessation prior to pregnancy is ideal, cessation at any time during pregnancy is associated with health benefits for patient and fetus, so ongoing discussions are encouraged. The pregnant patient will also need ongoing support to reduce the risk of remission after delivery.

Discussing the symptoms of nicotine withdrawal prior to cessation may decrease failure rates in nicotine-dependent patients. It is not uncommon for patients to avoid smoking cessation secondary to a previous experience or fear of withdrawal symptoms. Common nicotine withdrawal symptoms include mood changes (irritability, anxiety, frustrated), difficulty concentrating, increased hunger, and restlessness.

Pharmacologic Therapy

In addition to counseling and reviewing the risks and benefits of quitting, the use of pharmacologic aids can increase the likelihood of successful smoking cessation when a patient has decided to quit. There are two broad modalities approved by the FDA to assist with smoking cessation: nicotine replacement and nonnicotine medications. Nicotine replacement products include gum, patch, inhaler, nasal spray, and lozenge. The approved nonnicotine medications are bupropion sustained release (brand name: Zyban) and varenicline (brand name: Chantix).

Bupropion was the first nonnicotine treatment for smoking cessation approved by the FDA. It is thought to work by blocking uptake of norepinephrine and/ or dopamine. It is contraindicated in patients with eating disorders, monoamine oxidase (MAO) inhibitor use in the last 2 weeks, or a history of seizure disorder. The usual course of treatment is 7 to 12 weeks, but it can be used for up to 6 months as maintenance therapy. This treatment can be used alone or in combination with nicotine-based treatments. According to a Cochrane Review, individuals taking bupropion for smoking cessation were two times more likely to quit compared with individuals taking a placebo. Common side effects include insomnia and dry mouth. Caution should be used in patients with established coronary heart disease; doses above the recommended amount can be cardiotoxic and lead to widened QRS complexes and subsequently fatal arrhythmias.

By acting as a partial nicotinic receptor agonist, varenicline increases the rate of smoking cessation by threefold when compared with placebo. Varencline reduces cravings for nicotine, reduces nicotine withdrawal symptoms, and blocks some of the binding of nicotine from cigarettes. Doses are reduced in patients on hemodialysis or with creatinine clearance less than 30 mL/min. Varenicline has been associated with neuropsychiatric symptoms including changes in behavior, agitation, depression, and suicidal behaviors. It should be used with caution in anyone with a history of psychiatric disorders. Given recent studies showing a possible increased risk of cardiac events while taking varenicline, caution should be used in people with coronary artery disease. Common side effects include nausea, trouble sleeping, and abnormal, vivid, or strange dreams.

Nicotine replacement therapies as a group increase smoking cessation rates over placebo by diminishing cravings and reducing nicotine withdrawal. They can be used in combination therapy, which may increase cessation rates over monotherapy. Specifically, the combination of a daily nicotine patch and an as-needed nicotine replacement therapy (nicotine gum, inhaler, nasal spray, or lozenge) has been shown to be more effective than the patch alone.

Nicotine gum is available in 2 and 4 mg of nicotine per piece. The patient chews a piece of the gum until the patient feels a peppery taste in the mouth, "parks" the gum in a cheek until the sensation goes away, and then chews the gum again until the peppery sensation returns. The 4-mg dose is recommended for those who smoke more than 25 cigarettes per day and the 2-mg dose for those who smoke fewer than 25 cigarettes per day. Common pitfalls include not "parking" the gum (ie, chewing constantly) and not using enough pieces per day initially. Consider advising the patient to use the gum on a scheduled basis, rather than as needed, initially, and then slowly tapering the number of pieces per day. Common side effects, such as mouth soreness, hiccups, dyspepsia, and jaw ache, often are related to improper chewing technique.

The nicotine cartridge inhaler is available by prescription and has also been found to be effective in increasing smoking cessation rates. Each cartridge contains 4 mg of nicotine in 80 inhalations. The recommended dose is 6 to 16 cartridges per day. The inhaler can be used over several months, with a gradual tapering of the dose. For the gum, lozenge, and inhaler, acidic beverages (coffee, soda, or juices) can reduce absorption of the nicotine from the buccal mucosa, so the patient should avoid ingestion within 15 minutes of use of these products. Common side effects such as local irritation of the mouth and throat, coughing, and rhinitis usually declined with continued use.

Another therapeutic option is the nicotine nasal inhaler. The inhaler provides 0.5 mg of nicotine per inhalation and can be used at a starting rate of 1 to 2 doses per hour, for a maximum of 40 doses per day (5 doses per hour). The inhaler can also be used over months, with gradual tapering of the dose. Nasal irritation is the most common side effect. Of all the nicotine replacement products, the inhaler has the highest peak nicotine level and therefore also has the highest dependency potential.

The nicotine lozenge is available over the counter in 2 and 4 mg nicotine doses. The 4-mg nicotine lozenge is recommended for those who smoke their first cigarette within 30 minutes of waking and the 2-mg nicotine lozenge is for those who smoke their first cigarette more than 30 minutes after waking. The patient should allow the lozenge to dissolve in their mouth without swallowing or chewing. The recommended dose is 1 lozenge every 1 to 2 hours, not to exceed 20 lozenges a day, for the first 6 weeks and then a gradual 6 week taper for a total of 12 weeks of treatment. Common side effects include nausea, hiccups, and heartburn.

The nicotine patch is a passive nicotine replacement system, compared to the other methods outlined above. There are two common over-the-counter forms of the nicotine patch: Nicoderm CQ, which comes in multiple doses (21, 14, and 7 mg of nicotine per patch) and are meant to be worn for 24 hours a day, and Nicotrol, which has 15 mg of nicotine and is meant to be worn for 16 hours a day. The patch is replaced daily, and consideration should be given to starting with higher-dose patches in heavy smokers. Treatment with the patch for fewer than 8 weeks is as effective as longer treatment periods. The most common side effect is irritation of the skin at the site of the patch.

The use of electronic cigarettes (also called, e-cigarettes) for smoking cessation has gained popularity since introduced to the United States in 2007. These battery operated devices convert liquid nicotine into a vapor that is inhaled. Depending on the version of e-cigarettes used, flavors, additives, herbal extracts, or vitamins may be added and nicotine may or may not be present. Electronic cigarettes are safer than cigarettes because they are free from carcinogens and tar. It is still unclear if e-cigarettes are more effective for treating smoking cessation than traditional nicotine replacement modalities. In effort to halt the increased use of e-cigarettes among children and adolescents, in 2014, the FDA prohibited the sale of smokeless tobacco to individuals younger than 18 years. Caution should be used when suggesting smokeless tobacco as a means for quitting. Until further research is conducted, more familiar methods should be recommended.

There is insufficient evidence for the effectiveness of pharmacologic therapy to aid in quitting in the populations of smokeless tobacco users, light smokers (fewer than 10 cigarettes/d), adolescents, and pregnant women. The nicotine inhaler, nasal spray, patch, and gum are pregnancy category D drugs. Pregnant smokers should be encouraged to quit without the use of any pharmacologic agents. However, these products can be considered for use in the pregnant smoker if counseling is insufficient to promote cessation, and if, in discussion with the patient, it is determined that the risks of continued smoking outweigh the risks of the medication. Bupropion and varenicline are pregnancy category C. They have not been studied in pregnancy and should only be used if the benefit justifies the potential risk to the fetus.

The United States Preventive Services Task Force (USPSTF) strongly recommends screening all adults and pregnant patients for tobacco use and offering cessation intervention for those who use tobacco products (Level A recommendation). For adolescent smokers, counseling has been shown to be effective and counseling interventions should be provided to aid in quitting (Level B recommendation). The strongest risk factor for smoking initiation among children and adolescents is parental smoking.

COMPREHENSION QUESTIONS

7.1 A pregnant woman who smokes 1 pack of cigarettes a day asks for your advice regarding smoking cessation while she is pregnant. Which of the following statements is most appropriate?

A. Bupropion is pregnancy category C.

B. Varenicline is pregnancy category B and relatively safe in pregnancy.

C. Nicotine gum delivers a lower and safer dose of nicotine than the nasal spray.

D. The use of smoking cessation products during pregnancy frequently leads to adverse outcomes.

7.2 Which of the following statements regarding available treatments for smoking cessation is accurate?

A. Bupropion can be used in combination with nicotine supplements.

B. Nicotine gum is most effective if chewed continuously, to promote a constant release of the nicotine.

C. Nicotine supplements are most effective when used as needed for withdrawal symptoms.

D. All of the available agents are more effective when used in combinations with each other.

7.3 Which of the following counseling strategies is most likely to enhance your patients' smoking cessation rates?

A. Discuss smoking cessation techniques only with patients who ask for your advice, as others will resent your suggestions.

B. Emphasize primarily the health risks of smoking.

C. Note in each patient's chart that you have discussed cessation, so that you don't repeat the message to the same patient at subsequent visits.

D. Ask about smoking cessation at each encounter.

ANSWERS

7.1 **A.** Bupropion and varenicline are both pregnancy category C. Pregnant smokers should be encouraged to quit without the use of any pharmacologic agents. However, pharmacologic aids to increase the rate of smoking cessation during pregnancy can be used, after discussion with the patient of the risks and benefits of the medications and of continued smoking. Cessation of smoking at anytime during the pregnancy is likely to provide health benefits for the mother and fetus. Nicotine gum delivers higher doses of nicotine than its nasal spray counterpart.

7.2 **A.** Bupropion can be used in combination with any of the nicotine supplementation products. The nicotine products can also be used in combination with each other. Varenicline has not been studied for use with other smoking cessation agents. Two common pitfalls in using nicotine supplementation are using supplementation only when having withdrawal symptoms and failing to use nicotine gum correctly. The gum should be chewed briefly and then parked in the cheek. It is less effective if chewed continuously.

7.3 **D.** Asking patients about tobacco use is a key to promoting cessation. It is important to ask each patient at each visit and to be prepared to provide advice and assistance at anytime.

CLINICAL PEARLS

▶ Most smokers require multiple attempts before successfully quitting for good. Remind your patients of this if they become discouraged in their efforts.

▶ Use the five As—Ask, Advise, Assess, Assist, and Arrange follow-up—to help your patients quit smoking.

REFERENCES

Drew AM, Peters GL. Electronic cigarettes: cautions and concerns. *Am Fam Physician*. 2014 Sep 1;90(5):282-284.

Fiore MC, Bailey WC, Cohen SJ, et al. *Treating Tobacco Use and Dependence. Clinical Practice Guideline*. Rockville, MD: US Department of Health and Human Services, Public Health Service; May 2008.

Hughes JR, Stead LF, Hartmann-Boyce J, Cahill K, Lancaster T. Antidepressants for smoking cessation. *Cochrane Database of Syst Rev*. 2014 Jan 8;1:CD000031.

Larzelere MM, Williams DE. Promoting smoking cessation. *Am Fam Physician*. 2012 Mar 15;85(6):591-598.

United States Preventive Services Task Force (USPSTF). Counseling and interventions to prevent tobacco use and tobacco-caused diseases in adults and pregnant women: USPSTF reaffirmation recommendation statement. Clinical guidelines. Available at: http://www.uspreventiveservicestaskforce.org/uspstf09/tobacco/tobaccors2.pdf. Accessed February 12, 2015.

U.S. Department of Health and Human Services. *The Health Consequences of Smoking—50 Years of Progress: A Report of the Surgeon General*. Atlanta, GA: U.S. Department of Health and Human Services, Centers for Disease Control and Prevention, National Center for Chronic Disease Prevention and Health Promotion, Office on Smoking and Health, 2014: http://www.surgeongeneral.gov/library/reports/50-years-of-progress/. Accessed February 12, 2015.

U.S. Food and Drug Administration. Protecting teens and children from tobacco: restricting sale and distribution. Available at: http://www.fda.gov/syn/html/ucm2022622. Accessed February 26, 2015.

A 16-year-old adolescent girl presents to your office with the complaint of greenish vaginal discharge for the past 2 months and the recent onset of lower abdominal pain. She reports that her last period was about 2½ months ago. She is sexually active with two partners and has never used a condom or any other contraception with either. On physical examination, she is not febrile with normal blood pressure and pulse. She has greenish discharge from the cervix with friability and cervicitis. There is no cervical motion tenderness. Her urine pregnancy test is positive. A cervical sample is positive for *Chlamydia* and negative for *Neisseria gonorrhoeae.* Her rapid plasma reagin (RPR) is nonreactive and an HIV test is negative. The patient is treated with appropriate antibiotics and counseled concerning safer sex practices. You also inform the patient regarding her risk for HIV conversion, even though today's test was negative. The patient asks if you are going to tell her mother that she is pregnant and has this infection. You inform the patient that because of patient confidentiality and ethical considerations you will not disclose this information to her mother without her consent. She tells you that she does not want her mother and boyfriends to know that she is infected.

▶ What should you do?
▶ What should you tell the patient?
▶ What are the ethical considerations?
▶ What are the guidelines for reporting communicable diseases?

ANSWERS TO CASE 8:
Medical Ethics

Summary: The patient is a teen who is pregnant and has a sexually transmitted infection (STI). She engages in high-risk sexual behaviors.

- **What you should do and tell the patient:** You must inform the patient that you have to contact the state health department. The department will contact her and her partners without disclosing her identity. You might also advise the patient to cooperate fully with the health department to avoid phone calls or letters received at home. It is also important to stress to the patient the importance of protecting her partners by telling them her diagnosis. She may avoid further exposure if her partner(s) are adequately treated.

- **Ethical considerations:** Teenage pregnancy, confidentiality, sexually transmitted infection reporting, and emancipation.

- **Guidelines for reporting communicable diseases:** The guidelines for reporting communicable disease vary slightly from state to state. However, there is usually a formal mechanism for reporting to the state department of health. The physician may do it himself/herself or may elect to use an agent, such as a nurse or other medical facility staff member. It is a federal mandate to report communicable diseases; failure to do so may result in adverse legal, civil, and even criminal actions. For example, in the state of Texas, failure to report communicable diseases (HIV/AIDS, gonorrhea, chlamydia, chancroid, and syphilis) is considered a class B misdemeanor.

ANALYSIS
Objectives

1. Discuss confidentiality and its ethical and legal considerations when treating adolescent or pregnant adolescent patients.

2. Understand the legal obligations for reporting communicable diseases and informing partners.

Considerations

There are several considerations involved in this case. The first issue is pregnancy. In some states, the patient would be considered emancipated. Consequently, legally she can make decisions regarding her pregnancy-related health care (excluding abortion in most states) without notice to or the express consent of her parents. In addition, she has a sexually transmitted infection, which is a reportable condition; thus the physician or the physician's agent **must** report this to the state health department for surveillance and infection control. She is also very concerned about informing her partners about the infection. There are also issues of confidentiality.

APPROACH TO:
Medical Ethics

DEFINITIONS

EMANCIPATION: Emancipation is a legal process in which a person who is younger than 18 years petitions the court to have herself/himself declared a legal adult. Laws for emancipation vary by state. Emancipation ends the parents' legal duty to support the minor, and also ends the parents' right to make decisions about the minor's residence, education, health care, and to control the minor's conduct. However, this does not include the ability to consume alcohol, use tobacco, or exercise voting rights.

MATURE MINOR DOCTRINE/RULE (JUDICIAL BYPASS): The mature minor exception to the need for parental consent for medical care is based on the West Virginia Supreme Court case *Belcher v CAMC*. Statute and court decisions in many states may vary. A minor may consent to receive medical care without the consent of the parents or guardian if deemed "mature" by the judicial system.

CLINICAL APPROACH

According to the Society for Adolescent Medicine, "the overall goal in clinical practice is to deliver appropriate, high-quality health care to adolescent patients, while encouraging communication between parents or other trusted adults without betraying the adolescent's trust in the health-care professional." It is very important to gain the confidence of adolescent patients because if the patient does not believe that the health-care provider will keep the patient's health information confidential, the patient is less likely to seek health care when needed. Confidential health care should be provided for all adolescent patients; however, the physician must consider some very important issues: Is the teen self-supporting? Is the minor mature enough to make his or her own medical care decisions? Would disclosure without consent harm the patient?

Ethics

Ethical considerations when treating adolescent patients can be complex and one should use the **moral principles of ethics**, which include **autonomy, beneficence, nonmaleficence, and justice** to guide clinical decisions to maintain confidentiality. Respect for **autonomy** should involve respect for the patient's wishes, choices, and beliefs when deciding what is best for the patient. It is important to understand the dynamics of the parent-child relationship and why the teen does not want to disclose important medical information to parents. This type of dialogue may reveal very important things about the child's current situation and help to guide your decision making. Knowing the intricacies of the family dynamic may also help the clinician and the patient develop solutions to aid in disclosure of very important health-related issues.

Nonmaleficence implies that the physician will do nothing to harm the patient, which includes emotional and psychological harm. Failure to maintain confidentiality may result in some emotional distress for the patient. Moreover, the physician should not apply the same moral standards to every patient. Some teens are more mature than others and the physician should use his or her judgment with each adolescent patient.

In addition, the treating physician should apply the principle of **beneficence**, which requires action to further a patient's welfare. In other words, do the right thing for the patient. Maintaining confidentiality may aid in full disclosure of symptoms, life situations, and so on. Full disclosure of pertinent medical information can help the physician provide the most comprehensive care to the patient.

Justice implies the fair and unbiased treatment of the patient regardless of age, sex, or ethnicity. Consequently, adolescent patients should be given the same level of care as adults, without having the fear of disclosure, when they are mentally capable of receiving care.

In most cases, every attempt should be provided to ensure confidentiality. However, **there are instances when it would be in the best interest of the patient to disclose medical information.** Examples of these situations could include patients with homicidal or suicidal ideation or serious chemical dependence, and in suspected cases of abuse. Disclosure of medical information should only be considered when the life of the adolescent must be protected. It is also important to point out that, in most cases, adolescents are not responsible for payment of medical services. The parent or the guardian usually has to assume the responsibility for payment. Thus, the maintenance of confidentiality in these cases is an issue. Because there are no clear-cut guidelines in this situation, it is important to encourage open dialogue between the patient and the patient's parent. However, in instances when this is not possible the physician must use his or her own clinical judgment while considering ethical issues and must act in the best interest of the patient.

Legal Considerations

There are laws in place to protect the confidentiality of health-care information. In general, the law requires the consent of the parent when health care is provided to minors; there are, however, exceptions, such as emergencies, care for the "**mature minor,**" and when the minor is legally entitled to consent to their own medical treatment.

Laws that allow minors to consent to medical treatment vary from state to state. In some states minors are allowed to consent to medical therapy based on status, such as emancipation, marriage, pregnancy, living apart from parents, and when given the status of "mature minor." The mature minor rule was created in 1967 and is based on the West Virginia Supreme Court case *Belcher v CAMC*, which allowed health-care providers to treat a youth as an adult based on an assessment and documentation of the adolescent's maturity level. According to this decision, a court must determine that a minor is deemed mature, which determination is based on various factors, including age, ability, experience, education and/or training, degree of maturity and/or judgment exhibited conduct and demeanor, and capacity to understand the risk and benefits of medical treatment. The process to become a mature minor is known as judicial bypass and may vary from state to state. This exception to parental consent must be received from a court.

In addition, **adolescents may consent to medical care if they are considered emancipated.** Emancipation implies that a minor must be of a certain age (which varies by state), must live apart from his or her parents, and must be self-sufficient. Minors are also considered emancipated if they are self-supporting, not living at home, married, pregnant or a parent, in the military, or declared emancipated by the judicial system.

In some states, **consent to health care may be based on the type of care the adolescent is seeking.** Examples of the types of health-care services that may be obtained without parental consent may include maternity services, contraceptive management, treatment and diagnosis of sexually transmitted infections (including HIV) or other reportable diseases, treatment of drug or alcohol problems, and care related to sexual assault or mental health services. These provisions are very important because they allow the necessary assessment and treatment of important health-related issues. Moreover, research shows that adolescents are more likely to seek medical care if confidentiality is protected.

Reportable Diseases

Reporting STIs, HIV, and other reportable illnesses can be stressful for the patient. This may be particularly stressful for the adolescent. The **information may be reported by the physician or by the physician's designated appointee.** All those involved in the oversight of blood products, including clinical laboratories or blood banks, are also required to report STIs and other reportable conditions to the state's health department. It is state and federal law that these illnesses be reported in a timely fashion to the state health department.

In addition, it is **mandatory that the information be disclosed to partners.** Partner reporting is a way to control the spread of disease and to ensure prompt and proper diagnosis and treatment of all those who may be affected. Partner notification can occur in either of two ways: by patient referral or by the department of health staff. The patient can contact his/her partner(s) for referral, diagnosis, and treatment. Alternatively, the partner(s) may be notified and counseled by department of health staff, if the patient is unwilling to inform them. In the setting where a patient is unwilling to inform his/her partner(s) of a reportable illness that places the partner(s) at risk, the health-care provider has a legal and ethical obligation to inform the partner(s) (if known by the provider) that they are at risk.

Teenage Pregnancy and Confidentiality

Issues regarding teenage pregnancy and consent to disclose information regarding pregnancy are quite controversial. Laws for reporting vary by state and the specifics may become quite daunting. For the purposes of this case, focus is limited to generalities. One must understand the laws pertaining to this issue in the state in which he or she practices. In the state of Texas, as may be the case in other states, a clinician is not required to inform the parents of issues related to the pregnancy of a minor without the child's consent, but it is not mandatory for the adolescent to give consent for a physician to disclose information related to pregnancy to parents.

However, studies demonstrate that failure to maintain confidentiality in "sensitive" health-related issues may inhibit appropriate health-care delivery to the adolescent.

In Texas, the law does not allow state funds to be used for contraception without the consent of the parent. Moreover, in most states, an adolescent younger than 18 years cannot give consent to abortion services without the consent and/or notification of one or both parents. This issue has been the subject of political debate for many years. Proponents of mandatory consent laws believe that it is in the best interest of the minor for her parent(s) or guardian to be informed of her pregnancy and decision to obtain abortion services, stating that by doing so, communication among adult and child may be improved.

Opponents of these laws, however, see them as a threat to the well-being of young women by forcing them to seek abortion services from unlicensed facilities, crossing state lines to obtain abortions, and increasing medical risk. The risk to young women may be increased by enforcing mandatory wait periods. Young women are at greater risk of having abortions later in the pregnancy.

Currently, only twelve states and the District of Columbia do not require consent from and/or notification to parents to obtain abortion services. In a state in which consent is required, there are some legal alternatives for young women. For example, if an adolescent is considered emancipated, then consent from parents or guardians is not required. Waivers of consent (judicial bypass) may also be obtained through the judicial system.

Emergency contraception (EC) when taken after sexual intercourse can prevent pregnancy by disrupting or delaying ovulation or fertilization. Some states allow EC to be accessed without a prescription in individuals 17 years and older. Certain states require that EC be given or offered to sexually assaulted victims in emergency departments. There are significant discrepancies from state to state and future changes are expected.

Conclusion

Pregnancy-related care, abortion services, and reportable illnesses are complex issues and a clinician should seek legal advice when appropriate. However, in general, it is preferable to protect the confidentiality of the minor unless it is unreasonable or unsafe to do so. It is also important to educate teens and parents of the importance of open communication and issues related to confidentiality in medical care.

COMPREHENSION QUESTIONS

8.1 A 14-year-old adolescent girl is here to see you for complaints of greenish vaginal discharge. She is sexually active with one partner and does not use condoms. You do a culture and find that she has *Trichomonas* vaginitis. She asks you not to tell her mother about this diagnosis or that she is sexually active. Which of the following statements is most accurate regarding disclosure or nondisclosure of this information to her parents?

A. You can keep this information confidential. However, it is advisable to talk with the teen about her sexual history and discuss communication issues between her and her parents.

B. Since she is a minor, you must disclose this information to her parents.

C. You can only keep this confidential for today for enhancing therapy, but then disclosure to the parents must be demonstrated and documented.

D. You may keep this confidential from the parents but you must call the partner to notify him of the infection.

8.2 In which of the following situations may a physician keep information confidential from parents or other authorities?

A. The physician finds injuries consistent with physical abuse while examining a 13 years old, but the patient fears further injury if the abuse is reported.

B. A depressed teenager reports a strong desire to kill herself and that she has secretly obtained a gun that she keeps in her bedroom.

C. An undocumented immigrant patient has active tuberculosis and fears deportation if the illness is reported.

D. A 19-year-old female college student, who is still on her parents' insurance plan, reports a consensual sexual relationship with a 35-year-old man and requests contraception, but does not want her parents to know.

8.3 Which of the following is most accurate regarding the term "emancipation" as it applies to a minor?

A. Able to vote

B. Able to purchase and consume alcohol

C. Able to make their own medical decisions without parental consent

D. Legally financially independent

8.4 Which of the following statements regarding a minor's ability to consent for an abortion is most accurate?

A. Because of medical confidentiality, a minor is able to consent to any medical therapy she chooses without the consent of her parents or guardian.

B. Although consent requirements for abortion services vary depending on the state, most states either have some form of required consent for abortion services to minors or a mandatory wait period.

C. There are no states in which a minor can obtain an abortion without the consent of a parent or guardian.

D. A minor cannot consent to any medical therapy without her parents' approval unless she has received a court order.

ANSWERS

8.1 **A.** The law does not require the disclosure of sensitive medical information to parents. However, in some states it is not forbidden to disclose that information. A clinician must use his or her best judgment when deciding whether to disclose medical information. More importantly, the physician should recognize the importance of confidentiality when treating patients and encourage open communication between adolescents and parents when it is reasonable to do so. Partner notification can occur by patient referral or by health department staff.

8.2 **D.** All states have laws mandating the reporting of certain conditions, even if the patient objects. The specific conditions may vary from state to state, so the physician must be aware of the rules where he/she practices. Child abuse must be reported to appropriate authorities if suspected in all states. Similarly, certain infections, such as active tuberculosis, must be reported to public health officials. Active suicidal ideation, especially if there is a plan and access to agents necessary to implement the plan, may lead the physician to intervene to prevent the action. Of the scenarios listed, only D does not obligate the physician to act.

8.3 **C.** Emancipation implies that the patient is able to make decisions regarding health-related issues but does not give the patient the right to vote, consume alcohol, or use tobacco products if the patient is not of legal age.

8.4 **B.** The laws regarding the consent for abortion services vary from state to state. Only 12 states currently allow a minor to have an abortion without the consent of or notification to parents.

CLINICAL PEARLS

▶ Adolescent health care is a complex issue. However, the clinician should attempt to administer confidential health care to minors seeking care for sensitive medical issues when it is safe and appropriate to do so.

▶ It is very important for clinicians to know the laws regarding consent and confidentiality when treating adolescent patients of the states in which they practice.

REFERENCES

Boonstra H, Nash E. Minors and the rights to consent to health care. The Guttmacher Report on Public Policy, Volume 3, Number 4, August 2000. Available at: http://www.guttmacher.org/pubs/tgr/03/4/gr030404.html. Accessed March 1, 2015.

Center for Reproductive Rights. Mandatory parental consent and notification laws. Item F039. March 2001. Available at: http://www.reproductiverights.org. Accessed March 1, 2015.

Cundiff D. Clinical case. Available at: http://virtualmentor.ama-assn.org/2005/10/pdf/ccas1-0510.pdf. Accessed March 1, 2015.

Ford C, English A, Sigman G. Society for Adolescent Medicine position statement. Confidential health care for adolescents: position paper of the Society for Adolescent Medicine. *J Adolesc Med.* 2004;35:160-167.

Litt I. Adolescent patient confidentiality: whom are we kidding [editorial]? *J Adolesc Health.* 2001;29:79.

Maradiegue A. Minor's right's versus parental rights: review of legal issues in adolescent health care. *J Midwifery Womens Health.* 2003;48(3):170-177.

Parental consent and notification laws. *Planned Parenthood.* Available at: http://www.plannedparenthood.org/health-topics/abortion/parental-consent-notification-laws-25268.htm. Accessed March 1, 2015.

The Guttmacher Institute. State polices in brief: emergency contraception. Available at: http://www.guttmacher.org/statecenter/spibs/spib_EC.pdf. Accessed March 1, 2015.

A 65-year-old African-American woman presented to the emergency room complaining of worsening shortness of breath and palpitations for about 1 week. She reports feeling "dizzy" on and off for the past year; the dizziness is associated with weakness that has been worsening for the past month. She has been feeling "too tired" to even walk to her backyard and water her flower bed that she used to do "all the time." She has been so dyspneic walking up the stairs at her home that she moved downstairs to the guest room about a week ago. Review of systems is significant for knee pain, for which she frequently takes aspirin or ibuprofen; otherwise the review of systems is negative. She has no significant medical history and has not been to a doctor in several years. She had a normal well-woman examination and screening colonoscopy about 5 years ago. She occasionally has an alcoholic drink and denies tobacco or drug use. She is married and is a retired shopkeeper. On examination, her blood pressure is 150/85 mm Hg; her pulse is 98 beats/min; her respiratory rate is 20 breaths/min; her temperature is 98.7°F (37.1°C); and her oxygen saturation is 99% on room air. Significant findings on examination include conjunctival pallor, mild tenderness with deep palpation in the epigastric and left upper quadrant (LUQ) region of the abdomen with normal bowel sounds, and no organomegaly but a positive stool guaiac test. The remainder of the examination, including respiratory, cardiovascular, and nervous systems, was normal.

► What is the most likely diagnosis?
► What is your next diagnostic step?
► What is the next step in therapy?

ANSWERS TO CASE 9:
Geriatric Anemia

Summary: A 65-year-old woman with worsening dyspnea on exertion, fatigue, dizziness, and palpitations. She is found to have conjunctival pallor and guaiac-positive stool.

- **Most likely diagnosis:** Anemia secondary to gastrointestinal bleeding; other considerations should include new-onset angina, congestive heart failure, and atrial fibrillation.

- **Next diagnostic step:** A complete blood count (CBC) to evaluate for the anemia. To evaluate for the other conditions on your differential diagnosis list, you should perform an electrocardiogram (ECG) and cardiac enzymes. A prothrombin time (PT) and partial thromboplastin time (PTT) to look for coagulation abnormalities would be helpful as well.

- **Next step in therapy:** Further workup, including blood transfusion (if needed), completion of two more sets of cardiac enzymes, and ECGs. A gastroenterology consult for esophagogastroduodenoscopy (EGD) and colonoscopy is appropriate because of the positive guaiac findings.

ANALYSIS

Objectives

1. Know a diagnostic approach to anemia in geriatrics.

2. Be familiar with a rational workup for anemia of different origins.

Considerations

A 65-year-old woman who has developed worsening dyspnea and palpitations over 1-week period of time needs to be evaluated for cardiac and respiratory problems despite the gradual onset of symptoms. Specifically, in a postmenopausal woman, signs and symptoms of angina or acute myocardial infarction may not always have a typical presentation. That the patient has been feeling weak and has conjunctival pallor warrants testing for anemia. As evaluation with serial cardiac enzymes and ECGs is part of the workup, admission into the hospital is appropriate.

Assuming that the initial workup for cardiac and pulmonary causes is negative and that the hemoglobin and hematocrit levels are low, a thorough evaluation for the cause of the anemia is necessary. A CBC with peripheral smear, reticulocyte count, iron studies, vitamin B_{12}, and folic acid levels would provide clues to the type of anemia that this patient has. A gastroenterology consult for possible EGD and colonoscopy to further investigate the source of gastrointestinal bleeding should be considered. The presence of epigastric and LUQ pain, along with long-term use of nonsteroidal anti-inflammatory drugs (NSAIDs), should also raise a flag for testing to rule out a bleeding ulcer.

The presence of other findings may direct your workup toward other diagnoses. If this patient was from a developing country, the possibility of intestinal parasites would need to be considered. If the PT and PTT were abnormal, gastrointestinal (GI) bleeding from a coagulopathy or liver disease would be possibilities. Weight loss, lymphadenopathy, and coagulopathy may warrant evaluation for nongastrointestinal malignancies, such as leukemias or lymphomas. In younger patients, sickle cell disease, thalassemias, glucose-6-phosphate dehydrogenase (G6PD) deficiency, and other inherited causes of anemia would be on the differential diagnosis list. These are unlikely to manifest as an initial diagnosis at the age of 65.

APPROACH TO:
Anemia in Geriatric Population

DEFINITIONS

ANEMIA: According to the World Health Organization (WHO), a hemoglobin level of less than 12 g/dL in women and less than 14 g/dL in men.

NHANES: The National Health and Nutrition Examination Surveys.

CLINICAL APPROACH

Epidemiology

The prevalence of anemia in Americans older than 65 years is estimated at 9% to 45%. There is **a wide variation in the rates of anemia in different ethnic and racial groups**, with NHANES data showing the highest rates in non-Hispanic blacks and lowest rates in non-Hispanic whites. These differences are reportedly a result of biologic, not socioeconomic, differences. Most studies show the rate of anemia to be higher in men than women and there is increasing evidence for anemia as an independent risk factor for increased morbidity and mortality and decreased quality of life (Level B recommendation).

Clinical Presentation

Fatigue, weakness, and dyspnea are symptoms that are commonly reported by elderly persons with anemia. These vague and nonspecific symptoms are often ignored by both patients and physicians as symptoms of "old age." Anemia may result in worsening of symptoms of other underlying conditions. For example, the reduced oxygen-carrying capacity of the blood as a consequence of anemia may exacerbate dyspnea associated with congestive heart failure.

Certain signs found on examination may prompt a workup for anemia. **Conjunctival pallor is recommended as a reliable sign of anemia in the elderly and commonly noted in patients with hemoglobin** less than **9 g/dL**. Other signs may suggest a specific cause of anemia. Glossitis, decreased vibratory and positional senses, ataxia, paresthesia, confusion, dementia, and pearly gray hair at an early age are signs suggestive of vitamin B_{12}-deficiency anemia. Folate deficiency can cause similar signs, except for the neurologic deficits. Profound iron deficiency may produce koilony-chias (spoon nails), glossitis, or dysphagia. Other clinical manifestations of anemia include jaundice and splenomegaly. Jaundice can be a clue that hemolysis is a contributing factor to the anemia, whereas splenomegaly can indicate that a thalassemia or neoplasm may be present.

Initial workup of anemia should include a CBC with measurement of red blood cell (RBC) indices, a peripheral blood smear, and a reticulocyte count. Further laboratory studies would be indicated based on the results of the initial tests and the presence of symptoms or signs suggestive of other diseases.

The most common cause of anemia with a low mean corpuscular volume (MCV), microcytic anemia, is iron deficiency. Iron deficiency could be confirmed by subsequent testing that shows a low serum iron, low ferritin, and high total iron-binding capacity (TIBC). Other causes of microcytic anemia include thalassemias and anemia of chronic disease. In the elderly, iron deficiency is frequently caused by chronic gastrointestinal blood loss, poor nutritional intake, or a bleeding disorder. A thorough evaluation of the gastrointestinal tract for a source of blood loss, usually requiring a gastroenterology consultation for upper and lower GI endoscopy, should be undertaken, as iron-deficiency anemia may be the initial presentation of a GI malignancy.

Anemia with an elevated MCV, macrocytic anemia, is most often a manifestation of folate or vitamin B_{12} deficiency; other causes include drug effects, liver disease, and hypothyroidism. The presence of macrocytic anemia, with or without the symptoms previously mentioned, should lead to further testing to determine B_{12} and folate levels. An elevated methylmalonic acid (MMA) level can be used to confirm a vitamin B_{12} deficiency; an elevated homocysteine level can be used to confirm folate deficiency. Folate deficiency anemia is usually seen in alcoholics, whereas B_{12}-deficiency anemia mostly occurs in people with pernicious anemia, a history of gastrectomy, and diseases associated with malabsorption (eg, bacterial infection, Crohn disease, celiac disease). Under normal conditions, the body stores 50% of its B_{12} (2-5 mg total in adults) in the liver for 3 to 5 years. A minimal amount of B_{12} is lost daily through gastrointestinal secretions. B_{12} deficiency anemia is rare but possible in long-term vegans and vegetarians. B_{12} deficiency can be distinguished clinically from folic acid deficiency by the presence of neurologic symptoms.

In the elderly, anemia of chronic inflammation (formerly known as anemia of chronic disease) is the most common cause of a normocytic anemia. Anemia of chronic inflammation is anemia that is secondary to some other underlying condition that leads to increased inflammation and bone marrow suppression. Along with causing a normocytic anemia, anemia of chronic inflammation can also present as a microcytic anemia. This type of anemia can easily be confused with iron-deficiency anemia because of its similar initial laboratory picture. In anemia of chronic inflammation, the body's iron stores (measured by serum ferritin) are normal, but the capability of using the stored iron in the reticuloendothelial system becomes decreased. A lack of improvement in symptoms and hemoglobin level with iron supplementation are important clues indicating that the cause is chronic disease and not iron depletion, regardless of the laboratory picture. Another cause of normocytic anemia is renal insufficiency due to decreased erythropoietin production. Although

Table 9–1 • LABORATORY VALUES DIFFERENTIATING IRON-DEFICIENCY ANEMIA FROM ANEMIA OF CHRONIC INFLAMMATION

Test	Iron Deficiency	Anemia of Chronic Inflammation
Serum iron	Low	Low or normal
TIBC	High	Low
Transferrin saturation	Low	Low or normal
Serum ferritin	Low	Normal or high

bone marrow iron store remains the gold standard to differentiate between iron-deficiency anemia and anemia of chronic disease, simple serum testing is still used to diagnose and differentiate these two types of anemia (Table 9–1).

Treatment

The treatment of anemia is determined based on the type and cause of the anemia. Any cause of anemia that creates a hemodynamic instability can be treated with a red blood cell transfusion. A hemoglobin less than 7 g/dL is a commonly used threshold for transfusion; however, transfusion may be indicated at higher levels if the patient is symptomatic or has a comorbid condition such as coronary artery disease. Iron-deficiency anemia is treated first by identification and correction of any source of blood loss. Most iron deficiency can be corrected by oral iron replacement. Oral iron is given as ferrous sulfate 325 mg (contains 65 mg of elemental iron) three times a day. In uncomplicated anemia, it is considered first-line therapy given its low cost and easy accessibility. Adherence to oral iron may be poor due to gastrointestinal side effects (dark stools, nausea, vomiting, and constipation) and the required 6 to 8 weeks of treatment needed to correct the anemia. Individuals with malabsorptive conditions, malignancy, chronic kidney disease, heart failure, or significant blood loss may not benefit from oral iron replacement and therefore require parenteral iron preparations. It is recommended that patients requiring parenteral administration be given iron intravenously and not intramuscular (IM). Given the high risk of side effects, only trained clinicians should administer intravenous iron.

Vitamin B_{12} deficiency traditionally has been treated by intramuscular B_{12} therapy with a regimen of 1000 μg IM daily for 7 days, then weekly for 4 weeks, then monthly for the rest of the patient's life. Newer research shows that many patients can be successfully treated with oral B_{12} therapy using 1000 to 2000 μg PO in a similar regimen. Folate deficiency can be treated with oral therapy of 1 mg daily until the deficiency is corrected.

Anemia of chronic inflammation is managed primarily by treatment of the underlying condition in order to decrease inflammation and bone marrow suppression. When anemia of chronic inflammation is severe (hemoglobin <10 g/dL), the risks and benefits of two modalities of treatment, blood transfusion and erythropoiesis-stimulating agents, may be considered. To note, the goals of treatment of anemia of chronic inflammation in patients with chronic kidney disease undergoing dialysis are to maintain a hemoglobin level between 10 and 12 g/dL; higher hemoglobin levels in this patient population are associated with increased rates of death and cardiovascular events.

COMPREHENSION QUESTIONS

9.1 A 58-year-old woman comes to your office complaining of fatigue. She has also noticed a burning sensation in her feet over the past 6 months. A CBC shows anemia with an increased MCV. Which of the following is the most likely cause of her anemia?

A. Lack of intrinsic factor

B. Inadequate dietary folate

C. Strict vegetarian diet

D. Chronic GI blood loss

9.2 A 65-year-old man with a history of rheumatoid arthritis is found to have a microcytic anemia. He had a colonoscopy 1 year ago which was normal and stool guaiac is negative. Which of the following is the most likely cause of his anemia?

A. Iron deficiency

B. Chronic disease

C. Pernicious anemia

D. Folate deficiency

For questions 9.3 and 9.4, match the following laboratory pictures (A-D) of patients with anemia:

A. Normal MMA; decreased serum folate level

B. Elevated MMA; decreased serum B_{12} level

C. Elevated ferritin; normal MCV; decreased serum iron level

D. Decreased ferritin; decreased MCV; decreased serum iron level

9.3 A 68-year-old man is found to have an incidental finding of anemia while in the hospital for alcohol abuse.

9.4 A 67-year-old man with dizziness and a positive stool guaiac test.

9.5 A 68-year-old man is found to have an incidental finding of anemia while hospitalized with pneumonia. His physical examination is normal except for crackles in the left lower lobe. Serum laboratory examinations reveal a normal MMA and a decreased serum folate level. Which of the following is the best next step?

A. Administer CAGE questionnaire

B. Esophagogastroduodenoscopy

C. Serum iron assay

D. Neurology consultation

ANSWERS

9.1 **A.** The clinical presentation and CBC findings are consistent with macrocytic anemia due to B_{12} deficiency. Pernicious anemia (lack of intrinsic factor) is the most common cause. B_{12} deficiency can also be seen in patients who follow a strict vegetarian diet; however, the body's B_{12} stores can last several years before they are depleted.

9.2 **B.** Anemia of chronic disease can cause normocytic or microcytic anemia, and may be secondary to rheumatoid arthritis in the patient. Iron-deficiency anemia is less likely with a normal colonoscopy and negative stool guaiac, and serum iron studies could be used to help differentiate the two.

9.3 **A.** Alcohol abuse is a common cause of folate deficiency. A normal MMA level essentially rules out a concomitant vitamin B_{12} deficiency.

9.4 **D.** Low serum iron, low MCV, and low ferritin levels, along with a finding of blood in the stool, are consistent with iron-deficiency anemia. A workup for the source of the GI blood loss should ensue.

9.5 **A.** Alcohol abuse, which may be assessed by the CAGE questionnaire, is a common cause of folate deficiency. CAGE is an acronym which stands for Cut back, Annoyed, Guilty, and Eye-opener. A normal MMA level essentially rules out a concomitant vitamin B_{12} deficiency. Gastric endoscopy—to look for atrophic gastritis—would be indicated for pernicious anemia. A serum iron assay would likely be high because of increased turnover of iron in patients with megaloblastic anemia due to either B_{12} or folate deficiency. A neurology consultation would be needed if the patient had neurologic signs or symptoms of B_{12} deficiency.

CLINICAL PEARLS

▶ Conjunctival pallor is an indication for anemia workup in elderly patients.

▶ Clinical findings of anemia require investigation for underlying causes.

▶ GI bleeding is an important cause of iron-deficiency anemia in both female and male geriatric patients; this type of anemia mandates a GI workup in this patient population.

▶ Investigating for vitamin B_{12} and folate deficiency is of high importance in a patient with a history of heavy ethyl alcohol (EtOH) intake and/or abuse.

REFERENCES

Adamson JW. Iron deficiency and other hypoproliferative anemias. In: Kasper D, Fauci A, Hauser S, et al, eds. *Harrison's Principles of Internal Medicine*. 19th ed. New York, NY: McGraw-Hill Education; 2015. Available at: http://accessmedicine.mhmedical.com/. Accessed May 24, 2015.

Auerbach M, Ballard H, Glaspy J. Clinical update: intravenous iron for anaemia. *Lancet*. 2007;369:1502.

Bross MH, Sock K, Smith-Knuppel T. Anemia in older persons. *Am Fam Physician*. 2010;82(5): 480-487.

Killip S, Bennett JM, Chambers MD. Iron deficiency anemia. *Am Fam Physician*. 2007;75:671-678.

Smith D. Anemia in the elderly. *Am Fam Physician*. 2000;62:1565-1572.

Voet, D, Voet, JG. *Biochemistry*. New York, NY: J. Wiley & Sons; 2010:957.

A 40-year-old man presents to the clinic complaining of having 10 episodes of watery, nonbloody diarrhea that started last night. He vomited twice last night but has been able to tolerate liquids today. He has had intermittent abdominal cramps as well. He reports having muscle aches, weakness, headache, and low-grade temperature. He is here with his daughter, who started with the same symptoms this morning. On questioning, he states that he has no significant medical history, no surgeries, and does not take any medications. He does not smoke cigarettes, drink alcohol, use any illicit drugs, and has never had a blood transfusion. He and his family returned to the United States yesterday, following a week-long vacation in Mexico.

On examination, he is not in acute distress. His blood pressure is 110/60 mm Hg, his pulse is 98 beats/min, his respiratory rate is 16 breaths/min, and his temperature is 99.1°F (37.2°C). His mucous membranes are dry. His bowel sounds are hyperactive and his abdomen is mildly tender throughout, but there is no rebound tenderness and no guarding. A rectal examination is normal and his stool is guaiac negative. The remainder of his examination is unremarkable.

▶ What is the most likely diagnosis?
▶ What is your next step?
▶ What are potential complications?

ANSWERS TO CASE 10:
Acute Diarrhea

Summary: A 40-year-old man who recently returned from Mexico with profuse, acute, nonbloody diarrhea, and dry mucous membranes on examination, which are consistent with developing dehydration. An ill family member with identical symptoms suggests an infectious cause of this acute illness.

- **Most likely diagnosis:** Acute gastroenteritis

- **Next step:** Fecal leukocyte or fecal lactoferrin testing; rehydration with oral or IV fluids

- **Potential complication:** Dehydration and electrolyte abnormalities

ANALYSIS

Objectives

1. To clearly understand when and how to do a workup for acute diarrhea, considering the most probable etiologies of diarrhea such as virus, *Escherichia coli*, *Shigella*, *Salmonella*, *Giardia*, and *amebiasis*.

2. To understand the role of fecal leukocytes and stool occult blood in the evaluation of acute diarrhea.

3. To understand that volume replacement and correction of electrolyte abnormalities are a key component in the treatment and prevention of diarrhea complications.

Considerations

This 40-year-old man developed severe diarrhea, nausea, and vomiting. His **most immediate problem is volume depletion,** as evidenced by his dry mucous membranes. The priority is to **replace the lost intravascular volume, usually with intravenous normal saline.** Electrolytes and renal function should be evaluated and abnormalities corrected. While correcting and/or preventing further dehydration, you need to determine the etiology of the diarrhea. Up to **90% of acute diarrhea is infectious** in etiology. He does not have any history compatible with chronic diarrhea, causes of which include Crohn disease, ulcerative colitis, gluten intolerance, irritable bowel syndrome, and parasites. He had been in Mexico recently, which predisposes him to different pathogens: *E coli*, *Campylobacter*, *Shigella*, *Salmonella*, and *Giardia*. Bacterial infections are more likely to be the source of acute diarrhea in individuals who have recently traveled, ingested contaminated food, or have other medical conditions. He does not have bloody stools. The **presence of blood in the stool would suggest an invasive bacterial infection,** such as hemorrhagic or enteroinvasive *E coli* species, *Yersinia* species, *Shigella*, and *Entamoeba histolytica*.

Examination of the stool for leukocytes is an inexpensive test that helps to differentiate between the types of infectious diarrhea. If leukocytes are present in the stool, the suspicion is higher for *Salmonella, Shigella, Yersinia,* enterohemorrhagic and enteroinvasive *E coli, Clostridium difficile, Campylobacter,* and *E histolytica.* Fecal lactoferrin immunoassay testing kits have increased in popularity due to their ease of use and faster results compared to fecal leukocytes. Lactoferrin is an iron-binding protein that is found in polymorphonuclear neutrophils (PMN) and bodily secretions such as breast milk. Gastrointestinal inflammation causes immune activated PMNs to release lactoferrin. Lactoferrin elevations in stool can be seen with irritable bowel syndrome, intestinal bacterial infections, parasitic infections, and other conditions. Lactoferrin will be low in viral infections, making it a useful test for distinguishing viral from bacterial diarrhea. In general, ova and parasite evaluation is unhelpful, unless the history strongly points toward a parasitic source or the diarrhea is prolonged. The majority of the diarrheas are viral, self-limited, and do not need further evaluation. In this particular patient, because of his recent travel to Mexico, traveler's diarrhea (TD) should be strongly considered and treated with the appropriate antibiotic.

APPROACH TO:
Acute Diarrhea

DEFINITIONS

ACUTE DIARRHEA: Diarrhea presents for fewer than 2-week duration

CHRONIC DIARRHEA: Diarrhea presents for longer than 4-week duration

DIARRHEA: Passage of abnormally liquid or poorly formed stool in increased frequency (three or more times a day)

SUBACUTE DIARRHEA: Diarrhea presents for 2- to 4-week duration

CLINICAL APPROACH

Etiologies

Approximately 90% of acute diarrhea is caused by infectious etiologies, with the remainder caused by medications, ischemia, and toxins. Infectious etiologies often depend on the patient population. **Travelers to Mexico** will frequently contract **enterotoxigenic** *E coli* as a causative agent. **Traveler's diarrhea** is a common entity and can be induced by a variety of bacteria, viruses, and parasites (Table 10–1). Campers are often affected by *Giardia*. Contaminated food and water supplies account for the high incidence of diarrhea in developing countries.

Consumption of foods is also frequently a culprit. *Salmonella* or *Shigella* can be found in **undercooked chicken**, enterohemorrhagic *E coli* from undercooked hamburger, and *Staphylococcus aureus* or *Salmonella* from **creamy foods**. Raw seafood may harbor *Vibrio, Salmonella*, or hepatitis A. Sometimes, the **timing** of the **diarrhea** following food ingestion is helpful. For example, **illness within 6 hours of eating a salad containing mayonnaise suggests *S aureus*, within 8 to 12 hours suggests *Clostridium perfringens*, and within 12 to 14 hours suggests *E coli*.**

Table 10–1 • COMMON ETIOLOGIES OF TRAVELER'S DIARRHEA		
Bacteria	Viruses	Parasites
E coli (all types)	Rotavirus	Giardia lamblia
Salmonella	Norovirus	E histolytica
Shigella		Cryptosporidium parvum
Vibrio non-cholera		
Campylobacter		

Daycare settings are particularly common for *Shigella*, *Giardia*, and rotavirus to be transmitted. Patients in nursing homes, or who were recently in the hospital, may develop C *difficile* colitis from antibiotic use. Consuming cold meats, raw milk, and soft cheeses increases the risk of listeriosis. Pregnant women are advised to avoid foods associated with listeriosis because they are at a significantly higher risk of infection. Immunocompromised patients (AIDS) are more susceptible to parasitic gastrointestinal infections.

Clinical Presentation

Most patients with acute diarrhea have self-limited processes and do not require much workup. Exceptions to this rule include profuse diarrhea, dehydration, fever exceeding 100.4°F (38.0°C), bloody diarrhea, severe abdominal pain, duration of the diarrhea for more than 48 hours, and children, elderly patients, and immunocompromised patients. Traveler's diarrhea is characterized by more than three loose stools in a 24-hour period accompanied by abdominal cramping, nausea, vomiting, fever, or tenesmus. Most cases occur within the first 2 weeks of travel.

Past and recent medical history should include exposures to medications and foods, travel history, and coworkers, classmates, or family members with similar symptoms. A history of a viral illness may provide a clue to the etiology. The initial evaluation should determine if the patient can tolerate oral intake. The patient who is both vomiting and having diarrhea is more prone to dehydration and more likely to need hospital admission for IV hydration.

The physical examination should focus on the vital signs, clinical impression of the volume status, and abdominal examination. Volume status is determined by observing whether the mucous membranes are moist or dry, the skin has good turgor, and the capillary refill is normal or delayed. Stool cultures have limited benefit due to high cost and inefficient results. The use of stool cultures should be limited to individuals with bloody diarrhea, diarrhea lasting for more than 3 to 7 days, immunocompromised patients, and evidence of systemic disease or severe dehydration. Ova and parasite evaluation is generally unhelpful, except in selected circumstances of very high suspicion. Testing for C *difficile* toxins A and B is recommended in patients who develop diarrhea within 3 days of hospitalization, during antibiotic treatment, or within 3 months of discontinuing antibiotics. Although classically associated with clindamycin, **any antibiotic can cause pseudomembranous colitis.** A complete blood count, electrolytes, and renal function tests are sometimes indicated.

Treatment

Most cases of diarrhea resolve spontaneously in a few days without treatment. Replacement of fluids and electrolytes is the first step in treating the consequences of acute diarrhea. For mildly dehydrated individuals who can tolerate oral fluids, solutions such as the World Health Organization oral rehydration solution or commercially available drinks, such as Pedialyte or Gatorade, often are all that is needed. It is no longer recommended that patients avoid eating solid foods for 24 hours. Increased intestinal permeability caused by gastrointestinal infections can be limited by early refeeding. Those with more serious volume deficits, elderly patients, and infants generally require hospitalization and intravenous hydration.

If a parasitic infection is the cause of the diarrhea, prescription antibiotics may ease the symptoms. Antibiotics sometimes, but not always, help ease symptoms of bacterial diarrhea. However, antibiotics will not help viral diarrhea, which is the most common kind of infectious diarrhea. Over-the-counter antimotility or antisecretory medications may help to slow down the frequency of the stools, but they do not speed the recovery. Certain infections may be made worse by over-the-counter medications because they prevent your body from getting rid of the organism that is causing the diarrhea. Probiotics, supplements that contain live organisms such as *Lactobacillus* sp or *Saccharomyces Boulardii*, may reduce the incidence of antibiotic-related diarrhea and the duration/severity of all-cause infectious diarrhea (Level A recommendation). Zinc supplementation has shown promising results for decreasing the duration and severity of the diarrheal illnesses in children. Better relief of acute diarrhea with excessive gas may be possible with combined loperamide and simethicone compared to either medication alone.

Prevention

Hand washing is a simple and effective way to prevent the spread of viral diarrhea. Adults, children, and clinic and hospital personnel should be encouraged to wash their hands. Because viral diarrhea spreads easily, children with diarrhea should not attend school or child care until their illness has resolved.

To prevent diarrhea caused by contaminated food, use dairy products that have been pasteurized. Serve food immediately or refrigerate it after it has been cooked. Do not leave food out at room temperature because it promotes the growth of bacteria.

Travelers to locations, such as developing countries, where there is poor sanitation and frequent contamination of food and water, need to be cautious to reduce their risk of developing diarrhea. They should be advised to eat hot and well-cooked foods, and to drink bottled water, soda, wine, or beer served in its original container. Avoid drinks served over ice. Beverages from boiled water, such as coffee and tea, are usually safe. Recommend the use of bottled water even for teeth brushing. Also recommend avoiding raw fruits and vegetables unless they are peeled by the consumer immediately before being eaten. Patients should avoid tap water and ice cubes. In all, these recommendations may reduce but not completely eliminate one's risk of developing traveler's diarrhea.

Traveler's Prophylaxis and Treatment

The **best method for preventing TD is to avoid contaminated food and water.** Antibiotic prophylaxis is not indicated unless the patient is at increased risk for complications from diarrhea or dehydration, such as underlying inflammatory bowel disease, renal disease, or an immunocompromised state. Fluoroquinolones are typically used for prophylaxis. Studies have shown that the antibacterial and antisecretory effects of bismuth subsalicylate decrease the incidence of traveler's diarrhea. Bismuth subsalicylate should be avoided in persons allergic to aspirin, pregnant women, or those taking methotrexate, probenecid, or doxycycline for malaria prophylaxis.

When antibiotics are indicated, therapy with a quinolone antibiotic should be started as soon as possible after the diarrhea begins. Most commonly, **ciprofloxacin (500 mg twice daily) is given for 3 days.** Quinolones cannot be used in children or pregnant women. **Azithromycin,** given as a single 1000-mg dose in adults or 10 mg/kg daily for 3 days in children, is another effective drug for the treatment of TD. Azithromycin also can be used in pregnant women with traveler's diarrhea. **Rifaximin** given as 200 mg three times a day for 3 days can be used in TD caused by noninvasive strains of E coli. However, rifaximin is not effective against infections associated with fever or blood in the stool. Rifaximin is safe for use in children under the age of 12. Trimethoprim-sulfamethoxazole, doxycycline, and ampicillin were popular drugs used in the past to treat TD, but increased resistance now limits their use. The evidence is insufficient regarding the efficacy of probiotics as prophylaxis for TD.

COMPREHENSION QUESTIONS

10.1 Several friends develop vomiting and diarrhea 6 hours after eating food at a private party. Which of the following is the most likely etiology of the symptoms?

   A. Rotavirus

   B. *Giardia*

   C. E coli

   D. S aureus

   E. *Cryptosporidium*

10.2 A 40-year-old man travels to Mexico and develops diarrhea 1 day after coming back to the United States. Which of the following is the most likely etiology of the symptoms?

   A. Rotavirus

   B. *Giardia*

   C. E coli

   D. S aureus

   E. *Cryptosporidium*

10.3 A young woman eats raw seafood and 2 days later develops fever, abdominal cramping, and watery diarrhea. Which of the following is the most likely etiology of the symptoms?

A. Rotavirus

B. *Giardia*

C. *E coli*

D. *S aureus*

E. *Vibrio*

10.4 During the winter, a young daycare worker develops watery diarrhea. Which of the following is the most likely etiology of the symptoms?

A. Rotavirus

B. *Giardia*

C. *E coli*

D. *S aureus*

E. *Cryptosporidium*

10.5 A 45-year-old man presents with 3 days of watery diarrhea and abdominal cramping. He has no sick contacts and has not traveled recently. He is not currently taking any medications, but he was prescribed amoxicillin 2 weeks ago for a sinus infection. Which of the following tests is most likely to identify the cause of his diarrhea?

A. Stool guaiac

B. Evaluation of stool for fecal leukocytes

C. Evaluation of stool for ova and parasites

D. *C difficile* toxin immunoassay

10.6 In the patient described in question 10.5, which of the following is the treatment of choice for his diarrhea?

A. Ciprofloxacin

B. Azithromycin

C. Metronidazole

D. Loperamide

ANSWERS

10.1 **D.** *S aureus* toxin usually causes vomiting and diarrhea within a few hours of food ingestion.

10.2 **C.** *E coli* is the most common etiology for traveler's diarrhea.

10.3 **E.** *Vibrio* is a common cause of diarrhea among people who eat raw seafood.

10.4 **A.** Rotavirus is a common etiology for watery diarrhea, especially in the winter.

10.5 **D.** Although any antibiotic can cause *C difficile* colitis, clindamycin, cephalosporins, and penicillins are the most commonly implicated.

10.6 **C.** Metronidazole or oral vancomycin can be used to treat *C difficile*. Ciprofloxacin and azithromycin can be used for treatment of traveler's diarrhea. Loperamide can decrease the frequency of bowel movements but is contraindicated in any patient with suspected *C difficile* colitis.

CLINICAL PEARLS

▶ Most acute diarrheas are self-limited.

▶ Be cautious when assessing diarrhea in a child, elderly patient, or immunosuppressed host.

▶ Dehydration, bloody diarrhea, high fever, and diarrhea that do not respond to therapy after 48 hours are warning signs of possible complicated diarrhea.

▶ In general, acute, uncomplicated diarrhea can be treated with oral electrolyte and fluid replacement.

REFERENCES

Barr W, Smith A. Acute diarrhea in adults. *Am Fam Physician.* 2014;89(3):180-189.

Centers for Disease Control and Prevention. Travelers' health—2014 Yellow Book. Available at: http://wwwnc.cdc.gov/travel/page/yellowbook-home. Accessed May 24, 2015.

Kligler B, Cohrssen A. Probiotics. *Am Fam Physician.* 2008;18(9):1073-1078.

LaRocque RC, Ryan ET, Calderwood SB. Acute infectious diarrheal diseases and bacterial food poisoning. In: Kasper D, Fauci A, Hauser S, et al, eds. *Harrison's Principles of Internal Medicine.* 19th ed. New York, NY: McGraw-Hill Education; 2015. Available at: http://accessmedicine.mhmedical.com/content.aspx?bookid=1130&sectionid=79734063. Accessed May 24, 2015.

Yates J. Traveler's diarrhea. *Am Fam Physician.* 2005;71:2095-2100, 2107-2108.

A 55-year-old Caucasian woman, new to your practice, presents for an "annual physical examination." She reports that she is very healthy, generally feels well, and has no specific complaints. She has a history of having had a "total hyster-ectomy," by which she means that her uterus, cervix, ovaries, and fallopian tubes were removed. The surgery was performed because of fibroids. She has had a Pap smear every 3 years since the age of 21, all of which have been normal. She has had annual mammograms since the age of 50, all of which have been normal. She has no other significant medical or surgical history. She takes a multivitamin pill daily but no other medications. Her family history is significant for breast cancer that was diagnosed in her maternal grandmother at the age of 72. The patient is married, monogamous, and does not smoke cigarettes or drink alcohol. She tries to avoid dairy products because of "lactose intolerance." She walks 30 minutes a day five times a week for exercise. Her physical examination is normal.

▶ For this patient, how often should a Pap smear be performed?
▶ What could you recommend to reduce her risk of developing osteoporosis?
▶ According to the United States Preventive Services Task Force (USPSTF), what is the recommended interval for screening mammography?

ANSWERS TO CASE 11:
Health Maintenance in Adult Female

Summary: A 55-year-old woman with a history of having had a total hysterectomy for a benign indication comes to your office for a routine health maintenance visit.

- **Interval for cervical cancer screening:** Based on her history of having a hysterectomy with removal of the cervix and no history of cancerous lesions, cervical cancer screening can be discontinued in this patient (USPSTF, Level B recommendation).

- **Interventions to reduce her risk of developing osteoporosis:** As a 55-year-old postmenopausal woman with no risk factors for fractures and dwelling outside of any institutions, USPSTF does not recommend supplementation outside of adequate dietary intake calcium and vitamin D daily (Level D recommendation). Regular weight-bearing and muscle-strengthening exercise, avoidance of tobacco smoke (active or passive), and excessive alcohol intake (>3 drinks/d) should be discussed as factors that increase risk of developing osteoporosis.

- **USPSTF recommended interval for screening mammography in a 55-year-old woman:** Biennial (every 2 years), between ages of 50 and 74 (Level B recommendation).

ANALYSIS

Objectives

1. Discuss age-appropriate preventive health measures for adult women.

2. Review evidence in support of specific health maintenance measures.

Considerations

When evaluating patients for preventive health measures, there should not be a "one size fits all" approach to care. Some interventions are appropriate across age groups; some are age or risk-factor specific and should be tailored accordingly. Interventions to consider include screening for cardiovascular disease (CVD), breast cancer, cervical cancer, osteoporosis, and domestic violence. Other health maintenance measures, such as screening for colon cancer and routine adult immunizations, are discussed in Case 1 and tobacco use is discussed in Case 7. The interventions discussed in this chapter are primarily based on recommendations of the USPSTF; recommendations of other expert panels or advocacy organizations are included where appropriate.

APPROACH TO:
Health Maintenance in Women

DEFINITIONS

BRCA: Abbreviation for genes associated with breast cancer and ovarian cancer. Mutations in the *BRCA-1* or *BRCA-2* genes can be associated with a three- to seven-fold increased risk for breast cancer, along with increased risks of ovarian, tubal, peritoneal, and possibly other types of cancer.

WOMEN'S HEALTH INITIATIVE: A National Institutes of Health (NIH)– sponsored research program to address the most common causes of morbidity and mortality in postmenopausal women. This initiative included clinical trials of the effect of hormone therapy on the development of heart disease, fractures, and breast cancer.

CLINICAL APPROACH

Cardiovascular Disease in Women

Cardiovascular diseases are the number one killer of women in the United States. Many of the cardiovascular disease risk factors in women are the same as those in men: hypertension, high low-density lipoprotein (LDL)–cholesterol, tobacco use, diabetes mellitus, family history of cardiovascular disease. As such, the **USP-STF screening recommendations for cardiovascular disease for women are similar to those for men.** All women aged 18 and older should be screened for hypertension by the measurement of blood pressure (Level A recommendation). **However, because the 10-year risk for heart disease is low in women without risk factors as compared to their male counterparts of the same age, USPSTF recommendations on lipid screening differ between genders. Women more than age 45 with risk factors for heart disease, including diabetes, previous history of heart disease, family history of CVD, tobacco use, hypertension, and obesity, should be screened with a lipid panel (Level A recommendation).** Furthermore, women between the ages of 20 and 44 who have risk factors as listed previously are also recommended to undergo a one-time screening for lipid disorders (Level B recommendation). Other professional organizations, such as the American Heart Association and the American College of Obstetricians and Gynecologists (ACOG) recommend routine lipid screening for all women. Abnormally elevated blood pressure or serum lipids should be managed appropriately.

An area of cardiovascular disease risk unique to women is in postmenopausal hormone replacement. Many women have taken hormone replacement therapy for relief of vasomotor symptoms ("hot flashes") and reduction of risk of developing osteoporosis. Recent studies, most notably the Women's Health Initiative, have shown **increased rates of adverse cardiovascular outcomes in women taking either estrogen alone or combined estrogen and progesterone.** These risks include an increased risk of coronary heart disease, stroke, and venous thromboembolic disease. For this reason, the use of hormone replacement therapy for the prevention of chronic conditions is not advised (Level D recommendation) and **any use of hormone replacement should be of the lowest effective dose for the shortest effective time period.**

Screening for Breast Cancer

Breast cancer is second to lung cancer in number of cancer-related deaths in women. There are over 200,000 new cases and nearly 40,000 deaths per year from breast cancer in the United States each year. The incidence increases with age; other risk factors include having the first child after the age of 30, a family history of breast cancer (particularly if in the mother or sister), personal history of breast cancer or atypical hyperplasia found on a previous breast biopsy, or a known carrier of the BRCA-1 or BRCA-2 gene.

The process of screening for breast cancer generally includes consideration of three modalities: the breast self-examination (BSE), the clinical breast examination (CBE) performed by a health-care professional, and mammography. Other modalities, including ultrasonography and magnetic resonance imaging (MRI), are available but currently they are not widely recommended for screening purposes, and are most beneficial as follow-up studies to screening mammograms when indicated. Upon review of the available trials, the USPSTF has determined that, at this time, there is insufficient evidence to recommend CBE (Level I recommendation) and recommend against teaching BSE (Level D recommendation). These trials suggest that in teaching of BSE to patients, there is no mortality benefit and, in fact, this modality may lead to unnecessary anxieties, biopsies, and tests. The evidence regarding CBE suggests that while as the sole screening modality it may have good detection rates, its benefits in conjunction with mammography are limited.

Mammography screening every 12 to 33 months has been shown to reduce mortality from breast cancer, with the most benefit at 24-month intervals. The **benefits of routine mammographic screening increase with age**, as the incidence of breast cancer is higher in older women. However, beyond the age of 75 years, continuation of screening should be individualized based on the overall health status and probability of death from other conditions prior to the expected benefits from detection of breast cancer.

Part of the discussion regarding mammography also includes the risk of false-positive or false-negative (less common) results and need for additional interventions, such as breast biopsy. **Most abnormalities found on mammography are not breast cancer** but require further evaluation to make that determination. The USPSTF advises screening with mammography, beginning at the age of 50 for the general population, with a recommended interval of every 2 years (Level B recommendation). For women aged 40 to 49, biennial screening should be an individual decision and take into account patient's values regarding the benefits and harms (Level C recommendation). Recommendations are also available from other organizations, including the American Cancer Society (ACS), American Academy of Family Physicians, and ACOG, which advocate annual mammography after the age of 50. Their recommendations for women aged 40 to 49 vary, but generally advise screening every 1 to 2 years.

Screening for Cervical Cancer

Cervical cancer is the 10th leading cause of cancer death in women in the United States, with an incidence and mortality of over 12,000 and approximately 4000 cases, respectively, this year alone. Over the last several decades, however, this rate has decreased dramatically as a direct result of routine cervical cancer screening with Pap smear (cytology). Risk factors for cervical cancer include early onset of sexual intercourse, multiple sexual partners, human papilloma virus (HPV) infection with high-risk subtype of HPV (HPV viral types 16, 18, 45, 56), and tobacco use.

As per the USPSTF, for any woman with a cervix, cervical cancer screening with Pap smear should begin at age 21 (regardless of sexual activity) and be repeated at 3-year intervals. For women more than age of 30 desiring a longer interval between tests, cotesting for HPV can be used in conjunction with cytology once every 5 years (Level A recommendation). However, because the likelihood of a positive test result is higher with HPV cotesting, women should be made aware of the possibility of frequent and ongoing testing if they persistently test positive for HPV. Both ACOG and ACS recommend beginning cervical cancer screening at age 21 with 3-year intervals without HPV cotesting, and in women above 30 years, 5-year intervals with cotesting.

HPV infection is the most significant cause of all cervical cancers. A vaccine against high-risk HPV subtypes is available as a three-series. It is indicated for use in females aged 11 through 26. To date, there is no recommendation to alter the Pap smear screening intervals for women who have been vaccinated against HPV.

Most cases of cervical cancer occur in women who either have not been screened in over 5 years or did not have follow-up after an abnormal Pap smear. The optimal screening interval therefore is based upon providing the maximum benefit from treatment of precancerous lesions, while preventing overtreatment of lesions that may have otherwise resolved spontaneously. Since the development of a cancerous lesion is a prolonged process, and at times treatment of cervical abnormalities is not without harm in terms of future childbearing potential, screening prior to age 21 (regardless of sexual activity) is not recommended (Level D recommendation).

Women who have had a hysterectomy constitute a group in whom special considerations regarding cervical cancer screening must be made. The recommendation for this group of women takes into account those who have undergone a supracervical hysterectomy with retention of the cervix versus those who have had their cervix removed, and the indication for this removal. As per USPSTF, in women who have had a hysterectomy with cervix removal for any reason other than cervical cancer, screening should be discontinued (Level D recommendation). A woman who had a hysterectomy for cancerous indications falls out of the general screening parameters discussed here. Women who have had a hysterectomy with retention of cervix should follow the recommendation for age-appropriate routine screening.

The USPSTF recommends stopping Pap smears at age 65 in women who have had three consecutive negative Pap results or two consecutive negative HPV results within the last 10 years (Level D recommendation). However, an individualized approach should be implemented in women who have previously been treated for precancerous lesions or those who have never been tested before. Both The ACS and ACOG recommend that screening may be stopped at the age of 65 if a woman has had adequate screening in the last 10 years, which is defined as three consecutive negative Pap smears or two consecutive negative cotests, with the most recent negative Pap smear within the last 5 years. This recommendation excludes women who have a history of cervical cancer.

Screening for Osteoporosis

Osteoporosis is a condition of decreased bone mineral density (BMD) associated with an increased risk of fracture. **Half of all postmenopausal women will have an osteoporosis-related fracture in their lifetime.** These include hip fractures, which are associated with higher risks of loss of independence, institutionalization, and death. The risk of osteoporosis is increased with advancing age, tobacco use, low body weight, poor nutrition, Caucasian or Asian ancestry, family history of osteoporosis, low calcium intake, and sedentary lifestyle.

Osteoporosis may also occur in men, although with a lower incidence than it does in women. Along with the risk factors noted above, the prolonged use of corticosteroids, presence of diseases that alter hormone levels (such as chronic kidney or lung disease), and undiagnosed low testosterone levels increase the risk of osteoporosis in men.

Screening for osteoporosis is done by measurement of bone density. Measurement of the hip bone density by dual-energy x-ray absorptiometry (DXA) is the best predictor of hip fracture. Measurement of bone density is compared to the bone density of young adults and the result is reported as standard deviation from the mean bone density of the young adult (T-score). **Osteoporosis is present if the patient's T-score is at or below −2.5** (ie, measurement of the patient's bone density is more than 2.5 standard deviations below the young adult mean); osteopenia is present if the T-score is between −1.0 and −2.5. Other modalities, such as measurement of wrist or heel density, single-energy x-ray absorptiometry, and ultrasound are being evaluated and may have some short-term predictive value. The USPSTF recommends screening for osteoporosis via DXA in women over the age of 65 and considering screening in women younger than 65 with higher risk of osteoporosis-related fractures (Level B recommendation). There is no current recommendation on repeating screening if the initial test is normal. Although in theory repeated testing may improve the likelihood of predicting fracture risk, studies have not shown the benefit of repeated BMD measurements as opposed to a single BMD measurement.

The role of calcium and vitamin D intake in the prevention of osteoporosis is currently a controversial issue and one regarding which recommendations differ between organizations. The National Osteoporosis Foundation (NOF) believes in the role of supplementation in prevention of osteoporosis, recommending that women over the age of 51 consume 1200 mg of calcium daily, stressing the fact that there is no additional benefit of consuming calcium in excess of 1200 to 1500 mg/d. They also recommend 800 to 1000 IU of vitamin D daily for women over the age of 50. If dietary intake is not sufficient, supplements may be used. Weight-bearing and muscle-strengthening exercise is also recommended both for its direct effects on increasing bone density and for its benefits in strength, agility, and balance, which may reduce the risk of falls, as is tobacco cessation and avoidance of excess alcohol intake. Although NOF still recommends vitamin D and calcium supplementation for primary prevention of osteoporosis, USPSTF maintains that trials have not been able to show the benefit of vitamin D and calcium supplementation in women who are not at risk for fractures and do not have osteoporosis. For this reason, and in light of an increased incidence of renal stones with calcium and vitamin D intake, USPSTF recommends against daily supplementation for primary prevention of fractures in postmenopausal women residing in the community (Level D recommendation). However, taking into account the burden imposed by fractures on the health-care system and on patient's quality of life, and the relatively low cost of supplementation, USPSTF still holds by its recommendation for daily vitamin D intake in women above the age of 65 who are at increased risk of falls (Level B recommendation).

When osteoporosis is diagnosed, patients should be treated with calcium, vitamin D, and exercise and strategies should be implemented to reduce the risk of falls. These strategies include evaluation and treatment, if needed, of vision and hearing deficits, management of medical disorders that can promote falls (movement disorders, neurologic disorders, etc), and periodic evaluation of medications taken that may affect balance or movement. Hip protectors may be beneficial in those at high risk for falls. See Case 58 for a discussion of medications used for the prevention and treatment of osteoporosis.

Screening for Domestic Violence

Estimates indicate that between 1 and 4 million women are sexually, physically, or emotionally abused by an intimate partner each year. Women are also much more likely to be abused by an intimate partner than men. Multiple factors are associated with intimate partner violence and include young age, low income status, pregnancy, mental illness, alcohol or substance use by victims or partner, separated or divorced status, and a history of childhood sexual/physical abuse. USPSTF recommends that physicians should screen women between the ages of 14 and 46 for evidence of physical, sexual, or psychological abuse by a current or former partner and to appropriately refer those with positive screens to interventional services (Level B recommendation). There are many different screening tools available to physicians, including HITS (Hurt, Insult, Threaten, Screen), HARK (Humiliation, Afraid, Rape, Kick), and STaT (Slapped, Threatened, and Throw). Most of these are three to four item questionnaires with very high sensitivity and specificity and are available in both English and Spanish. Documentation and treatment of injuries, counseling, and information regarding protective services are part of the evaluation when domestic violence is suspected. Reporting of domestic violence is mandatory in several states; be aware of the requirements of your state.

CASE CORRELATION
- See also Case 1 (Health Maintenance, Adult Male).

COMPREHENSION QUESTIONS

11.1 A 21-year-old woman presents for her first Pap smear. She received the full HPV vaccine series at age 19. Assuming that her examination and Pap smear results are normal, when would you recommend that she return for a follow-up Pap smear?

   A. 6 months, as the first Pap smear should be followed up soon to reduce the false-negative rate associated with this screening test

   B. 1 year, as she is higher risk because of her age

   C. 3 years, as the Pap smear was normal

   D. 5 years, as she is at low risk because she received the HPV vaccine

11.2 Which of the following situations is associated with an increased risk of intimate partner violence?

   A. Pregnancy

   B. Older age

   C. Higher income

   D. Married status

11.3 Which of the following statements regarding breast cancer screening is true?

   A. Breast self-examination (BSE) has been shown to decrease mortality rates from breast cancer.

   B. Clinical breast examination (CBE) in conjunction with routine mammography is shown to improve mortality rates.

   C. Most abnormalities found on routine mammography are not breast cancer.

   D. Because breast cancer rates increase in older women, there is no upper age at which breast cancer screening may be discontinued.

11.4 A 48-year-old woman presents for a well-woman examination. She notes that she had a supracervical hysterectomy in the past. Your records reveal that she had her uterus removed, but the cervix and ovaries were left in place. You also note that she has had Pap smears with HPV cotesting every 5 years since her 20s and that all were normal. She read on the internet that women who have had a hysterectomy no longer need Pap smears. Which of the following would be your advice?

   A. "You no longer need to get Pap smears since you have had a hysterectomy."

   B. "You should continue to have Pap smears every 3 years since your hysterectomy is an indication to shorten the interval for testing."

   C. "You should continue to have Pap smears with HPV cotesting every 5 years since your hysterectomy does not exclude you from routine screening recommendation for your age group."

   D. "You should continue with annual Pap smears until the age of 50. If they are all normal, you can stop having them at that time."

ANSWERS

11.1 **C.** As per USPSTF, screening for cervical cancer should begin at age 21 and be repeated at 3-year intervals. Six months and 1-year intervals are inappropriate and not part of routine screening recommendations for women with normal Pap smears. The use of HPV vaccine is not an indication to alter cervical cancer screening recommendations at this time.

11.2 **A.** Intimate partner violence can occur in any relationship, but the risk is increased in certain situations, which include young age, low income status, pregnancy, mental illness, alcohol or substance use by victims or partner, separated or divorced status, and a history of childhood sexual/physical abuse.

11.3 **C.** Most abnormalities seen on mammography are not cancerous. They may, however, require further imaging studies, testing, or biopsy. Breast self-examination has not been definitively shown to reduce cancer mortality. Clinician breast examination may be of benefit but likely does not impact outcome if mammography is available. The age to consider discontinuation of mammography screening should be individualized, based on the woman's risk factors and overall health status.

11.4 **C.** Women who have had a hysterectomy with removal of the cervix for benign indications can discontinue Pap smear screening. Women who still have a cervix should continue with screening for cervical cancer as per screening recommendation for their age group. Cervical cancer screening can be discontinued at age 65, if she has had adequate screening for the last 10 years, which is defined as three consecutive normal Pap smears or two consecutive normal cotesting, with the most recent one being in the last 5 years.

CLINICAL PEARLS

▶ Women of childbearing age should be screened for intimate partner violence.

▶ The number one killer of women in America is cardiovascular disease. Risk factors for cardiovascular diseases in women need to be managed as aggressively as they are in men.

▶ HPV infection is the most significant cause of all cervical cancers. HPV vaccine is available as a three-dose series for females aged 11 to 26; however, vaccination status has no bearing on cervical cancer screening recommendations.

REFERENCES

American Cancer Society. *Cancer Facts & Figures*. Atlanta, GA: American Cancer Society; 2014.

American Congress of Obstetricians and Gynecologists. *Screening for Cervical Cancer*. Washington, DC: ACOG; 2013.

Centers for Disease Control and Prevention. *HPV Vaccine*. Atlanta, GA: CDC; 2014.

National Osteoporosis Foundation. *Clinician's Guide to Prevention and Treatment of Osteoporosis*. Washington, DC: National Osteoporosis Foundation; 2014.

United States Preventive Services Task Force (USPSTF). Genetic risk assessment and BRCA mutation testing for breast and ovarian cancer susceptibility. Available at: http://www.uspreventiveservices-taskforce.org/uspstf/uspsbrgen.htm. Accessed December 2014.

United States Preventive Services Task Force (USPSTF). Osteoporosis screening. Available at: http://www.uspreventiveservicestaskforce.org/uspstf/uspsoste.htm. Accessed December 2014.

United States Preventive Services Task Force (USPSTF). Screening for breast cancer. Available at: http://www.uspreventiveservicestaskforce.org/uspstf/uspsbrca.htm. Accessed December 2014.

United States Preventive Services Task Force (USPSTF). Screening for cervical cancer. Available at: http://www.uspreventiveservicestaskforce.org/uspstf/uspscerv.htm. Accessed December 2014.

United States Preventive Services Task Force (USPSTF). Screening for family and intimate partner violence. Available at: http://www.uspreventiveservicestaskforce.org/uspstf/uspsfamv.htm. Accessed December 2014.

Women's Health Initiative. Available at: http://www.nhlbi.nih.gov/whi/. Accessed December 2014.

A 25-year-old man presents to your office on a Monday morning with ankle pain. He was playing in his usual Saturday afternoon basketball game when he injured his right ankle. He says that he jumped for a rebound and landed on another player's foot. His right ankle "rolled over," he fell to the floor, and his ankle immediately started to hurt. He did not hear or feel a pop. He was able to stand and walk with a limp, but was unable to continue playing. His ankle swelled over the next day in spite of rest, icing, and elevation. He suffered no other injury from the fall. On examination, he is a healthy appearing man with normal vital signs. The lateral aspect of the right ankle is swollen. The right ankle has normal dorsiflexion and plantar flexion and there is no focal tenderness to palpation of the fibula, malleoli, or foot. No ligamentous laxity is noted on testing. He can bear weight with minimal pain. There is normal sensation and capillary refill in the foot. The remainder of his examination is normal.

▶ What is the most likely diagnosis of this injury?
▶ What further diagnostic testing is needed at this time?
▶ What is the most appropriate therapy?

ANSWERS TO CASE 12:
Musculoskeletal Injuries

Summary: A 25-year-old man presents with an inversion injury of his right ankle that occurred during a basketball game. His ankle is swollen, but he is able to bear weight, and has no focal tenderness and no ligament laxity.

- **Most likely diagnosis:** Sprain of the right ankle

- **Further diagnostic testing needed:** None at this time

- **Most appropriate initial therapy:** "PRICE" therapy: Protection, Rest, Ice, Compression, and Elevation; a nonsteroidal anti-inflammatory drug (NSAID) or acetaminophen as needed for pain and early mobilization

ANALYSIS

Objectives

1. Learn an approach to the diagnosis of musculoskeletal injuries.

2. Know when to order imaging tests and which test to order to evaluate musculoskeletal complaints.

3. Be able to manage common joint sprains and strains.

Considerations

Ankle sprains are the most common acute, sports-related injury, and are a common reason for visits to primary care physicians, urgent care centers, and emergency rooms. As in this case, **most ankle sprains are the result of landing on an inverted foot that is plantar flexed,** such as landing on another player's foot in basketball, stepping in a hole or on uneven ground when running, missing a curb while walking. More than 20,000 people sprain their ankles every day in the United States. The lateral ankle is injured much more commonly than the medial ankle, with around 85% of all sprains involving the lateral structures. This is because the bony anatomy of the tibiotalar joint and the very strong deltoid ligament complex protect the medial ankle from injury. The lateral ligaments responsible for resistance against inversion and internal rotation—anterior talofibular ligament (ATFL), calcaneofibular ligament (CFL), and posterior talofibular ligament (PTFL)—are relatively weaker and more commonly injured. The **ATFL is the most commonly injured ligament,** followed by the CFL. Some common risk factors include previous ankle fracture, excess body weight, and an unconditioned body.

Ankle sprains are graded as grade 1, 2, or 3 injuries according to degree of severity. A grade 1 sprain is characterized by a stretch of a single ligament, most commonly the ATFL, but with minor swelling, no mechanical instability, and without significant loss of function. The patient can usually bear weight with, at most, mild pain. The history and examination of the patient in the case presented is consistent with a grade 1 ankle sprain. A grade 2 sprain represents a partial ligamentous tear. This injury causes more severe pain, swelling, and bruising. There is mild to moderate joint instability, significant pain with weight bearing, and loss of range of motion. A grade 3 sprain is a complete ligamentous tear. This injury causes significant joint instability, swelling, loss of function, and inability to bear weight.

The Ottawa Ankle Rules are a decision model designed to aid a physician in determining which patients with ankle injuries need an x-ray. These decision rules have been validated for nonpregnant adults who have a normal mental status, no other significant concurrent injury, and who are evaluated within 10 days of the injury. When properly applied, the **Ottawa Ankle Rules have a sensitivity approaching 100% in ruling out significant malleolar and midfoot fractures.** These rules state that x-rays of the ankle should be performed if there is bony tenderness of the posterior edge or tip of the distal 6 cm of either the medial or lateral malleolus; tenderness in the midfoot coupled with point tenderness over the bony aspects of base on fifth metatarsal or the navicular; or if the patient is unable to bear weight immediately or when examined. Negative findings on Ottawa ankle rules safely eliminate the need for an x-ray. The patient presented, who has no bony tenderness, no limitation in weight bearing, and no contraindication to the application of the decision rules, does not need imaging of his ankle or foot. These rules, however, have a specificity of 30% to 50%, indicating that positive findings do not necessarily confirm a fracture, but confirms the need for x-ray to evaluate the possibility of a fracture.

Management of ankle sprains is geared toward decreasing pain and swelling, speed recovery, providing appropriate ankle support, and protecting against a recurrence of the sprain in the future. An easy way to remember the cornerstone of management of ankle sprains is by the mnemonic "PRICE."

Protection by appropriate splinting or casting can help to prevent further injury. Although initial rest during the acute phase marked by maximal pain and swelling is common sense, evidence has shown that prolonged rest is in fact inferior to early functional mobilization. Additionally range-of-motion exercises started early in the recovery period allow for a quicker recovery and return to activities than otherwise.

Ice applied as soon as possible after the injury helps to minimize swelling and relieve pain. Cryotherapy is now recommended in the first 3 to 7 days for short-term pain relief and improved functionality.

Compression and elevation with an air stirrup brace with an elastic compression wrap also promote reduction of swelling. In most cases, NSAIDs or acetaminophen are adequate for pain relief. Surgery is rarely needed for ankle sprains, and its use is controversial even in the presence of chronic pain or persistent functional instability. Surgery for ankle sprains has been shown to increase stiffness in the joint, lead to longer recovery times, and result in impaired mobility when compared to conservative treatment only. Therefore, surgical consideration should be a last resort when all else has failed and should be discussed in a case by case manner.

APPROACH TO:
Sprains and Strains

DEFINITIONS

SPRAIN: A stretching or tearing injury of a **ligament**.

STRAIN: A stretching or tearing injury of a **muscle** or **tendon**.

CLINICAL APPROACH

History

As in all areas of medicine, the history of the presenting illness will guide the diagnostic workup. In the history of a patient with musculoskeletal complaints, important information to gather includes whether the primary symptom is pain, limited movement, weakness, instability, or a combination of symptoms. The onset of the symptoms—whether acute, chronic, or an acute worsening of a chronic problem—can be significant. The location, severity, and pattern of radiation of pain should be delineated. Associated symptoms, such as numbness, should be identified. Efforts should be made to identify as specifically as possible the mechanism of any injury that led to the complaint. Interventions that have already been made, such as ice or heat, medications, splinting, and whether or not the interventions helped, should be noted.

Joint Examination

Examination of the musculoskeletal system should include documentation of inspection, palpation, range of motion, strength, neurovascular status, and, where appropriate, testing specific for the involved joint. Inspection should note the presence of swelling, bruising, deformity, and the use of any supports or assistive devices (eg, splints, crutches, bandages) that the patient is already using. **Examination of the unaffected limb can provide a good comparison and allow for subtle changes to be more easily identified.** Documentation should also be made of the patient's general functioning and mobility—does the patient walk with a limp, can the patient easily rise from a chair, is there difficulty getting on the examining table, is the patient's arm moving freely or held tightly to the patient's chest, and so on.

Palpation of the affected and surrounding areas can help to localize and confirm the presence of a specific injury. A focal area of bony tenderness may lead to the consideration of a fracture, whereas a tender, tight muscle may be more suggestive of a strain. The presence of joint effusions or soft-tissue swelling should be documented and may lead to consideration of specific injuries. Notation should be made of sensation, peripheral pulses, and capillary refill in the involved extremity. Absent pulses and delayed capillary refill, especially if the extremity is cool or cold, should prompt emergent evaluation and management of vascular insufficiency.

Range of motion should be tested both passively and actively. Active range of motion tests the patient's ability to move a joint. It tests the structural integrity of the joint, muscles, tendons, and neurologic impulses to the area and can be limited by problems with any of them or by the presence of pain. Passive range of motion tests the movement that an examiner can elicit in a relaxed patient. The presence of a dislocated joint or significant joint effusion may lead to limitations in both passive and active range of motion, where a torn tendon or muscle injury may have limited active, but preserved passive, range of motion.

Each joint or body area has specific examination maneuvers that can help to identify injury to specific structures. Reexamination 3 to 5 days after acute injury, when pain and swelling have improved, may help with diagnosis. Table 12–1 lists some common maneuvers that are used to examine the shoulder, knee, and ankle.

Imaging

Following the history and examination, the physician must decide when it is necessary to perform x-rays or other imaging tests. Validated decision rules are available to aid in some of these decisions. The Ottawa Ankle Rules for the determination of when an x-ray is necessary in an ankle injury were discussed earlier in this case. Similarly, the Ottawa Knee Rules can aid in the determination of when to perform an x-ray in a knee injury. The Ottawa Knee Rules recommend performing a knee x-ray on patients with a knee injury who have any one of the following five criteria: (1) age 55 or older, (2) isolated patella tenderness, (3) tenderness of the head of the fibula, (4) inability to flex the knee to 90°, and (5) inability to bear weight for four steps immediately and in the examination room (regardless of limping).

These rules were validated for, and should only be applied to, adults older than 18 years, although further study suggests that they may be valid in younger ages.

When a decision is made to perform an imaging test, whether to acutely rule out a fracture or to evaluate an injury that is failing to improve, the **initial imaging study of choice is the plain x-ray**. At minimum, an x-ray series should include at least two views at 90° angles to each other. In patients with normal x-rays and continued symptoms, or with suspected ligament or tendon injuries of the shoulder, ankle, knee, or hip, magnetic resonance imaging (MRI) has largely supplanted other modalities as the imaging method of choice. MRI is highly sensitive and specific for articular or soft-tissue abnormalities, including ligament, tendon, and cartilage tears.

Management Principles

The initial management of most acute sprains and strains is "PRICE"—Protection from further injury, relative Rest, Ice to reduce swelling and pain, Compression, and Elevation to reduce edema. In most cases, NSAIDs or acetaminophen are adequate for pain control, with narcotics used only when necessary.

Numerous studies show that early mobilization of injured ligaments actually promotes healing and recovery. Range-of-motion exercises should be started at 48 to 72 hours after injury in patients with sprains and strains. For lower-extremity injuries, protected weight bearing with orthotics is allowable, with advancement to unsupported weight bearing as tolerated. Crutches may be necessary initially because of painful weight bearing. Lace-up or semirigid ankle supports have been shown to be superior to tape and elastic bandages and provide stability to the injured ankle.

Table 12–1 • SPECIFIC TESTS FOR SHOULDER, KNEE, AND ANKLE EXAMINATIONS

Test	Structure Tested	Result Identified (compare to unaffected side)
Shoulder/Rotator Cuff		
Empty can test—with arm abducted, elbow extended, and thumb pointing down, patient elevates arm against resistance	Supraspinatus	Rotator cuff injury or tear
External rotation—with elbows at sides and flexed at 90°, patient externally rotates against resistance	Infraspinatus and teres minor	Rotator cuff injury or tear
Lift-off test—patient places dorsum of hand on lumbar back and attempts to lift hand off of back	Subscapularis	Rotator cuff injury or tear
Internal rotation—with elbows at sides and flexed at 90°, patient internally rotates against resistance		
Hawkins impingement—pain with internal rotation when the arm is flexed to 90° with the elbow bent to 90°	Subacromial impingement of the supraspinatus tendon	Rotator cuff injury or tear
Drop-arm rotator cuff—patient is unable to lower his arm slowly from a raised position		Large rotator cuff tears
Ankle		
Anterior drawer—examiner pulls forward on patient's heel while stabilizing lower leg with other hand	Anterior talofibular ligament	Excessive translation of joint suggests ATFL tear
Inversion stress test—examiner inverts ankle with one hand while stabilizing lower leg with other hand	Calcaneofibular ligament	Excessive translation or palpable "clunk" of talus on tibia suggests ligament tear
Squeeze test—examiner compresses tibia/fibula at midcalf	Syndesmosis	Pain at anterior ankle joint (below where examiner is squeezing) suggests syndesmotic ("high ankle") injury
Knee		
Lachman test—knee in 20° flexion, examiner pulls forward on upper tibia while stabilizing upper leg	Anterior cruciate ligament	Excessive translation with no solid end point suggests tear
Anterior drawer—knee in 90° flexion, examiner pulls forward on upper tibia while stabilizing upper leg	Anterior cruciate ligament	Excessive translation with no solid end point suggests tear
Valgus stress—in full extension and at 30° flexion, medial-directed force on knee, lateral-directed force on ankle	Medial collateral ligament	Excessive translation suggests tear
Varus stress—in full extension and at 30° flexion, lateral-directed force on knee and medial-directed force on ankle	Lateral collateral ligament	Excessive translation suggests tear

The **most common cause of persistently stiff, painful, or unstable joints following sprains is inadequate rehabilitation.** All patients with sprain or strain injuries should be educated on the importance of rehabilitative exercises. When possible, handouts with a specific exercise program should be given to the patient when the patient is evaluated. If the patient is unsuccessful in accomplishing this on his own, referral for a formal physical therapy program can be beneficial.

> ## CASE CORRELATION
> - See also Case 3 (Joint Pain, Gout).

COMPREHENSION QUESTIONS

12.1 Based on the Ottawa Ankle Rules, which of the following examination findings would make obtaining a radiograph most appropriate?

A. An 18-year-old athlete who injures his ankle during basketball but continues to play until the end of the game

B. A 33-year-old overweight woman who has multiple injuries, including ankle pain, following a motor vehicle accident

C. A 43-year-old man injured his ankle yesterday while playing volleyball and was unable to walk on it immediately afterwards

D. A 22-year-old woman seen in the emergency room (ER) immediately after falling while drunk and who falls asleep repeatedly during the examination

12.2 A 32-year-old man comes for evaluation of right shoulder pain that he has had for the past 3 weeks. He thinks that he injured it playing softball but does not remember a specific injury. There is no bruising or swelling. He gets pain in the joint on external rotation and abduction, but has preserved range of motion. Which of the following is the initial imaging test of choice?

A. X-ray

B. MRI

C. CT scan

D. Arthrogram

12.3 A 45-year-old woman comes in for follow-up of an ankle sprain that occurred while she was jogging 2 weeks ago. X-rays done at your initial visit were negative for fracture. She has been unable to run because of persistent stiffness. She is frustrated as she states she has tried everything including ice, NSAIDs, bracing, and weight bearing as tolerated. Examination reveals no joint instability or focal tenderness. Which of the following is the most appropriate management at this time?

A. Referral for therapeutic ultrasound as this has shown to benefit patients who have failed conservative treatment.

B. Referral to chiropractor for soft-tissue techniques to loosen up the stiff muscles.

C. Change to another NSAID as the current one may not be strong enough.

D. Urge immobilization of the ankle as she may be doing too much too soon.

E. Discuss importance of rehabilitative stretching, strengthening, and range-of-motion exercises to gain functionality.

ANSWERS

12.1 **C.** The Ottawa Ankle Rules state that radiography should be obtained if there is pain in the malleolar area with point tenderness over the tip of lateral or medial malleolus, bony tenderness over area of base of **fifth metatarsal** or **navicular bone**, or an inability to bear weight for four steps immediately after the injury (answer choice C). These decision rules are not validated in patients with multiple painful injuries or with an altered mental status.

12.2 **A.** Plain film x-rays are the diagnostic imaging test of choice for the initial evaluation of the painful joint. In patients who have normal x-rays and who have a suspected soft-tissue (ligament, tendon, or cartilage) injury, MRI scanning is usually the next most appropriate imaging study to perform.

12.3 **E.** The most common cause of a stiff or painful joint following a sprain is inadequate rehabilitation. At 2 weeks postinjury, the patient is considered to be out of the acute phase and the focus should be on regaining range of motion and strength instead of NSAIDs, immobilization, or alternative treatments (choices A, B, or C). Studies have not shown any benefit with therapeutic ultrasound or hyperbaric oxygen therapy for the treatment of acute ankle sprains.

CLINICAL PEARLS

▶ A complete history and physical is essential in diagnosing and treating musculoskeletal injuries.

▶ If you suspect that a patient's limited active range of motion is primarily a result of pain, you can numb the joint by injecting lidocaine into it and then reexamine the joint.

▶ Use the uninjured, contralateral extremity as a comparison for your examination of an injured extremity.

▶ An adequate x-ray series must include at least two views at 90° to each other.

REFERENCES

Brigham and Women's Hospital: Dept of Rehabilitation Services. Standard of Care: Ankle Sprain. 2010.

Burbank KM, Stevenson JH, Czarnecki GR, Dorfman J. Chronic shoulder pain: part I. Evaluation and diagnosis. *Am Fam Physician*. 2008;77:453-460.

Burbank KM, Stevenson JH, Czarnecki GR, Dorfman J. Chronic shoulder pain: part II. Treatment. *Am Fam Physician*. 2008;77:493-497.

Hockenberry RT, Sammarco GJ. Evaluation and treatment of ankle sprains. *Phys Sports Med*. 2001;29(2):57-64.

Tiemstra JD. Update on acute ankle sprains. *Am Fam Physician*. 2012 Jun 15; 85(12):1170-1176.

Trojian TH, McKeag DB. Ankle sprains: expedient diagnosis and management. *Phys Sports Med*. 1998;26(10):29-40.

A 45-year-old white woman presents to your office concerned about a "mole" on her face. She says that it has been present for years but her husband has been urging her to have it checked. She denies any pain, itching, or bleeding from the site. She has no significant past medical history, takes no medications, and has no allergies. She has no history of skin cancer in her family. She is an accountant by occupation.

On examination, the patient is normotensive, afebrile, and appears slightly younger than her stated age. A skin examination reveals a nontender, symmetric, 4-mm papule that is uniformly reddish-brown in color. The lesion is well circumscribed, and the surrounding skin is normal in appearance. There are no other lesions in the area.

▶ What is the most likely diagnosis?
▶ What features are reassuring of a benign condition?
▶ What is your next step?

ANSWERS TO CASE 13:
Skin Lesions

Summary: A 45-year-old healthy woman with no significant past medical history presents for evaluation of a skin lesion. She does not have a family history of skin cancer. The lesion is symmetric, with well-defined borders, relatively small (<6 mm), and uniform coloration. She is not able to assess whether the lesion has changed recently (ie, become larger), and does not give a history of itching or bleeding at the site of the lesion.

- **Most likely diagnosis:** Benign nevus

- **Reassuring features:** Size less than 6 mm, symmetric, uniform color, well-defined borders

- **Next step in treatment:** Reassurance and surveillance

ANALYSIS
Objectives

1. Describe an approach to the evaluation of skin lesions.

2. Be able to describe the features of a skin lesion in dermatologic terms.

3. Know which features of a lesion are typically benign and which are concerning for malignancy or potential malignancy.

Considerations

This case represents a typical scenario seen in primary care medicine: "I have this mole. Is it cancer?" Although simplified, this is what the patient is most concerned about and wants to know. The **role of the physician is to determine the likelihood of malignancy or premalignancy and to define a course of action that is appropriate.** In this particular case, there are several features that reassure a benign condition that can be monitored without the need for a biopsy. There was neither a family medical history of skin cancer nor history of skin cancer in the patient. She has an occupation that does not expose her to harmful chemicals or the sun on a regular basis. On examination, the lesion has typically benign features (size <6 mm, symmetric, uniform color, well-defined borders). In this case, it would be appropriate to make a note (or possibly even a photograph) in the patient's chart describing the characteristic features of the lesion and monitor for changes in the lesion at periodic health evaluations. The patient should also be educated in self-examination of the skin, with an emphasis on what to look for and when to come to the physician's office for an evaluation of a new or changing skin lesion. Finally, it should be understood that many otherwise benign-appearing moles might have an atypical characteristic that warrants further investigation. The **criteria that are used to predict the likelihood of a benign versus malignant lesion are only guidelines,** to be sure. Not all malignant skin lesions present in the same manner and a malignant melanoma is not always visibly pigmented. The bottom line is that the physician should use all of the tools at his disposal: the history of present illness (HPI), medical history of the patient, the family medical history (FMH), social and occupational history, and a pertinent review of systems so as to arrive at a conclusion that is consistent with the physical examination.

APPROACH TO:
Skin Lesions

DEFINITIONS

ABSCESS: A closed pocket containing pus

BULLA: A blister greater than 0.5 cm in diameter (plural: bullae)

CYST: A closed, saclike, membranous capsule containing a liquid or semisolid material

MACULE: A discoloration on the skin that is neither raised nor depressed

NODULE: A small mass of rounded or irregular shape that is greater than 1.0 cm in diameter

PAPULE: A small, circumscribed *elevated* lesion of the skin that is less than 1.0 cm in diameter

PLAQUE: A plateaulike, raised, solid area on the skin that covers a large surface area in relation to its height above the skin

ULCER: A lesion through the skin or mucous membrane resulting from loss of tissue

VESICLE: A small blister less than 0.5 cm in diameter

CLINICAL APPROACH

Incidence and Risk Factors

There has been an increase in the morbidity and mortality of skin cancer in the past few decades in the United States. American Academy of Dermatology estimates that almost 138,000 new cases of melanoma will be diagnosed in 2015 alone. When you consider nonmelanoma skin cancers, including basal cell carcinoma or squamous cell carcinoma, more than 3.5 million new cases of skin cancer are diagnosed annually. Skin cancers cause approximately 15,000 deaths per year, of which 75% are due to melanoma.

The **single most important risk factor for the development of skin cancer is exposure to natural and artificial ultraviolet radiation.** It is also one of the only risk factors that can be avoided, and avoiding it can potentially prevent millions of new cases of skin cancer every year. Other risk factors include a prior history of skin cancer, a family history of skin cancer, fair skin, red or blonde hair, a propensity to burn easily, chronic exposure to toxic compounds such as creosote, arsenic, or radium, and a suppressed immune system.

BASIC TYPES OF MELANOMA

Melanoma in Situ

No invasion has occurred in this type of melanoma, as the malignant melanocytes are localized to the epidermis. If diagnosed early, this type of lesion should be excised with 5-mm borders.

Superficial Spreading Melanoma

This is the **most common type of melanoma** in both sexes. As its name implies, this lesion spreads superficially along the top layers of skin before penetrating into the deep layers. The superficial, or radial, growth phase is slower than the vertical phase, which is when the lesion grows into the dermis and can invade other tissues or metastasize. Men are more commonly affected on the upper torso, whereas women are affected mostly on the legs. Common clinical features include raised borders and brown lesions with pinks, whites, grays, or blues.

Lentigo Maligna

Similar to the superficial spreading type, this lesion is **most often found in the elderly** (**commonly diagnosed in the seventh decade of life**), usually on chronic sun-damaged skin such as the face, ears, arms, and upper trunk. Although it is the **least common of the four types of melanoma**, this is the most common form of melanoma found in Hawaii. They are clinically characterized as tan to brown lesions with very irregular borders.

Amelanotic Melanoma

This is an uncommon (<5%) melanoma that is nonpigmented and can clinically present as many other types of noncancerous conditions, including eczema, fungal infections, basal or squamous cell carcinoma. Because of its lack of pigmentation, this type of melanoma usually remains undiagnosed until a more invasive stage as compared to other melanomas.

Acral Lentiginous Melanoma

Similar to the other two superficial melanomas in that it begins in situ, this lesion is different in many ways. This is the **most common melanoma found in African Americans and Asians**. This melanoma is usually found under the nails, on the soles of the feet, and on the palms of the hands; common clinical features include flat, irregular, dark brown to black lesions.

Nodular Melanoma

This melanoma, unlike the others, is usually invasive at the time of diagnosis. This is the **most aggressive and second most common type of melanoma** (**Figure 13–1**). They are clinically characterized as mostly black, but occasionally brown, blue, gray, red, or tan lesions that arise from nevi or normal skin.

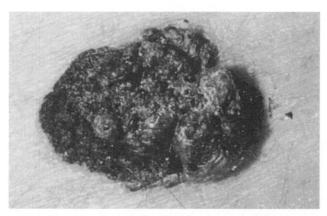

Figure 13–1. Nodular melanoma. (*Reproduced, with permission, from Kasper DL, Braunwald E, Fauci A, et al.* Harrison's Principles of Internal Medicine. *16th ed. New York, NY: McGraw-Hill; 2005:499.*)

PHYSICAL EXAMINATION

In 1985, it was noted by clinicians studying melanoma that there were several characteristic features of skin lesions that correlated with melanoma. Specifically, color variegation, border irregularity, asymmetry, and size greater than 6 mm in diameter were consistently observed with melanoma. This led to the **ABCD acronym**, which has been used extensively to determine the likelihood of a cancerous skin lesion (Table 13–1).

One other criterion that is often used is the change in the size or appearance of the skin lesion. This is sometimes cited as E in the above ABCD criteria, and referred to as Evolving and Elevation. Benign lesions may present at birth, or any time thereafter, and several benign lesions may also present near the same point in time. However, a benign lesion, once present, will usually remain stable in size and appearance, whereas a malignancy will present as increasing in size or changing in appearance. Thus, it is useful to ask whether a "mole" has recently changed in appearance or has grown in size.

The "Ugly Duckling Sign" may guide physical examination of skin lesions as it is easy to remember and teach. Simply, as the name suggests, this alludes to the

Table 13-1 • CLASSIC ABCD CRITERIA OF SUSPICIOUS SKIN LESIONS			
Acronym	Characteristic	More Likely Benign	More Likely Malignant
A	Asymmetry	Symmetric (right half looks like left half)	Asymmetric (in >2 axes)
B	Borders	Well defined	Ragged or blurred
C	Color	Uniform color	Variegated (2 or more colors)
D	Diameter	<6 mm	>6 mm
E	Elevation	Flat surface	Raised surface
	Evolving	Stable in size and appearance	Enlargement, changes in thickness, or bleeding

blatantly different appearance of the melanoma as compared to the other lesions the patient may have.

Another procedure that may aid the detection of melanoma in the family physician's office is dermoscopy. This is a magnification technique by which a skin lesion can be visualized for more detail regarding its pigment and structure. The dermoscopic properties of a lesion may guide the physician's management in terms of either observing its evolution or performing a biopsy to further evaluate it.

TREATMENT

Benign nevi need only be monitored visually. The patient can accomplish this after education on what to look for and when to come back for reevaluation. In general, any preexisting nevus that has changed or any new pigmented lesion that exhibits any of the ABCDE signs should be excised completely with a 2- to 3-mm margin around the lesion. Larger lesions that may be cosmetically difficult to completely excise may be biopsied in several areas. If the pathology indicates a malignancy, the lesion should then be completely excised with 5-mm margins by a physician trained in plastic surgical technique. Complete excision of malignant melanomas requires at least a 5-mm margin. Once a patient has been identified as having a malignant skin lesion, the patient should be observed on an annual basis for any new or changing skin lesions. Shave biopsy may be used for raised lesions, and punch biopsy or elliptical excision for flat lesions. If the entire lesion cannot be removed due to size or location, biopsies should be taken from the most suspicious parts of the lesion.

PROGNOSIS

The single most important piece of information for prognosis in melanoma is the thickness of the tumor, known as the Breslow measurement. **Melanomas less than 1-mm thick have a low rate of metastasis** and a high cure rate with excision. Thicker melanomas have higher rates of metastases and poorer outcomes.

PREVENTION

Prevention is aimed at reducing exposure to ultraviolet radiation. When possible, avoid the sun between 10 AM and 4 PM; wear sun-protective clothing when exposed to sunlight; wear a sunscreen with a sun protection factor (SPF) of at least 15; and avoid artificial sources of ultraviolet (UV) radiation. Due to the high risk of developing skin cancer in fair-skinned individuals, The United States Preventive Services Task Force (USPSTF) recommends behavioral counseling regarding minimizing exposure to UV radiation to reduce risk of skin cancer (grade B). This recommendation is targeted for age group between 10 and 24 years who are fair skinned. For individuals older than 24, this recommendation currently has insufficient evidence for effectiveness of behavioral counseling.

The USPSTF, however, does *not* recommend routine screening with whole body examination in the general population for the early detection of premalignant lesions as the evidence of benefit versus harm or routine screening in preventing malignancy is insufficient (grade I). It should be kept in mind that these recommendations are for the general population. Special population including those with family history of skin cancers, prior history of benign or malignant cancer, and other risk factors should be examined and managed appropriately on an individual basis.

NONMELANOMA SKIN CANCERS

Both basal cell and squamous cell carcinomas arise from the epidermal layer of the skin. The primary risk for these types of skin cancers is exposure to ultraviolet radiation, especially sun exposure but also tanning bed use. A history of actinic keratoses and human papillomavirus infection of the skin also raises the risk of squamous cell carcinomas.

Basal cell carcinomas are the most common of all cancers. They typically appear as pearly papules, often with a central ulceration or with multiple telangiectasias. Patients typically present with a growing lesion and sometimes complain that it bleeds or itches. Basal cell carcinomas rarely metastasize but can grow large and can be locally destructive. The primary treatment is excision.

Squamous cell carcinomas have a higher rate of metastasis than basal cell carcinomas, but the risk is still low. These lesions are often irregularly shaped plaques or nodules with raised borders. They are frequently scaly, ulcerated, and bleed easily. Complete excision is the treatment of choice.

COMPREHENSION QUESTIONS

13.1 A 36-year-old man is noted to have a bothersome "mole" that on biopsy reveals malignant melanoma. The pathologist comments that this histology is a very rare type of melanoma and usually escapes diagnosis until a more advanced stage. Which of the following is the most likely finding?

 A. Melanoma in situ

 B. Superficial spreading melanoma

 C. Amelanotic melanoma

 D. Nodular melanoma

 E. Acral lentiginous melanoma

13.2 A 73-year-old woman presents for concern about several tan-colored moles on her arms, face, and ears that have progressively grown over the past 6 months. Upon further examination, the moles are determined to be between 6 and 8 mm with very irregular borders. The physician decides to obtain an excisional biopsy. Which of the following skin lesions should the physician be most suspicious of based on history alone?

 A. Benign nevus

 B. Superficial spreading melanoma

 C. Lentigo maligna

 D. Nodular melanoma

 E. Acral lentiginous melanoma

13.3 A 23-year-old Caucasian woman presents to your office for a routine well-woman examination. She feels well without any concern/complaints. She is a non-smoker with no significant past medical history. Her last Pap smear with cotesting was last year. Her last tetanus shot was 2 years ago and she has received a flu shot for the current season already. She states that she has never been checked for skin cancer before and asks to be checked for it today. She denies excessive sun exposure and has never been to a tanning facility before. Based on the above information, which preventive services does she need at today's visit?

A. Pap smear and tetanus shot

B. Whole body examination to check for skin lesions based on age and race

C. Tetanus shot only

D. Mammogram and tetanus shot

E. Counseling to avoid excessive sun exposure and tanning booths

13.4 A 45-year-old African-American woman presents for a routine examination. You notice a 9-mm-diameter lesion on the palm of her right hand that is dark black, slightly raised, and has a notched border. When asked about it, she says that it has been present for about a year and is growing. A friend told her not to be concerned because, "black people don't get skin cancer." Which of the following is your advice?

A. Her friend is correct and this is nothing to worry about.

B. While anyone can get skin cancer, this lesion has primarily benign features and can be safely observed.

C. This lesion is suspicious for cancer but this is most likely a metastasis from another source, such as a breast cancer.

D. This lesion is suspicious for a primary melanoma and needs further evaluation immediately.

13.5 A 70-year-old woman presents for evaluation of a lesion on her left cheek. It has been present for several months. It is slowly enlarging and bleeds if she scratches it. On examination, you find a 7-mm-diameter pearly appearing papule with visible telangiectasias on the surface. Which of the following is the appropriate management of this lesion?

A. Close observation and reexamination in 3 months

B. Reassurance of the benign nature of the lesion

C. Excision

D. Local destruction by freezing with liquid nitrogen

ANSWERS

13.1 **C.** Amelanotic melanoma is an uncommon type of melanoma that due to its lack of pigmentation often goes undiagnosed until it is in a more invasive and advanced stage.

13.2 **C.** Lentigo maligna is most often found in the elderly usually on chronic sun-damaged skin such as the face, ears, arms, and upper trunk. Think of this type with tan-colored lesions on sun-damaged skin that has very irregular borders.

13.3 **E.** This patient is up-to-date on her cervical cancer screening and immunizations for her age. She is not yet of the age where screening mammography would be recommended. Per USPSTF recommendations, whole body skin cancer screening is not generally recommended but counseling to reduce the risk of development of skin cancer would be advised.

13.4 **D.** The lesion described is suspicious for an acral lentiginous melanoma and needs evaluation. While skin cancers are more common in persons with lighter skin, they can occur in persons with any skin color or tone.

13.5 **C.** The lesion is most likely a basal cell carcinoma and should be treated with excision. While the likelihood of metastatic spread is low, these lesions can grow and be locally destructive.

CLINICAL PEARLS

▶ The preventable risk factor common to all skin cancers is sun exposure. Recommend to your at-risk patients limiting exposure to sunlight in the middle of the day, wearing appropriate protective clothing, and using sunscreen.

▶ Contrary to popular belief, the use of tanning beds is also a risk factor for skin cancer.

▶ There is no such thing as a "healthy tan."

▶ Clinicians should be aware that fair-skinned men and women older than 65 years, patients with atypical moles, and those with more than 50 moles constitute known groups at substantially increased risk for melanoma.

▶ Excisional biopsy should be done for any lesion suspicious for melanoma. If the entire lesion cannot be removed due to size or location, full-thickness biopsies should be taken from the most suspicious parts of the lesion.

REFERENCES

Abbasi NR, Shaw HM, Rigel DS, et al. Early diagnosis of cutaneous melanoma: revisiting the ABCD criteria. *JAMA*. 2004;292:2771-2776.

American Academy of Dermatology. Excellence in dermatopathology. 2015. https://www.aad.org/media-resources/stats-and-facts/conditions/skin-cancer. Accessed October 24, 2015.

American Cancer Society. *Cancer Facts & Figures 2015*. Atlanta, GA: American Cancer Society; 2015.

American Skin Association. 2012. http://www.americanskin.org/resource/melanoma.php. Accessed October 24, 2015.

Ebell M. Clinical diagnosis of melanoma. *Am Fam Physician*. 2008;78(10):1205-1208.

Rager El, Bridgeford EP, Ollila DW. Cutaneous melanoma: update on prevention, screening, diagnosis and treatment. *Am Fam Physician*. 2005;72(2):269-276.

Rose LC. Recognizing neoplastic skin lesions: a photo guide. *Am Fam Physician*. 1998;4:58.

Shenenberger DW. Cutaneous malignant melanoma: a primary care perspective. *Am Fam Physician*. 2012 Jan 15;85(2):161-168.

Stern RS. Prevalence of a history of skin cancer in 2007: results of an incidence-based model. *Arch Dermatol*. 2010 Mar;146(3):279-282.

Stulberg DL, Crandell B, Fawcett RS. Diagnosis and treatment of basal cell and squamous cell carcinomas. *Am Fam Physician*. 2004;70:1481-1488.

U.S. Preventive Services Task Force. Skin cancer screening. 2009. Available at: http://www.uspreventiveservicestaskforce.org/Page/Topic/recommendation-summary/skin-cancer-screening. Accessed May 24, 2015.

U.S. Preventive Services Task Force. Skin cancer counseling. 2012. Available at: http://www.uspreventiveservicestaskforce.org/Page/Topic/recommendation-summary/skin-cancer-counseling. Accessed May 24, 2015.

Wolff K, Johnson R, Saavedra AP, et al. Melanoma precursors and primary cutaneous melanoma. In: Wolff K, Johnson R, Saavedra AP, et al, eds. *Fitzpatrick's Color Atlas and Synopsis of Clinical Dermatology*. 7th ed. New York, NY: McGraw-Hill; 2013. http://accessmedicine.mhmedical.com/content.aspx?bookid=682&Sectionid=45130143. Accessed May 24, 2015.

A 40-year-old man with no past medical history presents to the clinic to establish care. He reports that he had a prior urinalysis that revealed blood as an incidental finding. The urinalysis was done as a standard screening test by his former employer. He denies ever seeing any blood in his urine and denies any voiding difficulties, dysuria, sexual dysfunction, or any history or risk factors for sexually transmitted diseases (STDs). His review of systems is otherwise negative. He has smoked a half-pack of cigarettes per day for the past 10 years and exercises by jogging 15 minutes and lightweight training daily. On examination, his vital signs are normal and the entire physical examination is unremarkable. A complete blood count (CBC) and a chemistry panel (electrolytes, blood urea nitrogen [BUN], and creatinine) are normal. The results of a urinalysis done in your office are specific gravity, 1.015; pH 5.5; leukocyte esterase, negative; nitrites, negative; white blood cell count (WBC), 0; red blood cell count (RBC), 4 to 5 per high-power field (HPF).

▶ What is the most likely diagnosis?
▶ How would you approach this patient?
▶ What is the workup and plan for this patient?
▶ What are the concerns and how would you counsel the patient?

ANSWERS TO CASE 14:

Hematuria

Summary: A 40-year-old male smoker is found incidentally to have red blood cells in his urine sample on a urinalysis.

- **Current diagnosis:** Asymptomatic microscopic hematuria.

- **Initial approach:** Repeat the urinalysis, assess for risk factors and possible reversible causes such as urinary tract infection (UTI), vigorous exercise or recent urologic procedure, perform renal function testing, and then depending on low or high risk of malignancy, perform additional imaging of lower and/ or upper urinary tract.

- **Workup and plan:** Rule out infection by performing urine culture; obtain further history including exercise routine or recent urologic procedures; perform renal function testing to rule out renal disease. If all of this is negative, evaluate for malignancy by imaging of the upper urinary tract via computed tomography (CT) urography and the lower urinary tract via cystoscopy.

- **Concerns and counseling:** The primary concern is to rule out malignancy, including renal cell carcinoma and transitional cell carcinoma. Counsel the patient on the importance of an appropriate workup, but reassure the patient about the low prevalence of the condition.

ANALYSIS

Objectives

1. Learn about the significance of microscopic hematuria.

2. Learn an evidence-based approach to workup asymptomatic microscopic hematuria.

3. Be familiar with recommendations for follow-up on patients with hematuria after a negative workup.

Considerations

This patient has asymptomatic microscopic hematuria, as opposed to gross hematuria. The American Urological Association (AUA) defines significant microscopic hematuria as more than 3 RBCs per HPF on urinalysis with microscopy. Although he is asymptomatic, this patient deserves a thorough workup in order to determine an etiology, if possible, and to rule out malignancy. The management guidelines differ in the workup of microscopic hematuria with fewer than 3 RBCs per HPF versus more than 3 RBCs per HPF.

The patient's history should be reviewed with specific questions to determine any risks for STDs, occupational exposures to chemicals, strenuous exercise, drugs, medications, and herbal/nutritional supplements. For a result of fewer than 3 RBCs per HPF, a urine analysis (UA) should be repeated three times at 6-week intervals. If these are negative (consistently <3 RBCs per HPF), the workup is complete and the patient should be reassured. For a primary result of more than 3 RBCs per HPF, a urine culture should be sent to evaluate for UTI. If a source is found, a repeat UA with microscopy should be done 6 weeks after the etiology has been resolved (for UTI or STD) or offending agent has been removed (exposure, strenuous exercise, medications, etc).

At this point if the condition persists, renal function testing should be done to evaluate for possible renal disease. This may include a basic metabolic panel to check for BUN and creatinine as well as glomerular filtration rate (GFR). If there are abnormalities in renal function testing, a nephrology referral should be generated immediately. If, however, no renal abnormalities are found at this point, or the patient has risk factors for malignancy, imaging with CT urography and cystoscopy should be done. Inform the patient that a complete workup is necessary to evaluate for the presence of conditions such as infections or tumors, since as many as 30% to 40% of people with gross hematuria and about 5% of those with microscopic hematuria are positive for malignancy.

APPROACH TO:
Hematuria

DEFINITIONS

GROSS HEMATURIA: The presence of enough blood in a urine sample to be visible to the naked eye

LOWER URINARY TRACT: The urinary bladder and urethra

MICROSCOPIC HEMATURIA: The presence of 3 or more RBCs per HPF on two or more properly collected urinalyses

UPPER URINARY TRACT: The kidneys and ureters

CLINICAL APPROACH

Hematuria is divided into glomerular, renal (nonglomerular), and urologic etiologies. Glomerular hematuria typically is associated with significant proteinuria, erythrocyte casts, and dysmorphic RBCs. Renal (nonglomerular) hematuria is secondary to tubulointerstitial, renovascular, and metabolic disorders. Like glomerular hematuria, it often is associated with significant proteinuria; however, there are no associated dysmorphic RBCs or erythrocyte casts. Urologic causes of hematuria include tumors, calculi, infections, trauma, and benign prostatic hyperplasia (BPH). Urologic hematuria is distinguished from other etiologies by the absence of proteinuria, dysmorphic RBCs, and erythrocyte casts.

Hematuria in adults should first be defined as gross hematuria or microscopic hematuria. Gross hematuria denotes that the patient is able to visualize blood in his voided specimen. Patients most often describe their urine as having a reddish or brownish color. Patients are commonly concerned about malignancy or kidney stones. In contrast, microscopic hematuria is usually asymptomatic and often discovered incidentally. **Although malignancy is found in 5% of all patients with incidental asymptomatic microscopic hematuria, United States Preventive Services Task Force (USPSTF) currently does not recommend routine screening for bladder cancer in asymptomatic patients (Level I).**

Clinically significant microscopic hematuria is defined as 3 or more RBCs per HPF on microscopic evaluation of urinary sediment from a properly collected specimen. The initial determination of microscopic hematuria should be based on microscopic examination of urinary sediment from a freshly voided, early-morning, clean-catch, midstream urine specimen. Urine must be refrigerated if it cannot be examined promptly, as delays of more than 2 hours between collection and examination often cause unreliable results.

Hematuria can be measured quantitatively by any of the following methods:

- Determination of the number of red blood cells per milliliter of urine excreted (chamber count)

- Direct examination of the centrifuged urinary sediment (sediment count)

- Indirect examination of the urine by dipstick (the simplest way to detect microscopic hematuria).

Given the limited specificity of the dipstick method (65%-99% for 2-5 RBCs per HPF), the initial **finding of hematuria by the dipstick method should be confirmed by microscopic evaluation of urinary sediment.** The limited specificity is due to the fact that the urine dipstick lacks the ability to distinguish RBCs from myoglobin or hemoglobin.

Because of the possibility of bladder cancer, the AUA recommends that a single positive result for hematuria on UA with microscopy warrants further workup. There are certain risk factors that are associated with a higher probability of bladder cancer that should be explored and should serve as an impetus for timely and efficient workup and referrals. Risk factors include smoking, occupational exposure to chemicals or dyes (benzenes or aromatic amines), history of gross hematuria, older than age 40, history of urologic disorder or disease, history of irritative voiding symptoms, history of UTI, analgesic abuse, or history of pelvic irradiation.

The prevalence of asymptomatic microscopic hematuria is roughly 2% to 31%. in the males over the age of 60. There are a myriad of possible causes; risk factors should guide the specific workup for the individual patient. Although some elements of the workup are standard for everyone, other more detailed and expensive tests can be deferred for those at low risk. The presence of significant proteinuria, red cell casts, renal insufficiency, or a predominance of dysmorphic RBCs in the urine should prompt an evaluation for renal parenchymal disease or referral to a nephrologist. In general, glomerular bleeding is associated with more than 80% dysmorphic red blood cells, whereas lower urinary tract bleeding is associated with more than 80% normal red blood cells.

Evaluation

Evaluation of the **urinary sediment** can allow for the diagnosis of patients with renal parenchymal disease. This analysis **will often also allow for distinction between**

glomerular disease and interstitial nephritis. The presence of red cell casts and dysmorphic red blood cells is suggestive of renal glomerular disease. Interstitial nephritis, often caused by analgesics or other drugs, is suggested by the presence of eosinophils in the urine.

A complete evaluation for microscopic hematuria starts with a detailed history and physical examination, appropriate laboratory testing (including urinary cytology), and imaging of the upper and lower urinary tract. If the UA with microscopy is positive for significant microscopic hematuria, further history should be obtained to rule out benign causes such as menstruation, strenuous exercise, recent urologic procedure, medications, etc. If a probable cause is determined, UA with microscopy should be repeated after 6 weeks of discontinuation of the cause. If the repeat urinalysis is negative and the patient remains asymptomatic, no further workup is required for low-risk patients. Transient microscopic hematuria can be caused by sexual intercourse, heavy exercise, a recent digital prostate examination, other urologic procedures, or contamination by menses. The repeat urinalysis should be done after avoidance of any potential confounders such as menses, medications, exercise, drugs, and nutritional/herbal products. Exercise-induced hematuria usually resolves spontaneously in 72 hours in the absence of other coexisting conditions. In addition, careful attention should be taken in women to ensure the blood is not from the vaginal or rectal areas. In men, one should also exclude local trauma to the foreskin. If in doubt, a catheterized specimen should be obtained, taking care not to induce trauma during the procedure.

The laboratory studies should start with urinalysis with microscopy and evaluation of centrifuged urinary sediment. The urine should be examined for number of RBCs per HPF, dysmorphic RBCs, and presence of casts and eosinophils. UTI should be ruled out by urine culture. If an infection is present, it should be appropriately treated and the urinalysis repeated in 6 weeks. If the **hematuria resolves with treatment of the UTI, no further workup is needed.**

A serum creatinine should also be obtained to assess renal function, with comparison to old records if available. If the laboratory evaluation reveals elevated creatinine or red cell casts, workup should focus on renal parenchymal disease and possible etiologies such as hypertension, diabetes, or autoimmune diseases. Referral to a nephrologist should be considered. Renal biopsy may be appropriate for certain individuals. Patients with risk factors should also undergo cytologic evaluation of the urine to assess for transitional cell carcinoma. Although voided urine cytology may not pick up low-grade carcinoma, it is fairly reliable for high-grade lesions, especially if repeated.

Numerous options exist for imaging of the upper urinary tract. Despite many studies comparing the radiographic methods, there are no evidence-based guidelines on which modality is most efficient. Choice of imaging modality should take into account any contraindications the patient may have including renal insufficiency, contrast allergy, or pregnancy. CT urography (with and without IV contrast), given its high sensitivity and specificity for imaging upper urinary tract, should be the initial modality of choice unless a contraindication exists. Urine cytology and urine markers should only be used in patients with risk factors for bladder cancer as detailed earlier; these procedures are not a part of the routine evaluation of microscopic hematuria. The lower urinary tract should be examined for transitional cell carcinoma by cystoscopy in all patients who are older than 35 years or who present with risk factors for lower urinary tract malignancies. In the absence of risk factors in selected patients with a negative history, examination, laboratory workup, and upper tract imaging, and those younger than 35 years, cystoscopy may be deferred or individualized at the discretion of the treating physician.

In patients with a thorough but negative workup, UA with microscopy should be repeated annually for 2 consecutive years. For those with persistent asymptomatic microscopic hematuria, the AUA recommends repeat evaluation within 3 to 5 years of the initial evaluation. For those with two consecutively negative results on annual UA with microscopy, workup can be stopped. However, if the patient develops gross hematuria, voiding difficulties, pain, or any abnormal cytology, immediate urologic reevaluation and urologic consultation is warranted. Patients who develop hypertension, proteinuria, glomerular casts, or abnormal renal function should be referred to a nephrologist for consultation.

COMPREHENSION QUESTIONS

14.1 A 60-year-old man with past medical history of BPH presents to you with gross hematuria for 1 day. He states this has never happened before and denies strenuous exercise. Upon further questioning he does reveal that 2 days ago he had a bladder catheterization to evaluate his postvoid residual. He denies smoking, family history of cancers, or chemical exposures. Which of the following is the most appropriate management at this time?

A. Counsel the patient on the high likelihood of gross hematuria after a urologic procedure and that this will likely subside. Let him know no test is required today.

B. Do a urine dipstick first. If positive then proceed to urinalysis with microscopy and have the patient return in a few weeks for a repeat UA with microscopy.

C. Discuss with the patient the high likelihood of malignancy with gross hematuria especially given his age and past history and recommend imaging upper and lower urinary tracts.

D. Tell him that he likely needs urine cytology today to rule out malignancy.

14.2 A 54-year-old postmenopausal woman with past medical history of hypertension is incidentally found to have significant microscopic hematuria on a UA that was done as part of her annual hypertension laboratory tests. She denies dysuria, gross hematuria, fevers, chills, and nausea/vomiting. Her physical examination is negative for suprapubic tenderness and flank pain. What would be the next best step in the management of this patient?

A. Repeat UA with microscopy in 3 months at her next follow-up visit for hypertension.

B. Perform a urine culture and if positive, treat immediately. Repeat UA posttreatment.

C. Order renal function testing to rule out medical renal disease as an etiology.

D. Repeat UA with microscopy in 6 weeks.

14.3 A 65-year-old man with past medical history of hypertension, coronary artery disease, chronic kidney disease (CKD), and a pacemaker presents to your office with complaint of "dark urine" for many weeks now. He states he has been evaluated by several other physicians who had done "several tests" that all came back negative. He states he has never had any imaging done and would like you to "take a look at what is going on in there." Upon accessing his medical records you see that he has already had several UA with microscopy that were all positive for microscopic hematuria, renal function testing, which is significant for elevated BUN and creatinine and decreased GFR, and negative urine cultures. At this time, what would be the most appropriate imaging modality and management for this patient?

A. Counsel the patient against imaging at this time as any imaging may worsen his CKD.

B. Order magnetic resonance urography (MRU) as the patient is unable to undergo CT urography given his renal insufficiency, along with an urgent urology referral.

C. Order a combined renal ultrasound and retrograde pyelogram for maximum visualization of upper urinary tract, along with an urgent urology referral.

D. Order urine cytology and urine markers as these are the least invasive test of choice at this time.

ANSWERS

14.1 **B.** Although it is very likely that the patient's hematuria is secondary to the recent urologic procedure, it is not a good practice to simply assume the cause and not do appropriate initial evaluation for hematuria, like one would for any patient with that chief complaint. The initial step in this case would be to do a urine dipstick, which if positive in office, would warrant a UA with microscopy. If this shows 3 or more RBCs per HPF, one would immediately go to thorough workup. However, if UA with microscopy shows fewer than 3 RBCs per HPF, the patient should be asked to return in 6 weeks for a repeat. It is appropriate to discuss with the patient that his gross hematuria, given his lack of risk factors for malignancy, is most likely caused by the recent bladder catheterization; however, as stated earlier, this is not a reason to dismiss further evaluation. Since there is a probable cause for this patient's hematuria, one would not immediately begin workup to rule out malignancy. Certainly, if his gross hematuria continues after several weeks, it would be imperative to conduct further evaluation.

14.2 **D.** This patient does not have signs or symptoms of a UTI and additional workup looking for an infection is not going to change management, as asymptomatic bacteriuria need not be treated except in pregnancy. As per the current guidelines, this patient needs a repeat UA with microscopy in 6 weeks before beginning workup to rule out medical renal disease. A 3-month interval between repeat UA testing is not an appropriate interval.

14.3 **C.** This patient has two simultaneous contraindications to imaging modalities preferred in the workup of microscopic hematuria. Due to his renal insufficiency he should not get a CT urography, and due to his pacemaker, he should not undergo MRI/MRU. For this reason, the next best imaging modality would have to be done, a renal ultrasound, which when combined with a retrograde pyelogram would provide maximum information about the upper urinary tracts. This would have to be done with a concurrent urology referral. Urine cytology and urine markers, although noninvasive, are not currently recommended in the routine evaluation of microscopic hematuria.

CLINICAL PEARLS

▶ Hematuria in adults should always be evaluated. If no source is found on a thorough initial workup, patients should be followed for at least 3 years to monitor for an underlying condition.

▶ In every case of a first-time microscopic hematuria, a repeat urinalysis with microscopy is required at 6-week interval before any other management is done.

REFERENCES

Cohen RA, Brown RS. Microscopic hematuria. *N Engl J Med*. 2003;348:2330-2338.

Davis RJ, Jones S, Barocas DA, et al. Diagnosis, evaluation and follow-up of asymptomatic microhematuria (AMH) in adults: AUA guideline. 2012. American Urological Association. Available at: https://www.auanet.org/common/pdf/education/clinical-guidance/Asymptomatic-Microhematuria.pdf. Accessed May 24, 2015.

Grossfeld GD, Litwin MS, Wolf JS, et al. Evaluation of asymptomatic microscopic hematuria in adults: the American Urological Association best practice policy—part I: definition, detection, prevalence, and etiology. *Urology*. 2001;57(4):599-603.

Grossfeld GD, Litwin MS, Wolf JS Jr, et al. Evaluation of asymptomatic microscopic hematuria in adults: the American Urological Association best practice policy—part II: patient evaluation, cytology, voided markers, imaging, cystoscopy, nephrology evaluation, and follow-up. *Urology*. 2001;57(4):604-610.

Lin J, Denker BM, Bradley M. Azotemia and urinary abnormalities. In: Kasper D, Fauci A, Hauser S, Longo D, Jameson J, Loscalzo J, et al., eds. *Harrison's Principles of Internal Medicine*. 19th ed. New York, NY: McGraw-Hill Education; 2015. Available at: http://accessmedicine.mhmedical.com/. Accessed May 24, 2015.

McDonald MM, Swagerty D, Wetzel L. Assessment of microscopic hematuria in adults. *Am Fam Physician*. 2006;73(10):1748-1754.

O'Connor OJ, McSweeney SE, Maher MM. Imaging of hematuria. *Radiol Clin North Am*. 2008;46:113.

Sharp VJ, Barnes KT, Erickson BA. Assessment of asymptomatic microscopic hematuria in adults. *Am Fam Physician*. 2013 Dec 1;88(11):747-754.

Simerville JA, Maxted WC, Pahira JJ. Urinalysis: a comprehensive review. *Am Fam Physician*. 2005; 71(6):1153-1162.

A 27-year-old woman presents to your office complaining of progressing nervousness, fatigue, palpitations, and the recent development of a resting hand tremor. She also states that she is having difficulty concentrating at work and has been more irritable with her coworkers. The patient also notes that she has developed a persistent rash over her shins that has not improved with the use of topical steroid creams. All of her symptoms have come on gradually over the past few months and continue to get worse. Review of systems also reveals an unintentional weight loss of about 10 lb, insomnia, and amenorrhea for the past 2 months (the patient's menstrual cycles are usually quite regular). The patient's past medical history is unremarkable and she takes no oral medications. She is currently not sexually active and does not drink alcohol, smoke, or use any illicit drugs. On examination, she is afebrile. Her pulse varies from 70 to 110 beats/min. She appears restless and anxious. Her skin is warm and moist. Her eyes show evidence of exophthalmos and lid retraction bilaterally, although funduscopic examination is normal. Neck examination reveals symmetric thyroid enlargement, without any discrete palpable masses. Cardiac examination reveals an irregular rhythm. Her lungs are clear to auscultation. Extremity examination reveals an erythematous, thickened rash on both shins. Neurologic examination is normal except for a fine resting tremor in her hands when she attempts to hold out her outstretched arms. Initial laboratory tests include a negative pregnancy test and an undetectable level of thyroid-stimulating hormone (TSH).

▶ What is the most likely diagnosis?
▶ What imaging study is most appropriate at this time?
▶ What is the definitive nonsurgical treatment of this condition?

ANSWERS TO CASE 15:
Thyroid Disorders

Summary: A 27-year-old woman presents with progressively worsening anxiety, palpitations, tremor, menstrual irregularities, and weight loss. Her TSH level is suppressed, confirming the presence of hyperthyroidism.

- **Most likely diagnosis:** Hyperthyroidism secondary to Graves disease
- **Most appropriate imaging study:** Nuclear medicine thyroid scan with uptake
- **Definitive nonsurgical treatment:** Thyroid ablation with radioactive iodine

ANALYSIS
Objectives

1. Know the most common conditions that cause hyper- and hypothyroidism.
2. Be able to interpret the common tests used to evaluate thyroid function.
3. Learn the modalities of treatment for disorders of the thyroid.

Considerations

This patient has symptoms and signs consistent with hyperthyroidism, including warm, moist skin caused by excessive sweating and cutaneous vasodilation; a resting tremor; an enlarged thyroid gland; weight loss; and tachycardia. Her irregular heartbeat may be a manifestation of atrial fibrillation, which occurs in approximately 10% of hyperthyroid patients. Eye abnormalities are common in hyperthyroid states. Retraction of the upper lid, resulting in the "thyroid stare" is common. Graves disease has a unique ophthalmopathy that may cause a prominent exophthalmos (Figure 15–1). **The most common cause of noniatrogenic hyperthyroidism is Graves disease,** an autoimmune thyroid disorder. Autoantibodies to the TSH receptors on the thyroid gland result in hyperfunctioning of the gland, with the result that the

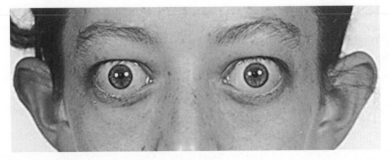

Figure 15–1. Exophthalmos and proptosis of Graves disease. (*Reproduced, with permission, from Kasper DL, Braunwald E, Fauci A, et al. Harrison's Principles of Internal Medicine. 16th ed. New York, NY: McGraw-Hill; 2005:2114.*)

thyroid gland functions outside the usual control of the hypothalamic-pituitary axis. Graves disease commonly occurs in reproductive-age females and is much more common in women than men. The treatment of Graves disease includes antithyroid drugs (such as propylthiouracil [PTU] and methimazole) and/or β-blockers to block some of the peripheral effects of excessive thyroxine. However, these are only temporary measures used to give patients symptomatic relief. The definitive treatment is radioactive iodine, which destroys the thyroid gland. **At least 40% of patients who receive radioactive iodine eventually become hypothyroid** and will need thyroid hormone replacement. Radioactive iodine therapy is contraindicated in pregnant women, as the isotope can cross the placenta and cause fetal thyroid ablation. Due to adverse effects on fetal development, methimazole is not used during first trimester of pregnancy. Most experts agree that PTU should be used in the first trimester, and methimazole can be safely used in second and third trimesters. Surgical removal of the thyroid gland is another option for the treatment of Graves disease, but it is often reserved for pregnant patients.

APPROACH TO:
Thyroid Disease

DEFINITIONS

GRAVES DISEASE: An autoimmune thyroid disorder in which autoantibodies to the TSH receptors on the thyroid gland result in hyperfunctioning of the thyroid gland. A prominent finding is also the "stare" due to the ophthalmic involvement.

THYROID STORM: An acute hypermetabolic state associated with the sudden release of large amounts of thyroid hormone into circulation, leading to autonomic instability and central nervous system dysfunction such as altered mental status, coma, or seizures. This condition has a significant mortality risk.

HYPERTHYROIDISM

Signs and Symptoms

Hyperthyroidism usually presents with progressive nervousness, palpitations, weight loss, fine resting tremor, dyspnea on exertion, and difficulty concentrating. Physical findings include a rapid pulse rate and elevated blood pressure, with the systolic pressure increased to a greater extent than the diastolic pressure, creating widened pulse-pressure hypertension. Examination findings can include atrial fibrillation and a fine resting tremor.

Thyroid storm is an acute hypermetabolic state associated with the sudden release of large amounts of thyroid hormone into circulation. It occurs most often in patients with Graves disease, but can also occur in acute thyroiditis conditions. Symptoms include fever, confusion, restlessness, and psychotic-like behavior. Examination may demonstrate tachycardia, elevated blood pressure, fever, and dysrhythmias. Patients can also have other signs of high-output heart failure, such as dyspnea on exertion and peripheral vasoconstriction, and may exhibit signs of cerebral or cardiac ischemia. **Thyroid storm is a medical emergency** that requires prompt attention and reversal of the metabolic demands of acute hyperthyroidism.

Pathogenesis

Graves disease is the most common cause of hyperthyroidism and is more commonly found in women. It is an autoimmune disorder caused by immunoglobulin (Ig) G antibodies that bind to TSH receptors, initiating the production and release of thyroid hormone. In addition to the usual findings, approximately **50% of patients with Graves disease also have exophthalmos.** The second most common cause of hyperthyroidism is an autonomous thyroid nodule that secretes thyroxine. These nodules do not rely on TSH stimulation and continue to excrete large amounts of thyroxine despite low or nonexistent, circulating TSH levels. Hyperthyroidism can also be caused by the acute release of thyroid hormone in the early stages of thyroiditis. In such cases, symptoms are generally transient and resolve within weeks of onset. Iatrogenic hyperthyroidism can occur secondary to the overuse of thyroxine supplementation.

Laboratory and Imaging Evaluation

Hyperthyroidism can be diagnosed by an elevated free thyroxine level, usually with a corresponding low TSH level. Once it has been identified, further testing for autoimmune antibodies and radionucleotide scanning of the thyroid can help to determine whether the problem is Graves disease, an autonomous nodule, or thyroiditis. Radionucleotide imaging provides a direct scan of the gland and an indication of its functioning. Imaging is performed using either an isotope of technetium-99 m (^{99m}Tc) or iodine-123 (^{123}I). After the administration of one of these agents, imaging the thyroid allows visualization of active and inactive areas, as well as an indication as to the level of activity in a particular area. In patients with Graves disease, there will be diffuse hyperactivity with large amounts of uptake. In contrast, thyroiditis demonstrates patchy uptake with overall reduced activity, reflecting the release of existing hormone rather than the overproduction of new thyroxine. The detection of serum thyroid-receptor antibodies is a specific diagnostic test for Graves disease.

Treatment

Radioactive iodine is the treatment of choice for Graves disease in adult patients who are not pregnant. It should not be used in children or breast-feeding mothers. Antithyroid drugs are also well tolerated and successful at blocking the production and release of thyroid hormone in patients with Graves disease. Some examples of these drugs include PTU, methimazole, and carbimazole. These drugs work by inhibiting the organification of iodine, and PTU also prevents the peripheral conversion of thyroxine (T_4) to triiodothyronine (T_3), its more active form. In April, 2010, the Food and Drug Administration (FDA) added a "black box" warning to the labeling of PTU because of the risk of hepatotoxicity. For this reason, methimazole should be considered the first-line agent except when the patient is pregnant. PTU Is preferred during first trimester of pregnancy. Another serious potential side effect of these drugs is agranulocytosis, which occurs in 3 per 10,000 treated patients per year. **Antithyroid drugs are especially useful in treating adolescents, in whom Graves disease may go into spontaneous remission after 6 to 18 months of therapy.** Surgery is reserved for patients in whom medications and radioactive iodine ablation are unacceptable treatment modalities, or in whom a large goiter is present that is either compressing nearby structures or is disfiguring. For patients presenting with thyroid storm, aggressive initial therapy is essential to prevent complications. Treatment should include the administration of high doses of PTU or methimazole and β-blockers (to control tachycardia and other peripheral symptoms of thyrotoxicosis). Hydrocortisone is given to prevent possible adrenal crisis.

HYPOTHYROIDISM

Signs and Symptoms

Patients with hypothyroidism can present with a wide range of symptoms, including lethargy, weight gain, hair loss, dry skin, slowed mentation or forgetfulness, constipation, intolerance to cold, and a depressed effect. **In older patients, hypothyroidism can be confused with Alzheimer disease** and other conditions that cause dementia. In women, it is often confused with depression. Physical findings that can present in hypothyroid patients include low blood pressure, bradycardia, nonpitting edema, hair thinning or loss, dry skin, and a diminished relaxation phase of reflexes.

Pathogenesis

Several different conditions can cause hypothyroidism. The **most common noniatrogenic condition causing hypothyroidism in the United States is Hashimoto thyroiditis,** an autoimmune thyroiditis. Iatrogenic causes include post-Graves disease thyroid ablation and surgical removal of the thyroid gland. Another cause is secondary hypothyroidism related to hypothalamic or pituitary dysfunction. These conditions are primarily found in patients who have received intracranial irradiation or surgical removal of a pituitary adenoma.

Laboratory and Imaging Evaluation

In primary hypothyroidism, the TSH level is elevated, indicating insufficient thyroid hormone production to meet metabolic demands. Free thyroid levels are low. In contrast, patients with secondary hypothyroidism have low or undetectable TSH levels. **Once the diagnosis of primary hypothyroidism is made, further imaging or serologic testing is unnecessary if the thyroid gland is normal on physical examination.** In cases of secondary hypothyroidism, however, further testing is needed to determine whether the cause is a hypothalamic or pituitary problem. This can be done by using a thyroid-releasing hormone (TRH) test. Endogenous TRH is released by the hypothalamus and stimulates the pituitary to release TSH. When TRH is injected intravenously, a normally functioning pituitary will result in an increase of TSH that can be measured in about 30 minutes. No increase in TSH after injection of TRH suggests a malfunctioning pituitary gland. In cases where pituitary dysfunction is suspected, imaging of the pituitary gland to detect microadenomas and testing of other hormones that are dependent on pituitary stimulation are indicated.

Treatment

Most healthy, nonpregnant adults with hypothyroidism require about 1.6 μg/kg of thyroid hormone replacement daily. The recommendation in patients over 50 years is to start with a dose between 25 and 50 μg daily, and increase by 25 μg every 3 to 4 weeks until optimal dose is reached. The same recommendation exists for those younger than 50 years with ischemic heart disease. In pregnancy, thyroid hormone replacement needs may increase by approximately 30%. This can be met by having the woman take nine doses of her prepregnancy dose of levothyroxine weekly. A referral to an endocrinologist may also be indicated.

Thyroxine is usually dosed once daily, although some evidence suggests that weekly dosing may also be effective. In patients with an intact hypothalamic-pituitary axis, the adequacy of thyroid replacement can be followed with serial TSH measurements. Evaluation of TSH levels should be performed 4 to 6 weeks after an adjustment in medication has been made. If TSH is greater than 5, underreplacement or nonadherence to medication should be suspected. If underreplaced, increase the levothyroxine dose by 12.5 to 25 μg per day. If TSH less than 0.35, patient is being overreplaced and a daily dose decrease by 25 μg is required. With increased age, thyroid binding decreases as a consequence of a drop in serum albumin level and the medication dosage may need to be reduced by up to 20%. Annual monitoring of the TSH level in the elderly is necessary to avoid overreplacement.

Screening

Screening asymptomatic adults for thyroid disorder is controversial. The United States Preventive Services Task Force (USPSTF) reports insufficient evidence for or against routine screening. The American Academy of Family Physicians (AAFP) does not recommend screening in asymptomatic adults. The American Thyroid Association recommends screening of all adults age 35 and more every 5 years.

NODULAR THYROID DISEASE

Thyroid nodules, both solitary and multiple, are common and are often found incidentally on physical examination, ultrasonography, or computed tomography. They are more prevalent in women and increase in frequency with age. Although their pathogenesis is not clear, nodules are known to be associated with iodine deficiency, higher gravidity, and the ingestion of goitrogens. **Further workup of identified nodules is indicated, as the incidence of malignancy in solitary nodules is estimated at 5% to 6%.** The incidence of malignancy is higher in children, adults younger than 30 or older than 60 years, and patients with a history of head or neck irradiation. Other historical risk factors include a family history of thyroid cancer, the presence of cervical lymphadenopathy, and the recent development of hoarseness of the voice, progressive dysphagia, or shortness of breath.

Initial assessment of thyroid nodules should include evaluation of thyroid function and ultrasonography to assess for the size of the nodule. Thyroid function can be assessed by measuring the TSH level. Ultrasonography is the imaging test of choice for assessment of the size of a thyroid nodule, its characteristics (solid or cystic), the overall size of the thyroid, and for the presence of other nodules that may not have been previously identified.

Functional adenomas that present with hyperthyroidism are rarely malignant. These represent less than 10% of all nodules. A patient who has a thyroid nodule and is found to be hyperthyroid should have a radioactive iodine uptake study to confirm functionality of the nodule. Hyperfunctioning nodules are treated with surgery or radioactive ablation therapy, depending on the level of hyperthyroidism.

Nodules measuring greater than 1 cm by ultrasonography in a person with a normal or elevated TSH require biopsy. This can be done by fine-needle aspiration (FNA), which is a highly sensitive test. Ultrasound findings suggestive of malignancy include irregular margins, intranodular vascular spots, and microcalcifications. Results of the FNA determine further management and treatment. Cytologic evaluation of FNA specimens are reported as being nondiagnostic, benign, follicular lesion of undetermined significance, follicular neoplasm, suspicious for malignancy, or malignant. **Follicular cell malignancy cannot be distinguished cytologically from its benign equivalent**, and thus is often read as follicular lesion of undetermined significance. These patients should be referred to surgery to obtain a definitive evaluation. Papillary, medullary, and anaplastic thyroid carcinomas can be diagnosed accurately by FNA. Patients with thyroid malignancy are treated by thyroidectomy followed by radioactive ablation. These patients will require long-term follow-up by an endocrinologist.

Thyroid nodules discovered during pregnancy are handled similarly, except that radioisotope scanning is contraindicated. FNA is safe during pregnancy, and thyroidectomy can be performed relatively safely during the second and third trimester. However, because thyroid cancer is relatively indolent, it may be wise to defer definitive diagnosis and treatment until the postpartum period in patients with indeterminate lesions on FNA.

COMPREHENSION QUESTIONS

15.1 A 28-year-old woman is noted to have had 10-lb unintended weight gain, hair loss, dry skin, and fatigue. She is diagnosed with probable hypothyroidism. Which of the following laboratory test results is most consistent with hypothyroidism?

A. Normal TSH and elevated T_4/T_3 levels

B. Elevated TSH levels and low T_4/T_3

C. Elevated TSH levels and normal T_4/T_3

D. Low TSH and elevated T_4/T_3 levels

15.2 A 35-year-old G2P1001 at 11 weeks' gestational age presents with complaint of palpitations, weight loss, nervousness and tremor. She denies prior history of thyroid problems. Laboratory studies confirm that TSH is severely suppressed. Which of the following is the best treatment for this patient at this time?

A. PTU

B. β-blockers

C. Levothyroxine

D. Methimazole

15.3 A 24-year-old woman who is 8 weeks pregnant is found to have a thyroid nodule. Biopsy is performed and malignancy of the thyroid is diagnosed. Which of the following management options is most appropriate?

A. Confirm the diagnosis of cancer using radioisotope scanning.

B. Perform an immediate thyroidectomy.

C. Follow clinically until after delivery of child.

D. Treat with radioactive iodine ablation in the second or third trimester.

15.4 A 28-year-old man presents to his physician for a health maintenance visit. He feels well and does not report changes in his appetite, weight, energy, or bowel movements. A firm nodule is palpated in the left lobe of his thyroid. The nodule is confirmed on ultrasound and measures 0.8 cm. Which of the following is the next step in the workup of this nodule?

A. Radioactive iodine uptake study

B. Fine-needle aspiration

C. Repeat ultrasound in 6 months

D. Referral to surgeon for open biopsy

ANSWERS

15.1 **B.** Hypothyroidism is marked by low levels of circulating thyroid hormones. When this happens, the negative feedback to TSH is stunted, and it in turn increases. Therefore hypothyroidism presents with an increased TSH and low T_3/T_4.

15.2 **A.** Experts agree that due to adverse effects of methimazole on fetal development, PTU should be used in first trimester of pregnancy, and methimazole in second and third trimesters.

15.3 **C.** Thyroid cancer detected during pregnancy can usually be observed until after the pregnancy is complete. If needed, thyroid surgery can be performed safely in the second and third trimesters. The use of radioactive iodine is contraindicated in pregnancy.

15.4   **C.** For thyroid nodules that are less than 1 cm, benign appearing, and no presence of positive clinical history of thyroid cancers, observation and repeat
thyroid ultrasound in 6 months is appropriate. Thyroid nodules greater than
1 cm should undergo FNA, as this is a sensitive and specific test for thyroid
nodules and can help to determine whether it is malignant.

CLINICAL PEARLS

▶ The most common forms of both hyper- and hypothyroidism are autoimmune: Graves disease and Hashimoto thyroiditis causing hypothyroidism.

▶ Once thyroid nodule is palpated on examination, the first steps are to
obtain a TSH level and a thyroid ultrasound.

▶ Thyroid disease in pregnancy needs to be evaluated and treated appropriately as both hypothyroidism and hyperthyroidism can have serious
effects on fetal development.

REFERENCES

Baloch ZW, LiVolsi VA, Asa SL, et al. Diagnostic terminology and morphologic criteria for cytologic
diagnosis of thyroid lesions: a synopsis of the National Cancer Institute Thyroid Fine-Needle Aspiration State of the Science Conference. *Diagn Cytopathol.* 2008;36:425.

Davis A, Shahla N. A practical guide to thyroid disease in women. *The Female patient* (Primary care ed).
2005;30(9):38-47.

Donangelo I, Braunstein GD. Update on subclinical hyperthyroidism. *Am Fam Physician.* 2011 Apr
15;83(8):933-938.

Gaitonde DY, Rowley KD, Sweeney LB. Hypothyroidsm: an update. *Am Fam Physician.* 2012 Aug
1;86(3):244-251.

Garber JR, Cobin RH, Hennessey JV, et al. Clinical practice guidelines for hypothyroidism in adults:
cosponsored by the American Association of Clinical Endocrinologists and the American Thyroid
Association. *Endocr Pract.* 2012 Nov-Dec;18(6):988-1028.

Jameson J, Mandel SJ, Weetman AP, et al. Disorders of the thyroid gland. In: Kasper D, Fauci A, Hauser
S, Longo D, Jameson J, Loscalzo J, eds. *Harrison's Principles of Internal Medicine.* 19th ed. New York,
NY: McGraw-Hill Education; 2015. Available at: http://accessmedicine.mhmedical.com/. Accessed
May 24, 2015.

Knox MA. Thyroid nodules. *Am Fam Physician.* 2013 Aug 1; 88(3):193-196.

A 25-year-old G2P1 woman at 39-week estimated gestational age presents to the labor and delivery triage unit stating that her "water has broken." She reports having had a large gush of clear fluid followed by a constant leakage of fluid from her vagina. She subsequently started having uterine contractions approximately every 4 minutes. She has had an uncomplicated prenatal course with good prenatal care since 8-week gestation. Her prenatal records are available for review in the triage unit. Her first pregnancy resulted in the full-term delivery of a 7-lb 8-oz, healthy boy.

In the triage unit, she is placed on an external fetal monitor. Her blood pressure is 110/70 mm Hg, her pulse is 90 beats/min, and her temperature is 98.7°F (37.0°C). Her general examination is normal. Her abdomen is gravid, with a fundal height of 38 cm. The fetus has a cephalic presentation by Leopold maneuvers and an estimated fetal weight of 8 lb.

▶ What signs and tests could confirm the presence of rupture of membranes?
▶ On the fetal monitoring strip shown (Figure 16–1), what is the approximate baseline fetal heart rate? How often is she having uterine contractions?
▶ Her prenatal records reveal that she had a positive group B *Streptococcus* (GBS) vaginal culture at 36-week gestation. What therapy should be instituted at this time?

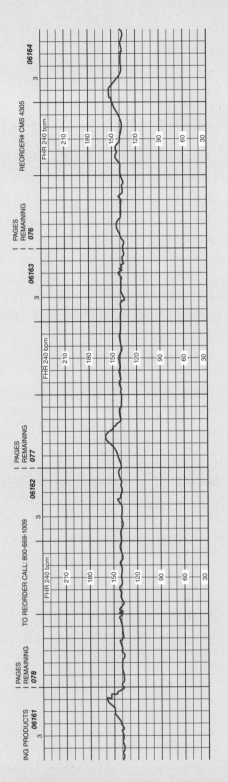
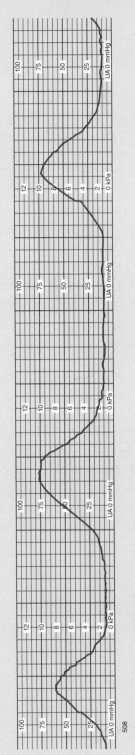

508

Figure 16–1. External Fetal Monitoring Strip.

ANSWERS TO CASE 16:
Labor and Delivery

Summary: A 25-year-old pregnant woman at term presents with the spontaneous rupture of membranes and subsequent uterine contractions, signaling the onset of labor.

- **Signs that could confirm the rupture of membranes:** Visualization of amniotic fluid leaking from the cervix; the presence of pooling of amniotic fluid in the posterior vaginal fornix; demonstration of a pH above 6.5 in fluid collected from the vagina using Nitrazine paper; or visualization of "ferning" on a sample of fluid on an air-dried microscope slide

- **Baseline fetal heart rate:** 140 beats/min

- **Contraction interval:** Approximately every 3 minutes

- **Recommended antibiotic prophylaxis for GBS colonization during labor:** Penicillin 5 million units IV loading dose followed by 2.5 million units IV every 4 hours; alternative treatments include IV ampicillin, cefazolin, clindamycin, and vancomycin

ANALYSIS

Objectives

1. Know the definition of labor, including the three stages of labor, understand the definitions and differences in the categories of fetal heart tracings, and know the normal progression of labor in nulliparous and multiparous women.

2. Understand the types of fetal monitoring that are routinely performed during labor and how monitoring correlates with the physiologic processes occurring during labor.

3. Be familiar with the abnormal progression of labor and some of the interventions that can be made to address these problems.

Considerations

This woman arrives at the labor and delivery triage unit in need of evaluation for the possibility that she is in labor and that she has ruptured her membranes (broken her bag of water). The accurate and appropriate diagnosis of labor is extremely important in obstetrical care. Incorrectly diagnosing a woman as being in labor may result in unnecessary interventions, whereas not diagnosing labor may result in complications or delivery occurring without access to appropriate personnel and facilities. Furthermore, the diagnosis of rupture of membranes is critical for several reasons. First, especially at term, the spontaneous rupture of membranes may signify the impending onset of labor. Second, if the presenting part is not well applied in the pelvis, prolapse of the umbilical cord with resultant compression of the cord and disruption of the oxygen supply to the fetus may occur. Finally, the prolonged rupture of membranes, especially after 24 hours or longer, may predispose to the development of infection.

The physician also must promptly make assessments of both maternal and fetal well-being. A careful history and physical examination should be performed. When available, prenatal records should be reviewed to evaluate for any problems during this, or previous, pregnancies and to confirm the gestational age of the pregnancy. In this case, the presence of GBS colonization requires the institution of appropriate antibiotic prophylaxis to reduce the risk of fetal infection with GBS, a common cause of neonatal morbidity and mortality. In GBS-colonized women, the recommended antibiotic prophylaxis is IV penicillin. When this is not available, ampicillin is often substituted. In penicillin-allergic women, cefazolin, clindamycin, or vancomycin can be used. Fetal well-being is most commonly monitored using external, electronic fetal-monitoring equipment, although other options are available. With this equipment, the baseline fetal heart rate, heart rate variability, accelerations and decelerations, along with the presence and frequency of uterine contractions, may be evaluated. Determination of the presentation of the fetus (cephalic, breech, or shoulder [ie, transverse lie]) is also critical, as this may play a significant role in the determination of route of delivery (vaginal or cesarean).

APPROACH TO:
Labor and Delivery

DEFINITIONS

FETAL LIE: The relationship of the long axis of the fetus to the long axis of the mother; either longitudinal or transverse

FETAL PRESENTATION: The part of the fetus that is either foremost in the birth canal or in closest proximity to the birth canal

LABOR: Regular uterine contractions that lead to the effacement and dilation of the cervix

PREMATURE RUPTURE OF MEMBRANES: Rupture of the fetal membranes prior to the onset of labor

CLINICAL APPROACH

Labor usually begins spontaneously and occurs normally within 2 weeks of the estimated date of confinement (280 days after the first day of the last menstrual period). The onset of labor more than 3 weeks before the estimated date of confinement (EDC) is considered preterm labor. If labor has not started spontaneously by 2 weeks after the EDC, the pregnancy is considered postterm.

Stages of Labor

Labor is typically divided into three stages. The **first stage of labor is from the onset of labor until the cervix is completely dilated**. This stage can further be divided into a latent phase and an active phase. During the latent phase of labor, the contractions become stronger, longer lasting, and more coordinated. The active phase of labor, which usually starts at 3 to 4 cm of cervical dilation, is when the rate of cervical dilation is at its maximum. Contractions are usually strong and regular. In active labor in a woman without an epidural, the minimum expected rates of cervical dilation are 1.2 cm per hour for a nulliparous woman and 1.5 cm per hour for a parous woman. The **second stage of labor is from complete cervical dilation (10 cm) through the delivery of the fetus.** The combination of the force of the uterine contractions and the pushing efforts of the mother results in the delivery of the baby. A normal second stage lasts less than 2 hours in a nulliparous patient and less than 1 hour in a parous patient. The presence of epidural anesthesia can prolong these times by up to 1 hour. The **third stage of labor begins after the delivery of the baby and ends with the delivery of the placenta and membranes.** The third stage is typically short and is considered prolonged if it lasts longer than 30 minutes.

The Progress of Labor

The progress of labor usually depends on the **"three Ps."** The **Power** is the strength of the uterine contractions during the active phase of labor and of the maternal pushing efforts during the second stage of labor. The power of the contractions can be assessed subjectively by an examiner palpating the uterus during a contraction or objectively by placing an intrauterine pressure catheter, which directly measures pressure within the uterine cavity. The **Passenger** is the fetus. Its size, lie, presentation, and position within the birth canal all play a role in the progression of labor and rate of fetal descent. Finally, the shape and size of the **Pelvis** can result in delay or failure of descent of the fetus because of the relative disproportion between the fetal and pelvic sizes.

The diagnosis of active labor is an indication for admission to the birthing unit for labor management and monitoring. The presence of ruptured membranes is also an indication for admission. The rupture of membranes can be confirmed by a careful vaginal examination performed with a sterile speculum and gloves. The visualization of fluid leaking from the cervical os, either spontaneously or with the patient performing a Valsalva maneuver, and the presence of amniotic fluid pooling in the posterior vaginal fornix are confirmatory. The detection of fluid in the vagina with a pH more than 6.5 is consistent with amniotic fluid, as normal vaginal secretions typically have a pH less than 5.5. Using a sterile applicator to sample vaginal fluid and applying it to Nitrazine paper can make this determination. The presence of semen, blood, or bacterial vaginosis can cause elevated pH in vaginal secretions and a false-positive Nitrazine test. The visualization of ferning of vaginal fluid under microscopic magnification of an air-dried sample also suggests the presence of amniotic fluid.

When the pregnant patient is admitted to the labor and delivery unit, **fetal well-being is assessed by either continuous or intermittent fetal heart rate monitoring.** Continuous external fetal heart rate monitoring is the more commonly used procedure in the United States. A Doppler ultrasound device is used to continuously trace the fetal heart rate. Continuous monitoring can also be accomplished using an internal device (fetal scalp electrode), by attaching an electrode to the fetal scalp that directly measures and amplifies fetal cardiac electrical activity. This procedure requires that the membranes are ruptured. With either of these two techniques, a continuous graphic recording of the fetal heart rate is recorded. Alternatively, intermittent auscultation using a stethoscope or handheld Doppler can be performed. The American College of Obstetricians and Gynecologists (ACOG) recommends that in intermittent auscultation of low-risk pregnancies, the fetal heart should be monitored after a contraction at least every 30 minutes during the first stage of labor and every 15 minutes in the second stage. In at-risk pregnancies, the monitoring frequency is increased to at least every 15 minutes during the first stage and to every 5 minutes in the second stage.

Important considerations in interpreting fetal heart rate data are the **baseline heart rate, variability,** and **periodic heart rate changes.** The baseline heart rate is the approximate average heart rate during a 10-minute tracing. A baseline heart rate of 110 to 160 beats/min is considered normal, less than 110 beats/min is considered to be bradycardia, and greater than 160 beats/min is considered to be tachycardia. Fetal bradycardia may occur with maternal hypothermia, certain medications given to the mother, congenital heart block, or may be a sign of significant fetal distress. Bradycardia may also be a normal variant. The most common cause of fetal tachycardia is maternal fever. Other common causes include medications and fetal arrhythmias.

Variability is regulated by the balance of sympathetic and parasympathetic control of the sinoatrial node. **Short-term variability** is the change in fetal heart rate from one beat to the next and can only be accurately determined when an internal scalp electrode is placed. Normal short-term variability is 6 to 25 beats/min. **Long-term variability** is the waviness of the baseline heart rate over 1 minute, with normal oscillations occurring at a rate of 3 to 5 cycles per minute. As variability is largely a manifestation of the autonomic nervous system, anything that affects nervous system functioning can affect it. Common causes of decreased variability are fetal sleep cycles, central nervous system (CNS) depressant drugs (such as narcotic analgesics) given to the mother, congenital neurologic abnormalities, and prematurity. Fetal acidemia secondary to hypoxemia can impair CNS function and reduce variability. The presence of normal variability makes fetal acidemia unlikely.

Periodic heart rate changes are the **accelerations** and **decelerations** from the baseline heart rate that occur, often related to uterine contractions. An acceleration is an increase in the fetal heart rate of 15 beats/min or more for 15 seconds or longer and is a reassuring finding. The presence of accelerations, whether occurring spontaneously or in response to contractions, fetal movement, or stimulation of the fetus (either scalp stimulation during a cervical examination or vibroacoustic stimulation using an artificial larynx) virtually ensures that the fetal arterial pH is greater than 7.2.

Decelerations are generally defined as **early, late,** or **variable** based on the timing of the deceleration in relation to a contraction. An **early deceleration** coincides with a contraction in onset of the fetal heart rate decline and return to the baseline. Early decelerations are thought to be a result of increased vagal tone caused by compression of the fetal head and are not associated with fetal hypoxia or acidemia. A **late deceleration** is a gradual reduction in the fetal heart rate that starts at or after the peak of a contraction and has a gradual return to the baseline. Late decelerations are a manifestation of uteroplacental insufficiency and can be caused by numerous circumstances. Common among these are maternal hypotension, as is often seen with epidural anesthesia and uterine hyperstimulation caused by oxytocin administration. Conditions that impair placental circulation, including maternal hypertension, diabetes, prolonged pregnancy, and placental abruption, often contribute to late decelerations. A **variable deceleration** is an abrupt decrease in fetal heart rate, usually followed by an abrupt return to baseline that occurs variably in its timing, relative to a contraction. Variable decelerations are the most common types of decelerations seen during fetal heart monitoring and are considered to be due to umbilical cord compression during contractions. Variable decelerations, particularly when there is also the presence of normal variability and accelerations, are usually not associated with fetal hypoxemia.

Current fetal monitoring equipment also allows for contraction monitoring along with the fetal heart rate assessment. An external tocodynamometer is most commonly used. It allows for evaluation of the presence and timing of contractions but does not measure the strength of the contractions. To assess the strength of contractions, an internal intrauterine pressure catheter (IUPC) can be placed. Like the fetal scalp electrode, this requires the presence of ruptured membranes. An IUPC can be useful when the first stage of labor is not progressing at an expected rate, as the frequency and power of contractions can be directly measured. Contractions that are inadequate in frequency or power may be augmented with an oxytocic agent. Intravenous oxytocin is the drug of choice, as it is effective, inexpensive, and most practitioners are familiar with its usage. Oxytocin has a short half-life, which allows it to be given by continuous infusion and allows for the rapid cessation of its activity when it is discontinued. Labor augmentation with oxytocin can cause uterine hyperstimulation, defined as the presence of six or more contractions in a 10-minute period that causes nonreassuring fetal heart rate abnormalities (such as late decelerations). This would be managed by reduction in dose or discontinuation of the oxytocin, repositioning of the patient, and providing oxygen via face mask to the mother.

Fetal heart tracings (FHT) can be categorized into three categories: I, II, and III, the determination of which further guides management. It is simplest to learn the definitions of categories I and III as category II tends to be everything in between. A category I FHT is considered normal and includes each of the five characteristics: a baseline heart rate of 110 to 160 beats/min, moderate baseline FHR variability, no late or variable decelerations, and both accelerations and early decelerations maybe absent or present. A category III FHT is considered abnormal and includes *either* absent baseline FHR variability plus any one of the following three: repeated late decelerations, variable decelerations or bradycardia, *or* a sinusoidal pattern. A category II FHT is considered indeterminable. This category includes a variety of findings, none of which can be categorized into I or III.

During labor, the fetal head descends through the birth canal and undergoes four **cardinal movements.** During initial descent, the head undergoes **flexion,** bringing the fetal chin to the chest. As descent progresses, **internal rotation** occurs, causing the fetal occiput to move anteriorly toward the maternal symphysis pubis. As the head approaches the vulva, it undergoes **extension,** to allow the head to pass below the symphysis pubis and through the upward-directed vaginal outlet. Further extension leads to the delivery of the head, which then restitutes via **external rotation** to face either to the maternal right or left side. This corresponds with rotation of the fetal body, aligning one shoulder anteriorly below the symphysis pubis and the other posterior toward the sacrum. Maternal pushing, along with gentle downward traction on the fetal head, will deliver the anterior shoulder, and upward traction similarly delivers the posterior shoulder. Delivery of the remainder of the body will quickly follow. Occasionally, the anterior shoulder will not readily pass below the pubic symphysis. This is called a **shoulder dystocia** and is an obstetrical emergency, requiring a coordinated effort by the entire medical team to reduce the dystocia. Maneuvers, including hyperflexion of the hips (McRoberts maneuver), suprapubic pressure, cutting an episiotomy, or rotation of the fetal body in the vaginal canal, are attempted and are usually successful.

Of deliveries in the United States, 20% or more are accomplished via cesarean delivery. The most common indications are a history of prior cesarean delivery, arrest of labor or descent, fetal distress necessitating immediate delivery, and breech presentation. Operative vaginal delivery can be performed using either forceps or vacuum assistance. These can only be used when the cervix is completely dilated, membranes are ruptured, the presenting part is the vertex of the scalp, and there is no disproportion between the size of the fetal head and maternal pelvis. If any of these conditions are not met and delivery must be accomplished urgently, a cesarean delivery is indicated.

GBS PROPHYLAXIS

GBS testing is routinely done between 35 and 37 weeks' gestational age. Testing is done by swabbing the vagina, perineum, and anus with a sterile culture applicator.

Current indications for GBS prophylaxis at the time of labor include the following:

- Positive GBS screen collected at 35+ weeks' gestational age
- History of invasive GBS infection in previous infant
- GBS bacteriuria at any time during the current pregnancy
- Unknown GBS status at time of labor plus one of the following:
  - Preterm labor (prior to 37 weeks)
  - Amniotic membrane rupture more than 18 hours
  - Intrapartum fever (temperature >100.4°F)
  - Intrapartum nucleic acid amplification test positive for GBS

Once the need for GBS prophylaxis is determined, an appropriate antibiotic must be given. If no allergy exists, penicillin is the recommended first-line agent. Alternatively, ampicillin could also be used, and this is often institution dependent. If there is no true allergy but intolerance to penicillin, cefazolin should be used. If the patient has a true allergy to penicillin, marked by urticaria, respiratory distress, angioedema, or anaphylaxis, susceptibility of the isolate to erythromycin or clindamycin should be tested. For isolates susceptible to the above alternatives, clindamycin is appropriate; in cases of resistance, vancomycin should be used.

> ## CASE CORRELATION
> - See also Case 4 (Prenatal Care).

COMPREHENSION QUESTIONS

16.1 A 21-year-old G1 woman is admitted to the labor unit with spontaneous rupture of membranes. On initial examination, her cervix is 5 cm dilated. Four hours later, her cervix remains unchanged. Which of the following is the most likely diagnosis?

A. Prolonged latent phase

B. Arrest of active phase

C. Arrest of descent

D. Prolonged third stage of labor

16.2 Which of the following is thought to be a result of compression of the fetal head?

A. Early decelerations

B. Variable decelerations

C. Late decelerations

D. Sinusoidal heart rate pattern

16.3 A pregnant woman with an estimated gestational age of 34 weeks presents to the labor triage unit with a clear vaginal discharge. On sterile speculum examination, you see a pool of watery fluid in the vagina. Microscopic examination reveals "ferning." She states she thinks her "water broke" about 4 hours ago. You determine that this patient is in preterm labor and have to make a decision regarding GBS prophylaxis. Her records indicate that she has had no prior infant with GBS disease and has never tested positive for GBS bacteriuria in current pregnancy. Which of the following is the best step in management of this patient?

A. Since she has no risk factors for GBS, she requires no prophylaxis.

B. She is in preterm labor and would automatically qualify for GBS prophylaxis.

C. A STAT vaginal-rectal GBS swab needs to be done at this time; if positive, GBS prophylaxis would need to be started.

D. Since it has not been more than 18 hours since rupture of membranes, the patient is not at risk for GBS colonization, and therefore nothing needs to be done at this time.

ANSWERS

16.1 **B.** The cervical dilation beyond 4 cm means active phase. No cervical change for 2 hours is defined as arrest of active phase.

16.2 **A.** Early decelerations are thought to be caused by fetal head compression. Variable decelerations are caused by cord compression and late decelerations by uteroplacental insufficiency.

16.3 **B.** One of the indications for GBS prophylaxis is unknown GBS status plus preterm labor. Since this patient is not 35 weeks yet, her GBS status is unknown as routine screening is done between 35 and 37 weeks. Rupture of membranes for less than 18 hours does not preclude her from receiving prophylaxis as she already has the indication of preterm labor that justifies beginning prophylaxis.

CLINICAL PEARLS

▶ The presence of accelerations on a fetal heart tracing is very reassuring and consistent with a fetal pH of greater than 7.2.

▶ The use of universal, prenatal screening for GBS and provision of intrapartum antibiotics to women who are colonized can reduce the risk of GBS disease in infants by approximately 50%. Routine screening is recommended at 35 to 37 weeks' gestation.

▶ Fetal heart rate tracings must be interpreted within the overall clinical situation. Reduction in variability shortly after giving a narcotic pain medication may represent fetal sleep cycle; reduction in variability along with repetitive late decelerations may be an ominous sign of fetal distress.

REFERENCES

Centers for Disease Control and Prevention. 2010 guidelines for the prevention of perinatal group B Streptococcal disease: recommendations and reports. *MMWR*. 2010;59(RR-10):14-36

Garite TJ. Intrapartum fetal evaluation. In: Gabbe SG, Niebyl JR, Simpson JL, eds. *Obstetrics: Normal and Problem Pregnancies*. 5th ed. New York, NY: Churchill Livingstone; 2007.

Parer JT, Ikeda T, King TL. The 2008 NICHD standard terminology of fetal heart rate monitoring. *Obstet Gynecol*. 2009 Jul;114(1):136-138.

Rouse DJ, St. John E. Normal labor, delivery, newborn care, and puerperium. In: Scott JR, Gibbs RS, Karlan BY, Haney AF, eds. *Danforth's Obstetrics and Gynecology*. 10th ed. Philadelphia, PA: Lippincott Williams & Wilkins; 2008.

A 58-year-old woman presents to your office for follow-up of an emergency department visit. She was seen 1 week earlier in the emergency department for abdominal pain and was diagnosed with nephrolithiasis. Ultimately, she was sent home with pain medications and given instructions to strain her urine for stones and to follow up with her primary care physician. Today, she is asymptomatic. She takes no medications on a regular basis. Her family history is significant only for a father with high blood pressure. She had several routine laboratory tests drawn in the emergency department, copies of which she brings with her. Upon your review of the laboratory values, you note the following (normal values are in parenthesis): sodium 142 mEq/L (135-145); potassium 4.0 mEq/L (3.5-5.0); chloride 104 mg/dL (95-105); bicarbonate 28 mEq/L (20-29); blood urea nitrogen (BUN) 20 mg/dL (7-20); creatinine 0.9 mg/dL (0.8-1.4); calcium 12.5 mg/dL (8.5-10.2); albumin 4.2 g/dL (3.4-5.4). The complete blood count (CBC) was within normal limits.

The renal calculus was detected by helical computed tomography (CT) scanning without contrast and was located in the right mid ureter.

Your patient has brought with her the stone that she has strained from the urine. Upon questioning, you learn that she has had multiple episodes of "kidney stones" in the past 2 years. You send the stone to the laboratory for analysis and order a repeat serum calcium level. The results show that the stone is made of calcium oxalate; the serum calcium is still elevated at 11.9 mg/dL.

▶ What is your diagnosis?
▶ What is the most likely cause?
▶ What is the next step?

ANSWERS TO CASE 17:
Electrolyte Disorders

Summary: This is a 58-year-old woman with a history of recurrent nephrolithiasis, presenting for follow-up and found to have calcium oxalate stones. She had an initial serum calcium level that was elevated, as was the repeat serum calcium 1 week later. At the time of her follow-up, she was completely asymptomatic. She takes no medications, and has a family history only significant for hypertension.

- **Diagnosis:** Hypercalcemia and recurrent nephrolithiasis
- **Most likely cause:** Hyperparathyroidism
- **Next step:** Further laboratory workup, including serum parathyroid hormone (PTH) level

ANALYSIS
Objectives

1. Be able to list common causes of calcium, sodium, and potassium disorders.
2. Describe the workup and management of common electrolyte disorders.

Considerations

This patient illustrates one common presentation of hypercalcemia. Many times, patients with hypercalcemia are asymptomatic and an elevated calcium level is found unexpectedly on routine laboratory studies. The diagnostic workup begins with a careful review of the patient's history, as clues to its etiology may often be elicited here. The diagnostic workup is designed to distinguish parathyroid dysfunction from other etiologies so that optimal treatment and management can be pursued.

APPROACH TO:
Electrolyte Disorders

DEFINITIONS

HYPERPARATHYROIDISM: Condition of elevated parathyroid hormone usually due to excessive production by the parathyroid glands, leading to hypercalcemia.

SECONDARY HYPERPARATHYROIDISM: Condition as the parathyroid glands overproduce PTH to respond to low serum calcium levels. This may occur as a response to low dietary calcium intake or a deficiency of vitamin D.

TERTIARY HYPERPARATHYROIDISM: Elevated PTH in patients who have renal failure.

CLINICAL APPROACH

Pathophysiology of Calcium Homeostasis

Before discussing the differential diagnosis of hypercalcemia, it is essential to review the basic mechanism by which normal calcium levels are maintained in the body. **Most of the calcium in the body is found in the skeleton** (approximately 98%). The remaining calcium is found in circulation. Of this remaining 2%, about half is bound to albumin and other proteins, and half is "free," or ionized. It is the ionized calcium that has physiologic effects. Because the serum calcium is partially bound to albumin, abnormally low serum albumin levels will affect the measurement of calcium, thus causing a misinterpretation of an abnormal calcium level. With patients found to have a concomitant hypoalbuminemia, the ionized calcium can be measured directly. However, there is a useful formula that can correct this error. A "corrected" serum calcium is provided by the formula:

$$\text{"Corrected" serum calcium} = [0.8 \times (\text{Normal albumin}) - (\text{Patient's albumin level})] + (\text{Serum calcium})$$

PTH, calcitonin, and 1,25-dihydroxyvitamin D_3 (calcitriol) are responsible for regulating calcium levels and maintaining calcium homeostasis. **Causes of hypercalcemia include an increase in calcium resorption from bone, decreased renal excretion of calcium, or an increase in calcium absorption from the gastrointestinal tract.** When calcium levels increase, calcitonin, produced by the thyroid parafollicular cells, attempts to lower calcium levels through renal excretion of calcium and by opposing osteoclast activation. When calcium is excreted through this pathway, phosphate is also excreted. Conversely, low levels of circulating calcium normally result in PTH secretion. This promotes osteoclast activation, which mobilizes calcium from bone and effects calcium resorption at the kidneys, thereby retaining circulating calcium. While PTH will increase the calcium in the blood, it has the opposite effect on serum phosphate levels. PTH also increases calcitriol levels, which act at the gastrointestinal tract to promote both calcium and phosphate absorption.

HYPERCALCEMIA

Etiology

Any process that increases gastrointestinal calcium absorption, decreases renal excretion, or activates osteoclastic activity will raise serum calcium levels. If this occurs beyond the normal bounds of maintaining calcium homeostasis, hypercalcemia will occur. **The most common cause of hypercalcemia in the ambulatory patient is hyperparathyroidism.** Cancer is the second leading cause. Hyperparathyroidism and cancer combined account for 90% of hypercalcemia cases. It is useful to categorize the etiologies of hypercalcemia into five main areas: parathyroid hormone-related, malignancy, renal failure, high bone turnover, and those related to vitamin D (Table 17–1).

Clinical Manifestations of Hypercalcemia

Normal values of serum calcium range from 8 to 10 mg/dL. Levels of serum calcium between 10.5 and 12 mg/dL are classified as mild hypercalcemia and patients

Table 17–1 • COMMON CAUSES OF HYPERCALCEMIA

Condition	Specific Example	Pathophysiology
Increased Bone Resorption		
Primary hyperparathyroidism	Sporadic or familial; multiple endocrine neoplasia (types 1 and II)	
Malignancy	Solid tumors of lung; squamous carcinoma of head and neck; renal carcinoma	Tumor secretion of **PTH-rP**
	Breast cancer; multiple myeloma; prostate cancer	Direct osteolysis
Hypervitaminosis A (vitamin A intoxication)	Includes both vitamin A and its analogs (used to treat acne)	Increased bone resorption
Immobilization	Less common than above causes	Increased risk when underlying disorder of high bone turnover (eg, Paget disease)
Increased Calcium Absorption		
Hypervitaminosis D (vitamin D intoxication)		Increased calcitriol level leads to increased GI absorption of calcium and phosphate
Granulomatous disease	Tuberculosis; sarcoidosis; Hodgkin disease	Increase extrarenal conversion of 25-hydroxyvitamin D_3 to calcitriol
Milk alkali syndrome		Excessive intake of calcium-containing antacids
Miscellaneous		
Medications	Thiazide diuretics lithium	Reduced urinary excretion of calcium; increased PTH secretion
Rhabdomyolysis		Calcium released from injured muscle
Adrenal insufficiency		Increased bone resorption and increased protein binding of calcium
Thyrotoxicosis (usually mild hypercalcemia)		Increased bone resorption

Abbreviation: PTH-rP, parathyroid hormone-related peptide.

are typically asymptomatic at these levels. As calcium levels increase, physical manifestations may become apparent. The classic mnemonic "stones, bones, psychic groans, and abdominal moans" is useful to categorize the constellation of physical symptoms associated with hypercalcemia (Table 17–2). Other clinical manifestations include the cardiac sequelae of shortening QT interval and arrhythmias.

Diagnostic Approach

The first step in the evaluation is a careful history to try to establish a cause and to assess for manifestations. The history should include family history of calcium disorders, such as renal stones or malignancy. The patient's risk factors for malignancy, such as smoking, should be investigated. The chronicity of symptom should

Table 17–2 • PHYSICAL MANIFESTATIONS OF HYPERCALCEMIA	
	Symptoms/Signs
Stones	Renal calculi
Bones	Bone pain, including arthritis and osteoporosis
Psychic groans	Poor concentration, weakness, fatigue, stupor, coma
Abdominal moans	Abdominal pain, constipation, nausea, vomiting, pancreatitis, anorexia

be taken in account; more acute symptoms suggest malignancy over hyperparathyroidism and vice versa. A careful review of medications should also take place, to include not only prescription medications but also over-the-counter supplements. Dietary intake of vitamin D and calcium should be questioned. Furthermore, history of immobilization secondary to hospital stay or recent injury should be looked into as prolonged immobilization can cause massive bone demineralization and hypercalcemia. At this point, if the hypercalcemia is mild and the patient is asymptomatic, it is acceptable to stop any suspect medication(s) and repeat the serum calcium level.

If a causative medication is not found, serum intact PTH level should be measured. This level will either be suppressed, normal, or elevated. As with many endocrine disorders, **it is useful not to think of normal or abnormal values; rather, one should understand what is appropriate for a given situation.** For example, in normal subjects, an increased calcium load will normally depress the PTH hormone level, thus a low PTH level in this situation is *normal*, or appropriately suppressed. If a patient has an elevated calcium level and the PTH is "normal," it is said to be inappropriately normal, because in the face of hypercalcemia it should be low, or suppressed.

If a patient with hypercalcemia has a normal or elevated PTH level, then the normal feedback loop is not responding. This defines hyperparathyroidism. Primary hyperparathyroidism occurs when the parathyroid gland overproduces PTH and does not respond to the negative feedback of elevated calcium levels. **The vast majority of primary hyperparathyroidism is caused by an adenoma (benign tumor) of one of the four parathyroid glands.**

Secondary hyperparathyroidism occurs as the parathyroid glands overproduce PTH to respond to low serum calcium levels. This may occur as a response to low dietary calcium intake or a deficiency of vitamin D. Tertiary hyperparathyroidism occurs in patients who have renal failure. Patients in renal failure initially present with *hypo*calcemia, hyperphosphatemia, and low vitamin D levels. If untreated, it leads to hyperplasia of the parathyroid glands, an increased PTH secretion, and subsequent hypercalcemia.

There is a condition that can produce inappropriately high PTH levels unrelated to the parathyroid production. This is familial hypocalciuric hypercalcemia (FHH), a genetic disorder related to a defect in a gene that codes for a calcium-sensing receptor. Consequently, simply measuring PTH alone may confound this diagnosis, which may be mistaken for primary hyperparathyroidism. To distinguish these entities, a 24-hour urinary calcium level is obtained. In hyperparathyroidism, the kidneys spill calcium into the urine at a normal or elevated level. With FHH, the urinary calcium level is low.

A PTH level that is low with elevated serum calcium suggests that the parathyroid gland is responding appropriately to the high calcium environment. This is seen when tumors produce a hormone that mimics the active site of the PTH molecule. This molecule is called parathyroid hormone-related peptide (PTH-rP). PTH-rP is produced by lung cancers, squamous cell cancers of the head and neck, and renal cell cancer. PTH-rP effects osteoclastic bone resorption, increases calcitriol, and promotes calcium resorption from the kidneys, resulting in increased levels of serum calcium. The continued production of PTH-rP effectively takes the parathyroid gland out of the loop in calcium homeostasis. Because cancer is a common etiology for hypercalcemia, the **search for malignancy is paramount at this step in diagnosis, before other, less common, disorders are considered.**

If a malignancy is not found, other etiologies must be considered. These fall into the category of endocrine disorders other than parathyroid and include hyperthyroidism, adrenal insufficiency, and acromegaly. The workup thus includes thyroid-stimulating hormone (TSH), a cortisol level, and a pituitary imaging study, respectively.

TREATMENT OF HYPERCALCEMIA

The **treatment of hypercalcemia is directed at the underlying disorder.** Patients with mild hypercalcemia may be treated with preventative measures aimed at avoiding aggravating factors. These measures include adequate hydration (dehydration aggravates nephrolithiasis), avoiding thiazide diuretics or other offending medications, encouraging physical activity, and avoiding prolonged inactivity.

For the treatment of primary hyperparathyroidism, surgical parathyroidectomy is the definitive treatment. Surgery is appropriate for patients with symptomatic hyperparathyroidism. Surgery may be an option for selected asymptomatic patients, including those who have developed osteoporosis or renal insufficiency, who have markedly elevated calcium levels, or who are younger than age 50.

Approach to Urgency in Acute Hypercalcemia

The most serious manifestations of hypercalcemia occur in the form of dysrhythmias and coma. In situations like these, it is imperative to correct the hypercalcemia while simultaneously doing workup to understand the etiology. Management includes rehydration as the first step with IV 0.9% saline 4 to 6 L in 24 hours. After rehydration, IV bisphosphonates should be used, keeping in mind that the dose and time over which these are administered must be decreased in renally impaired patients.

SODIUM DISORDERS

Hyponatremia

Hyponatremia is defined as a plasma [Na+] less than 135 mEq/L. It is a disorder of water balance that primarily causes neurologic symptoms due to a lowered serum osmolality that promotes water movement into brain cells. In hyponatremic states, total body sodium and total body water can be low, normal or high, so assessment of the patient's overall volume state and osmolality is critical to the diagnosis and management. Although most patients with hyponatremia are asymptomatic, early symptoms may manifest as nausea, vomiting, lethargy in acute cases. As most cases of hyponatremia present with a low serum osmolality (<280 mOsm), evaluation of the patient's volume status will help determine possible causes and guide therapy, as presented below:

1. Hypovolemic hyponatremia—Exhibits signs of volume depletion on physical examination with urinary sodium levels less than 20 mEq/L. Common causes include cerebral salt wasting, skin loss, diuretic use, gastrointestinal (GI) losses, mineralocorticoid deficiency, and third-spacing of fluids. The treatment is volume repletion with normal saline and addressing the underlying condition. Severe symptomatic hyponatremia, which can manifest as confusion, coma, or seizures, are usually observed with serum sodium less than 125 mEq/L and warrants urgent treatment with hypertonic (3%) saline. Often, very small corrections in serum sodium will improve the symptoms. It is recommended to correct the sodium level slowly to avoid the risk of osmotic demyelination, which can result in permanent neurologic injury and death.

2. Hypervolemic hyponatremia—Exhibits signs of volume expansion on examination due to decreased renal excretion of water. Common causes include heart failure, cirrhosis, and nephrosis. The treatment is use of diuretics and restriction of fluid and sodium intake.

3. Euvolemic hyponatremia—Antidiuretic hormone (ADH) is normally secreted in response to low volume states, resulting in retention of free water. The syndrome of inappropriate antidiuretic hormone secretion (SIADH) occurs when ADH is secreted independently of volume status, resulting in the inappropriate retention of free water with resultant hyponatremia and hypotonicity. SIADH is a common complication of many conditions, including infections, malignancies, medications, and central nervous system disorders (See Table 17–3). The treatment of SIADH involves fluid restriction and, when possible, correction of the underlying condition. Other, less common causes of euvolemic hyponatremia include water intoxication, hypothyroidism, and low solute intake.

Another cause of low plasma [Na+] that should also be considered is pseudohyponatremia. In this scenario, the observed low sodium levels may be appropriate for the given clinical situation, such as in the setting hyperglycemia, hypertriglyceridemia, hyperproteinemia, laboratory errors, or mannitol use. In this situation, patients usually have a normal volume status with normal osmolality.

Hypernatremia

Hypernatremia is defined as a plasma [Na+] greater than 145 mEq/L, and reflects a state of increased serum osmolality that promotes water movement out of cells. The condition is usually due to net water loss that is often associated with an impaired thirst response or restricted access to water (eg, in the elderly, young infants, and intubated patients). Symptoms are primarily neurologic, just like hyponatremia,

Table 17-3 • CAUSES OF SYNDROME OF INAPPROPRIATE ADH SECRETION

Central nervous system disorders
  Head trauma
  Stroke
  Subarachnoid hemorrhage
  Hydrocephalus
  Brain tumor
  Encephalitis
  Guillain-Barré syndrome
  Meningitis
  Acute psychosis
  Acute intermittent porphyria
Pulmonary lesions
  Tuberculosis
  Bacterial pneumonia
  Aspergillosis
  Bronchiectasis
  Neoplasms
  Positive-pressure ventilation
Malignancies
  Bronchogenic carcinoma
  Pancreatic carcinoma
  Prostatic carcinoma
  Renal cell carcinoma
  Adenocarcinoma of colon
  Thymoma
  Osteosarcoma
  Lymphoma
  Leukemia
Drugs
  Increased ADH production
    Antidepressants: tricyclics, monoamine oxidase inhibitors, SSRIs
    Antineoplastics: cyclophosphamide, vincristine
    Carbamazepine
    Methylenedioxymethamphetamine (MDMA; Ecstasy)
    Clofibrate
    Neuroleptics: thiothixene, thioridazine, fluphenazine, haloperidol, trifluoperazine
  Potentiated ADH action
    Carbamazepine
    Chlorpropamide, tolbutamide
    Cyclophosphamide
    NSAIDs
    Somatostatin and analogs
    Amiodarone
Others
  Postoperative
  Pain
  Stress
  AIDS
  Pregnancy (physiologic)
  Hypokalemia

Abbreviations: ADH, antidiuretic hormone; NSAIDs, nonsteroidal anti-inflammatory drugs; SSRIs, selective serotonin reuptake inhibitors.
Reproduced, with permission, from Papadakis MA, McPhee SJ, Rabow MW. Current Medical Diagnosis & Treatment. New York, NY: McGraw-Hill Education; 2015. Table 21-2.

and manifest as anorexia, muscle weakness, nausea, vomiting, and lethargy, which may lead to seizures and coma in severe cases.

The most important first step in assessing patients with hypernatremia is to check the urine osmolality. A high urine osmolality (>400 mOsm/kg) suggests the body's ability to conserve water is intact and that water losses are due to hypotonic fluid loss (eg, excessive sweating, GI losses, etc). A low urine osmolality (<300 mOsm/kg) suggests pure water loss as seen in diabetes insipidus (DI), which is further broken down into nephrogenic DI (renal resistance to action of antidiuretic hormone) and central DI (lack of antidiuretic hormone production). Treatment involves correcting the underlying condition and the deficit in water. As with hyponatremia, hypernatremia should be cautiously corrected, as rapid correction leads to cerebral edema due to intracellular fluid shifts.

POTASSIUM DISORDERS

Hypokalemia

Hypokalemia is defined as a plasma [K+] less than 3.5 mEq/L. The potential causes of hypokalemia are numerous, but are generally broken down into several categories: decreased net intake, intracellular shifts (eg, alkalosis, excess insulin), and renal losses or extrarenal losses (see Table 17–4).

Patients present with fatigue, muscle aches, ascending muscular weakness, or cramps that, in severe cases, can lead to paralysis or rhabdomyolysis. ECG changes may be seen in hypokalemia but are not well-correlated with serum potassium concentration. Hypokalemia can lead to ST-segment depression, flattened T waves, and prominent U waves. The therapeutic goals are to prevent life-threatening complications (eg, arrhythmias, respiratory failure), to correct the potassium deficit, and to identify and treat the underlying condition. In most cases, potassium deficits are best corrected by oral potassium replacement. IV potassium should be reserved for profound deficits and for persons unable to take oral medications.

Hyperkalemia

Hyperkalemia is defined as a plasma [K+] greater than 5.0 mEq/L. Causes of hyperkalemia are commonly caused by the following:

- Medications including angiotensin-converting enzyme inhibitors, angiotensin receptor blockers, and potassium-sparing diuretics
- Shifts from intracellular to extracellular spaces including acidosis, insulin deficiency, and burns
- Reduced renal excretion of potassium including renal insufficiency/failure, Addison disease, and renal tubular acidosis type IV

It is also important to consider pseudohyperkalemia as a possible cause of elevated plasma potassium, especially in the setting of possible laboratory error, hemolysis, or traumatic venipuncture.

Symptoms that may be present in true hyperkalemia include weakness, ascending flaccid paralysis, paresthesias, areflexia, ileus, and in severe cases, can lead to

Table 17–4 • CAUSES OF HYPOKALEMIA

Decreased potassium intake
Potassium shift into the cell
  Increased postprandial secretion of insulin
  Alkalosis
  Trauma (via β-adrenergic stimulation?)
  Periodic paralysis (hypokalemic)
  Barium intoxication
Renal potassium loss
  Increased aldosterone (mineralocorticoid) effects
    Primary hyperaldosteronism
    Secondary aldosteronism (dehydration, heart failure)
    Renovascular hypertension
    Malignant hypertension
    Ectopic ACTH-producing tumor
    Gitelman syndrome
    Bartter syndrome
    Cushing syndrome
    Licorice (European)
    Renin-producing tumor
    Congenital abnormality of steroid metabolism (eg, adrenogenital syndrome, 17-α-hydroxylase
      defect, apparent mineralocorticoid excess, 11-β-hydroxylase deficiency)
  Increased flow to distal nephron
    Diuretics (furosemide, thiazides)
    Salt-losing nephropathy
  Hypomagnesemia
    Unreabsorbable anion
    Carbenicillin, penicillin
  Renal tubular acidosis (type I or II)
    Fanconi syndrome
    Interstitial nephritis
    Metabolic alkalosis (bicarbonaturia)
  Congenital defect of distal nephron
    Liddle syndrome
Extrarenal potassium loss
  Vomiting, diarrhea, laxative abuse
  Villous adenoma, Zollinger-Ellison syndrome

Reproduced, with permission, from Papadakis MA, McPhee SJ, Rabow MW. Current Medical Diagnosis & Treatment. New York, NY: McGraw-Hill Education; 2015. Table 21–3.

respiratory failure. The most serious effect of hyperkalemia is the risk of cardiac arrhythmias. ECG changes that are characteristic to hyperkalemia include peaked T waves, flattening of P waves, and widening of QRS complexes.

Acute management of hyperkalemia in the setting of ECG changes, rapid rise in plasma potassium levels, and the presence of significant acidosis include (1) stabilizing the myocardium with IV calcium to decrease the risk of arrhythmias; (2) shifting potassium into cells to decrease plasma concentration by the administration of glucose and insulin; and (3) eventually lowering total body K+ with Kayexalate, loop diuretics, or dialysis. Long-term treatment of hyperkalemia should address the underlying cause (such as discontinuation of a suspect medication), patient counseling on low-potassium diets, and use of diuretics to promote excretion of potassium.

> ## CASE CORRELATION
> - See also Case 10 (Acute Diarrhea).

COMPREHENSION QUESTIONS

17.1 A 56-year-old Asian woman with history of hypertension, diabetes, and newly diagnosed polycystic kidney disease presents for follow-up for hypertension. Routine laboratory work shows elevated calcium of 13 mg/dL and an elevated phosphate level. The patient denies weight loss, is taking only metoprolol for her blood pressure, and denies recent history of immobilization. Given as above, which etiology of hypercalcemia would you be most concerned about in this patient?

A. Primary hyperparathyroidism as this is the most common etiology of hypercalcemia

B. Iatrogenic hypercalcemia secondary to medications

C. A primary vitamin D deficiency given her age

D. Secondary hyperparathyroidism due to renal disease

17.2 A 48-year-old man presents for follow-up of an elevated calcium level of 12.3 mg/dL found on routine screening laboratory tests at his last well-man visit. He takes no medications other than an occasional antihistamine for allergies. He recently started smoking a half-pack of cigarettes per day. He was prompted to attend to his well-man visit by his wife who claims that he has become forgetful, has a decreased appetite, and has had a 10-lb weight loss over the past 2 months. As part of his follow-up laboratory tests, you obtain a serum PTH, which comes back within the normal range. Which of the following is the next step in diagnosis?

A. Chest x-ray

B. Repeat calcium after hydration

C. Measurement of PTH-rP levels

D. Measurement of urinary calcium excretion

17.3 An 80-year-old woman is brought to the emergency room (ER) with altered mental status and fever. She is awake and cooperative but is not oriented to time or place. Her blood pressure is normal, her pulse is normal, and her temperature is 101°F. She is found to have pneumonia. Laboratory testing reveals a sodium level of 130 mEq/L but otherwise normal electrolytes. Which of the following is the most appropriate treatment for her?

A. IV antibiotic only

B. IV antibiotic and aggressive rehydration with IV normal saline

C. IV antibiotic and fluid restriction

D. IV antibiotic and IV 3% saline

17.4 A 65-year-old dialysis patient is found to have a serum potassium level of 6.8 mEq/L, which is verified on a STAT repeat level. An ECG shows peaked T waves and a widened QRS complex. What is the first intervention that should be made at this point?

A. IV glucose and insulin administration

B. Arrangement for a dialysis treatment

C. Oral Kayexalate given

D. IV furosemide

E. IV calcium

ANSWERS

17.1 **D.** Secondary hyperparathyroidism occurs in patients with early renal disease when due to hyperphosphatemia, hypocalcemia, and impaired production of 1,25-dihydroxyvitamin D by the failing kidneys, PTH levels increase abnormally, causing in turn elevated levels of calcium. In this disorder therefore you would see increased PTH and increased calcium, signaling a disruption of the normal feedback cycle.

17.2 **D.** This patient has symptomatic hypercalcemia. He has an inappropriately normal PTH level, which should be suppressed with this degree of hypercalcemia. The next step is to measure a 24-hour urinary calcium excretion to determine if this condition represents primary hyperparathyroidism (most common) or familial hypocalciuric hypercalcemia (rare).

17.3 **C.** This is a common presentation of SIADH due to pneumonia. This patient is euvolemic, so aggressive rehydration is not necessary. Treatment of the underlying pneumonia is key, so antibiotics must be given. With a sodium level of 130 mg/dL, the use of 3% saline is not necessary. The electrolyte abnormality should correct with treatment of the pneumonia and with fluid restriction.

17.4 **E.** This patient has hyperkalemia with cardiac changes—an acute, life-threatening condition. The first intervention should be to give IV calcium to stabilize the cardiac membranes and reduce the risk of arrhythmia. After this, interventions can be made to lower the potassium level.

CLINICAL PEARLS

▶ Be sure to question any patient with hypercalcemia regarding all medications—both prescription and over-the-counter—as both megadose vitamins (A and D) and excessive use of calcium carbonate antacids may play a role.

▶ Hypercalcemia with a suppressed PTH should be considered malignancy until you can prove otherwise.

▶ Assess the volume status in patients with hyponatremia to help determine the cause and guide therapy.

▶ ECG Changes in the setting of hyperkalemia require urgent treatment.

REFERENCES

Bartstow C, Braun M, Psyzocha N. Diagnosis and management of sodium disorders: hyponatremia and hypernatremia. *Am Fam Physician.* 2015;91(5):299-307.

Calvert J, Hollander-Rodriguez J. Hyperkalemia. *Am Fam Physician.* 2006;73:283-290.

Carroll M, Schade D. A practical approach to hypercalcemia. *Am Fam Physician.* 2003;67:1959-1966.

Chow KM, Szeto CC. An unusual cause of hypercalcemia. *South Med J.* 2004;97(6):588-589.

Potts JT, Jüppner H. Disorders of the parathyroid gland and calcium homeostasis. In: Kasper D, Fauci A, Hauser S, Longo D, Jameson J, Loscalzo J, eds. *Harrison's Principles of Internal Medicine.* 19th ed. New York, NY: McGraw-Hill Education; 2015. Available at: http://accessmedicine.mhmedical.com. Accessed May 9, 2015.

Society for Endocrinology, Emergency Endocrine Guidance. Acute hypercalcaemia. Available at: http://www.endocrinology.org/policy/docs/13-02_EmergencyGuidance-AcuteHypercalcaemia.pdf. Accessed May 9, 2015.

Taniegra ET. Hyperparathyroidism. *Am Fam Physician.* 2004;69:333-340.

A 75-year-old white man presents for a health maintenance checkup. The patient has stable hypertension but has not seen a physician in more than 2 years. He denies any particular problem. He lives alone. He takes an aspirin a day and is compliant with his blood pressure medication (hydrochlorothiazide). His son fears that his father is either experiencing a stroke or getting Alzheimer disease because he is having trouble understanding what family members are saying, especially during social events. The son reported no noticeable weakness or gait impairment. On physical examination, the patient's blood pressure was 130/80 mm Hg. Examination of the ears showed no cerumen impaction and normal tympanic membranes. His general examination is normal. Laboratory studies, including thyroid-stimulating hormone (TSH), are normal.

▶ What is the most likely diagnosis?
▶ What is the next step?

ANSWERS TO CASE 18:
Geriatric Health Maintenance

Summary: A 75-year-old man who presents with loss of speech discrimination and complains of difficulty understanding speech and conversation in noisy areas.

- **Most likely diagnosis:** Presbycusis.

- **Next step:** Presbycusis is a diagnosis of exclusion. Hearing aids are underused in presbycusis, but are potentially beneficial for most types of hearing loss, including sensorineural hearing loss. Consequently, referral to an audiologist for testing and consideration of amplification with a hearing aid may be an important next step.

ANALYSIS

Objectives

1. Be familiar with geriatric health maintenance.

2. Be aware of the importance of geriatric screening.

Considerations

The patient described in this case is a 75-year-old man who has difficulty with speech discrimination and complains of difficulty understanding speech and conversation in noisy areas. He most likely has presbycusis, which is an age-related sensorineural hearing loss typically associated with both selective high-frequency loss and difficulty with speech discrimination. Physical examination of the ears in patients with presbycusis is normal. Other conditions in the differential diagnosis include cerumen impaction, otosclerosis, and central auditory processing disorder. Cerumen impaction and otosclerosis can be diagnosed by otoscopy. Central auditory processing disorder is diagnosed when the patient can hear sounds without difficulty, but has difficulty in understanding spoken words.

APPROACH TO:
Health Maintenance in the Elderly

DEFINITIONS

PRESBYCUSIS: An age-related sensorineural hearing loss typically associated with both selective high-frequency loss and difficulty with speech discrimination.

FUNCTIONAL ASSESSMENT: An evaluation process that gauges a patient's ability to manage tasks of self-care, household management, and mobility.

CLINICAL APPROACH

By the year 2030, the number of people aged 65 and older is expected to double from what it was in 1999, increasing from 34 to 69 million. Geriatric health maintenance provides screening and therapy with the goal of enhancing function and preserving health in the elderly. Screening is not indicated unless early therapy for the screened condition is more effective than late therapy or no therapy. **Preventive services for the elderly include as goals the optimization of quality of life, satisfaction with life, and maintenance of independence and productivity.** Most recommendations for patients older than age 65 overlap with recommendations for the general adult population. Certain categories are unique to older patients, including sensory perception and fall. The primary care physician can perform effective health screening using simple and relatively easily administered assessment tools (Figure 18–1).

Functional Assessment

Functional assessment gauges a patient's ability to manage tasks of self-care, household management, and mobility. Impairment in activities of daily living (ADL) results in an increased risk of falls, hip fracture, depression, and institutionalization. An estimated **25% of patients older than 65 years have impairments in their**

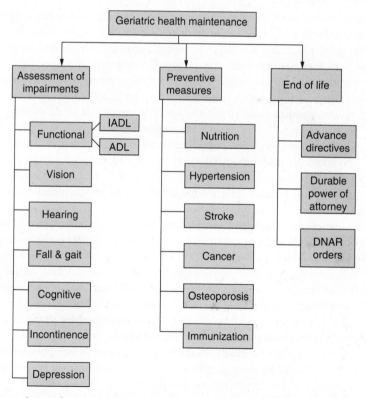

Figure 18–1. Approach to geriatric health maintenance. ADL, activities of daily living; DNAR, do not attempt resuscitation; IADL, instrumental activities of daily living.

Table 18–1 • INSTRUMENTAL ACTIVITIES OF DAILY LIVING (IADL) AND ACTIVITIES OF DAILY LIVING (ADL)	
IADL	**ADL**
Transportation	Bathing
Shopping	Dressing
Cooking	Eating
Using the telephone	Transferring from bed to chair
Managing money	Continence
Taking medications	Toileting
Housecleaning	Grooming
Laundry	

instrumental activities of daily living (IADL) or ADL (Table 18–1). Persons who are unable to perform IADL independently are far more likely to have dementia than their independent counterparts.

Vision Screening

Visual impairment is an independent risk factor for falls, which has a significant impact on quality of life. The majority of conditions leading to vision loss in the elderly are presbyopia, macular degeneration, glaucoma, cataract, and diabetic retinopathy. For older patients with risk factors for cataracts and age-related macular degeneration (AMD) including vision changes, smoking, diabetes, steroid use and family history, visual acuity testing with Snellen chart would be of benefit for identifying visual impairment and is a reasonable initial test to do in the primary care setting. However, United States Preventive Services Task Force (USPSTF) has found insufficient evidence regarding beneficial functional outcomes in the elderly who routinely undergo visual acuity testing. Visual acuity testing does not accurately identify ocular diseases that affect the elderly including cataracts, glaucoma and AMD, so routine referrals for ophthalmologic examination should be considered.

The incidence of presbyopia increases with age. Patients have difficulty focusing on near objects while their distant vision remains intact. **AMD is the leading cause of severe vision loss in the elderly.** AMD is characterized by atrophy of cells in the central macular region of the retinal pigment epithelium, resulting in the loss of central vision. Treatment options for exudative AMD include laser photocoagulation, and intravitreal injections of vascular endothelial growth factor.

Glaucoma is characterized by a group of optic neuropathies that can occur in all ages. Although glaucoma is most often associated with elevated intraocular pressure, it is the optic neuropathy that defines the disease. For patients who are asymptomatic, USPSTF found insufficient evidence to routinely screen for glaucoma. However, for elderly patients with risk factors including increased intraocular pressure, family history, vision changes, or African-American race, screening would be of benefit.

Cataract is any opacification of the lens. Age-related, or senile, cataracts account for 90% of all cataracts. **Cataract disease is the most common cause of blindness worldwide.** The definitive treatment for cataracts is surgery. Diabetic retinopathy is the leading cause of blindness in working-age adults in the United States. It is important to consider diabetic retinopathy in geriatric vision screening.

Hearing Screening

More than one-third of persons older than age 65 and half of those older than age 85 have some hearing loss. This deficit is correlated with social isolation and depression. The whispered voice test has sensitivities and specificities ranging from 70% to 100%. The initial office screening for general hearing loss can be reliably performed with questionnaire such as the HHIE-S (Hearing Handicap Inventory for the Elderly). Limited office-based pure-tone audiometry is more accurate in identifying patients who would benefit from a more formal audiometry.

The majority of patients with hearing impairment will present with complaints unrelated to their sensory deficit. In a quiet examination room with face-to-face conversation, patients can overcome significant hearing loss and avoid detection from a physician. Family members are often more concerned about the hearing loss than the patient. **Common causes of geriatric hearing impairments are presbycusis, noise-induced hearing loss, cerumen impaction, otosclerosis, and central auditory processing disorder.** Presbycusis is age-related sensorineural hearing loss usually associated with both selective high-frequency loss and difficulty with speech discrimination. Presbycusis is the most common form of hearing loss in the elderly. Because it often goes unrecognized, exact prevalence data are lacking. Presbycusis is a diagnosis of exclusion. Complete deafness is not an expected end result of presbycusis. Noise-induced hearing loss is essentially a wear and tear phenomenon that can occur with either industrial or recreational noise exposure. Patients will typically present with tinnitus, difficulty with speech discrimination, and problems hearing background noise. Cerumen impaction in the external auditory canal is a common, frequently overlooked problem in the elderly that may produce a transient, mild conductive hearing loss. It is estimated that 25% to 35% of institutionalized or hospitalized elderly are affected by impacted cerumen. Otosclerosis is an autosomal dominant disorder of the bones in the inner ear. It results in progressive conductive hearing loss with onset most commonly in the late twenties to the early forties. Speech discrimination is typically preserved. Geriatric patients with hearing loss may have otosclerosis complicating their presentation. Central auditory processing disorder (CAPD) is the general term for conditions involving hearing impairment that results from central nervous system (CNS) dysfunction. The patient with CAPD will have difficulty understanding spoken language, but may be able to hear sounds well.

Just as with visual acuity testing, USPSTF did not find sufficient evidence to justify the use of routine screening tests for hearing loss in the elderly. Since the last recommendation, evidence of routine screening has become available that shows that the widespread use of hearing aids after objective hearing loss was identified via in-office tests did not benefit those who did not self-report hearing loss. In other words, only those who had subjective hearing loss seemed to benefit from hearing aids, therefore raising the question of the benefit of routine hearing loss screening in a population in which this problem is so prevalent secondary to the natural process of aging. However, this recommendation does not apply to elderly patients with symptoms of hearing loss, cognitive impairment, or psychosocial complaints indicating other diagnoses.

Fall Assessment

Falls are the leading cause of nonfatal injuries in the elderly. The associated complications are the leading cause of death from injury in those older than age 65. Hip fractures are common precursors to functional impairment and nursing home placement. Approximately **30% of the noninstitutionalized elderly fall each year.** The annual incidence of falls approaches 50% in patients older than 80 years. Factors contributing to falls include age-related postural changes, alterations in visual ability, certain medications, and diseases affecting muscle strength and coordination. Due to the far-reaching consequences that falls have on both the patient and the health-care system, the American Geriatric Society recommends that physicians ask their elderly patients about history of falls and balance problems. Additionally, USPSTF recommends incorporation of exercise and physical therapy, including aerobic and strength training, as well as vitamin D supplementation to prevent falls.

Cognitive Screening

The prevalence of dementia doubles every 5 years after age 60, so that by age 85 approximately 30% to 50% of individuals have some degree of impairment. Patients with mild or early dementia frequently remain undiagnosed because their social graces are retained. **The combination of the "clock draw" and the "three-item recall" is a rapid and fairly reliable office-based screening for dementia.** When patients fail either of these screening tests, further testing with the Folstein Mini-Mental State questionnaire should be performed.

Incontinence Screening

Incontinence in the elderly is common. Incontinence is estimated to affect 11% to 34% of elderly men and 17% to 55% of elderly women. Continence problems are frequently treatable, have major social and emotional consequences, but are often not raised by patients as a concern.

Depression Screening

Depressive symptoms are more common in the elderly despite major depressive disorder being slightly lower in prevalence when compared with younger populations. **Unlike dementia, depression is usually treatable.** Depression significantly increases morbidity and mortality, and is often overlooked by physicians. A simple two-question screen (*Have you felt down/depressed/hopeless in the last 2 weeks? and Have you felt little interest or pleasure in doing things?*) shows high sensitivity. Positive responses can be followed up with a Geriatric Depression Scale, a 30-question instrument that is sensitive, specific, and reliable for the diagnosis of depression in the elderly.

Nutrition Screening

Approximately 15% of older outpatients and half of the hospitalized elderly are malnourished. **A combination of serial weight measurements obtained in the office and inquiry about changing appetite is likely the most useful method of assessing nutritional status in the elderly.** Adequate calcium intake for women is advised. Supplementation with a multivitamin formulated at about 100% daily value can decrease the prevalence of suboptimal vitamin status in older adults and improve their micronutrient status to levels associated with reduced risk for several chronic diseases. Malnutrition is common in nursing homes, and protein undernutrition has a prevalence of 17% to 56% in this setting. Protein undernutrition is associated with an increased risk of infections, anemia, orthostatic hypotension, and decubitus ulcers.

Hypertension Screening

Treatment of hypertension is of substantial benefit in the elderly. Heart disease and cerebrovascular disease are leading causes of death in the elderly. Treatment of hypertension has contributed to a reduction in mortality from both stroke and coronary artery disease. Lifestyle modifications are recommended for all hypertensive patients. Thiazides are the drugs of choice unless a comorbid condition makes another choice preferable.

Stroke Prevention

The incidence of stroke in older adults roughly doubles with each 10 years of age. The greatest risk factor is hypertension followed by atrial fibrillation. Anticoagulation with warfarin or newer agents, including dabigatran and apixaban, reduces the risk of strokes in people with atrial fibrillation. However, many elderly patients are not anticoagulated because of the fear of injuries from falls. In most instances, the benefits of anticoagulation are likely to outweigh the increased risk of fall-related bleeding, unless the patient has multiple falls, high-risk falls, or a very low risk of stroke. Aspirin use in women between the ages of 55 and 79 is recommended to decrease risk of ischemic stroke in a patient with no preexisting risk factors for gastrointestinal bleeding (USPSTF recommendation, Level A).

Cancer Screening

Screening elderly men for prostate cancer is not routinely recommended, as it has not been definitively shown to prolong life and because of the risk of incontinence or erectile dysfunction caused by the treatments. An older woman should undergo annual mammography until her life expectancy falls below 5 to 10 years, although the USPSTF states that there is insufficient evidence for or against screening in women over the age of 75. Screening for colon cancer is not generally recommended after the age of 75 although there may be some cases where it is appropriate (Level C) and is not recommended after the age of 85 (Level D). Screening for cervical cancer can be stopped in women older than 65 who have had adequate prior screening and are not at high risk for cervical cancer.

Osteoporosis Screening

The prevalence of low bone mineral density in the elderly is high, with osteopenia found in 37% of postmenopausal women. Primary prevention of osteoporosis begins with identification of risk factors (older age, female gender, white or Asian race, low calcium intake, smoking, excessive alcohol use, and chronic glucocorticoid use). Calcium carbonate (500 mg three times daily) and vitamin D (400-800 IU/d) reduce the risk of osteoporotic fractures in both men and women. Bone mineral density testing using dual-energy x-ray absorptiometry (DEXA) of patients with multiple risk factors may uncover asymptomatic osteoporosis. USPSTF recommends osteoporosis screening for women of 65 years and older and those younger than 65 years with risk for fracture equal to or greater than a 65-year-old Caucasian woman with no risk factors besides age.

Immunizations

Everyone over the age of 6 months should receive annual influenza vaccination. Persons older than age 65 should receive at least one pneumococcal immunization and a single booster dose of tetanus, diphtheria, and pertussis vaccine. The herpes zoster vaccine carries a Food and Drug Administration (FDA) indication for use starting at the age of 50, but the Advisory Committee on Immunization Practices recommends one dose of herpes zoster vaccine at age 60 or older.

END-OF-LIFE ISSUES

Advance Directives

Well-informed, competent adults have a right to refuse medical intervention, even if refusal is likely to result in death. To further patient autonomy, physicians are obligated to inform patients about the risks, benefits, alternatives, and expected outcomes of end-of-life medical interventions such as cardiopulmonary resuscitation, intubation and mechanical ventilation, vasopressor medication, hospitalization and intensive care unit (ICU) care, and artificial nutrition and hydration. **Advance directives are oral or written statements made by patients when they are competent that are intended to guide care should they become incompetent.** Advance directives allow patients to project their autonomy. Although oral statements about these matters are ethically binding, they are not legally binding in all states. Written advance directives are essential so as to give effect to the patient's wishes in these matters.

Durable Power of Attorney for Health Care

A durable power of attorney for health care (DPOA-HC) allows the patient to designate a surrogate decision maker. The responsibility of the surrogate is to provide "substituted judgment" to decide as the patient would, not as the surrogate wants. In the absence of a designated surrogate, physicians turn to family members or next of kin, under the assumption that they know the patient's wishes.

Do Not Attempt Resuscitation Orders

Physicians should encourage patients to express their preferences for the use of cardiopulmonary resuscitation (CPR). Despite the favorable portrayal of CPR in the media, **only approximately 15% of all patients who undergo CPR in the hospital survive to hospital discharge.** DNAR ("do not attempt resuscitation") is the preferred term over DNR ("do not resuscitate") to emphasize the low likelihood of successful resuscitation. In addition to mortality statistics, patients deciding about CPR preferences should also be informed about the possible consequences of surviving a CPR attempt. CPR may result in fractured ribs, lacerated internal organs, and neurologic disability. There is also a high likelihood of requiring other aggressive interventions if CPR is successful. For some patients at the end of life, decisions about CPR may not be about whether they will live but about how they will die.

CASE CORRELATION

- See also Cases 1 (Health Maintenance, Adult Male) and 11 (Health Maintenance, Adult Female).

COMPREHENSION QUESTIONS

18.1 A third-year medical student is researching various recommendations for the care of the geriatric patient. Which of the following statements is most accurate?

A. USPSTF recommends routine screening for colorectal cancer in all adults starting at the age of 50.

B. USPSTF recommends stopping screening for cervical cancer with Pap smear in all women past the age of 65.

C. The USPSTF recommends that all men should be screened for prostate cancer with prostate-specific antigen (PSA) testing annually starting at the age of 50.

D. Herpes zoster vaccination is recommended for all adults over the age of 50.

18.2 A 70-year-old man is having difficulty hearing his family members' conversations. He is diagnosed with presbycusis. Which of the following statements regarding his condition is most accurate?

A. Presbycusis does not respond to hearing aid use.

B. Presbycusis is usually caused by a conductive disorder.

C. Presbycusis usually results in loss of speech discrimination.

D. Presbycusis usually results in unilateral hearing loss.

E. Presbycusis usually results in low-frequency hearing loss.

18.3 Which one of the following recommendations is accurate regarding the current USPSTF recommendation for osteoporosis screening in the elderly?

A. All women with strong risk factors, regardless of age, should be screened for osteoporosis.

B. Only women above the age of 65 should be screened for osteoporosis.

C. Men and women above the age of 65 should be screened for osteoporosis.

D. African-American race is an independent risk factor for osteoporosis and should warrant screening regardless of other risk factors.

ANSWERS

18.1 **A.** The only accurate answer among the choices is that regarding colorectal screening. There is no recommendation for annual routine PSA testing for prostate cancer screening. Pap smears can be safely discontinued in women over the age of 65 who have had adequate prior screening. The herpes zoster vaccine is recommended for routine use at age 60 or older.

18.2 **C.** Up to one-third of people older than age 65 suffer from hearing loss. Presbycusis typically presents with symmetric high-frequency hearing loss. There is loss of speech discrimination, so that patients complain of difficulty understanding rapid speech, foreign accents, and conversation in noisy areas. The mechanism is sensorineural rather than a conductive problem.

18.3 **A.** USPSTF recommends screening for osteoporosis in women above 65 years and younger than 65 years with risk factors. Therefore, considering age as a risk factor, essentially *all* women with risk factors must be screened for osteoporosis with bone mineral density test or DEXA scan. The current recommendation applies only to women, as there is insufficient evidence to support screening in men, and the race mostly at risk is Caucasian.

CLINICAL PEARLS

▶ Protein undernutrition is associated with an increased risk of infections, anemia, orthostatic hypotension, and decubitus ulcers.

▶ Smoking is associated with osteoporosis.

▶ If "osteoporotic" fractures, such as vertebral compression fractures, occur in conjunction with osteopenia on x-ray, the diagnosis of osteoporosis is almost certain.

▶ Hearing loss and sensory impairments, in general, can be confused with cognitive impairment or an affective disorder.

▶ Presbyopia, macular degeneration, glaucoma, cataracts, and diabetic retinopathy account for the majority of conditions leading to vision loss in the elderly.

REFERENCES

Centers for Disease Control. Recommended adult immunization schedule, United States—2015. Available at: http://www.cdc.gov/vaccines/schedules/downloads/adult/adult-combined-schedule.pdf. Accessed April 19, 2015.

Harper G, Johnston C, Landefeld C, et al. Geriatric disorders. In: Papadakis MA, McPhee SJ, Rabow MW, eds. *Current Medical Diagnosis & Treatment.* New York, NY: McGraw-Hill; 2014. Available at: http://accessmedicine.mhmedical.com. Accessed May 24, 2015.

Kudrimoti AM, Perman SE. Hearing and vision impairment in the elderly. In: South-Paul JE, Matheny SC, Lewis EL, et al., eds. *Current Diagnosis & Treatment: Family Medicine.* 4th ed. New York, NY: McGraw-Hill; 2015. Available at: http://accessmedicine.mhmedical.com. Accessed May 24, 2015.

Rabow MW, Pantilat SZ. Palliative care and pain management. In: Papadakis MA, McPhee SJ, Rabow MW, eds. *Current Medical Diagnosis & Treatment.* New York, NY: McGraw-Hill; 2014. Available at: http://accessmedicine.mhmedical.com. Accessed May 24, 2015

Rosenfeld KE, Wenger NS, Kagawa-Singer M, et al. End-of-life decision making: a qualitative study of elderly individuals. *J Gen Intern Med.* 2000;15:620.

Spalding MC, Sebesta SC. Geriatic screening and preventive care. *Am Fam Physician.* 2008 Jul 15;78(2):206-215.

State-specific advance directives forms. Available at: http://www.caringinfo.org/stateaddownload. Accessed April 19, 2015.

Tulsky JA, Fischer GS, Rose MR, et al. Opening the black box: how do physicians communicate about advance directives? *Ann Intern Med.* 1998;129:441.

United States Preventive Services Task Force Published Guidelines. Available at www.uspreventiveservicestaskforce.org/Browse. Accessed April 19, 2015.

A 45-year-old man presents to the clinic with a cough productive of purulent sputum of 3-week duration. He says that he had just gotten over a cold a few weeks prior to this episode. He occasionally has fevers and he coughs so much that he has chest pain. He reports having a mild sore throat and nasal congestion. He has no history of asthma or of any chronic lung diseases. He denies nausea, vomiting, diarrhea, and any recent travel. He denies any smoking history. On examination, his temperature is 98.6°F (37.0°C), his pulse is 96 beats/min, his blood pressure is 124/82 mm Hg, his respiratory rate is 18 breaths/min, and his oxygen saturation is 99% on room air. Head, ears, eyes, nose, and throat (HEENT) examination reveals no erythema of the posterior oropharynx, tonsillar exudates, uvular deviations, or significant tonsillar swelling. Neck examination is negative. The chest examination yields occasional wheezes but normal air movement is noted.

▶ What is the most likely diagnosis?
▶ What is your next step?
▶ What are some common noninfectious causes of cough?

ANSWERS TO CASE 19:
Upper Respiratory Infections

Summary: A 45-year-old man, who has no history of lung disease and does not smoke, with 3 weeks of productive cough following an upper respiratory infection.

- **Most likely diagnosis:** Acute bronchitis.

- **Next step:** Bronchodilators, analgesics, and antitussives. Antibiotics have not been consistently shown to be beneficial. The illness is usually self-limited.

- **Common noninfectious causes of cough:** Asthma, chronic obstructive pulmonary disease (COPD), malignancy, postnasal drip, gastroesophageal reflux disease (GERD), medication side effect (eg, angiotensin-converting enzyme [ACE] inhibitors), congestive heart failure.

ANALYSIS

Objectives

1. Develop a differential diagnosis of cough persisting for 3 weeks or more.

2. Understand that most upper respiratory infections are self-limited illnesses.

3. Develop an approach for rational prescription of antibiotics for respiratory infections.

Considerations

The patient described in the case is a 45-year-old man with no prior history of lung disease, immunocompromised state, or tobacco use. These risk factors are important considerations since respiratory complaints in the setting of COPD or HIV or a smoking history require a higher index of suspicion of lower respiratory tract infections such as pneumonia. As with any respiratory complaint, the ABCs should be considered; that is airway, breathing, and circulation. In the ambulatory setting, a very quick assessment of the patient's distress level, respiratory use or nonuse of accessory muscles, anxiety level, stridor, and ability to speak sentences helps to triage to acute emergency versus more relaxed assessment. The individual described is afebrile, has a normal respiratory rate, and appears to be comfortable. The lung examination reveals some slight wheezes, but otherwise normal breath sounds and air movement. The most likely diagnosis in this setting is acute bronchitis. Chest radiograph is not necessarily indicated; however, since the complaint has persisted for 3 weeks, any other abnormal finding such as dullness on percussion of the chest, history of fever, or clinical suspicion would be sufficient reason for chest x-ray. Most acute bronchitis is caused by viruses and antibiotic therapy is not helpful. It is important to remember that acute bronchitis is a diagnosis of exclusion and by definition should not be made in the presence of clinical or radiographic evidence of pneumonia and only after ruling out other etiologies such as GERD, asthma, and the common cold. This patient with true acute bronchitis is best treated by bronchodilator therapy such as albuterol and antitussive agents and follow-up in 2 to 3 weeks.

APPROACH TO:
Upper Respiratory Infections

DEFINITIONS

ACUTE BRONCHITIS: Inflammation of the tracheobronchial tree.

PNEUMONIA: Inflammation or infection of the lower respiratory tract, involving the distal bronchioles and alveoli.

CLINICAL APPROACH

Acute Bronchitis

Acute bronchitis refers to inflammation of the tracheobronchial tree. The inflammatory response to the trigger, whether infectious, allergic, or irritant, leads to increased mucous production and airway hyperresponsiveness. As bronchitis most commonly occurs in the setting of an upper respiratory illness, it is seen more frequently in the winter. Influenza, parainfluenza, adenovirus, rhinovirus, other viruses, *Mycoplasma pneumoniae*, and *Chlamydia pneumoniae* have been implicated as causes.

As the primary symptoms are nonspecific, other etiologies can be mistakenly diagnosed as acute bronchitis. In one study, one-third of patients who had been determined to have recurrent bouts of acute bronchitis were eventually identified as having asthma. Occupational history may be important in determining whether irritants play a role.

There are no specific diagnostic criteria for acute bronchitis, although cough productive of purulent sputum is the most common presentation. Other symptoms are often present, including fever, malaise, rhinorrhea or nasal congestion, sore throat, wheezing, dyspnea, chest pain, myalgias, or arthralgias. The sputum produced can be of variable color and consistency; **the color of sputum is not diagnostic of the presence of a bacterial infection.**

The physical examination in bronchitis is typically nonspecific and, frequently, is normal. The presence of fever, tachypnea, tachycardia, and blood pressure abnormalities should be noted. In persons with underlying pulmonary or cardiac conditions, or in persons with more severe symptoms, oxygen saturation by pulse oximetry may be warranted. Examination of the lungs may reveal rales, rhonchi, or wheezes, but in most cases is unremarkable.

Occasionally, findings on examination may suggest a particular etiology or an alternate diagnosis. Prolonged fever, tachycardia, tachypnea, hypotension, and signs of consolidation on pulmonary examination may suggest a diagnosis of pneumonia. When pneumonia is suspected, a chest radiograph should be obtained to confirm the diagnosis. Conjunctivitis and adenopathy suggest adenoviral infection, although these findings are not specific.

There is no requirement for obtaining viral cultures, serologic testing, or sputum analyses in a suspected case of acute bronchitis as the organism responsible is rarely identified, and more importantly, these tests have no effect on the subsequent management.

Bronchitis is nearly always self-limited in an otherwise healthy individual. Although most acute bronchitis lasts for less than 2 weeks, in some cases the cough can last for 2 months or more. Severe cases occasionally produce deterioration in patients with significant comorbid conditions.

Treatment

The use of antibiotics has not been shown consistently to alter the natural history of acute bronchitis, except in the case of infection with *Bordetella pertussis*. Patients with abnormal vital signs (pulse ≥100 beats/min, respiration ≥24 breaths/min, temperature ≥100.4°F [38.0°C]) and examination findings consistent with pulmonary consolidation should be evaluated further for the diagnosis of pneumonia and treated appropriately, if confirmed. Pneumonia may present atypically in the elderly and in persons with chronic lung disease. Physicians must have a higher index of suspicion in these populations.

As some of the symptoms of bronchitis are caused by airway hyperreactivity, bronchodilator therapy has been shown in some studies to offer benefit in reducing symptoms. Antitussives, such as dextromethorphan and codeine, may have modest benefits in reducing the cough associated with this illness. Mucokinetic agents have not shown to be of benefit and are therefore not recommended.

OTHER INFECTIONS OF THE UPPER RESPIRATORY TRACT

The most common cause of chronic cough in healthy, nonsmokers with a normal chest x-ray is the encompassing diagnosis of upper airway cough syndrome (UACS). This diagnosis encompasses a variety of upper respiratory conditions, which are distinguished from one another by physical examination findings, signs and symptoms, and sometimes after a trial of therapy. Some conditions under this umbrella diagnosis are allergic rhinitis and bacterial sinusitis.

Rhinosinusitis

Rhinosinusitis is the inflammation/infection of the nasal mucosa and of one or more paranasal sinuses. Sinusitis occurs with obstruction of the normal drainage mechanism. It is traditionally subdivided into acute (symptoms lasting <4 weeks), subacute (symptoms lasting 4-12 weeks), chronic (symptoms lasting >12 weeks), recurrent acute rhinosinusitis (four or more episodes of acute rhinosinusitis per year, with interim resolution of symptoms), and acute exacerbation of chronic sinusitis.

The signs and symptoms of rhinosinusitis are nonspecific and similar to other general upper respiratory tract infection symptoms. As most viral upper respiratory tract infections improve in 7 to 10 days, expert opinion suggests considering a diagnosis of bacterial rhinosinusitis after 7 days of symptoms in adults and 10 days in children. The diagnosis is suggested by the presence of purulent nasal discharge, maxillary tooth or facial pain, unilateral maxillary sinus tenderness, and worsening of symptoms after initial improvement.

Streptococcus pneumoniae and *Haemophilus influenzae* are the organisms most commonly responsible for acute bacterial sinusitis in adults; *S pneumoniae*, *H influenzae*, and *Moraxella catarrhalis* are most common in children. In chronic sinusitis, the infecting organisms are variable, with a higher incidence of anaerobic organisms seen (eg, *Bacteroides*, *Peptostreptococcus*, and *Fusobacterium* species).

Treatment of acute sinusitis should be directed at the likely causative agents. Amoxicillin and trimethoprim-sulfamethoxazole are widely used first-line agents, typically for 10- to 14-day regimens. Second-line antibiotics, for those who fail to improve on the initial regimen or who have recurrent or severe disease, include amoxicillin-clavulanic acid, second- or third-generation cephalosporins (cefuroxime, cefaclor, cefprozil, and others), fluoroquinolones, or second-generation macrolides (azithromycin, clarithromycin). Adjunctive therapy with oral or topical decongestants may provide symptomatic relief. Topical decongestants should not be used for more than 3 days to avoid the risk of rebound vasodilation with resultant worsening of symptoms. Nonsteroidal anti-inflammatory drugs (NSAIDs) and acetaminophen may provide symptomatic relief of pain and fever.

Pharyngitis

Pharyngitis is an inflammation or irritation of the pharynx and/or tonsils. In adults, the **vast majority of pharyngitis is viral**. It can also be bacterial or allergic in origin; trauma, toxins, and malignancy are rare causes. As most cases of pharyngitis in adults are benign and self-limited, a focus of the examination of a patient with symptoms of pharyngitis should be to rule out more serious conditions, such as epiglottitis or peritonsillar abscess, and to diagnose group A β-hemolytic *Streptococcus* (GAS) infection.

Pharyngitis occurs with much greater frequency in the pediatric population, with a peak incidence between 4 and 7 years of age. *M pneumoniae*, *C pneumoniae*, and *Arcanobacterium haemolyticus* are common causes of pharyngitis in teens and young adults. GAS causes 15% of all adult pharyngitis and approximately 30% of pediatric cases.

The cause of pharyngitis cannot always be distinguished based on history or examination. Sore throat associated with cough and rhinorrhea is more likely to be viral in origin. The presence of tonsillar exudates does not distinguish bacterial from viral causes, as GAS, Epstein-Barr virus (infectious mononucleosis), mycoplasma, *Chlamydia*, and adenoviruses, among others, can all cause exudates. **Findings frequently associated with GAS infections include an abrupt onset of sore throat and fever, tonsillar and/or palatal petechiae, tender cervical adenopathy, and absence of cough.** GAS can also cause an erythematous, sandpaper-like (scarlatiniform) rash.

Infectious mononucleosis, caused by infection with Epstein-Barr virus, is extremely difficult to distinguish clinically from GAS infection. Exudative pharyngitis is prominent. Features suggestive of mononucleosis include retrocervical or generalized adenopathy and hepatosplenomegaly. Atypical lymphocytes can be seen on peripheral blood smear. The associated splenomegaly can be significant, as it predisposes to splenic rupture in response to trauma (even minor trauma). A patient with splenomegaly from mononucleosis should be restricted from activities, such as sports participation, in which abdominal trauma may occur.

On examination, the **patency of the airway must be addressed first.** The presence of stridor, drooling, and a toxic appearance suggest epiglottitis. Patients with epiglottitis are sometimes seen leaning forward on their outstretched arms, the so-called tripod position. Patients with suspected epiglottitis need to be managed in a setting where the airway can be emergently secured, via intubation or cricothyroidotomy. Epiglottitis is a rare infection and is becoming even rarer, with near-universal immunization for *H influenzae*, type B.

Swelling of the peritonsillar region, with the associated tonsil pushed toward the midline and with contralateral deviation of the uvula, is consistent with a peritonsillar abscess. This can be seen either as the initial complaint of sore throat, frequently with associated trismus (pain with chewing), or as a complication of streptococcal pharyngitis. Suspicion of peritonsillar abscess should prompt immediate referral for surgical drainage of the abscess.

The diagnosis of GAS infection can be made by rapid antigen testing or throat culture. **Rapid antigen tests** can be conducted in a few minutes in the office or emergency department setting. They are **highly specific but have a lower sensitivity than throat culture.** A positive rapid antigen test would prompt antibiotic treatment; a negative test should be followed by a throat culture. **Throat cultures are considered the gold standard** for diagnosis of GAS infections. Cultures can take 24 to 48 hours; this is acceptable in most instances, as the risk of complication from GAS infections is low if treatment is instituted within 10 days of onset of symptoms.

Several clinical guidelines have been proposed to aid in the rapid diagnosis and management of patients presenting with pharyngitis. One of the most widely used is the modified Centor criteria. In this guideline, a patient is given a point for each of the following criteria: absence of cough; enlarged/tender anterior cervical adenopathy; fever of 100.4°F or higher; and tonsillar swelling/exudates. One point is also awarded if the patient is age 3 to 14 and one point deducted for the age of 45 or higher. Based on the number of points assessed, the following decision guidelines are proposed:

Points	Recommendation
0-1	No further testing and no antibiotic indicated
2-3	Perform rapid strep or throat culture and treat with antibiotic if positive
4 or more	Consider empiric antibiotic treatment

Complications from untreated GAS infections are rare, but include rheumatic fever, glomerulonephritis, toxic shock syndrome, peritonsillar abscess, meningitis, and bacteremia. Rheumatic fever, which may complicate up to one in 400 untreated cases of GAS pharyngitis, can cause permanent cardiac and neurologic sequelae. Glomerulonephritis results from antigen/antibody complex deposition in the glomeruli. **Poststreptococcal glomerulonephritis may occur whether or not the patient receives appropriate antibiotic treatment.**

Penicillin is the antibiotic of choice for GAS pharyngitis. Oral therapy requires a 10-day course of penicillin V. Intramuscular therapy of penicillin G benzathine for adults and children weighing greater than 27 kg is 1.2 million units. Children who weigh less than 27 kg can receive 600,000 units of penicillin IM. In penicillin-allergic patients, treatment options include cephalosporins and macrolides.

Other Common Causes of Chronic Cough

Asthma remains a significant cause of chronic cough across all age groups, but especially in the pediatric population. The pathophysiology of asthma is characterized by reversible airflow obstruction as well as inflammation and hyperreactivity of the airway. Symptoms besides cough include chest tightness, exacerbation by particular triggers, and improvement with inhaled bronchodilators and corticosteroids, which remain the mainstay of treatment. Spirometry must be done to diagnose asthma, and management is based on the variant determined by factors such as duration of symptoms, nighttime occurrences, and medication requirement to keep symptoms at bay.

Another leading cause of a chronic cough is GERD. The afferent limb of the cough reflex is activated by the acid interfering with the upper respiratory system. GERD presents with a cough that gets worse in a supine position, heartburn and increased symptoms after meals. Although the definitive test is 24-hour esophageal pH monitoring, GERD is usually a clinical diagnosis. A trial of proton pump inhibitor is both diagnostic and therapeutic.

ACE Inhibitor–Related Cough

It is important to mention this etiology as medication-related cough could be an easily overlooked cause of a nonproductive cough. ACE inhibitor–related cough usually appears 1 week to 6 months from initiation of therapy. The management is quite simply to discontinue the medication and assess response. Because it may take several weeks for the cough to go away after discontinuation of medication, response should be at the 4-week mark at the earliest. A good substitute for ACE inhibitor is an angiotensin receptor blocker (ARB).

INFECTIONS OF THE EAR

Otitis externa (OE) is an infection of the external auditory canal. Patients with OE complain of ear pain and, sometimes, itching. The pain from OE can be severe. Examination shows an inflamed, swollen, external ear canal, often with exudates and discharge. Movement of the external ear is usually quite painful. The tympanic membrane may be uninvolved. The most common pathogens include staphylococci, streptococci, and other skin flora. Some cases have been associated with the use of swimming pools or hot tubs. This infection (swimmer's ear) is usually caused by *Pseudomonas aeruginosa*. Irrigation and administration of topical antibiotics, frequently combined with steroid, is usually successful. **Patients with diabetes mellitus are at risk for an invasive external otitis** (malignant OE) caused by *P aeruginosa*. Treatment for this condition involves surgical debridement of necrotic tissue and 4 to 6 weeks of IV antibiotics, if cranial bones are involved.

Otitis media (OM) is an infection of the middle ear seen primarily among preschool children, but occasionally in adults as well. Infection of the middle ear space, caused by upper respiratory tract pathogens, is promoted by obstruction to drainage through edematous, congested eustachian tubes. Viral infection with serous otitis may predispose to acute bacterial otitis media. Fever, ear pain, diminished hearing, vertigo, and tinnitus are common presenting symptoms. On examination, the tympanic membrane may appear red, but the presence of decreased membrane mobility or fluid behind the tympanic membrane is necessary for the diagnosis. *S pneumoniae*, *H influenzae*, and *M catarrhalis* are the most common bacterial pathogens. **Most cases of acute OM will resolve spontaneously.** Indications for treatment with antibiotics include prolonged, recurrent, or severe symptoms. Numerous antibiotics can be used for treatment. Amoxicillin remains the recommended initial therapy. Alternative treatments include amoxicillin-clavulanic acid, trimethoprim-sulfamethoxazole, or second- and third-generation cephalosporins. Complications are uncommon, but include mastoiditis, bacterial meningitis, brain abscess, and subdural empyema.

> ## CASE CORRELATION
> - See Cases 2 (Dyspnea, COPD) and 6 (Allergic Disorders).

COMPREHENSION QUESTIONS

19.1 A 30-year-old woman with no past medical history presents with a productive cough of 2-week duration. She states she also has a runny nose, body aches, congestion, and fevers for the past week. In office she is normotensive, with a normal pulse, and temperature of 101.2°F. Her physical examination is significant for sinus tenderness, boggy nasal turbinates, and crackles in the left lower lobe lung fields. Which one of the following is the best initial step in management?

A. Reassure the patient that she likely has a viral infection and it will resolve on its own.

B. Order a rapid strep test and treat if positive

C. Prescribe amoxicillin for a likely bacterial infection

D. Order chest x-ray to rule out possible pneumonia

19.2 A 55-year-old man with history of hypertension and diabetes presents with intermittent nighttime cough for a few months. He states he often has a "weird taste" in his mouth a couple of hours after eating and is afraid of eating dinner because he gets terrible heartburn during the night. He states he has tried over the counter antacid and this has worked to somewhat alleviate his symptoms; however, his nighttime cough is still very bothersome. His vitals in office are within normal limits and physical examination is positive for epigastric tenderness upon palpation. Which one of the following is true regarding the most likely etiology of this patient's cough?

A. It is the second leading cause of chronic cough.

B. The most sensitive and specific test for this condition is a 24-hour esophageal pH monitoring.

C. The first line of treatment for this condition is a trial of 4 weeks of H$_2$ blocker.

D. This condition always requires a diagnostic test for confirmation and should not be diagnosed clinically.

19.3 A 13-year-old adolescent girl presents with fever and sore throat of 48-hour duration. She has a temperature of 101°F in office and is tachycardic with a pulse of 118 beats/min. Her physical examination is positive for tender, enlarged left cervical lymphadenopathy and tachycardia. Her pharynx is erythematous but without tonsillar enlargement or exudate. She has had no cough. What is the best step in management?

A. Treat empirically with antibiotics.

B. Order rapid strep test and, if positive, treat with antibiotics.

C. Neither further testing nor antibiotics.

D. Order throat culture and, if positive, treat with antibiotics.

ANSWERS

19.1 **D.** Acute bronchitis is a diagnosis of exclusion in the absence of clinical or radiographic findings concerning for pneumonia. In this patient with fevers, productive cough, and rales on lung examination, it is important to rule out pneumonia. If there is a strong clinical suspicion of community-acquired pneumonia, a chest x-ray is not necessary, and outpatient treatment with antibiotics can be initiated. The diagnosis of streptococcal pharyngitis is made with rapid strep test or throat culture and the decision to order these in office is guided by modified Centor criteria based on the following factors: age, presence of tonsillar exudates, fever, absence of cough.

19.2 **B.** This patient's cough is most likely secondary to GERD. The most definitive test to diagnose this condition is a 24-hour pH monitoring test, however, this is not required for diagnosis. GERD is almost always a clinical diagnosis and a 4-week trial of proton pump inhibitor is both diagnostic and therapeutic. Lastly, GERD is the third leading cause of chronic cough, after upper airway cough syndrome and asthma.

19.3 **A.** Management of strep pharyngitis is frequently guided by modified Centor criteria, which calculates a probability of strep throat based on a scoring system (presented earlier in the chapter). This patient gets one point for the presence of fever, tender cervical adenopathy, absence of cough, and age. You could reasonably consider an empiric antibiotic treatment for GAS in her.

CLINICAL PEARLS

▶ The main concerns with pharyngitis are to rule out more serious conditions, such as epiglottitis or peritonsillar abscess, and to diagnose group A β-hemolytic streptococcal infections.

▶ Upper airway cough syndrome (UACS) is an umbrella term that encompasses a variety of upper respiratory conditions including rhinitis and sinusitis.

▶ A tonsillopharyngeal exudate does not differentiate viral and bacterial causes.

▶ Asthma and GERD are the second and third leading cause of chronic cough, respectively, after UACS, which is the most common cause of cough.

REFERENCES

Aring AM, Chan MM. Acute rhinosinusitis in adults. *Am Fam Physician.* 2011 May 1;83(9):1057-1063.

Benich JJ, Carek PJ. Evaluation of the patient with chronic cough. *Am Fam Physician.* 2011 Oct 15;84(8):887-892.

Choby BA. Diagnosis and treatment of streptococcal pharyngitis. *Am Fam Physician.* 2009 Mar 1;79(5):383-390.

Gonzales R, Bartlett JG, Besser RE, et al. Principles of appropriate antibiotic use for treatment of uncomplicated acute bronchitis: background. *Ann Intern Med.* 2001;134(6):521-529.

Irwin RS, Baumann MH, Bolser DC, et al. Diagnosis and management of cough executive summary: ACCP evidence-based clinical practice guidelines. *Chest.* 2006 Jan;129(suppl 1):1-S23.

Knutson D, Braun C. Diagnosis and management of acute bronchitis. *Am Fam Physician.* 2002;65: 2039-2044, 2046.

Rosenfeld RM, Andes D, Bhattacharyya N, et al. Clinical practice guideline: adult sinusitis. *Otolaryngol Head Neck Surg.* 2007;137(suppl 3):S1-S31.

A 56-year-old man is brought to the emergency department (ED) complaining of chest discomfort for about 90 minutes. He has had occasional symptoms for a month, but it is worse today. Today's symptoms began while he was walking his dog and decreased slightly with rest, but have not resolved. He describes the feeling as a pressure sensation in the left substernal area of his chest associated with shortness of breath and mild diaphoresis. He does not have any radiation of the discomfort today, but has experienced radiation to the left upper extremity in the past. The patient denies any health problems, but his wife reports that he has not seen a physician in years. His wife made him come in because his younger brother had a heart attack 6 months ago. He is a vice president of a bank and lives with his wife and three daughters. He has smoked 1½ pack of cigarettes per day for more than 30 years and denies drinking alcohol or any drug use.

On physical examination he is an anxious, obese gentleman who appears pale and has a moist brow. His temperature is 98.8°F (37.1°C), his pulse is 105 beats/min, his respirations is 18 breaths/min, his blood pressure is 190/95 mm Hg, his height is 74 in, and his weight is 250 lb. Cardiac examination reveals regular rhythm without murmur, but he has an S_4 gallop. Lungs are clear to auscultation. Neck is without carotid bruits or jugular venous distension. Abdomen is normal. He does have a right femoral bruit. Extremities reveal trace edema but no clubbing or cyanosis. He has 2+ pulses in radial and dorsal pedalis arteries. Rectal examination has no masses or tenderness with a normal prostate, and is guaiac negative.

▶ What is your most likely diagnosis?
▶ What is your next diagnostic step?
▶ What is the next step in therapy?

ANSWERS TO CASE 20:
Chest Pain

Summary: A 56-year-old obese man presents to the ED with chest discomfort. He has a pressure sensation in the left substernal area of his chest associated with shortness of breath and diaphoresis. His symptoms began with minimal exertion. The patient is without prior medical care. He has a family history of coronary artery disease (CAD) and a history of tobacco abuse. He is hypertensive and tachycardic. He has a cardiac gallop. Lower extremities have trace edema and a femoral bruit.

- **Most likely diagnosis:** Unstable angina pectoris; must rule out myocardial infarction (MI)

- **Next diagnostic step:**
  Initial studies in the emergency room: complete blood count (CBC), electrolytes, blood urea nitrogen (BUN), creatinine, prothrombin time (PT), partial thromboplastin time (PTT), international normalized ratio (INR), glucose, 12-lead electrocardiography (ECG), and chest x-ray (CXR); markers of myocardial damage including creatine kinase (CK) and MB isoenzyme (CK-MB), troponin T and troponin I to be done STAT and every 6 to 10 hours for three cycles; oxygen saturation must be monitored, as well
  Studies that can be performed later: fasting lipids, liver function tests, magnesium, homocysteine level, urine drug screen, urinalysis, and myoglobin

- **Next step in therapy:** MONA therapy: Morphine, Oxygen, Nitroglycerin, Aspirin
  Morphine can achieve adequate analgesia which decreases levels of circulating catecholamines, thus reducing myocardial oxygen consumption. It must be initiated rapidly if nitroglycerin cannot alleviate the discomfort.
  Oxygen 2 to 4 L/min by nasal cannula; may be discontinued after 6 hours if oxygen saturation remains normal without other complications.
  Nitroglycerin must be given sublingually initially every 5 minutes for a total of three doses (in the absence of hypotension or contraindications such as sildenafil [Viagra] use), then advanced to IV or transdermal routes.
  Aspirin 325 mg should be chewed and swallowed (clopidogrel may be used if allergy to aspirin exists).
  β-Adrenergic antagonist reduces myocardial damage and may limit infarct size.
  Glycoprotein (GP) IIb/IIIa inhibitors reduce end point of death or recurrent ischemia when given in addition to standard therapy for patients with high-risk unstable angina or non–ST-elevation MI treated with percutaneous coronary intervention, or who are refractory to prior treatment.

ANALYSIS

Objectives

1. Understand a diagnostic approach to chest pain and how to reduce potential damage to myocardium by implementing rapid evaluation.

2. Know the acute evaluation of chest pain and how to best implement the primary and secondary treatment of chest pain.

3. Identify the risks and the need to educate patients to reduce their risks.

4. Be familiar with the differential diagnosis of chest pain and how to best rule in and out the more life-threatening problems.

Considerations

This 56-year-old man has unstable angina with a variety of risk factors for CAD. All patients who present to primary care physicians with chest pain are immediate challenges. Most resources emphasize the life-threatening etiologies; however, the non–life-threatening etiologies are far more common in presentation. Physicians must master a cost-effective approach to diagnosing the various etiologies of chest pain, determining which patients warrant further evaluation, putting a large emphasis on thorough history and physical examination. The cause of this patient's symptoms must be determined as soon as possible. If the etiology is determined to be cardiac, there are medications and interventions that can dramatically reduce both morbidity and mortality. A complete history and physical examination can give information that can guide if and when other more expensive and invasive tests are necessary. The patient's most immediate problem is his acute symptoms. His anxiety will decrease slightly when he perceives that he is getting adequate care and information.

Nearly 1½ million people in the United States experience an MI each year. This is fatal approximately one-third of the time. However, there has been a continuous decline in the mortality rate over the past three decades because of a better understanding of the etiology and pathophysiology of MI, and because of advances in therapeutic treatments.

The first priority is to obtain ECG and CXR, while giving medications to decrease the damage caused to his myocardium and simultaneously reducing his blood pressure. Nitroglycerin and β-adrenergic antagonists will begin achieving these goals. He will need constant monitoring and continuous telemetry. Oxygen needs to be continued as well. Before the ECG and CXR have been completed, aspirin, oxygen, nitroglycerin, morphine, and β-adrenergic antagonist should be given. The providers must assume cardiac etiology until it has been effectively ruled out to limit possible morbidity and mortality to the patient.

The laboratory tests previously listed need to be drawn, at which time IV access can be started in two places. The results of the tests will determine if the patient has other risk factors in addition to his known hypertension, family history of CAD, tobacco abuse, and obesity. If he routinely walks his dog, his lifestyle contains at least minimal physical activity.

The changes seen in an ECG that are indicative of angina include ST-segment elevation or depression and/or T-wave inversion. MIs include these changes plus elevated CK-MB and/or troponin levels. Pathologic Q waves may also indicate cardiac pathology, but typically represent myocardial tissue necrosis from a completed infarction. When Q waves are present, the benefits of thrombolytic therapy are uncertain. **Not all MIs will have ECG changes.** A normal ECG reduces the likelihood of MI but does not rule out cardiac pathology. Any person with symptoms of angina who has a left bundle branch block (LBBB) on ECG must have serum cardiac enzymes drawn, because there is a high degree of correlation between LBBB and organic heart disease, especially CAD. LBBB can mask signs of myocardial pathology, as it can mimic both acute and chronic ischemic changes. All of the listed ECG changes have a differential diagnosis that includes MI. The clinical picture is of utmost importance, again demonstrating the need for complete history and physical examination.

APPROACH TO:
Chest Pain

DEFINITIONS

ANGINA PECTORIS: Severe pain around the heart caused by a relative deficiency of oxygen supply to the heart muscle.

MYOCARDIAL INFARCTION: Cardiac muscle death caused by partial or complete occlusion of one or more of the coronary arteries.

NEW YORK HEART ASSOCIATION FUNCTIONAL CLASSIFICATION OF ANGINA:

Class I—Angina only with unusually strenuous activity

Class II—Angina with slightly more prolonged or slightly more vigorous activity than usual

Class III—Angina with usual daily activity

Class IV—Angina at rest

UNSTABLE ANGINA: Angina of new onset, angina at rest or with minimal exertion, or a crescendo pattern of angina with episodes of increasing frequency, severity, or duration.

CLINICAL APPROACH

Etiologies

Atherosclerosis leading to plaque rupture and then cascading to coronary artery thrombosis is the cause of an acute MI approximately 90% of the time, but **many different conditions can be the culprit for angina.** Coronary artery spasm, including cocaine-induced injury, can cause angina. Aortic dissection extending into a coronary artery will cause extensive damage. An embolus to a coronary artery can be caused by endocarditis, prosthetic heart valves, or myxoma. Embolism can also cause cerebral vascular accidents, increasing the extent of the initial evaluation that is warranted.

Chest pain or discomfort is one of the most common complaints in both the outpatient and emergency setting. Assessing the cause of such symptoms in a rapid fashion is of utmost importance. **If the patient is experiencing myocardial ischemia or infarction, time is myocardium.** Initial evaluation should be done within 10 minutes of presentation and the goal of this evaluation should be to determine the need for further testing such as cardiac enzymes, stress test, or angiography. Ischemic heart disease remains the leading cause of morbidity and mortality in the United States. It is important to identify risk factors for coronary artery disease in patients, the presence of which would indicate an increased suspicion for an acute MI. Male gender, age older than 60 years, diaphoresis, radiation of pain to neck, arm, shoulder, or jaw, and a past history of angina or acute MI are all considered risk factors.

TREATMENT

Primary Treatment

All patients who rule in for MI should receive aspirin and an antithrombotic treatment, if there are no contraindications. Aspirin and heparin reduce the risk of subsequent MI and cardiac death in patients with unstable angina. Studies present different recommendations for using clopidogrel in addition to aspirin and heparin. Current American College of Cardiology/American Heart Association recommendations advise withholding clopidogrel for 5 to 7 days before planned bypass surgery. It is reasonable to give clopidogrel 300 mg orally to patients with suspected acute coronary syndrome (ACS) (without ECG or cardiac marker changes) who are either allergic to or have gastrointestinal intolerance of aspirin.

Heparin usually should be continued for 48 hours or until angiography is performed. Patients suffering from unstable angina with ECG changes should also be given platelet glycoprotein IIb/IIIa receptor inhibitors because the composite risk of death, MI, and recurrent ischemia is significantly reduced with these medications.

Nitroglycerin is best given IV initially because of the ability to achieve predictable blood levels rapidly. Once stabilized after 24 hours, the asymptomatic patient should be switched to a long-acting oral or transdermal nitrate. A β-adrenergic antagonist should also be given, unless contraindicated. The **combination of nitroglycerin and β-adrenergic antagonist reduces the risk of subsequent MI.** β-Adrenergic antagonists decreased mortality and reduced infarct size in many clinical trials.

Angiotensin-converting enzyme (ACE) inhibitors reduce short-term mortality when started within 24 hours of acute MI. Postinfarction ACE inhibitors prevent left ventricular remodeling and recurrent ischemic events. It is reasonable to recommend their indefinite use in the absence of any contraindications. All trials with oral ACE inhibitors have shown benefit from their early use, including those in which early entry criteria included clinical suspicion of acute infarctions. Magnesium sulfate should be given if levels are low, as hypomagnesemia can increase the incidence of *torsade de pointes*–type ventricular tachycardia.

Despite the widespread use of calcium channel blockers both during and after myocardial ischemia, no evidence exists supporting any benefit when taking these medications. Rapid release, short-acting dihydropyridines (eg, nifedipine) are contraindicated because they increased mortality in multiple trials.

Patients who are asymptomatic after 48 hours of drug therapy can perform a modified Bruce protocol stress test. Patients who have a markedly positive stress test should be referred for angiography. There is some debate concerning when angiography should be done. One approach shows that an early invasive approach with angiography within 24 to 48 hours is beneficial, whereas others recommend a more conservative approach, doing angiography only if recurrent ischemia is present or a stress test was positive. There is no clear consensus as to which approach is superior.

All patients admitted for angina or MI should receive a reduced saturated fat and cholesterol diet. These patients may benefit from nutrition counselors to help them develop healthy lifestyle changes.

Secondary Treatment

Primary prevention of CAD must be encouraged for all patients. **Risk factors for CAD include diabetes mellitus, dyslipidemia, age, hypertension, tobacco abuse, family history of premature CAD, male gender, postmenopausal status, left ventricular hypertrophy, and homocystinemia** (Table 20–1). Modification of these risk factors has a direct link to reduce morbidity and mortality. Patient education is particularly important.

Aspirin, nitrates, and β-adrenergic antagonist have proven benefits for both primary and secondary treatment. Prolonged treatment with aspirin reduces risks for

Table 20–1 • RISK FACTORS FOR CAUSES OF CHEST PAIN	
Risk Factor	Event
Age/gender: male >40 y old	CAD
Hypertension	CAD and aortic dissection
Tobacco abuse	CAD, thromboembolism, aortic dissection, pneumothorax, and pneumonia
Diabetes mellitus	CAD
Cocaine use	MI
Hyperlipidemia Increasing TC, TG, LDL Decreasing HDL	MI
Left ventricular hypertrophy	MI
Family history of premature CAD	MI
Blunt trauma to chest	Pneumothorax, myocardial or pulmonary contusion, chest wall injury

Abbreviations: CAD, coronary artery disease; HDL, high-density lipoprotein; LDL, low-density lipoprotein; MI, myocardial infarction; TC, total cholesterol; TG, triglyceride.

both CAD and cerebrovascular disease. β-Adrenergic antagonist reduces first-year mortality. If no adverse effects are experienced, patients should continue β-adrenergic antagonist 2 to 3 years or longer. Long-acting nitrates can treat angina symptoms.

β-Hydroxy-β-methylglutaryl-coenzyme A (HMG-CoA) reductase inhibitors (statins) have documented a consistent decrease in the incidence of major adverse cardiovascular events when given within a few days after onset of ACS. There are few data on patients treated within 24 hours of the onset of symptoms. It is safe and feasible to start statin therapy early (within 24 hours) in patients; once started, continue statin therapy uninterrupted. The American College of Cardiology/American Heart Association recommendations are for all persons with known atherosclerotic cardiovascular disease (ASCVD) to be treated with high-intensity statin therapy.

Hypertension must be treated using agents that reduce cardiac complications, as previously discussed. If further reduction is necessary, many medications treat hypertension and angina. Blood pressure and coronary pathology have a linear relationship; as blood pressure is reduced, the risk, morbidity, and mortality of cardiac disease are also reduced. Agents used often depend on a patient's comorbid conditions.

Physical activity is an important component of lifestyle change. Recommendation of a minimum goal of 30 minutes of exercise on most days should be given to all patients. Weight management is also encouraged, but often requires numerous interventions. A minimum of a 5% reduction in weight will provide benefits to the patient. Body mass index needs to become part of the vital signs examined every visit.

CLINICAL PRESENTATION

The history should focus on onset and evolution of the chest pain. The cardinal features of all chief complaints should be followed, paying attention to patient's description of the pain/discomfort, location, radiation of pain, quality of pain, severity of pain, duration, associating factors, and aggravating and/or alleviating factors (Table 20–2). **Many people do not describe angina as chest pain.** It is more effective to ask the patient to describe the discomfort. Some describe it as pressure, squeezing, crushing, or smothering. Some may use a "Levine sign," a fist held firmly against the chest. The discomfort is usually central and substernal. It may radiate to the jaw, shoulder, arm, or hand, usually to the left side. Cardiogenic nausea and vomiting are associated with larger MIs.

The relationship of the symptoms to exertion is very important. Exertion, emotional stress, or other situations that either increase myocardial oxygen demand or decrease oxygen supply can increase symptoms. **Angina usually responds promptly to measures that reduce myocardial oxygen demand**, such as rest. Pain typically resolves in less than 5 minutes. If angina persists for longer than 20 to 30 minutes, a MI is more likely. In this setting, hospitalization and further evaluation are warranted.

The targeted history in patients with angina needs to ascertain whether the patient has had prior episodes of myocardial ischemia (stable or unstable angina, MI, interventions such as bypass surgery or angioplasty). Evaluation of the patient's complaints should focus on chest discomfort, associated symptoms, gender and

Table 20–2 • DIFFERENTIAL DIAGNOSIS OF CHEST PAIN		
Disorder	Symptoms/Findings	Studies
Angina	Substernal pressure for duration <30 min	ECG, CXR, serum values
	Radiation to arm, neck, jaw ± dyspnea, N/V, diaphoresis ↑ with exertion; ↓ with rest and NTG	
MI	Anginal symptoms but duration >30 min	ECG, CXR, serum values
Pericarditis	Sharp pain radiates to trapezius ↑ with respiration; ↓ with sitting forward	Friction rub, ECG, ± pericardial effusion
Aortic dissection	Sudden onset of tearing pain with radiation to back	CXR, widened mediastinum CT, TEE, MRI
Heart failure	Exertional chest pain and dyspnea (uncommon cause of angina, but often patients may also have CAD)	CXR, displaced apical impulse, edema (pulmonary, lower extremities), JVD, cardiac gallop, murmurs
Pneumonia	Dyspnea, fever, and cough; pleuritic pain	CXR, egophony, dullness to percussion
Pneumothorax	Unilateral sharp pleuritic pain of sudden onset, CXR findings	Unilateral ↓ breath sounds and/or hyperresonance
Pulmonary embolism	Sudden onset of pleuritic pain, tachycardia, tachypnea, hypoxemia	D-dimer, V/Q scan, CT chest, pulmonary angiogram
Gastroesophageal reflux	Burning epigastric/substernal pain, acid taste in mouth, ↑ with meals; ↓ with PPIs or antacids	Endoscopy, esophageal pH probe
Peptic ulcer disease	Epigastric pain ↓ with antacids and PPIs	Endoscopy Helicobacter pylori test
Pancreatitis	Severe epigastric and back pain	↑ amylase and lipase, abdominal CT
Costochondritis	Localized pain that is easily reproducible, tender to palpation	Tenderness to palpation
Anxiety	"Tightness" sensation of chest, SOB, tachycardia	Ask screening questions for anxiety and panic
Herpes zoster	Pain often presents prior to rash	Unilateral pain in dermatomal distribution

Abbreviations: ↓, decreasing; ↑, increasing; CAD, coronary artery disease; CT, computed tomography; CXR, chest x-ray; ECG, electrocardiogram; JVD, jugular venous distension; MI, myocardial infarction; MRI, magnetic resonance imaging; NTG, nitroglycerin; N/V, nausea and vomiting; PPI, proton pump inhibitor; SOB, shortness of breath; TEE, transesophageal echocardiogram.

age-related differences in presentation, hypertension, diabetes mellitus, possibility of aortic dissection, risk of bleeding, and clinical cerebrovascular disease (amaurosis fugax, face/limb weakness or clumsiness, face/limb numbness or sensory loss, ataxia, or vertigo).

The physical examination needs to concentrate on evidence that supports or disproves a diagnosis of cardiovascular disease. General appearance and vital signs can reveal much about the patient and the patient's stability. Hypertension, evidence of elevated lipids, changes consistent with diabetes mellitus, and signs of peripheral vascular disease all increase the risk of CAD.

Funduscopic examination can show signs of chronic hypertension or diabetes mellitus. All blood vessels must be auscultated for bruits, a direct sign of atherosclerotic disease. Diminished peripheral pulses are also a sign of atherosclerotic disease. Signs of heart failure include pulmonary edema, rales, jugular venous distension, and hepatojugular reflux. New gallops or murmurs can signal myocardial ischemia. Shallow, painful breathing suggests chest pain with a pleural cause. Asymmetric expansion of the chest with unilateral hyperresonance to percussion and diminished breath sounds are indicative of a possible pneumothorax.

The cardiac examination requires careful evaluation. **Unequal carotid pulses or upper extremity pulses can indicate aortic dissection, but most patients with dissection will not have pulse deficit.** The murmur of aortic stenosis can be significant, as aortic stenosis can present with angina, which can then lead to syncope and heart failure.

The patient's chest wall should be palpated. If this examination reproduces the chest pain, costochondritis becomes more likely. **Musculoskeletal causes of chest pain are the most common etiology in an outpatient setting.** Abdominal examination is also important, as gastrointestinal etiology is the second most common culprit for chest pain in an outpatient setting. Careful examination of both upper quadrants and epigastric area must be done. The abdominal aorta warrants careful examination. Additionally, panic disorder and anxiety can cause chest pain, tightness and shortness of breath. Physicians should use a questionnaire to evaluate any possible psychogenic causes when this is suspected.

COMPREHENSION QUESTIONS

20.1 A 58-year-old man presents to his physician for follow-up of his hypertension and hyperlipidemia. He also reports chest pain and feeling short of breath after climbing two flights of stairs or walking three to four blocks. The symptoms resolve after several minutes of rest. Which of the following drugs is contraindicated as a first-line agent in the treatment of this patient's new condition?

A. Labetalol

B. Nitroglycerin

C. Enalapril

D. Nifedipine

E. Aspirin

20.2 Which one of the following patients presenting with chest pain is at the highest risk for an acute myocardial infarction?

A. A 40-year-old woman on proton pump inhibitor for reflux disease

B. A 75-year-old man with parasternal chest pain, lipid abnormalities, and no past history or cardiac disease

C. A 23-year-old man recently diagnosed with hypertrophic cardiomyopathy

D. A 67-year-old man with a history of a prior angioplasty, with chest pain radiating to the neck and complaint of diaphoresis

20.3 Which of the following ECG changes makes the determination of acute MI the most difficult?

A. Q wave

B. ST-segment elevation

C. Left bundle branch block

D. First-degree atrioventricular block

E. T-wave inversion

20.4 A 64-year-old woman with a history of hypertension and angina pectoris presents with chest pain for the last 3 hours. She describes the pain as "sharp," it is worse when she inhales deeply, and it is not relieved by sublingual nitroglycerin. Her ECG shows ST elevation in most leads. Which of the following is the most likely diagnosis in this patient?

A. Unstable angina pectoris

B. Myocardial infarction

C. Aortic dissection

D. Congestive heart failure

E. Pericarditis

ANSWERS

20.1 **D.** This patient has new onset of angina. Rapid release, short-acting dihydropyridines (nifedipine) are contraindicated because they increased mortality in multiple trials. β-Blocking agents are the agents of choice since they increase survival; nitroglycerin helps to abate chest pain, but has not been shown to impact survival.

20.2 **D.** Risk factors for increased likelihood of acute MI are male gender, age older than 60 years, chest pain radiating to neck, jaw, arm, or shoulder, and a prior history of angina or acute MI.

20.3 **C.** The changes of left bundle branch block make the determination of an acute MI by an ECG extremely difficult. In these patients, it is particularly important to obtain serum markers of myocardial damage.

20.4 **E.** This patient likely has pericarditis. The pain is described as sharp in nature rather than dull, aching, pressure. The pain is exacerbated by inspiration, and finally there is global ST-segment elevation noted on the ECG.

CLINICAL PEARLS

▶ Angina pectoris is the most frequent symptom of intermittent ischemia.

▶ Targeted history and physical examinations of patients with angina are vital to expedite proper diagnosis and treatment of patients. The patient's description of their discomfort is key; history must be given attention because it is the most important diagnostic factor.

▶ Physical examination may be normal in many patients with angina.

▶ Aspirin, nitrates, β-adrenergic antagonists, and statins are the backbone in treatment and prevention of myocardial pathology, having proven benefit for both primary and secondary treatment.

▶ Time is myocardium. Initial diagnosis and treatment must be done as soon as possible.

▶ Be mindful of polypharmacy, as many drugs have side effects that can exacerbate myocardial damage.

▶ The most common etiology of chest pain in the primary care setting is musculoskeletal. However, it is imperative to rule out cardiac cause of chest pain before making a musculoskeletal-related diagnosis.

REFERENCES

American Heart Association. 2005 International consensus conference on cardiopulmonary resuscitation and emergency cardiovascular care science with treatment recommendations. Dallas, Texas. January 23-30, 2005.

Bosker G. *Textbook of Adult and Pediatric Emergency Medicine.* 2nd ed. Atlanta, GA: American Health Consultants; 2002.

Braunwald E, Antman EM, Beasly JW, et al. ACC/AHA guidelines for the management of patients with unstable angina and non–ST-segment elevation myocardial infarction: executive summary and recommendations. *Circulation.* 2000 Sep 5;102(10):1193-1209.

Elliott A. ACC/AHA guidelines for the management of patients with ST-elevation myocardial infarction—executive summary. A report of the American College of Cardiology/American Heart Association Task Force on Practice Guidelines. *Circulation.* 2004;110:588-636.

Marshall S. *On Call Principles and Protocols.* 3rd ed. Philadelphia, PA: WB Saunders; 2000.

McConaghy JR, Oza RS. Outpatient diagnosis of acute chest pain in adults. *Am Fam Physician.* 2013 Feb 1;87(3):177-182.

Sabatine M. Pocket medicine. *The Massachusetts General Hospital Handbook of Internal Medicine.* Baltimore, MD: Lippincott Williams & Wilkins; 2000.

Shubhada A, Kellie F, Subramanian P. *The Washington Manual of Medical Therapeutics.* 30th ed. Baltimore, MD: Lippincott Williams & Wilkins; 2001.

Wiviott S, Braunwald E. Myocardial infarction. *Am Fam Physician.* 2004;70:535-538.

A 46-year-old woman presents to the clinic for the first time, complaining of decreased urinary output for 5 months with a foamy appearance. She also complains of swelling in both legs and nonbloody, nonbilious emesis a few times a week. She was diagnosed with diabetes 10 years ago and has been taking insulin for 2 years. She does not check her sugars at home because she does not like to "stick" herself. When asked about her diet she states that she eats the best she can for what she can afford but often has very little appetite. The patient last saw her physician 8 months ago and insulin is her only medication. On examination, the patient is an obese woman. Her temperature is 99°F (37.2°C), her heart rate is 108 beats/min, her blood pressure is 198/105 mm Hg, her respiration is 19 breaths/min, and her oxygen saturation is 94% on room air. A head, ears, eyes, nose, and throat (HEENT) examination reveals periorbital edema. Her skin is hyperpigmented on both lower extremities. Her heart is tachycardic with an S_1, S_2, S_4 gallop auscultated with no murmur or rub. When palpating the heart's point of maximal impulse (PMI), it is lateral to the left midclavicular line. There are vesicular breath sounds in both lungs throughout. Her neck reveals no jugular venous distension and there are no carotid bruits. Her abdomen is nontender, with no bruits or masses palpated. The lower extremities reveal pitting pretibial edema with a pit recovery time less than 40 seconds. Laboratory studies in your office include a urinalysis showing hyaline casts, 3+ proteinuria, and glucose, but negative for ketones. Her hemoglobin is 10.9 g/dL and her hematocrit is 32% with a mean corpuscular volume (MCV) of 82.3 g/dL.

▶ What is the most likely diagnosis?
▶ What is your next diagnostic step?
▶ What is the next step in therapy?

ANSWERS TO CASE 21:
Chronic Kidney Disease

Summary: This is a 46-year-old woman with chronic kidney disease (CKD). She has a history of uncontrolled diabetes and currently has uncontrolled hypertension. She presents with periorbital edema, long-standing lower-extremity edema, an S_4 and displaced PMI, and central obesity. The urinalysis shows hyaline casts, 3+ proteinuria and glucose, negative ketones, and hemoglobin 10.9 g/dL with an MCV of 82.3 g/dL.

- **Most likely diagnosis:** Acute worsening of CKD

- **Next diagnostic step:** Measurement of serum electrolytes, blood urea nitrogen (BUN), and creatinine; imaging of the kidneys

- **Next step in therapy:** Further history to identify and remove any offending agents (such as nonsteroidal anti-inflammatory drugs [NSAIDs]), and control of blood pressure and diabetes; may require dialysis if she develops complications such as pulmonary edema, severe hyperkalemia, or anuria

ANALYSIS

Objectives

1. Know the risks for developing CKD.

2. Learn to evaluate for CKD.

3. Be familiar with the management of CKD.

4. Recognize the complications associated with CKD.

Considerations

This 46-year-old patient presents with a concerning symptom of a decrease in urination with a change in the appearance of the urine. The most immediate concern is how often she is urinating and to what degree she is urinating less. A significant reduction requires immediate evaluation of creatinine function and volume status. Volume status is assessed by skin turgor, mucous membranes, specific gravity in the urinalysis, and orthostatic blood pressure, which also measures heart rate in the lying, sitting, and standing positions. A low volume status with an elevated creatinine requires that the patient be given IV fluids to see if there can be any recovery of kidney function. The patient's uncontrolled diabetes and hypertension predispose her to kidney damage. Another common offender is a patient with this history who is taking NSAIDs. This will increase the patient's already high risk of damage.

With CKD, patients are often able to compensate for the metabolic imbalances that occur such as hyper- or hyponatremia, hyperkalemia, elevated uric acid levels, and metabolic acidosis. Patients also experience secondary hyperparathyroidism. Significantly elevated potassium levels require treatment with sodium polystyrene sulfonate (Kayexalate), insulin with glucose, and retention enemas, depending on the degree of elevation. When the patient is no longer compensating, there are symptoms of pulmonary edema, which include shortness of breath, lower-extremity edema, jugular venous distension, and abnormal lung sounds (rales). This patient was compensating and mostly demonstrated the result of a hypoalbuminemic state from the loss of protein in the urine. She had lower-extremity edema with a long pit time that reflected her low albumin state. Her occasional emesis reflects high levels of urea and other toxins. Persistent emesis mandates treatment. Her normocytic anemia was the result of reduced erythropoietin from the kidneys. In this setting, treatment with exogenous erythropoietin improves prognosis for cardiovascular mortality. The hyaline casts reflect the long-standing damage to the kidneys.

Increasing the patient's chance of improved kidney function requires glucose and blood pressure control, removing offenders such as NSAIDs and diuretics (if allowable), maintaining normal volume status (which is difficult with a low albumin state), and adding agents that both treat blood pressure and improve kidney and cardiovascular function such as angiotensin-converting enzyme (ACE) inhibitors and angiotensin receptor blockers (ARBs). CKD itself is a cardiovascular risk factor. Patients are more likely to die from cardiovascular disease than to develop end-stage renal disease (ESRD) requiring dialysis. The patient's gross proteinuria of 3+ reflects her high risk for cardiovascular disease.

APPROACH TO:
Chronic Kidney Disease

DEFINITIONS

CKD: A spectrum of processes associated with abnormal kidney function and progressive decline in glomerular filtration rate (GFR).

ESRD: The irreversible loss of kidney function such that the patient is permanently dependent on renal replacement therapy (dialysis or transplantation). It is also defined as a GFR of less than 15 mL/min.

CLINICAL APPROACH

Etiologies

CKD is becoming more common in the United States. **The most common etiologies are diabetes, hypertension, and glomerulonephritis.** Diabetic kidney disease occurs in 30% to 40% of type I diabetics, in 25% of type II diabetics, and in 24% of hypertensive patients. Within the diabetic patient population, 20% to 60% have hypertension. Many patients present at a later stage of CKD and it is then difficult to determine the etiology.

Evaluation

The Kidney Disease Outcomes Quality Initiative (KDOQI) from the National Kidney Foundation (NKF) recommends both a serum creatinine (Cr) to estimate

GFR and random urinalysis for albuminuria in those groups at risk for CKD. The stage of CKD is based on GFR, which can be estimated with a random Cr level calculated with one of two commonly used equations:

Modification of Diet in Renal Disease (MDRD) equation:

$$\text{GFR (mL/min/1.73 m}^2) = 186 \times (\text{Scr})^{-1.54} \times (\text{age})^{-0.203} \times (0.742, \text{ if female}) \times (1.210, \text{ if black})$$

Cockcroft-Gault equation:

$$\text{Ccr (mL/min)} = ([140 - \text{age}] \times \text{weight [kg]})/(72 \times \text{Scr}) \times (0.85, \text{ if female})$$

(Scr = serum creatinine concentration; Ccr = creatinine clearance)

A normal GFR is between 90 and 120 mL/min. Stage 1 of CKD correlates with a GFR more than 90 mL/min in the presence of signs of kidney disease, such as proteinuria, hematuria, or abnormal renal structure; stage 2 correlates with a GFR of 60 to 89 mL/min; stage 3 correlates with a GFR of 30 to 59 mL/min; stage 4 correlates with a GFR of 15 to 29 mL/min; and stage 5 correlates with a GFR less than 15 mL/min or dialysis. The Cockcroft-Gault equation is preferred for older patients and in renal dosing of medications. It is important to note that these equations do not give an accurate calculation of GFR in the setting of an acute change in renal function, such as acute kidney injury. Serial measurements of renal function are recommended for newly diagnosed cases to determine the pace of renal deterioration and whether the disease is truly chronic, as opposed to acute or subacute. A 24-hour urine collection is recommended for persons with extremes of age and weight, malnutrition, skeletal muscle disease, paraplegia or quadriplegia, or a vegetarian diet.

The evaluation in all patients with CKD includes renal imaging (typically with renal ultrasound) and microscopic evaluation of urine. Treatment may be more successful in patients with normal-size kidneys. Small kidneys show irreversible disease. Asymmetry suggests renovascular disease. Evidence of proteinuria or microalbuminuria should be evaluated in all patients with CKD. If the urine dipstick does not reveal gross proteinuria, a sample should be sent to evaluate for microalbumin. A test is positive if there is more than 30 mg of microalbumin per gram Cr. It is recommended in the case of less than 200 mg of protein per gram Cr that the test be repeated yearly. Any patient with more than 200 mg of protein per gram Cr will need diagnostic evaluation and treatment. The protein-to-creatinine ratio in an early-morning random urine sample may be used instead of a 24-hour urine protein excretion.

Underlying causes may be ascertained through clinical presentation, symptomatology, and past medical and family history. Some common laboratory studies include antinuclear antibody (ANA), antiphospholipid antibodies, C3, C4, erythrocyte sedimentation rate (ESR) and/or C-reactive protein (CRP) (looking for lupus nephritis), hepatitis panel and HIV test (looking for infectious etiologies), serum and urine protein electrophoresis (looking for multiple myeloma) for those patients older than age 35, hemoglobin A1c, fasting blood sugar, and analysis of urine sediment. Renal biopsy, if not contraindicated by comorbidities, is indicated in patients with unknown etiology after history and laboratory evaluation, if parenchymal disease is suspected, or if treatment or prognosis will be based on the biopsy. However biopsy is contraindicated if bilateral small kidneys are seen on imaging, as there is a low likelihood of improving outcome due to the presence of late-stage disease. Common conditions associated with CKD, such as anemia and hyperphosphatemia should be tested for.

Management

Managing CKD includes treatment of reversible causes. Hypovolemia, hypotension, infection leading to sepsis, and drugs that lower the GFR all reduce renal perfusion. History and physical examination allow for this diagnosis, and a trial of fluids may improve kidney function. Drugs such as NSAIDs, aminoglycosides at full strength, and radiographic contrast material can affect kidney function. Urinary tract obstruction, commonly caused by prostate enlargement in elderly men, is a potentially reversible cause.

Nonproteinuric renal disease requires strict blood pressure control. JNC 8 guidelines recommend blood pressure goal of less than 140/90 mm Hg in all patients age 18 or older with CKD. Multiple guidelines recommend blood pressure goal of less than 130/80, especially if there is diabetes or proteinuria. Another goal is the reduction of protein excretion to less than 500 to 1000 mg/d (or at least 60% of the baseline value). JNC 8 guidelines recommend starting with an ACE inhibitor or an ARB for blood pressure control in patients with CKD, followed by a thiazide diuretic or calcium channel blocker if the blood pressure goal is not achieved. β-Blockers may also be considered as second- or third-line treatment for blood pressure control. Combining both an ACE inhibitor and an ARB is not recommended.

Other treatments may be beneficial in CKD. Dietary protein restrictions of 0.8 to 1.0 mg/kg/d may be beneficial. Statins are recommended for treatment of hyperlipidemia in most CKD patients not on dialysis. The volume overload associated with CKD responds well to sodium restriction and loop diuretics. This lowers the intraglomerular pressure. Hyperkalemia may be prevented by a low-potassium diet and avoiding drugs such as NSAIDs and, sometimes, ACE inhibitors. Metabolic acidosis may be treated with sodium bicarbonate, with a goal to maintain a concentration of 22 mEq/L. Dietary phosphate restriction may limit the development of secondary hyperparathyroidism in these patients. Vitamin D supplementation has moderate evidence for reduction in all-cause mortality. Patients should also have influenza, pneumococcal vaccinations. Those with high risk of progression should also receive hepatitis B vaccination.

When the GFR is below 25 to 30 mL/min, oral phosphate binders are usually required. Caution is used when treating hyperphosphatemia in stages 3 to 5 CKD. It is suggested that calcium intake not exceed 2000 mg/d, as this may contribute to cardiovascular disease.

Guidelines suggest evaluation of anemia with hemoglobin less than 12 g/dL in females and 13.5 g/dL in adult males. This should include evaluation for nonrenal causes of anemia.

Treating patients with CKD with erythropoietin if hemoglobin is less than 10 g/dL to goal less than 12 g/dL in low-risk patients and less than 13 mg/dL in those at risk for stroke and cardiovascular events may reduce symptoms of anemia, show cardiovascular improvement, and possibly decrease mortality. Ultimately, the patient that is going toward ESRD must be identified and adequately prepared for renal replacement therapy. It is recommended that patients with a GFR less than 30 mg/dL, difficult to control comorbidities, significant proteinuria, or sudden worsening of renal function be referred to a nephrologist for evaluation and preparation for possible dialysis.

> ## CASE CORRELATION
> - See also Case 14 (Hematuria).

COMPREHENSION QUESTIONS

21.1 A 56-year-old man with known CKD presents with a 3-day history of shortness of breath and rapid weight gain. On examination, you are able to auscultate an S_3, hear crackles at the bases, and see moderate jugular venous distension (JVD). Which of the following is your next step in evaluation?

A. Perform an echocardiogram.

B. Order a chest x-ray.

C. Measure a Cr to calculate GFR.

D. Check for cardiac enzymes.

21.2 A 39-year-old woman with multiple medical problems has been noted to have progressively worsening renal insufficiency. Which of the following measures is most important in the prevention of end-stage renal disease?

A. Tobacco cessation

B. Triglyceride control

C. Glycemic control

D. Weight control

E. Dietary sodium restriction

21.3 A 72-year-old man, with a long history of hypertension, presents to the emergency department (ED) complaining of a 2-day history of emesis and 36 hours of no urination. On examination, the abdomen is firm and tender, and the prostate is enlarged. His serum creatinine level is 3.4 mg/dL. Which the following is the best next step?

A. Give him IV fluids and see if he begins to make urine.

B. Perform a renal ultrasound in the ED.

C. Maintain tight control of his blood pressure.

D. Place an indwelling Foley catheter.

21.4 A 45-year-old woman with type 2 diabetes presents to the clinic with decreased vision in the left eye for 1 year, 1+ proteinuria, a baseline Cr of 1.6 mg/dL, an low-density lipoprotein (LDL) of 135 mg/dL, blood pressure of 145/92 mm Hg, and occasional chest pain for the past 2 months. Which of the following is the best medication to start the patient on at this time?

A. ACE inhibitor

B. β-Blocker

C. Oral nitrate

D. Thiazide diuretic

ANSWERS

21.1 **B.** The patient has CKD with volume overload as evidenced by symptoms and physical examination. A simple first step is to do a chest x-ray to confirm what you already suspect—pulmonary edema. After initiating furosemide (Lasix), the chest x-ray may be repeated to see to what degree the diuresis has improved the overload. Cardiac workup is also indicated but would not be the first test done.

21.2 **C.** Optimal control of high blood pressure, acidosis, volume depletion, and cholesterol are all important to prevent worsening renal function. Diabetes is a leading cause of end-stage renal disease. Tight glycemic control can prevent the microvascular complications of diabetes such as diabetic nephropathy, though it has not been shown to decrease significantly the occurrence of macrovascular complications of diabetes such as coronary artery disease (CAD) or peripheral vascular disease (PVD). Treating secondary hyperparathyroidism prevents complications such as renal osteodystrophy. The patient's weight does not impact on renal function substantially. Smoking has numerous health risks but does not tend to impact kidney function directly; nevertheless, its effect on cardiovascular system may impact on the kidneys.

21.3 **D.** The patient has an enlarged prostate that has caused urinary obstruction and potentially reversible renal failure, depending on at which point the obstruction is resolved. Placing the Foley catheter will usually allow for significant reversal of an elevated Cr. Following catheter placement, the urine output needs to be carefully monitored and the Cr repeated later. Another clue is the tense lower abdomen that is caused by a very enlarged bladder. It is especially important to rely on clinical examination skills in elderly patients who have less-than-optimal communication skills as a consequence of dementia or who have a history of stroke when evaluating for a cause.

21.4 **A.** ACE inhibitors would help in hypertension treatment and to protect renal function in this patient. Both diabetes and CKD are known to be cardiovascular risk equivalents. Other factors, such as uncontrolled blood pressure and cholesterol, add to the patient's high risk, which is why it is so important for all diabetics and CKD patients to improve all modifiable risk factors. The goals become much more stringent when looking at these two groups of patients.

CLINICAL PEARLS

▶ Small kidneys on imaging usually reflect irreversible disease. Small kidneys should rarely be biopsied, as the result of the biopsy usually will not alter the treatment or prognosis of the condition.

▶ Calculation of the estimated GFR using the Cockcroft-Gault formula is an important process as, especially in older persons, a seemingly normal serum creatinine could reflect a significant reduction in GFR and could affect dosing of medications.

REFERENCES

Bargman JM, Skorecki K. Chronic kidney disease. In: Kasper D, Fauci A, Hauser S, et al., eds. *Harrison's Principles of Internal Medicine*. 19th ed. New York, NY: McGraw-Hill; 2015. Available at: http://accessmedicine.mhmedical.com. Accessed May 25, 2015.

Fowler M. Microvascular and macrovascular complications of diabetes. *Clin Diabetes*. 2008;26:2. Available at: http://clinical.diabetesjournals.org/content/26/2/77.full.pdf+html. Accessed May 2009.

James PA, Oparil S, Carter BL, et al. 2014 evidence-based guideline for the management of high blood pressure in adults: report from the panel members appointed to the eighth Joint National Committee (JNC 8). *JAMA*. 2014;311(5):507-520.

Kidney Disease Improving Global Outcomes clinical practice guideline for lipid management in chronic kidney disease: 2013 update. *Kidney Int Suppl*. 2013;3:263-264.

National Kidney Foundation. NKF-KDOQI clinical practice guidelines and clinical practice recommendations for anemia in chronic kidney disease. *Am J Kidney Dis*. 2006;47(suppl 3):S26.

National Kidney Foundation. KDOQI clinical practice guideline for diabetes and CKD: 2012 update. *Am J Kidney Dis*. 2012;60(5):850-886.

Patel A, MacMahon S, Chalmers J, et al. Intensive blood glucose control and vascular outcomes in patients with type 2 diabetes. *N Engl J Med*. 2008 June 6;358(24):2560-72. Available at: http://dx.doi.org/10.1056/NEJMoa0802987. Accessed June 2009.

Rivera JA, O'Hare AM, Harper GM. Update on the management of chronic kidney disease. *Am Fam Physician*. 2012 Oct 15;86(8):749-754.

A 25-year-old woman presents to the office with a 1-week history of vaginal discharge. She describes the discharge as being green-yellow in color with a bad odor. She has never had this type of discharge in the past. She complains of increased vaginal soreness and discharge after she has intercourse. She denies any itching, abdominal pain, nausea, vomiting, fever, chills, or sweats. She is currently sexually active and is using an intrauterine device (IUD) as her contraceptive method. She has been with one male partner for the past 3 months and he has no symptoms. She does state that she first had intercourse at age 15 and has had multiple sexual partners. She had a chlamydial infection 2 years ago that was treated with oral antibiotics. Her last menstrual period was 2 weeks ago and was normal. She also denies any recent antibiotic treatment. On examination, she is afebrile, has normal vital signs, and appears to be in no acute distress. Her general physical examination is normal. On pelvic examination, she has normal external genitalia. She has a small amount of frothy, homogenous green-gray discharge at the introitus. The cervix has a "strawberry"-red appearance with a slight amount of discharge noted in the os. The IUD string is in place. *Chlamydia* and gonorrhea specimens are obtained from the os and a sample of the vaginal discharge is collected for microscopic evaluation. Bimanual examination shows no cervical motion tenderness, and a normal uterus and adnexa.

▶ What organism is the most likely cause of her symptoms?
▶ What would you expect to see on microscopic examination of the vaginal discharge?
▶ What is the recommended treatment for this infection?

ANSWERS TO CASE 22:
Vaginitis

Summary: A 25-year-old woman presents with a foul-smelling vaginal discharge. She has a greenish, frothy discharge and a "strawberry cervix" noted on examination.

- **Organism most likely to cause this infection:** *Trichomonas vaginalis.*

- **Expected microscopic examination findings:** Motile, flagellated trichomonads, and many white blood cells.

- **Recommended treatment:** Metronidazole 2 g by mouth in a single dose for both the patient and her sexual partner. Metronidazole 500 mg twice a day for a week is an alternate regimen.

ANALYSIS
Objectives

1. Be able to differentiate among common presentations of vaginitis on the basis of clinical information and laboratory testing.

2. Know the current guidelines for treatment of the various etiologies of vaginitis.

Considerations

Women with vaginitis may present with a variety of symptoms, including vaginal discharge, itching, odor, and dysuria. There are many potential causes of vaginitis, including sexually transmitted pathogens and overgrowth of organisms found in the normal vaginal flora. Common among the causes of vaginitis are *Candida albicans, T vaginalis*, and polymicrobial (*Gardnerella vaginalis* predominant) mix of bacterial vaginosis.

Certain historical information may lead a clinician to suspect a specific cause of vaginitis in a given patient. For example, a history of recent antibiotic use may predispose to a *Candida* vaginitis, as the antibiotic may alter the normal vaginal flora and allow the overgrowth of a fungal organism. Women with diabetes mellitus are also more predisposed to developing yeast infections. A history of multiple sexual partners may raise the likelihood of a sexually transmitted infection, such as trichomoniasis.

The patient's symptoms and signs may also suggest a specific organism as the cause of her vaginitis. Fungal infections tend to have thick discharge and cause significant pruritus. The discharge of bacterial vaginosis is often thinner and patients complain of a "fishy" odor. *Trichomonas* produces a discharge that is usually frothy and the patient's cervix is frequently very erythematous.

The key test to determining the cause of vaginal discharge, which guides the specific treatment, is microscopic examination of the discharge. A sample of the discharge is examined both as a "wet mount" (ie, mixed with a small amount of normal saline) and as a "KOH prep" (ie, mixed with a small amount of 10% potassium hydroxide). On wet mount, the examiner can evaluate the normal epithelial cells and look for white blood cells, red blood cells, clue cells, and motile trichomonads. The hyphae or pseudohyphae of *Candida* are best seen on KOH prep.

APPROACH TO:
Vaginal Infections

DEFINITIONS

BACTERIAL VAGINOSIS: Condition of excessive anaerobic bacteria in the vagina, leading to a discharge that is alkaline.

CANDIDA VULVOVAGINITIS: Vaginal and/or vulvar infection caused by *Candida* species, usually with heterogenous discharge and inflammation.

TRICHOMONAS VAGINITIS: Infection of the vagina caused by the protozoa *T vaginalis*, usually associated with a frothy green discharge and intense inflammatory response.

CLINICAL APPROACH
ETIOLOGIES

Vulvovaginal Candidiasis

This infection is typically caused by *C albicans*, although other species are occasionally identified. **More than 75% of women have at least one episode during their lifetime.** The presenting symptom is a thick, whitish discharge that has no odor and the patient complains of significant pruritus of the external and internal genitalia. On physical examination, the vaginal area can be edematous with erythema present. The discharge has a pH between 4.0 and 5.0. The diagnosis is confirmed by wet mount or KOH preparation showing budding yeast or pseudohyphae. **Fungal cultures are not needed to confirm the diagnosis,** but they are useful if the infection recurs or is unresponsive to treatment. Numerous treatment options are available for patients with vulvovaginal candidiasis, including over-the-counter and prescription medications. Uncomplicated candidiasis can be treated effectively with short-term intravaginal preparations (creams or vaginal suppositories) or single-dose oral therapies (fluconazole 150 mg). Treatment of complicated or recurrent infection should begin with an intensive regimen for 10 to 14 days followed by 6 months of maintenance therapy to reduce the likelihood of recurrence. Treatment of sexual partners is not indicated unless symptomatic (eg, male partners with balanitis).

Trichomoniasis

This infection is caused by the protozoan *T vaginalis* and is classified as a sexually transmitted disease (STD). The incubation period is 3 to 21 days after exposure.

Certain factors predispose to infection, such as multiple sexual partners, pregnancy, and menopause. The presenting complaint is copious amounts of a thin, frothy, green-yellow or gray malodorous vaginal discharge. Women can also have vaginal soreness or dyspareunia. Symptoms may start or be exacerbated during the time of their menses. Vaginal examination may reveal that the cervix has a "strawberry" appearance (red and inflamed with punctations) or that redness of the vagina and perineum is present. Microscopically, the wet mount preparation can demonstrate motile trichomonads and many white blood cells, although cultures may be necessary because of the significant number of false-negative results. The recommended treatment for trichomoniasis is oral metronidazole, given in a single, 2-g oral dose or 1-week regimen of 500 mg twice a day to both the patient and her sexual partner. It is important to screen for other STDs and to remember to treat the partner to ensure better cure rates.

Bacterial Vaginosis

Bacterial vaginosis (BV) arises when normal vaginal bacteria are replaced with an overgrowth of anaerobic bacteria and G vaginalis. Although not an STD, it is associated with having multiple sexual partners. Diagnosis can be based on the presence of three of four clinical criteria: (1) a thin, homogenous vaginal discharge; (2) a vaginal pH more than 4.5; (3) a positive KOH "whiff" test (a fishy odor present after the addition of 10% KOH to a sample of the discharge); and (4) the presence of clue cells in a wet mount preparation (Figure 22–1). Culture is generally not needed. Treatment options include both oral and topical vaginal preparations of metronidazole or clindamycin. There are no advantages to any of these regimens with regard to cure rates or recurrence, although patients do report more satisfaction with the vaginal preparations. Treatment of BV in asymptomatic pregnant women may reduce the incidence of preterm delivery. Treatment of sexual partners is not necessary and does not reduce the risk of recurrent infection.

Mucopurulent Cervicitis

This infection is characterized by purulent or mucopurulent discharge from the endocervix, which may be associated with vaginal discharge and/or cervical bleeding. The diagnostic evaluation should include testing for *Chlamydia trachomatis* and *Neisseria gonorrhoeae*, although the etiologic agent is not always found. Absence of symptoms should not prevent additional evaluation and treatment, as approximately 50% of gonococcal infections and 70% of chlamydial infections are asymptomatic in women. The gold standard for establishing the diagnosis is a culture of the cervical discharge. Empiric treatment should be considered in areas of high prevalence of infection or if follow-up is unlikely. The first-line treatment recommendation for gonorrhea is ceftriaxone 125 mg intramuscularly. Because of the growing problem of antibiotic resistance, quinolone antibiotics (ciprofloxacin, ofloxacin) and oral cephalosporin antibiotics are no longer recommended for treatment of gonorrhea. The recommended treatment for *Chlamydia* infections is azithromycin in a single 1-g oral dose or doxycycline 100 mg orally twice daily for 7 days. Typical treatment regimens will cover for both gonorrhea and chlamydia and the treatment of sexual partners is advised.

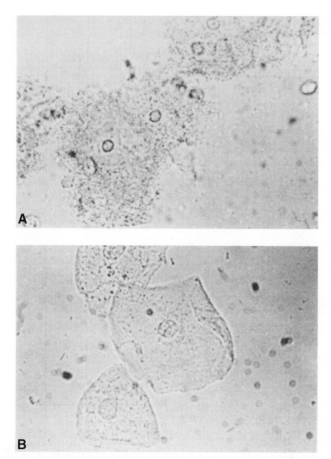

Figure 22–1. Bacterial vaginosis. (A) "Clue cells." (B) Normal epithelium. (*Reproduced, with permission, from Kasper DL, Braunwald E, Fauci A, et al. Harrison's Principles of Internal Medicine. 16th ed. New York, NY: McGraw-Hill; 2005:767.*)

Pelvic Inflammatory Disease

Pelvic inflammatory disease (PID) is defined as inflammation of the upper genital tract, including pelvic peritonitis, endometritis, salpingitis, and tubo-ovarian abscess caused by infection with gonorrhea, *Chlamydia*, or vaginal and bowel flora. **The presence of lower abdominal tenderness with both adnexal and cervical motion tenderness, without other explanation of illness, is enough to diagnose PID.** Other criteria that enhance the specificity of the diagnosis include temperature more than 101°F, abnormal cervical or vaginal discharge, elevated sedimentation rate, elevated C-reactive protein, and cervical infection with gonorrhea or *Chlamydia*. **Because of the clinical similarity between PID and ectopic pregnancy, a serum pregnancy test should be performed on all patients suspected of having PID.**

Determination of appropriate treatment should consider pregnancy status, severity of illness, and compliance. Less-severe disease can generally be treated on an outpatient basis. Women who are pregnant, have HIV, or have severe disease

Table 22–1 • TREATMENT REGIMENS FOR PID
Oral and Intramuscular
Regimen A • Ceftriaxone 250 mg IM single dose *or* cefoxitin 2 g IM with probenecid 1 g PO given concurrently • *Plus* doxycycline 100 mg PO BID for 14 d • *With or without* metronidazole 500 mg PO BID for 14 d Regimen B • Cefotaxime 1 g IM single dose *or* ceftizoxime 1 g IM single dose • *Plus* doxycycline 100 mg PO BID for 14 d • *With or without* metronidazole 500 mg PO BID for 14 d
Parenteral
Regimen A • Cefotetan 2 g IV every 12 h *or* cefoxitin 2 g IV every 6 h • *Plus* doxycycline 100 mg PO *or* IV every 12 h Regimen B • Clindamycin 900 mg IV every 8 h • *Plus* gentamicin 2 mg/kg loading dose (IV or IM) followed by 1.5 mg/kg IV every 8 h. Single daily dosing (3-5 mg/kg) can be substituted Regimen C • Ampicillin/sulbactam 3 g IV every 6 h *plus* doxycycline 100 mg PO or IV every 2 h

generally require inpatient therapy and treatment with parenteral antibiotics. Table 22–1 lists PID treatment regimens.

Patients who have PID need to be aware of potential complications, including the potential for recurrence of disease, the development of tubo-ovarian abscess, chronic abdominal pain, infertility, and the increased risk of ectopic pregnancy. It is important to discuss these potential problems with patients who are given a diagnosis of PID. All patients with STDs or who are at risk for developing STDs should be counseled on safer sexual practices, including abstinence, monogamy, and the use of latex condoms.

CASE CORRELATION

- See also Case 11 (Health Maintenance, Adult Female).

COMPREHENSION QUESTIONS

22.1 A 24-year-old nulliparous woman is noted to have a bothersome vaginal discharge. On examination, she is found to have a homogenous discharge with a fishy odor. Which of the following characteristics is likely to be noted on examination of the discharge?

A. Motile protozoa on wet mount

B. pH more than 4.5

C. Strawberry cervix on speculum examination

D. Budding hyphae on KOH examination

22.2 A 38-year-old woman complains of a new-onset vaginal discharge and irritation. She notes having had a urinary tract infection 10 days previously, with subsequent resolution of her symptoms following treatment. Which of the following is the best empiric therapy for her condition?

A. Oral metronidazole

B. Vaginal metronidazole

C. Oral fluconazole

D. Oral clindamycin

E. Oral estrogen and progestin therapy

22.3 A 24-year-old woman is noted to have lower abdominal tenderness, cervical motion tenderness, and a vaginal discharge. She has a low-grade fever of 100.5°F (38.0°C). Which of the following is the best therapy for her condition?

A. Ceftriaxone intramuscularly and doxycycline orally

B. Ampicillin orally and azithromycin orally

C. Metronidazole orally as a single dose

D. Ciprofloxacin orally as a single dose

ANSWERS

22.1 **B.** This discharge of homogenous and fishy odor is most likely bacterial vaginosis associated with an alkaline pH. Partner treatment is not necessary for bacterial vaginosis. Oral metronidazole is one treatment.

22.2 **C.** This patient most likely has *Candida* vulvovaginitis, since her discharge appeared after her cystitis, likely treated with antibiotics. A treatment for *Candida* vulvovaginitis includes fluconazole or topical azole agents such as miconazole.

22.3 **A.** An option for outpatient therapy of salpingitis (PID) is IM ceftriaxone and oral doxycycline. Oral metronidazole as a single dose is a treatment for *Trichomonas* vaginitis. Fluoroquinolones are not recommended in the United States for the treatment of gonorrhea or associated conditions, such as PID, due to increasing rates of resistance.

CLINICAL PEARLS

▶ Remember to treat sexual partners when you diagnose a sexually transmitted infection and to test for other sexually transmitted infections that may initially be asymptomatic, such as HIV, hepatitis B and C, and syphilis.

▶ Single-dose therapy is available for many types of infections, including *Trichomonas*, gonococcal and chlamydial cervicitis, and *Candida* vaginitis. Providing single-dose therapy in your office will improve your patient's compliance, as well as rates of successful treatment.

REFERENCES

Centers for Disease Control and Prevention (CDC). Sexually transmitted diseases treatment guidelines. *MMWR Morb Mortal Wkly Rep.* 2010;59(RR-12):63-66.

Centers for Disease Control and Prevention (CDC). Update to CDC's sexually transmitted diseases treatment 2010 guidelines: oral cephalosporins no longer a recommended treatment for gonococcal infections. *MMWR Morb Mortal Wkly Rep.* 2012 August 10;61(31):590-594.

Gradison M. Pelvic inflammatory disease. *Am Fam Physician.* 2012 Apr 15;85(8):791-796.

Maier R, Katsufrakis PJ. Sexually transmitted diseases. In: South-Paul JE, Matheny SC, Lewis EL, et al., eds. *Current Diagnosis & Treatment: Family Medicine.* 4th ed. New York, NY: McGraw-Hill; 2015. Available at: http://accessmedicine.mhmedical.com. Accessed May 25, 2015.

A 62-year-old man presents to your office for a routine evaluation. His only complaint is of fatigue over the past 2 to 3 months despite no changes in diet or lifestyle. On questioning, the patient reports that he has never smoked and admits to an increase in his consumption of alcohol upon retiring, to about two to three beers per day. He has occasional headaches on the day after a night of heavy drinking, which are easily relieved by the use of over-the-counter nonsteroidal anti-inflammatory drug (NSAID) preparations. While talking to the patient and examining his chart, you note no distress and proceed with your examination. You note a 4-lb weight loss since his last visit 6 months ago and a relative increase in his pulse with a blood pressure of 129/81 mm Hg. Remarkable to this visit is the paleness of his conjunctivae, but the rest of his general examination is unchanged from the previous examination. You perform a digital rectal examination and find a smooth, normal-size prostate and some soft, reducible protrusions within the internal sphincter, along with guaiac-positive stools. You decide on a more direct approach and delve into his drinking, bowel habits, and NSAID use. His only addition is the occasional production of bloody stools accompanied by some diffuse abdominal discomfort.

► What is the most likely diagnosis?
► What is your next diagnostic step?
► What is the next step in therapy?

ANSWERS TO CASE 23:
Lower Gastrointestinal Bleeding

Summary: A 62-year-old man presents to your office for a routine checkup. He reports having occasional bloody stools and you discover guaiac-positive stools. He is a bit pale, but hemodynamically stable at the moment. You decide that further evaluation of this bleeding is necessary, but most of it can be carried out on an outpatient basis with close follow-up.

- **Most likely diagnosis:** Hemorrhoids.

- **Next diagnostic step:** Complete blood count (CBC) and colonoscopy.

- **Next step in therapy:** Discontinue NSAID use and decrease alcohol consumption.

ANALYSIS

Objectives

1. Know how to recognize the subtle signs and symptoms of lower gastrointestinal (GI) bleeding.

2. Understand the etiologies of lower GI bleeding.

3. Understand how to correctly evaluate and treat patients with lower GI bleeding in outpatient settings.

Considerations

This 62-year-old man presented to your office for a routine examination but was found to have some type of lower gastrointestinal bleeding that needs further evaluation. During his office visit there are no signs of hemodynamic instability or active bleeding that require immediate referral to an emergency room (ER) or inpatient treatment, so you decide on close outpatient follow-up during his workup. His immediate identifiable and modifiable risk factors for GI bleeding include the regular consumption of alcohol and NSAIDs. You counsel him on both these matters and send him to the laboratory for a CBC, chemistry panel, liver function tests, and coagulation profile prior to his discharge home from your office. Barring any abnormal laboratory values that require emergent management, you schedule him for an outpatient colonoscopy later in the week. Your differential diagnosis at this time is wide but you start to consider the most frequent offenders in his age group, which include diverticular disease, hemorrhoids, tumors, and ulcerative colitis. For the time being, you modify those factors that may contribute to any of these etiologies and await the results of his laboratory tests.

> # APPROACH TO:
> ## Lower Gastrointestinal Bleeding

DEFINITIONS

HEMATOCHEZIA: Bright red blood visible in the stool.

LOWER GI BLEEDING: Bleeding that comes from a source distal to the ligament of Treitz.

CLINICAL APPROACH

The manifestations of GI bleeding depend on the source, rate of bleeding, and underlying or coexisting disease. An older patient, or someone with significant comorbidities, such as coronary artery disease, would be at a higher risk of presenting in shock. A younger, healthier individual may present with symptoms such as fatigue or dyspnea on exertion, or may complain directly of seeing blood in the stool. Signs and symptoms of anemia are common and include weakness, easy fatigability, pallor of the conjunctivae or skin, chest pain, dizziness, tachycardia, hypotension, and orthostasis.

A history of blood in the stool or finding guaiac-positive stool on examination should prompt further evaluation to determine the source of the bleeding. Depending on a patient's history and hemodynamic status, more immediate and invasive measures may be necessary once GI bleeding is identified. For example, **hematochezia is usually pathognomonic of lower GI bleeding, but can also be found in patients with heavy upper GI bleeding.** In this setting, a nasogastric aspirate may help differentiate this small subset of patients.

It is critical to transport unstable patients who present with GI bleeding to the ER for hospitalization. Intensive care unit (ICU) admission should not be delayed in those with severe bleeding and a team approach, consisting of a gastroenterologist, a surgeon with expertise in GI surgery, and skilled nursing, should always be anticipated. Major causes of morbidity and mortality in patients with GI bleeding include blood aspiration and shock. To prevent these complications, endotracheal intubation should always be considered to protect the airway of patients with altered mental status. Most cases of lower GI bleeding do not warrant emergency therapy, but be prepared for decompensation in the elderly and in those with borderline normal hemodynamic parameters.

Diagnosis

The test of choice for the determination of the source of lower GI bleeding is colonoscopy. Adequate bowel preparation with an oral sulfate purge to clear the bowel of blood, clots, and stool increase the yield in diagnosing colonic bleeding sites. Angiography and technetium-labeled colloid or red blood cell scans may be of value if colonoscopy cannot be performed or if heavy bleeding prevents adequate visualization of the colon. However, the magnitude of bleeding required to show the bleeding site limits their usefulness. Sigmoidoscopy with air-contrast barium enema x-rays may be an alternative when colonoscopy is unavailable or if the patient refuses colonoscopy. If the initial sigmoidoscopy is negative, a colonoscopy must be performed. If both of these studies are negative, panendoscopy should be carried out. Capsule endoscopy has a diagnostic yield of 61% to 74% and can be done when source of bleeding is still elusive after both upper and lower GI endoscopy.

Always consider the possibility of upper GI bleeding as a source of hematochezia. An aspirate from a nasogastric tube can help to make this determination. An aspirate that shows bile but not blood will help to confirm that the bleeding is from a lower GI source.

ETIOLOGIES

The most common causes of lower GI bleeding include hemorrhoids (59%), colorectal polyps (38%-52%), diverticulosis (34%-51%), colorectal cancer (8%), ulcerative colitis, arteriovenous malformations, and colonic strictures. Percentages vary among age groups and most serious causes are expected in the elderly.

Hemorrhoids

Hemorrhoids are dilated veins in the hemorrhoidal plexus of the anus. They are defined as "internal" if they arise above the dentate line and "external" if they arise below the dentate line. Both can be the cause of hematochezia. Chronic constipation, straining for bowel movements, pregnancy, and prolonged sitting (eg, truck drivers) are risk factors. Along with bleeding, external hemorrhoids can cause pain, irritation, and a palpable lump. Internal hemorrhoids can cause bleeding and can prolapse through the anus. Conservative treatment with a high-fiber diet, stool softeners, and precautions against prolonged straining are usually successful. When necessary, various surgical procedures can be performed for definitive treatment.

Diverticular Disease

Diverticula are outpouchings of the colonic mucosa through weakened areas of the colon wall. They occur most often where blood vessels penetrate through the muscles of the colon. They are **most often asymptomatic and found on endoscopy or bowel imaging studies**. They can cause symptomatic, and occasionally massive, bleeding that is usually painless. Diverticular bleeding occurs in 10% to 20% of cases of lower GI bleeding, with most cases being increased by NSAID or aspirin use. In diverticular disease, bleeding is often self-limited and ceases approximately 75% of the time, while recurring at a rate of approximately 38%. When the bleeding is extremely heavy or fails to stop, surgical resection of the affected portion of the colon may be necessary. Asymptomatic diverticulosis is managed with dietary modification, primarily a high-fiber diet.

Diverticulitis is a painful inflammation and infection of a diverticulum. Diverticulitis frequently causes left lower quadrant abdominal pain along with fever, nausea, diarrhea, and constipation. Perforation of a diverticulum resulting in peritonitis or intra-abdominal abscess formation can be a complication. Diverticulitis is typically treated with bowel rest and antibiotics effective against gut flora. A combination of a quinolone and an agent for anaerobic organisms, such as metronidazole, is one commonly used regimen. In severe cases, recurrent cases, or when perforation occurs, surgery is indicated.

Inflammatory Bowel Disease

Ulcerative colitis and Crohn disease are the two primary diagnoses considered in the category of inflammatory bowel disease (IBD). **Ulcerative colitis causes continuous inflammation of the large bowel**, starting from the rectum and extending proximally. Severe disease can cause pancolitis, affecting the entire colon. **Crohn disease causes areas of focal inflammation, but can occur anywhere in the gastrointestinal tract.** Both diseases can cause recurrent episodes of abdominal pain, diarrhea, weight loss, rectal bleeding, fistulas, and abscesses. The definitive etiology of IBD is not known, but these are autoimmune syndromes and a family history of IBD is a major risk factor. Along with GI symptoms, **numerous extraintestinal manifestations may occur, most frequently arthritis.** Other extraintestinal manifestations include sclerosing cholangitis, cirrhosis, fatty liver, pyoderma gangrenosum, and erythema nodosum. Ulcerative colitis is a significant risk factor for the development of colon cancer. Patients with ulcerative colitis require frequent surveillance colonoscopic examinations. IBD can be managed with symptomatic therapy, such as antidiarrheal medications, along with anti-inflammatory medications (aminosalicylates, corticosteroids) given orally or as enemas, and immunosuppressive medications. Ulcerative colitis can be definitively treated with a total colectomy, which is usually reserved for severe pancolitis, failure to respond to medical therapy, or because of the risk of colon cancer.

Colon Neoplasms

Polyps are benign neoplasms of the colon. Hyperplastic polyps tend to be small, smooth growths found incidentally during endoscopy and are of no prognostic significance. Adenomatous polyps are benign growths that have a potential to become malignant. Listed in order of potential for becoming cancerous (from least to most), the three types of adenomas are tubular adenomas, tubulovillous adenomas, and villous adenomas. Larger polyps have a higher risk of causing bleeding and becoming malignant than smaller polyps. Polyps can be identified and removed during endoscopic procedures.

Colon cancer is the third most common cancer and the second leading cause of cancer deaths in men and women. The risk of colon cancer increases with age, with a history of colon polyps, a family history of colon cancer, or a personal history of ulcerative colitis. **Any patient older than age 50, who has lower GI bleeding, must be evaluated for the presence of colon cancer.** Because of the presence of premalignant lesions (polyps) that can be identified and removed in asymptomatic patients, colon cancer screening is recommended for all adults older than age 50, and at younger ages for those with increased risks. The treatment and prognosis of colon cancer depends on the stage in which it is found. The Dukes System stages colon cancer from A to D, depending on the penetration through the bowel wall layer, the presence of lymph node spread, and distant metastases. Dukes A colon cancer has an excellent prognosis with surgical resection; Dukes D cancer is usually not curable and is treated with combinations of surgery, chemotherapy, and radiation.

> **CASE CORRELATION**
> • See also Case 9 (Geriatric Anemia).

COMPREHENSION QUESTIONS

23.1 A 52-year-old man presents with bright red blood per rectum. He states that he has been bleeding heavily for a couple of hours. In the ER, his pulse is 110 beats/min, blood pressure is 90/50 mm Hg, he is cool and clammy appearing, and he has blood present on rectal examination, although he does not appear to be bleeding at the present. Which of the following is the best initial next step?

A. Colonoscopy.

B. Flexible sigmoidoscopy.

C. Place a nasogastric tube.

D. Start a bolus of IV normal saline.

E. Give a transfusion of type O-negative blood.

23.2 On a screening colonoscopy, a patient is noted to have several diverticuli in the sigmoid colon. He has never had any complaints of constipation, diarrhea, abdominal pain, or rectal bleeding. Which of the following is the best step in the management of this patient?

A. Annual colonoscopy

B. Sigmoid colectomy

C. High-fiber diet

D. Proton pump inhibitor

23.3 A 25-year-old man has a colonoscopy for diagnostic evaluation of abdominal pain, weight loss, diarrhea, and blood in the stool. The colonoscopy shows diffuse mucosal inflammation in the anus and descending colon. Which of the following is the most likely diagnosis?

A. Ulcerative colitis

B. Crohn disease

C. Pseudomembranous colitis

D. Colon cancer

ANSWERS

23.1 **D.** The initial evaluation of this acutely ill patient is "ABC"—airway, breathing, and circulation. As he appears to be in hypovolemic shock, with tachycardia and hypotension, a bolus of a crystalloid fluid, such as normal saline or lactated Ringer solution, is necessary before proceeding with any of the other evaluations.

23.2 **C.** Asymptomatic diverticuli are a common finding on screening colonoscopies. The initial management of this is a high-fiber diet. Diverticulosis by itself does not increase one's risk of developing colon cancer. Surgery is typically reserved for severe or recurrent symptomatic cases.

23.3 **A.** Ulcerative colitis causes continuous inflammation of the colon anywhere from rectum only to the entire colon, whereas Crohn disease causes patchy inflammation with skip areas throughout the alimentary canal but often the ileum and right side of colon. Pseudomembranous colitis is a complication of *Clostridium difficile* infection of the colon.

CLINICAL PEARLS

▶ Lower GI bleeding is usually suspected in lesions or pathology that is distal to the ligament of Treitz. Simple measures like nasogastric lavage can aid in ruling out upper GI bleeding as a cause of hematochezia.

▶ In a patient with acute lower GI bleeding, consider performing colonoscopy. Other diagnostic procedures that may be useful include radionuclide imaging and mesenteric angiography.

▶ Any patient older than 50 years should be screened for colon cancer. If a patient has a family history of colon cancer, colonoscopy screening should be performed 10 years prior to the age of diagnosis in the relative, or at age 50, whichever comes first.

REFERENCES

Ahmed R, Gearhart SL. Diverticular disease and common anorectal disorders. In: Kasper D, Fauci A, Hauser S, et al., eds. *Harrison's Principles of Internal Medicine*. 19th ed. New York, NY: McGraw-Hill; 2015. Available at: http://accessmedicine.mhmedical.com. Accessed May 25, 2015.

Anthony T, Penta P, Todd RD, et al. Rebleeding and survival after acute lower gastrointestinal bleeding. *Am J Surg*. 2004;188:485-490.

Bull-Henry K, Al-Kawas FH. Evaluation of occult gastrointestinal bleeding. *Am Fam Physician*. 2013 Mar 15;87(6):430-436.

Fargo MV, Latimer KM. Evaluation and management of common anorectal conditions. *Am Fam Physician*. 2012 Mar 15;85(6):624-630.

Friedman S, Blumberg RS. Inflammatory bowel disease. In: Kasper D, Fauci A, Hauser S, et al., eds. *Harrison's Principles of Internal Medicine*. 19th ed. New York, NY: McGraw-Hill; 2015. Available at: http://accessmedicine.mhmedical.com. Accessed May 25, 2015.

A 61-year-old woman presents to the emergency room (ER) complaining of cough for 2 weeks. The cough is productive of green sputum and is associated with sweating, shaking chills, and fever up to 102°F (38.8°C). She was exposed to her grandchildren who were told that they had upper respiratory infections 2 weeks ago but now are fine. Her past medical history is significant for diabetes for 10 years, which is under good control using oral hypoglycemics. She denies tobacco, alcohol, or drug use. On examination, she looks ill and in distress, with continuous coughing and chills. Her blood pressure is 100/80 mm Hg, her pulse is 110 beats/min, her temperature is 101°F (38.3°C), her respirations are 24 breaths/min, and her oxygen saturation is 97% on room air. Examination of the head and neck is unremarkable. Her lungs have rhonchi and decreased breath sounds, with dullness to percussion in bilateral bases. Her heart is tachycardic but regular. Her extremities are without signs of cyanosis or edema. The remainder of her examination is normal. A complete blood count (CBC) shows a high white blood cell (WBC) count of 17,000 cells/mm^3, with a differential of 85% neutrophils and 20% lymphocytes. Her blood sugar is 120 mg/dL.

▶ What is the most likely diagnosis?
▶ What is your next diagnostic step?
▶ What is the next step in therapy?
▶ What are potential complications to this condition?

ANSWERS TO CASE 24:
Pneumonia

Summary: This is a 61-year-old woman with fever, chills, and productive cough. She has an abnormal pulmonary examination and is found to have a high white cell count. Her significant medical history is diabetes mellitus.

- **Most likely diagnosis:** Community-acquired pneumonia.

- **Next diagnostic step:** Chest x-ray, sputum Gram stain and culture, and blood cultures.

- **Next therapeutic step:** Determine whether the patient requires in-patient or out-patient therapy and start antibiotics.

- **Potential complications:** Bacteremia, sepsis, parapneumonic pleural effusion, and empyema.

ANALYSIS
Objectives

1. Recognize the differential diagnosis of pneumonia.

2. Be familiar with widely accepted decision-making strategies for the diagnosis and management of different kinds of pneumonia.

3. Learn about the treatment and follow-up of pneumonia.

4. Recognize the effects of comorbid conditions.

Considerations

This 61-year-old patient presents with a common diagnostic dilemma: productive cough with green sputum and fever. The first priority for the physician is to assess whether the patient is more ill than the complaint would indicate. Helpful clues to the patient's overall condition include a toxic appearance, using accessory muscles to breathe, and low oxygen saturation. Tachycardia, hypotension, and altered mental status are signs of more critical illness. **Cardiopulmonary stabilization must always be addressed.**

Fortunately, this patient does not have those alarming symptoms. If a patient has respiratory distress, the physician may need to check arterial blood gases. If the patient has low oxygen saturation, give oxygen by nasal cannula and then proceed to your history and physical examination.

The most common etiology of cough is an upper respiratory tract infection. This patient has several features that make pneumonia more likely, including her **age, cough with green sputum, fever with chills, and exposure to close contacts with respiratory infections.** The gold standard for diagnosis of pneumonia is the presence of an infiltrate on chest x-ray, although normal x-ray does not exclude the diagnosis. X-rays may be normal early in the course of disease and a patient who is dehydrated may not demonstrate an infiltrate until the patient is adequately rehydrated.

APPROACH TO:
Pneumonia

DEFINITIONS

PNEUMONIA: Infection of lung parenchyma caused by agents that include bacteria, viruses, fungi, and parasites.

PNEUMONITIS: An inflammation of the lungs from a variety of noninfectious causes such as chemicals, blood, radiation, and autoimmune processes.

CLINICAL APPROACH

Bronchitis and pneumonia represent a continuum of lower respiratory infection. The extent of involvement of adjacent lung parenchyma determines whether there is an infiltrate on x-ray.

Pneumonia is defined as an infection of lung parenchyma caused by agents that include bacteria, viruses, fungi, and parasites. It should be distinguished from pneumonitis, which is an inflammation of the lungs from a variety of noninfectious causes such as chemicals, blood, radiation, and autoimmune processes. The occurrence and severity of pneumonia depends on both the state of the body's defense mechanism against infection and the characteristics of the infectious agent. The **most common mechanism triggering pneumonia is upper airway colonization** by potentially pathogenic organisms that are subsequently aspirated. The type of organism involved depends, in part, on host characteristics.

Community-Acquired Pneumonia

Pneumonia that occurs in persons who are not hospital in-patients or residents of long-term care facilities is defined as community acquired. Community-acquired pneumonias can be either viral or bacterial in etiology, and both can range from a mild to severe presentation. Common viral causes of pneumonia include influenza A and B, adenoviruses, respiratory syncytial viruses, and parainfluenza viruses. The most common bacterial cause of community-acquired pneumonia is *Streptococcus pneumoniae* (pneumococcus). Other common bacterial etiologies are *Mycoplasma pneumoniae*, *Haemophilus influenzae*, and *Moraxella cararrhalis*. Pneumococcal pneumonia classically causes an illness of acute onset with cough productive of rust-colored sputum, fever, shaking chills, and a lobar infiltrate on chest x-ray. *H influenzae* is often seen in patients with underlying chronic obstructive pulmonary disease.

M pneumoniae, *Chlamydia pneumoniae*, and *Legionella pneumophila* are bacteria that cause what is classified as "atypical" pneumonia. Atypical pneumonia is also caused by several different viruses. The **typical pneumonia organisms are more**

common in the very young and in the older patient. Atypical pneumonias occur more commonly in adolescent or young adult patients. Atypical organisms tend to cause bilateral, diffuse infiltrates, rather than focal, lobar infiltrates, on x-ray.

Health-Care–Associated Pneumonia

Health-care–associated pneumonia includes infections that develop in hospitals, nursing homes, skilled nursing facilities, or other long-term care facilities. The pathogens found in these types of facilities may have multidrug resistance, so the recommended treatments may include extended spectrum antibiotics until sensitivity of causative organism is found. Health-care–associated pneumonia is a major source of morbidity, mortality, and prolonged hospitalization. **Risk factors include hospitalization within 90 days, home infusion therapy, dialysis, and being a resident at a nursing home.** Risks for drug-resistant organisms include being hospitalized for more than 5 days, antibiotics within the last 90 days, immunosuppresion, and high rates of antibiotic resistance in the community. The causative organisms include the pathogens involved in community-acquired pneumonia as well as aerobic gram-negative bacteria (*Pseudomonas, Klebsiella, Acinetobacter*) and gram-positive cocci such as *Staphylococcus aureus*. The incidence of drug-resistant organisms, such as methicillin-resistant *S aureus* (MRSA), is increasing. Avoiding intubation when possible, using oropharyngeal intubation as opposed to nasopharyngeal intubation, keeping the head of the patient's bed elevated during tube feedings, and utilizing infection control techniques, such as careful hand washing and use of alcohol-based hand disinfectants, can reduce risks.

Diagnosis

Patient history in cases of pneumonia commonly includes the symptoms of productive cough, fever, pleuritic chest pain, and dyspnea. The symptoms can be very nonspecific in the very old and very young. In young children, rapid breathing is commonly seen; in the elderly, pneumonia may present as altered mental status.

Sometimes, the history may assist in determining the specific organism involved. An abrupt onset or abruptly worsening illness is seen frequently in pneumococcal pneumonia. *Legionella* often causes diarrhea, hyponatremia, and elevated liver enzymes along with pneumonia in older patients. *S aureus* is a common cause of postinfluenza pneumonia.

Physical examination findings can include fever, tachycardia, tachypnea, hypotension, and reduced oxygen saturation. Auscultation of the lungs may reveal rhonchi or rales. Egophony (E to A change) can be a sign of focal lung consolidation, and dullness to percussion may be the result of a pulmonary effusion.

All patients with suspected pneumonia should have a chest x-ray. The presence of an infiltrate can confirm the diagnosis. Absence of an infiltrate does not rule out pneumonia as a diagnosis. A chest x-ray can also identify a pleural effusion, which may be a complication of pneumonia (parapneumonic effusion).

Specific x-ray findings may also lead to consideration of certain etiologic agents or types of pneumonia. As noted previously, lobar infiltrates are more common with typical infections and diffuse infiltrates are more likely with atypical infections. A bilateral, "ground glass"–appearing infiltrate is associated with *Pneumocystis jiroveci* (formerly known as *Pneumocystis carinii*) infections, which are seen most often in patients with AIDS. Apical consolidation may be seen with tuberculosis. Pneumonia caused by the aspiration of gastrointestinal contents commonly is seen in the right lower lobe because of the branching of the bronchial tree.

Other testing indicated in patients with pneumonia includes a CBC and a chemistry panel. Specific microbiologic diagnosis is possible with blood or sputum cultures. **Cultures have a low sensitivity** (many false negatives), but a positive culture can help to guide treatment. *Legionella* can be confirmed in suspected cases by urine antigen testing.

Treatment

When pneumonia is diagnosed, the initial decision to be made is whether the patient can be treated safely as an outpatient or is hospitalization required. This prediction should be based primarily on mortality and severity prediction scores. **Commonly used prediction scoring systems include the CURB-65 mortality prediction tool for patients with community-acquired pneumonia, and the pneumonia severity index (PSI/PORT score)**, which is the most validated risk assessment tool. It assigns patients to a risk category based on their age, comorbid illnesses, specific examination, and laboratory findings. High-risk comorbidities include neoplastic disease, liver disease, renal disease, congestive heart failure, and diabetes. Physical examination findings taken into consideration are tachypnea, fever, hypotension, tachycardia, and altered mental status. Laboratory findings include a low pH, low serum sodium, low hematocrit, low oxygen saturation, high glucose, high blood urea nitrogen (BUN), and pleural effusion on x-ray. Based on the patient's demographics and individual findings, a risk class and mortality risk is assigned. Low-risk classes (classes 1 and 2) can be safely treated as an outpatient; higher-risk classes (classes 3, 4, and 5) should be hospitalized.

The emergence of drug-resistant pneumococci and the development of new antimicrobials have changed the empiric treatment of community-acquired pneumonia. In healthy persons suitable for outpatient treatment, a macrolide (clarithromycin or azithromycin) or doxycycline is recommended empiric therapy. If the patient has chronic comorbidities such as diabetes or heart and lung disease, treatments with fluoroquinolones (levofloxacin, moxifloxacin) or the combination of a β-lactam (high-dose amoxicillin, amoxicillin/clavulanate, cefpodoxime, or cefuroxime) plus a macrolide would be recommended.

For hospitalized patients with community-acquired pneumonia who do not require intensive care unit (ICU) treatment, an intravenous β-lactam (cefotaxime, ceftriaxone, or ampicillin/sulbactam) and an intravenous macrolide (erythromycin or azithromycin) are recommended. An IV fluoroquinolone with activity against *S pneumoniae* can be substituted. If the patient is suitable to begin outpatient treatment, the follow-up visit to the office 3 to 4 days later will help to assess response to therapy. Early follow-up chest x-rays are mandatory in those who fail to show clinical improvement by 5 to 7 days, as bronchogenic carcinoma can present with the picture of a typical pneumonia.

Health-care–associated pneumonias require broader antibiotic coverage of the likely pathogens, many of which have developed multiple-drug resistance.

If *Pseudomonas* is considered a likely cause, such as in a patient with immuno-compromise or recent hospitalization with intubation, treatment with an antipneu-mococcal and antipseudomonal β-lactam (piperacillin/tazobactam, cefepime, imipenem, or meropenem) plus a fluoroquinolone (levofloxacin, moxifloxacin) and/or an aminoglycoside (amikacin or tobramycin and azithromycin) is advised. Methicillin-resistant *S aureus* may require treatment with vancomycin.

The duration of the treatment is influenced by the severity of illness, the etiologic agent, response to therapy, the presence of other medical problems, and complications of the infection. Community-acquired pneumonia therapy lasts from 5 to 10 days or until the patient is afebrile for at least 72 hours. Two to three weeks of therapy is appropriate for hospital-acquired pneumonias caused by *S aureus*, *Pseudomonas aeruginosa*, *Klebsiella*, anaerobes, *M pneumoniae*, *C pneumoniae*, or *Legionella* species.

Complications

Bacteremia occurs in approximately 25% to 30% of patients with pneumococcal pneumonia. Mortality rates for patients with bacteremia range from 20% to 30%, but can be as high as 60% in the elderly. Parapneumonic pleural effusion develops in 40% of hospitalized patients with pneumococcal pneumonia. Fewer than 5% of cases progress to empyema. If more than a minimal amount of fluid is present, as evidenced by significant blunting of the costophrenic angle on x-ray, it may be necessary to perform a thoracentesis with Gram stain and culture of the pleural fluid. The presence of an empyema usually requires drainage with a chest tube or surgical procedure.

Prevention

Pneumococcal vaccine is recommended for all persons aged 65 and older, all adults with chronic cardiopulmonary diseases, cigarette smokers, and all immunocompromised persons. In addition to the traditional immunization with the 23-valent pneumococcal polysaccharide vaccine for all adults aged 65 and older, the Advisory Committee on Immunization Practices (ACIP) now recommends routine use of the 13-valent pneumococcal conjugate vaccine in a series with the original 23-valent vaccination. Revaccinate 5 years after the initial dose in patients known to be immunocompromised or without a functioning spleen.

Influenza vaccination is recommended in the late fall and winter months for all individuals aged 6 months and older. The association between influenza virus infection and pneumonia is well recognized. The number of cases of invasive pneumococcal disease from influenza peaks in mid-winter, when influenza is prevalent. Influenza virus infection can lead to a secondary pneumonia by facilitating bacterial colonization and impairing host defense mechanisms. *S aureus* is the most common causative organism in these cases. A prospective study of patients of 65 years and older demonstrated the effectiveness of influenza and pneumococcal vaccination at reducing hospitalizations for pneumonia and at preventing invasive pneumococcal disease.

> ## CASE CORRELATION
> - See also Case 2 (Dyspnea, COPD) and Case 19 (Upper Respiratory Infections).

COMPREHENSION QUESTIONS

24.1 A 17-year-old adolescent boy presents to the ER with a temperature of 101.0°F (38.3°C), a deep nonproductive cough, and generalized malaise for 3 days. He doesn't recall being around any particular sick contacts but is around many people in his after-school job in sales and at school. He states that he never had the chicken pox and is unaware of what immunizations he received as a child. He was diagnosed at age 12 with leukemia but has since been healthy. He is worried that his cancer may no longer be in remission. A chest x-ray reveals bilateral, diffuse infiltrates. Which of the following is the most likely cause of illness?

   A. Pneumonia caused by *S pneumoniae*

   B. Pneumonia caused by *P jiroveci*

   C. Pneumonia caused by *L pneumophila*

   D. Pneumonia caused by *M pneumoniae*

   E. Pneumonia caused by *H influenzae*

24.2 A 35-year-old morbidly obese woman returns to clinic with sudden onset of night sweats, chills, shortness of breath, and cough productive of yellowish-green sputum. Her vital signs show a temperature of 104.0°F, with a respiratory rate of 30 breaths/min, heart rate of 100 beats/min, pulse oximetry is 93% on room air. She was seen 8 days ago for headache, fever of 102.0°F, nonproductive cough, and myalgias. She was prescribed a dose of oseltamivir for 5 days. She felt better after taking the medication initially but now feels she is getting worse. She is sent to the emergency room for expedited evaluation. Assuming admission for pneumonia, which of the following is the best empiric antibiotic treatment for this patient?

   A. A 14-day trial of oseltamivir

   B. Azithromycin

   C. Penicillin

   D. Levofloxacin

   E. Ceftriaxone with vancomycin

24.3 A 76-year-old widowed man who lives alone presents to clinic with increasing shortness of breath and chest pain at rest for the past 2 weeks. He has had chronic hypertension and coronary artery disease (CAD) for 20 years for which he takes hydrochlorothiazide (HCTZ), enalapril, and aspirin 81 mg daily. Other medical problems include hyperlipidemia, peripheral vascular disease, and gastroesophageal reflux disease (GERD) which are controlled by lovastatin, warfarin, and omeprazole. Two years ago, he suffered a cerebrovascular accident that was localized to the brain stem. He now has dysphagia and is noted to cough frequently at night. He has no cough at present and has not been able to take his temperature at home. Which of the following is the best next step?

A. Upper endoscopy

B. Removal of angiotensin-converting enzyme (ACE) inhibitor

C. Nitroglycerine patch

D. Chest radiograph

ANSWERS

24.1 **D.** Bilateral, diffuse infiltrates are more likely to be seen in patients with pneumonia caused by atypical agents, such as *Mycoplasma*, than in patients with typical pneumonia or aspiration pneumonia. *Legionella*, another atypical pneumonia, usually is in older patients and the patient did not have diarrhea. It is more likely that the patient contracted an atypical pneumonia than having a relapse of leukemia with such profound immunodeficiency as to have contracted a *Pneumocystis* infection, with no prior symptoms.

24.2 **E.** This patient is most likely suffering from postinfluenza pneumonia. Due to the higher risk of mortality associated with morbid obesity and some vital signs indicating risk of sepsis, this patient should be evaluated quickly for possible admission. If admitted for pneumonia, antibiotic coverage should cover for *Pneumococcus* and *S aureus*. Levofloxacin would be reasonable for community-acquired pneumonia but does not provide good coverage for staph infections.

24.3 **D.** This patient most likely has aspiration pneumonia. With impairment of the gag reflex after cerebrovascular accident (CVA), he is more likely to aspirate during sleep, indicated by his cough. His GERD is well controlled by medication, so upper endoscopy is not warranted at this time. Nitroglycerine patches may be indicated if he described symptoms more related to angina. An ACE inhibitor would cause a cough unrelated to the time of day.

CLINICAL PEARLS

▶ Elderly patients often have fewer or less-severe symptoms or atypical presentations of pneumonia. Consider pneumonia in the differential diagnosis of altered mental status in the elderly.

▶ Appropriate use of influenza and pneumococcal vaccination reduces the risk of pneumonia in susceptible populations. New vaccination guidelines now recommend both the 23-valent and 13-valent pneumococcal vaccines given in series to all patients 65 and older.

▶ Consider the diagnosis of empyema in patients with pneumonia and a pleural effusion, especially if the patients continue to have fever despite appropriate antibiotic therapy.

REFERENCES

Chesnutt MS, Prendergast TJ. Pulmonary disorders. In: Papadakis MA, McPhee SJ, Rabow MW, eds. *Current Medical Diagnosis & Treatment 2015*. New York, NY: McGraw-Hill; 2014.

Mandell LA, Wunderink RG. Pneumonia. In: Kasper D, Fauci A, Hauser S, et al., eds. *Harrison's Principles of Internal Medicine*. 19th ed. New York, NY: McGraw-Hill; 2015. Available at: http://accessmedicine.mhmedical.com. Accessed May 25, 2015.

Marrie TJ. Pneumonia. In: Halter JB, Ouslander JG, Tinetti ME, Studenski S, High KP, Asthana S, eds. *Hazzard's Geriatric Medicine and Gerontology*. 6th ed. New York, NY: McGraw-Hill; 2009.

Tomczyk S, Bennett NM, Stoecker C, et al. Use of PCV-13 and PPSV-23 vaccine among adults aged 65 and older: recommendations of the Advisory Committee on Immunization Practices (ACIP). *MMWR Morb Mortal Wkly Rep*. 2014;63(37):822-825.

Watkins RR, Lemonovich TL. Diagnosis and management of community-acquired pneumonia in adults. *Am Fam Physician*. 2011 Jun 1;83(11):1299-1306.

A 38-year-old woman presents to the office with complaints of weight loss, fatigue, and insomnia of 3-month duration. She feels tired most of the time and frequently does not want to get out of bed. Despite feeling so tired, she has been staying up late at night because she cannot fall to sleep. She does not feel that she is doing well in her occupation as a secretary and states that she has trouble remembering things. She does not go outdoors as much as she used to and cannot recall the last time she went out with friends or enjoyed a social gathering. She denies any recent medication, illicit drug, or alcohol use. She feels intense guilt regarding past relationships because she feels that it was her fault they failed. She states she has never thought of suicide, but has begun to feel increasingly worthless.

Her vital signs and general physical examination are normal, although she becomes tearful while discussing her symptoms. Her mental status examination is significant for depressed mood, psychomotor retardation, and difficulty attending to questions. Laboratory studies reveal a normal metabolic panel, normal complete blood count (CBC), and normal thyroid functions.

▶ What is the most likely diagnosis?
▶ What is your next step?
▶ What are important considerations and potential complications of management?

ANSWERS TO CASE 25:

Major Depression

Summary: This is a 38-year-old woman with depression. She meets at least five of the *Diagnostic and Statistical Manual of Mental Disorders, 5th edition (DSM-V)* diagnostic criteria during a 2-week period that represents a change from her previous level of functioning. At least one of the symptoms must be either depressed mood or loss of interest or pleasure.

- **Most likely diagnosis:** Major depression.

- **Next step:** Evaluate the patient for suicidal risk; begin pharmacologic and psychotherapeutic management.

- **Important considerations and potential complications:** Rule out other medical diagnoses such as hypothyroidism, anemia, and infectious processes that could mimic some symptoms of depression; review any recent medication changes for agents that may contribute to these symptoms (eg, β-blockers, steroids, sedatives, chemotherapy agents), verify that no substance abuse or use is taking place; screen for bipolar disorder and inquire about a family history of mood disorders; investigate and address suicidal ideation.

ANALYSIS

Objectives

1. Recognize the common presenting signs and symptoms of depression.

2. Understand the multifactorial pathogenesis of depression.

3. Learn about the treatment of depression and the sequelae of this condition.

4. Be familiar with the appropriate follow-up of this condition.

5. Recognize the importance of assessing for risk of suicide.

Considerations

The case presented represents a common presentation of depression. The patient often does not come in with a complaint of depression. However, the symptoms of fatigue, insomnia, and mood swings are frequently seen. It then becomes incumbent on the physician to address the topic of depression with the patient. The symptoms of depression, such as memory disturbance or inability to concentrate, might limit your patient's ability to provide a good history. If the patient gives permission, it could be helpful to speak to a close contact of the patient, such as the spouse, to gather information that will confirm the diagnosis.

Once the diagnosis of depression is suspected, it is critical to determine the most appropriate level of care for the patient. The clinician must specifically and directly address the patient's risk of harming herself or others. If she is actively suicidal, such as describing the desire to hurt herself and having a plan to do so, then hospitalization may be necessary. Similarly, if the patient is unable to care for herself then hospitalization should be considered. If the patient does not have suicidal ideations, is not assessed as a risk to her or others, and has support at home, then outpatient therapy with close follow-up is usually appropriate.

APPROACH TO:
Depression

DEFINITIONS

MAJOR DEPRESSION: One or more episodes of mood disorder each lasting at least 2 weeks. The most prominent symptoms of major depressive disorder are depressed mood and loss of interest or pleasure. Insomnia and weight loss often accompany major depression, but depressed patients may also have weight gain or hypersomnia.

DYSTHYMIC DISORDER: Chronically depressed mood occurring most of the day, more than half the time, for at least 2 years, but does not meet the criteria for major depression, in terms of either severity or duration of individual episodes.

CLINICAL APPROACH

Background

Depression has a lifetime prevalence of 7% to 12% in men and 20% to 25% in women, with a **greater incidence in the elderly and patients with coexisting chronic medical conditions.** To meet the DSM-V criteria for major depressive disorder, the patient must experience at least five of the nine following symptoms nearly every day during the same 2-week time period. This must represent a change from previous functioning and include one of the first two symptoms: either depressed mood or anhedonia:

1. Depressed mood

2. Anhedonia: Diminished interest or pleasure

3. Change in appetite or weight: Decreased appetite, or increased appetite associated with specific food cravings; significant weight loss or weight gain

4. Change in sleep patterns: Insomnia or hypersomnia

5. Change in activity: Psychomotor agitation or retardation

6. Fatigue or loss of energy

7. Feelings of worthlessness or excessive or inappropriate guilt

8. Change in cognition: Diminished ability to think or concentrate; indecisiveness

9. Recurrent thoughts of death, suicidal ideation, suicide attempt, or specific plan

Also,

- Symptoms cause clinically significant distress or impairment of functioning.

- Symptoms are not a result of the direct physiologic effects of a substance or a generalized medical condition.

- There has never been a manic or hypomanic episode.

- Symptoms are not better explained by schizoaffective disorder, schizophrenia, schizophreniform disorder, delusional disorder, or other psychotic disorders.

It is noted in the DSM-V that responses to a significant loss, such as the death of a loved one, financial ruin, losses from a natural disaster, or serious medical illness can lead to symptoms very similar to that of major depression, and this may be considered a normal response, but it is still important to evaluate for a major depressive episode.

Risk factors for developing depression are family or personal history of depression, female sex, younger age, traumatic brain injury, chronic medical illnesses, chronic pain, low income, low self-esteem, poor social support, chronic minor daily stress, and being single, divorced, or widowed.

The differential diagnosis of depression includes many other psychiatric and medical disorders. Psychiatric disorders include dysthymic disorder, seasonal affective disorder, anxiety disorders, and bipolar disorder. Anxiety and depression often coexist. **Numerous medical conditions can cause depressive symptoms.** Common among these are dementia in older patients, hypothyroidism, and anemia. The role of pharmacologic agents and substance use, abuse, or dependence also should be investigated, as these can cause significant mood changes. This is especially true of alcohol, sedatives, narcotics, and cocaine.

Screening for depression is recommended by the United States Preventive Services Task Force (USPSTF) for adults and children 12 to 18 years old when there are systems to ensure accurate diagnosis, treatment, and follow-up. Patients with depression should be assessed for suicide risk, but there is no recommendation for screening the general population for risk of suicide. Adult screening can be completed using the 2-question or 9-question Patient Health Questionnaires (PHQ-2 or PHQ-9). For older adults, there is a Geriatric Depression Scale that can be used, and for children the Beck Depression Inventory and Children's Depression Inventory can be used.

Pathophysiology

The etiology of depression is thought to be multifactorial, due to a complex interaction of genetic, psychosocial, and neurobiologic factors. Theoretical psychosocial contributors include stressful life events, particularly involving loss of a loved one, early childhood stress, and lack of positive reinforcement. Depression does run in families, but the mode of inheritance is unknown. Multiple neurotransmitter systems are involved, including the serotonergic, noradrenergic, and dopaminergic systems. Evidence of the effects of neurotransmitters on mood disorders is supported by the mechanism of action of antidepressant medications: all currently available antidepressant agents appear to work by increasing the amount of neurotransmitter available to the postsynaptic nerve. This is accomplished by (1) enhancing neurotransmitter release, (2) reducing neurotransmitter breakdown, or (3) inhibiting the reuptake of the neurotransmitter by the presynaptic neuron.

Clinical Findings

On presentation, patients may complain of sadness, irritability, or mood swings. Difficulty concentrating or loss of energy and motivation are common. Thinking is often negative, and frequently accompanied by feelings of worthlessness, hopelessness, or helplessness. Some may complain of poor memory or concentration. Women are more likely to experience seasonal depression and atypical symptoms such as hypersomnia, hyperphagia, carbohydrate craving, weight gain, and evening mood exacerbations. Some patients with depression may present to the physician with various somatic complaints and decreased energy level rather than a complaint of depression. **The diagnosis of depression needs to be considered in scenarios where a patient presents with multiple unrelated physical symptoms.** Some typical non-specific symptoms of depression include headache, neck or back pain, joint pain, abdominal pain, constipation, poor sleep, change in weight or appetite, weakness, and fatigue. The elderly may present with confusion or a general decline in function.

Most patients with depression have no significant physical abnormalities on examination. A mental status examination is very important, including mood, affect, appearance, behavior, speech, thought process, and content, etc. Those who have more severe symptoms may reveal decline in grooming or hygiene along with weight changes. Speech may be normal, slow, monotonic, or lacking in content. Pressured speech is suggestive of mania, whereas disorganized speech suggests the need to evaluate for psychosis. The thought content of patients with depression includes feelings of inadequacy, helplessness, or hopelessness. Sometimes patients complain of being overwhelmed. Psychomotor retardation can manifest as slowing of movements or reactions, especially in the elderly. The physical examination should include evaluation for possible underlying causes of depressed mood, and a cognitive examination may be helpful in older adults.

Morbidity and Mortality

Depression causes significant morbidity and mortality in numerous ways. The World Health Organization states that depression is the fourth leading cause of disability in the world, and it causes more disability and social impairment than diabetes, arthritis, hypertension, or coronary artery disease. Depression is frequently reported in persons with underlying medical conditions, such as stroke, Parkinson disease, traumatic brain injury, diabetes, coronary atherosclerotic disease, pancreatic cancer, and other terminal illnesses. Patients with depression are more likely to develop atherosclerotic coronary artery and cerebrovascular disease, diabetes, and osteoporosis. It is a common occurrence following myocardial infarctions and cerebrovascular accidents. Persons with depression and preexisting cardiac disease have three times greater risk of dying after a heart attack than do patients without depression, and patients with coexisting depression and diabetes have more microvascular and macrovascular complications. Studies also show that **persons with depression have a greater chance of developing or dying from cardiovascular disease,**

Table 25–1 • RISK FACTORS FOR SUICIDE	
Demographic, Social, and Environmental Factors	Males More Likely to Complete; Females More Likely to Attempt
	Age >65 more likely to complete; age <30 more likely to attempt
	American Indian, Alaska Native, non-Hispanic white
	Social isolation (divorced, widowed, living alone)
	Lesbian, gay, bisexual, or transgender
	Stressful life events
	Access to firearms
Historical factors	Family history of suicide
	History of suicide attempt and lethality of prior attempt
	Concurrent chronic medical illness
Psychiatric and behavioral factors	Major depression, substance abuse (especially alcohol), schizophrenia, panic disorder, borderline personality disorder
	Symptoms: hopelessness, anhedonia, insomnia, severe anxiety, panic attacks, impaired concentration, psychomotor agitation

Data from American Psychiatric Association. Diagnostic and Statistical Manual of Mental Disorders. 5th ed. Washington, DC: American Psychiatric Association Press; 2013; Sernyak MJ, Jr., Rohrbaugh RM. Emergency psychiatry. In: Ebert MH, Loosen PT, Nurcombe B, Leckman JF, eds. Current Diagnosis & Treatment: Psychiatry. 2nd ed. New York, NY: McGraw-Hill; 2008; U.S. Preventive Services Task Force. Screening for suicide risk in adolescents, adults, and older adults in primary care: recommendation statement. Am Fam Physician. 2015 Feb 1;91(3):190F-190I.

even after controlling for risk factors such as smoking, gender, weight, activity, blood pressure, and cholesterol. Depression also contributes to the disruption of interpersonal relationships, the development of substance abuse, and absenteeism from work and school.

All depressed patients should be screened for suicidal and homicidal/violent ideations. A history of suicide attempts or violence is a significant risk factor for future attempts. Major depression plays a role in more than half of all suicide attempts. **Women, especially those younger than age 30, attempt suicide more frequently than men, but men are more likely to complete suicide.** Firearms are the most commonly used method in completed suicides. Table 25–1 lists the risk factors for suicide attempts and completed suicides.

TREATMENT

Initial pharmacotherapy should be based on physician familiarity with medication, anticipated safety and tolerability, anticipation of adverse effects, and history of prior treatments. **Pharmacotherapy with psychotherapy is more effective than either pharmacotherapy or psychotherapy alone.** Physicians should encourage their patients to pursue both therapies to improve chances of success. A helpful tool is the PHQ-9, which can be used to assess symptom severity and track improvement over time. An adequate trial of an antidepressant requires a minimum of 4 to 6 weeks on an appropriate dose. Up to half of patients may not respond to the first antidepressant they try, and will need to be switched to another agent. Treatment failures typically result from medication noncompliance, inadequate duration of therapy, or inadequate dosing. No class of medication has been proven to be more effective than other classes. Once in remission, patients treated for a first episode of major depression should be treated for at least 4 to 9 months. At least 60% of patients will experience a relapse at some point, and recurrent depression needs to be treated for longer periods of time. The need for lifelong therapy is higher with increasing number of episodes of depression. **All antidepressants carry a Food and Drug Administration (FDA) "black box" warning that they increase the risk of suicidal thoughts and behaviors in children, adolescents, and young adults, especially in the first months of treatment.** Women may have more side effects from antidepressants because absorption of these medications may be higher due to decreased gastric acid secretion, slower gastrointestinal transit, and higher body fat-to-muscle ratio (which increases volume of distribution) in women.

CLASSES OF MEDICATIONS

Table 25–2 lists the medications used in the treatment of depression.

Selective Serotonin Reuptake Inhibitors

Selective serotonin reuptake inhibitors (SSRIs) increase the amount of the neurotransmitter serotonin (5-hydroxytryptamine) available to the postsynaptic neuron by blocking the presynaptic neuron's ability to reabsorb serotonin. Because it can take 3 to 6 weeks of therapy before significant improvement in mood occurs, dosage adjustments of these medications should occur no more often than monthly. These agents have a low risk of toxicity if taken as an overdose (either accidentally or intentionally), making them very safe to use. Common side effects include sexual dysfunction, weight gain, nausea/gastrointestinal disturbance, insomnia or somnolence, and agitation. Because of their efficacy and safety, SSRIs are frequently used as first-line agents for the treatment of depression. SSRIs are first-line treatment

Table 25–2 • MEDICATIONS USED IN THE TREATMENT OF DEPRESSION				
SSRI	**SNRI**	**TCA**	**Atypical**	**MAOI**
Fluoxetine (Prozac)	Venlafaxine (Effexor)	Amitriptyline (Elavil)	Bupropion (Wellbutrin)	Phenelzine (Nardil)
Paroxetine (Paxil)	Duloxetine (Cymbalta)	Nortriptyline (Pamelor)	Amoxapine (Asendin)	Tranylcypromine (Parnate)
Sertraline (Zoloft)	Mirtazapine (Remeron)	Desipramine (Norpramin)	Trazodone (Desyrel)	Selegiline transdermal (Emsam)
Fluvoxamine (Luvox)	Desvenlafaxine (Pristiq)	Clomipramine (Anafranil)		
Citalopram (Celexa)		Doxepin (Sinequan)		
Escitalopram (Lexapro)		Imipramine (Tofranil)		

for depression in children, and fluoxetine (Prozac), citalopram (Celexa), sertraline (Zoloft), and escitalopram (Lexapro) have been approved for use in children.

However, when used in combination with other serotonergic agent the clinician should be aware of the possibility of developing serotonin syndrome. There may also be a slight increase risk of bruising, nosebleeds, and other bleeding episodes. Patients who are on nonsteroidal anti-inflammatory drugs (NSAIDs) or antiplatelet medications may be at increased risk for significant bleeding.

Serotonin-Norepinephrine Reuptake Inhibitors

Serotonin-norepinephrine reuptake inhibitors (SNRIs) affect both the serotonergic and noradrenergic systems. They act primarily on the serotonergic system at lower dosages and have a more balanced effect on the serotonergic and noradrenergic systems at higher dosages. Their side effects are similar to SSRIs. They can be used as first-line treatment for depression and because of their effects on two neurotransmitter systems, may be used as second-line agents in SSRI failure.

Tricyclic Antidepressants

Tricyclic antidepressants (TCAs) are older agents that affect, to varying degrees, the reuptake of norepinephrine and serotonin. They are effective for the treatment of depression and because they have been in use for many years, they are inexpensive. However, they have numerous side effects from antimuscarinic effects (dry mouth, blurry vision, constipation, urinary retention, and sinus tachycardia), histamine blockade (sedation, drowsiness, weight gain), and α-1 receptor blockade (orthostatic hypotension and sedation). Because of the side effects and risks, TCAs have largely been replaced by SSRIs as the first-line treatment of depression.

Monoamine Oxidase Inhibitors

Monoamine oxidase inhibitors (MAOIs) cause increased amounts of serotonin and norepinephrine to be released during nerve stimulation. Patients taking MAOIs must be on a tyramine-restricted diet to reduce the risk of severe, and sometimes fatal, hypertensive crisis. MAOIs also interact with numerous other medications, including SSRIs and meperidine (Demerol). These interactions can also be fatal. Because of the risks, MAOIs should only be used by experienced practitioners and only when the benefits outweigh the risks.

Atypical Agents

The different atypical agents may act similarly to SSRIs, TCAs, and MAOIs, in varying degrees. Their primary benefit is a lower incidence of sexual disturbance as a side effect. Bupropion is associated with increased risk of seizure at higher doses and is contraindicated in patients with a history of seizure disorders. Trazodone carries the risk, although rare, of causing priapism. It is also highly sedating and is frequently used as a sleep aid. Mirtazapine can be a good choice for patients with insomnia or anorexia, as it can improve sleep latency and duration and stimulate appetite. It is also less likely to cause sexual dysfunction or gastrointestinal (GI) side effects, has little α-1 blocking effects (like orthostatic hypotension), and can also help reduce anxiety.

INPATIENT MANAGEMENT

Inpatient management is indicated when the patient presents a significant risk to self (suicide, inability to care for self) or others (risk of violence), or the symptoms are sufficiently severe to initiate treatment in controlled settings. Involvement of a psychiatrist is warranted in the care of patients in whom more severe symptoms require more intensive care (suicidal ideations, psychosis, mania, and severe decline in physical health).

ELECTROCONVULSIVE THERAPY

Electroconvulsive therapy (ECT) is typically reserved for treatment-resistant depression. It may also be used for patients who cannot tolerate medications or in cases of severe or psychotic depression. It has been found to be more effective than placebo, simulated ECT, and antidepressants, but long-term efficacy is not known. The primary adverse effect of ECT is short-term memory loss or cognitive impairment which usually resolves in a few days to a few weeks.

OTHER MOOD DISORDERS

Anxiety Disorders

Anxiety disorder is a classification of mood disorders that are common in the population such as **panic disorder, obsessive-compulsive disorder (OCD), generalized anxiety disorder, posttraumatic stress disorder (PTSD), and phobia.** Patients with generalized anxiety disorder have excessive and difficult-to-control worry and anxiety that causes physical symptoms, including restlessness, irritability, sleep disturbance, and difficulty concentrating. Panic disorder is characterized by recurrent panic attacks, which are defined as periods of intense fear of abrupt onset. OCD manifests as either obsessions (recurrent, intrusive, and inappropriate thoughts) or compulsions (repetitive behaviors) that are unreasonable, excessive, and cause much distress to the patient. PTSD is a response to a severe traumatic event in which the patient suffers fear, helplessness, or horror. A phobia is an irrational fear that causes a conscious avoidance of a situation, subject, or activity. **Patients with anxiety disorders are at high risk for developing comorbid depression.**

Bipolar Disorder (Manic Depression)

This mood disorder affects genders equally but often presents in young people. Symptoms of mania include the abrupt onset of elevated or irritable mood, inflated self-esteem, decreased need for sleep, pressured speech, racing thoughts, distractibility, increased goal-directed activity, and engaging in pleasurable activities with potentially painful consequences. Concomitant substance abuse should always be investigated. Episodes of mania must last at least 1 week (or any duration if hospitalization is needed) and occur during a distinct period, not continuously. Continuous behavior of this type suggests personality disorders or schizophrenia. A single episode of mania is sufficient for the diagnosis of bipolar disorder. **All patients diagnosed with depression should be questioned about mania**, as the treatments are different. Bipolar disorder is typically treated with mood stabilizers, which include valproate, carbamazepine, and lithium. The use of antidepressant agents in bipolar disorder may precipitate acute manic behaviors.

Dysthymic Disorder

This mood disorder presents with continuous low mood as the primary symptom, lasting at least 2 years. Dysthymia is less acute but longer in duration than major depression It often includes at least two of the following: change in appetite or weight, change in sleep patterns, low energy or fatigue, poor concentration or difficulty making decisions, and feelings of hopelessness. If a major depressive episode takes place during an episode of dysthymia, then by definition, the patient suffers from major depression.

CASE CORRELATION

- See also Case 15 (Thyroid Disorders).

COMPREHENSION QUESTIONS

25.1 A 62-year-old man presents for a follow-up visit for severe depression. His symptoms have included crying episodes, insomnia, and decreased appetite. He has suicidal ideations and states that he has a gun in his home that he might use. He has had auditory hallucinations, saying he hears a voice telling him that his wife is the devil. His symptoms have not been relieved by maximum doses of sertraline (Zoloft), venlafaxine (Effexor), or citalopram (Celexa). He is currently taking duloxetine (Cymbalta), which has also failed to improve his symptoms. Which of the following would most likely provide the quickest relief of his symptoms?

A. Electroconvulsive therapy (ECT)

B. Bupropion (Wellbutrin)

C. Stopping duloxetine and starting on an MAO inhibitor

D. Behavioral modification

25.2 A 40-year-old woman sees you in follow-up of treatment for recurrent depression. Her symptoms are improved a little after 2 months of fluoxetine (Prozac) 10 mg a day and weekly counseling sessions with a psychologist. She is having no medication side effects and both she and her husband state that she is taking her medication regularly. Which of the following would be the most appropriate next step?

A. Continue with your current plan and give it more time.

B. Increase the fluoxetine dose to 20 mg daily and continue counseling.

C. Discontinue fluoxetine and start paroxetine 10 mg daily.

D. Continue fluoxetine and add bupropion as adjunctive therapy.

E. Discontinue medications and arrange for psychiatric consultation for ECT.

25.3   Three weeks after starting a 22-year-old man on an SSRI for a first episode of depression, you receive a call from his mother stating that he hasn't slept in days, is speaking very rapidly, and has maxed-out his credit card buying electronic equipment. Which of the following is the most likely explanation for this situation?

A.   He is having a medication side effect.

B.   He is secretly taking too much of his SSRI.

C.   His SSRI has unmasked underlying bipolar disorder.

D.   His SSRI has precipitated a hyperthyroid state.

ANSWERS

25.1   **A.** This patient has psychotic depression with suicidal ideation and has not responded to maximum doses of several antidepressants. He is more likely to respond to electroconvulsive therapy than to counseling or a change in medication.

25.2   **B.** The most common causes of treatment failure or poor response to therapy are inadequate medication dosing, inadequate length of treatment, or noncompliance. In this setting, where the patient is compliant and has had adequate time for response, increasing the dose of medication from 10 mg (a low starting dose) to 20 mg would be your first step. Typically, antidepressant medication dosages can be increased after 4 weeks of treatment if the response is inadequate.

25.3   **C.** In bipolar patients, the use of an SSRI can precipitate a manic state. It is critically important to assess for a history of manic episodes prior to starting antidepressant therapy. In some cases, bipolar disorder may initially present as major depression, so the institution of antidepressant medication may unmask an undiagnosed bipolar condition. Another condition to assess for in this situation is the concomitant use of recreational drugs, such as cocaine or methamphetamine.

CLINICAL PEARLS

▶ While working up depression, other medical diagnoses such as hypothyroidism, anemia, or infectious processes that could mimic some symptoms of depression must be ruled out.

▶ Always investigate the use of alcohol and drugs when evaluating for mood disorders.

▶ Suicidal and homicidal ideation should always be investigated and thoroughly addressed when diagnosing depression.

▶ The addition of any new medication should be investigated to ensure it is not contributing to the patient's symptoms.

REFERENCES

American Psychiatric Association. *Diagnostic and Statistical Manual of Mental Disorders.* 5th ed. Arlington, VA: American Psychiatric Publishing; 2013.

Bhatia SC, Bhatia SK. Childhood and adolescent depression. *Am Fam Physician.* 2007;75(1):73-80.

Douglas DM. Screening for depression. *Am Fam Physician.* 2012 Jan 15;85(2):139-144.

Eisendrath SJ, Cole SA, Christensen JF, Gutnick D, Cole M, Feldman MD. Depression. In: Feldman MD, Christensen JF, Satterfield JM, eds. *Behavioral Medicine: A Guide for Clinical Practice.* 4th ed. New York, NY: McGraw-Hill; 2014.

Guck TP, Kavan MG, Elsasser GN, et al. Assessment and treatment of depression following myocardial infarction. *Am Fam Physician.* 2001;64:641-648, 651-652.

Lisanby SH. Electroconvulsive therapy for depression. *N Engl J Med.* 2007;359(19):1939-1945.

Little A. Treatment-resistant depression. *Am Fam Physician.* 2009 Jul 15;80(2):167-172.

Shim RS, Primm A. Depression in diverse populations and older adults. In: South-Paul JE, Matheny SC, Lewis EL, eds. *Current Diagnosis & Treatment: Family Medicine.* 4th ed. New York, NY: McGraw-Hill; 2015. Available at: http://accessmedicine.mhmedical.com. Accessed May 25, 2015.

A 26-year-old G1P1001 woman presents for a routine postpartum visit 6 weeks following the vaginal delivery of a 7-lb baby girl. She had an uncomplicated prenatal course. She went into labor spontaneously at 39 2/7-week gestation. Her labor was augmented with oxytocin (Pitocin). The first stage of labor lasted for 9 hours, the second stage for 45 minutes, and the third stage for 15 minutes. She had a second-degree perineal laceration that was repaired without difficulty. She started breast-feeding her baby immediately after delivery. Her postpartum course was uncomplicated and she was discharged from the hospital on the second postpartum day. She is exclusively breast-feeding her baby and reports that it is going well. She says that she felt "stressed, sad, and overwhelmed" during her first week at home, but that those feelings resolved after a week or so. She is now in excellent spirits and has strong support at home from her husband and her mother. She had some light vaginal bleeding that stopped about a week after delivery. She had minimal to moderate, white discharge for a couple of weeks that has also stopped and she has had no vaginal discharge since. On examination, she appears well and has normal vital signs. Her general physical examination is normal. A pelvic examination shows a well-healed laceration repair, no cervical or vaginal discharge, and no cervical motion tenderness. Her uterus is normal size, firm, and nontender, and there are no adnexal masses.

▶ What are the maternal benefits of breast-feeding?
▶ If the patient had been using a diaphragm for contraception prior to her pregnancy and wishes to use one again, what counseling should be given?
▶ If she prefers oral contraception, which type would be most appropriate for this patient?

ANSWERS TO CASE 26:
Postpartum Care

Summary: A 26-year-old first-time mother presents for a routine, 6-week postpartum examination. She is breast-feeding her baby. Her examination is normal. She had a brief period in which she felt sad and overwhelmed, but this has resolved. She requests counseling about contraception.

- **Maternal benefits of breast-feeding:** Along with benefits to the baby, the maternal benefits include (but are not limited to) a more rapid return of uterine tone with reduced bleeding and a quicker return to nonpregnant size; a more rapid return to prepregnancy body weight; a reduced incidence of ovarian and breast cancer; contraceptive effects; the convenience of always having a readily available feeding supply for baby; and lower cost (no need to purchase formula).

- **Counseling regarding use of diaphragm:** There is no contraindication to using a diaphragm but she should have a new fitting.

- **Recommended oral contraception:** In breast-feeding women, the progestin-only "minipill" is recommended, as combined hormonal contraceptives can interfere with milk supply.

ANALYSIS

Objectives

1. Know the normal changes that occur in the postpartum period.

2. Be familiar with the diagnosis and management of common postpartum complications.

3. Be able to counsel patients on common postpartum issues such as contraception, breast-feeding, and postpartum depression.

Considerations

The postpartum period is defined as the time starting after the delivery of the placenta and lasting for 6 to 12 weeks. The postpartum period is a time of great change for the woman and her family. There are numerous normal physiologic changes that occur during the change from the pregnant to the nonpregnant state. Just as important are the many personal, social, and family changes that occur, which can be magnified for first-time parents or when there are unforeseen complications.

The immediate postpartum period, while still in the delivery suite, is usually focused on the medical conditions of both the neonate and the mother. The delivery attendant examines the mother, repairs any lacerations or episiotomy, and monitors uterine tone and vital signs so that complications such as postpartum hemorrhage can be diagnosed and treated quickly. Simultaneous to this, the neonate is assessed and cared for during his or her initial transition to extrauterine life.

The baby is often quite alert during this time, making it an ideal time to start breast-feeding efforts. Rh D-negative women who are not isoimmunized and whose infant is Rh D-positive should receive Rh D immunoglobulin shortly after delivery.

Expected postdelivery hospital stay is 24 to 48 hours for an uncomplicated vaginal delivery and 72 to 96 hours for a cesarean delivery. This time allows for recovery from the delivery or surgery, allows further monitoring for both maternal and neonatal problems, and can be used to provide education and support for the new mother and family. Only 3% of vaginal deliveries and 9% of cesarean deliveries result in complications that require a prolonged hospital stay. Goals of postpartum care include early ambulation, resuming a healthy regular diet, perineal and bladder care, bowel regimen, addressing postpartum blues, and breast-feeding support. Typical maternal problems that occur during this time frame include pain, bleeding, lactation problems, and urinary difficulties (infections, incontinence, and retention). Postpartum fever is most often a sign of endometritis (infection of the uterus), but can also be caused by urinary tract or wound infections, thromboembolic disease, and mastitis.

Prior to discharge, women should be instructed on normal physiologic changes after delivery, including lochia, diuresis, and milk letdown, as well as what to do in the case of alarming symptoms such as fever, excessive vaginal bleeding, leg pain or swelling, persistent headaches, shortness of breath, and chest pain. Women who are not already immune to rubella or rubeola should receive combined measles-mumps-rubella vaccination. A tetanus, diphtheria, and acellular pertussis (Tdap) vaccine is recommended for women who were not vaccinated during their pregnancies. Influenza vaccine is also recommended for women who have not yet been vaccinated.

The time following discharge from the hospital and for the subsequent 6 to 12 weeks usually represents the period of greatest adjustment. There are normal changes that occur, along with many potential medical and emotional complications. Future family planning and contraceptive issues need to be addressed as well. A 6-week postpartum examination is usually scheduled, but many of the issues that can occur during this time frame should be addressed prior to discharge from the hospital.

APPROACH TO:
Postpartum Care

DEFINITIONS

ENDOMETRITIS: A polymicrobial infection of the endometrium, myometrium, and parametrial tissues of the uterus, usually caused by ascending infection from the vagina.

LOCHIA: Normal postpartum vaginal discharge which is initially reddish in color and consists of blood, decidua and epithelial cells, then becomes thicker and yellow-white as leukocytes predominate.

CLINICAL APPROACH

Normal Changes

The uterus increases significantly in size and weight during pregnancy. Immediately after delivery, it weighs approximately 1 kg and is the size of a 20-week pregnancy (fundus palpable at the umbilicus), and begins the process of involution, the return to its nonpregnant size. Regular contractions of the uterine musculature (which cause "afterpains"), promoted by endogenous oxytocin secretion, improve hemostasis by compressing the uterine blood vessels. Oxytocin release increases during breast-feeding, so early breast-feeding is encouraged to assist involution. Supplemental oxytocin (Pitocin) given by intravenous infusion during or immediately after the third stage of labor will also aid in increasing uterine tone. By the end of the first postpartum week, the uterus will be about the size of a 12-week gestation, palpable at the symphysis pubis and in most cases it will return to normal size (weighing <100 g) by the time of the 6-week follow-up visit. If the normal process of involution does not occur, the patient should be evaluated for infection and retained placenta.

Vaginal bleeding is usually heaviest in the hours following delivery, then decreases significantly. Brown or blood-tinged lochia occurs for about the next week. This is followed by white or yellow lochia, which continues for approximately 4 to 6 more weeks. **In women who are not breast-feeding, menstruation usually restarts by the third postpartum month.** In women who are breast-feeding, ovulation and menstruation can be suppressed for much longer. Anovulation will persist for longer periods of time in women who exclusively breast-feed their babies.

Breast engorgement, signaling increased milk production, typically occurs 1 to 4 days after delivery and can cause breast pain, milk leakage, and fever. In breast-feeding women, this is best managed by increased frequency of feedings. In women who are not breast-feeding, the use of ice packs, supportive bras, and nonsteroidal anti-inflammatory drugs (NSAIDs) can reduce discomfort.

MEDICAL COMPLICATIONS

Hemorrhage

Postpartum hemorrhage is defined as loss of more than 500 mL of blood after delivery and occurs in about 4% of vaginal deliveries. Early postpartum hemorrhage occurs within 24 hours of delivery, most often immediately postpartum; late postpartum hemorrhage occurs between 24 hours and 12 weeks after delivery and is usually the result of abnormal placental site involution. The causes of most cases of postpartum hemorrhage can be remembered with the mnemonic "The Four Ts" (Table 26–1). Careful examination focused on the likely causes should be performed promptly to identify the source of the bleeding in both early and late postpartum hemorrhage.

Risk factors for postpartum hemorrhage include prolonged third stage of labor, multiple delivery, episiotomy, fetal macrosomia, and history of postpartum hemorrhage, but any patient can develop postpartum hemorrhage so it is important to prepare for prevention and early management at all deliveries. Active management

Table 26-1 • THE FOUR Ts OF POSTPARTUM HEMORRHAGE	
Tone	Uterine atony
Trauma	Cervical, vaginal, or perineal lacerations; uterine inversion
Tissue	Retained placenta or membranes
Thrombin	Coagulopathies

of the third stage of labor is the best way to prevent postpartum hemorrhage. This involves administration of a uterotonic agent, such as oxytocin or misoprostol, coinciding with delivery of the anterior shoulder, gentle cord traction, and uterine massage.

As with all emergency situations, the **first priority in managing postpartum hemorrhage is assessment of cardiopulmonary stability.** It is important to ensure that adequate IV access is available, preferably two large-bore IV catheters. Fluid resuscitation with a crystalloid solution (normal saline, lactated Ringer solution) should be given as necessary and massive hemorrhage may require transfusion with packed red blood cells.

Uterine atony causes approximately 70% of postpartum hemorrhage. Failure of the uterus to contract adequately results in continued bleeding from uterine vasculature. Risks include prolonged labor, prolonged use of oxytocin during labor, a large baby, and grand multipara (five or more previous children). **Initial management of uterine atony includes initiating bimanual uterine compression and massage, and administration of oxytocin, which may be given intravenously or intramuscularly.** Additional options for continued bleeding include methylergonovine (Methergine), carboprost (Hemabate), and misoprostol (Cytotec). Methylergonovine is contraindicated in patients with preeclampsia or hypertension, as it may cause an abrupt increase in blood pressure. Carboprost is contraindicated in women with asthma. Misoprostol has limited use due to high gastrointestinal and other side effects.

Trauma (lacerations, hematomas, and inverted uterus) causes approximately 20% of bleeds and is managed procedurally. **Retained placenta** causes approximately 10% of bleeds and is also managed procedurally. **Coagulopathies** cause approximately 1% of bleeds and require clotting factor replacement for management.

Fever

Postpartum fever, especially if associated with uterine tenderness and foul-smelling lochia, is often a sign of endometritis. Endometritis complicates approximately 10% cesarean and 1% to 2% of vaginal deliveries, even with antibiotics given prophylactically. When it does occur, endometritis following vaginal delivery should be treated with broad-spectrum antibiotics that cover vaginal and gastrointestinal flora, such as a combination of ampicillin and gentamicin. Following cesarean deliveries, antibiotics must also cover for anaerobes, and a combination of clindamycin and gentamicin may be used.

Urinary tract infections (UTIs) are another common cause of fever after both vaginal and cesarean deliveries. Urinary frequency, urgency, and burning are typical presenting symptoms. Catheterization of the urinary bladder, which occurs routinely during a cesarean delivery and frequently during vaginal deliveries, raises the risk of introducing bacteria into the normally sterile environment of the bladder.

Breast infections such as mastitis may occur as well. Symptoms include breast engorgement, erythema, induration, and tenderness. Prompt treatment with continued breast-feeding or pumping from the affected breast and antibiotics that cover staph infections are helpful in preventing breast abscess development. Mastitis should not result in discontinuation of nursing.

Other causes of fever in the postpartum period, especially in women delivered by cesarean, are identical to causes of fever in other postsurgical patients. These include atelectasis, wound infections, and venous thromboembolic disease.

Mood Disorders

Up to three-fourths of women develop some type of psychological reaction following the delivery of a child. In most cases, the symptoms are mild and self-limited. However, a smaller but significant percentage can have a reaction of such severity as to require medical or psychiatric intervention.

Approximately 30% to 70% of women develop a temporary state known as the "maternity blues" or "baby blues." This condition **develops within the first week after delivery and typically resolves by the 10th postpartum day.** Symptoms include tearfulness, sadness, and emotional lability. The etiology is not entirely clear, but may be multifactorial and include hormonal changes following delivery, nutritional deficiencies, stress, sleep deprivation, and adjustment to the new role of mother.

Postpartum depression occurs following 10% to 20% of pregnancies and can occur following gestations of any length—term, preterm, miscarriages, or abortions. The onset is defined by the DSM-V as occurring within 4 weeks' postpartum, but may occur as late as 1 year postpartum, and 50% of "postpartum" major depressive episodes may actually begin prior to delivery. **The symptoms of postpartum depression are the same as in major depression.** The severity can vary from mild to severe and suicidal. There is a **high recurrence rate in subsequent pregnancies** and an increased risk in women with a history of depression unrelated to pregnancy. Untreated, postpartum depression can last for 6 months or more and can be a significant cause of morbidity.

All women should be screened for a history of psychiatric disorders during their prenatal care and should be questioned about symptoms of depression at 2- and 6-week postpartum visits. **Treatment is similar to the treatment of nonpregnancy-related depression.** Women who are a risk to themselves, or to others, or who are unable to care for themselves should be admitted to the hospital. Selective serotonin reuptake inhibitors (SSRIs) are first-line therapy because of their efficacy and safety. They also are considered safe in breast-feeding. Counseling and general supportive measures at home are also important adjuncts to treatment.

Postpartum psychosis is a rare, but potentially devastating, complication following pregnancy. Manic or frankly delusional behaviors may present within a few days to a few weeks of delivery in up to 1 in 1000 postpartum patients. All women with postpartum psychosis should be hospitalized and comanaged with a psychiatrist.

Without proper treatment, there is a high risk of suicide and infanticide associated with this diagnosis.

BREAST-FEEDING

Counseling and encouragement regarding both the maternal and infant benefits of breast-feeding should start during the prenatal period. Neonatal benefits include ideal nutrition, increased resistance to infection, and a reduced risk of gastrointestinal tract infections and atopic dermatitis. Maternal benefits include improved mother-child bonding, more rapid uterine involution, quicker return to prepregnant body weight, convenience, decreased costs, contraception while the mother remains amenorrheic, and long-term reduced risks of ovarian and breast cancer. Breast-feeding promotion and education can increase the rate of breast-feeding and the duration for which women breast-feed their babies (See Table 26–2).

Women should be allowed to nurse their newborns as soon as possible following delivery. During this time, the newborns are often very alert and have strong rooting and sucking reflexes, which promote latching on to the nipple. Initial feedings provide colostrum, a yellow fluid which is rich in immunoglobulin A, minerals, amino acids, and proteins. Breast engorgement and milk letdown commonly occurs between the second and fourth postpartum days. Mature milk contains fats, proteins, carbohydrates, vitamins, minerals, and hormones.

There are few contraindications to breast-feeding. HIV infection, miliary tuberculosis, acute hepatitis B, herpetic breast lesions, and chemotherapy are contraindications. Abuse of substances, such as cocaine, heroin, PCP, and alcohol are contraindications. Women who have had breast-reduction surgery with nipple transplantation will be unable to breast-feed.

Common maternal complications of breast-feeding include sore or cracked nipples and mastitis. Sore nipples can be managed by ensuring proper latch-on, frequent position changes, alternating breasts during feedings, nipple shields,

TABLE 26–2. • TEN STEPS FOR SUCCESSFUL BREAST-FEEDING
1. Have a written breast-feeding policy that is regularly communicated to all health-care staff.
2. Train all staff in skills necessary to implement this policy.
3. Inform all pregnant women about the benefits and management of breast-feeding.
4. Help mothers initiate breast-feeding within an hour of birth.
5. Show mothers how to breast-feed and sustain lactation, even if they should be separated from their infants.
6. Feed newborn infants nothing but breast milk, unless medically indicated, and under no circumstances provide breast milk substitutes, feeding bottles, or pacifiers free of charge or at low cost.
7. Practice rooming-in, which allows mothers and infants to remain together, 24 hours a day.
8. Encourage breast-feeding on demand.
9. Give no artificial pacifiers to breast-feeding infants.
10. Help start breast-feeding support groups and refer mothers to them.

Reproduced, with permission, from Cunningham F, Leveno KJ, Bloom SL, et al. Williams Obstetrics. 24th ed. New York, NY: McGraw-Hill; 2013, Table 36–3.

keeping the nipples clean and dry between feedings, and applications of lanolin or the patient's own breast milk as a salve. Vitamin E, herbal rubs, and other creams and topical agents should be avoided because of risk of absorption by the infant.

FAMILY PLANNING

Most women resume sexual activity by 3 months' postpartum. Numerous options are available to women for contraception and family planning. Discussion of these options ideally should occur in the prenatal period and again before discharge from the hospital.

Oral contraceptive pills (OCPs) are the most widely used reversible form of contraception. Available OCPs contain both estrogen and progestin or are progestin only. **In breast-feeding women, the progestin-only pills are preferred** because combination OCPs might reduce lactation. Both the American College of Obstetricians and Gynecologists and the World Health Organization recommend waiting for 6 weeks' postpartum to start oral contraceptives in breast-feeding women. Injectable long-acting depot medroxyprogesterone (Depo-Provera) may also be used in breast-feeding women and should also be given at or after 6 weeks' postpartum. **Non–breast-feeding women should wait 3 weeks after delivery to start combined OCPs,** as the risk of thromboembolic disease is higher in those who start at earlier times.

Barrier methods of contraception may also be used regardless of breast-feeding status. An intrauterine device (IUD) may be placed at the 6-week postpartum visit; earlier placement is associated with an increased rate of expulsion of the device. **Diaphragms and cervical caps can be used, but should be refitted at the 6-week visit** to ensure an appropriate fit.

Lactation-induced amenorrhea provides a high level of natural contraception in the first 6 months; postpartum. Women who breast-feed exclusively and who are amenorrheic have a 99% contraceptive protection for 6 months. After 6 months, if menses restart, or if breast-feeding is reduced, the risk of pregnancy increases and alternate forms of contraception should be used.

> ## CASE CORRELATION
> - See also Cases 4 (Prenatal Care) and 16 (Labor and Delivery).

COMPREHENSION QUESTIONS

26.1 You are called by the postpartum nurse to see a 20-year-old woman who delivered an 8-lb 9-oz newborn boy approximately 6 hours ago. The nurse noted that the patient is continuing to bleed more than expected. The patient is awake and talking, but feels dizzy. Her blood pressure is 90/40 mm Hg and her pulse is 110 beats/min. You see that her perineal pad is soaked with blood. Which of the following is your most appropriate initial intervention?

A. Add 20 units of oxytocin (Pitocin) to the IV of 0.45% saline that is currently running at 125 mL/h.

B. Perform bimanual uterine massage.

C. Place a large-bore IV and give a 1 L bolus of 0.9% saline.

D. Give an IM injection of methylergonovine (Methergine).

26.2 A 29-year-old first-time mother comes to you for her routine 6-week postpartum visit. Her husband, who accompanied her to the visit, reports that his wife is tearful much of the time. She has not been sleeping well, has little energy, and a reduced appetite. She denies any suicidal thoughts, hallucinations, or feelings that she wants to harm her baby. Which of the following is the most appropriate intervention?

A. Reassurance that these feelings will pass within a week or so

B. Referral to a psychiatrist for outpatient management

C. Institution of SSRI therapy and close follow-up

D. Admission to the hospital and urgent psychiatric consultation

26.3 You see a 30-year-old woman for an acute visit 16 days' postpartum. She has been nursing her baby daughter, but has developed a very sore left breast. On examination, the patient has a temperature of 101.3°F (38.5°C). The breast is diffusely tender, but primarily in the upper inner quadrant. The skin overlying the area of most tenderness is erythematous and warm. There is no nipple discharge and the remainder of the examination is normal. Which of the following is the best treatment?

A. This condition is self-limited, but she should stop nursing the baby on the left breast until this condition resolves.

B. She may nurse from the unaffected breast, but should simply pump and discard the milk from the painful breast.

C. The patient should receive oral dicloxacillin or clindamycin.

D. She should have a fine-needle aspiration.

26.4 A 19-year-old woman is seen in the office 3 weeks' postpartum. She is exclusively breast-feeding and has not had a menstrual cycle since her delivery. She would like to have an IUD placed for contraception, as she would like to wait several years before having another baby. Which of the following actions would be most appropriate at this time?

A. Plan to insert the IUD at a 6-week postpartum visit.

B. Prescribe progestin-only minipills until she is no longer breast-feeding and then insert the IUD.

C. Advise that she needs no contraception until she is no longer breast-feeding and she should return after that time for the IUD.

D. Insert the IUD today.

ANSWERS

26.1 **C.** This patient is symptomatically hypovolemic, with dizziness, hypotension, and tachycardia. Fluid resuscitation must be your first intervention. Once you have started the management of this critical issue, you should turn your attention to identifying and correcting the source of the bleeding.

26.2 **C.** This is a picture of postpartum depression. The symptoms are identical to those of a major depressive episode. The maternity blues is a self-limited condition that starts in the first postpartum week and resolves in the second. Fortunately, this patient does not have signs of postpartum psychosis—mania, hallucinations, and delusions. Appropriate management includes the use of an SSRI, counseling, and close follow-up.

26.3 **C.** Mastitis is a common complication of breast-feeding. It is caused by gland obstruction and sometimes, as in this case, there also are signs of infection. Treatment is directed at relieving the obstruction, so increased breast-feeding or pumping is helpful. The antibiotics typically used for this complication are considered safe to use while nursing. Empiric staphylococcal coverage is recommended. Dicloxacillin, and cephalexin are appropriate for areas with low rates of methicillin-resistant staphylococcus aureus (MRSA). Clindamycin or sulfamethoxazole-trimethoprim is good choice for areas with high rates of MRSA.

26.4 **A.** IUDs provide highly effective, reversible contraception and are very useful for women who wish to space out pregnancies for several years. Postpartum insertion prior to 6 weeks is associated with a higher risk of expulsion of the IUD from the uterus as it involutes. Breast-feeding–induced amenorrhea provides a high degree of protection against pregnancy for about the first 6 months' postpartum, but an alternate form of contraception should be used after 6 months or when menses restart.

CLINICAL PEARLS

▶ Many of the important postpartum issues—mood problems, contraception, and breast-feeding—are best managed by addressing them in the prenatal course first, and then readdressing or reinforcing them in the postpartum period.

▶ Most causes of postpartum hemorrhage can be remembered with the four Ts: tone, trauma, tissue, and thrombin.

REFERENCES

Anderson JM, Etches D. Prevention and management of postpartum hemorrhage. *Am Fam Physician*. 2007 Mar 15;75(6):875-882.

Blenning CE, Paladine H. An approach to the postpartum office visit. *Am Fam Physician*. 2005 Dec 15;72(12):2491-2496.

Conti TD, Patel M, Bhat S. Breastfeeding and infant nutrition. In: South-Paul JE, Matheny SC, Lewis EL, eds. *Current Diagnosis & Treatment: Family Medicine*. 4th ed. New York, NY: McGraw-Hill; 2015. Available at: http://accessmedicine.mhmedical.com. Accessed May 25, 2015.

Cunningham F, Leveno KJ, Bloom SL, et al. The puerperium. In: Cunningham F, Leveno KJ, Bloom SL, et al., eds. *Williams Obstetrics*. 24th ed. New York, NY: McGraw-Hill; 2013.

Cunningham F, Leveno KJ, Bloom SL, et al. Puerperal complications. In: Cunningham F, Leveno KJ, Bloom SL, eds. *Williams Obstetrics*. 24th ed. New York, NY: McGraw-Hill; 2013.

Pessel C, Tsai MC. The normal puerperium. In: DeCherney AH, Nathan L, Laufer N, Roman AS, eds. *Current Diagnosis & Treatment: Obstetrics & Gynecology*. 11th ed. New York, NY: McGraw-Hill; 2013.

A 66-year-old woman presents to your office complaining of shortness of breath and bilateral leg edema that have been worsening for 3 months. She emphatically tells you, "I get out of breath when I do housework and I can't even walk to the corner." She has also noticed difficulty sleeping secondary to a dry cough that wakes her up at night and further exacerbation of her shortness of breath while lying flat. This has forced her to use three pillows for a good night's sleep. She denies any chest pain, wheezing, or febrile illness. She has no past illnesses and takes no medications. She's never smoked and drinks socially. On examination, her blood pressure (BP) is 187/90 mm Hg, her pulse is 97 beats/min, her respiratory rate is 16 breaths/min, her temperature is 98°F (36.6°C), and her oxygen saturation is 93% on room air by pulse oximetry. She has a pronounced jugular vein. Cardiac examination reveals a pansystolic murmur. Examination of her lung bases produces dullness bilaterally. You find 2+ pitting edema of both ankles. An electrocardiogram (ECG) shows a normal sinus rhythm and a chest x-ray demonstrates mild cardiomegaly with bilateral pleural effusions. You decide she needs further workup, so you call the hospital where you have admitting privileges and arrange for a telemetry bed.

▶ What is the most likely diagnosis?
▶ What is the next diagnostic step?
▶ What is the initial step in therapy?

ANSWERS TO CASE 27:
Congestive Heart Failure

Summary: A 66-year-old woman presents to your office with worsening shortness of breath, bilateral leg edema, and three-pillow orthopnea. She is not known to be hypertensive, but her BP is 187/90 mm Hg and her oxygen saturation is 93% on room air. Her examination reveals jugular venous distension (JVD), a cardiac murmur, and decreased breath sounds at both lung bases. On a chest x-ray, you find bilateral pleural effusions and decide to admit her for further workup and management.

- **Most likely diagnosis:** New-onset congestive heart failure (CHF)

- **Next diagnostic step:** Serial cardiac enzymes and ECGs; blood work to include a CBC, electrolytes, and renal function; echocardiogram

- **Initial therapy:** Telemetry monitoring, IV diuretics, and oxygen

ANALYSIS
Objectives

1. Know how to clinically recognize congestive heart failure (CHF).

2. Understand the classification of CHF.

3. Understand the mechanism of action of the drugs used in the treatment of acute and chronic CHF.

4. Understand the underlying pathophysiology that occurs in CHF and the rationale for treatment options.

5. Be familiar with the outpatient management of CHF and the importance of patient education.

Considerations

This 66-year-old woman presented with CHF. Her most immediate problem is oxygenation and volume overload on her weakened heart. The **first priority is optimizing oxygen exchange** by administering oxygen via nasal cannula, dilating pulmonary vasculature, and decreasing cardiac preload and afterload. Most cases of CHF are caused by either coronary artery disease or hypertension, so it is imperative to evaluate these patients for acute coronary syndrome and coronary arterial disease. The overloading of fluid in the lungs is a common cause of anxiety and distress in patients with acute CHF because of the continuous struggle to oxygenate adequately. This anxiety activates sympathetic pathways and mounts catecholamine-induced responses, which produce further worsening of acute heart failure by causing tachycardia and increasing peripheral vascular resistance, leading to greater stress on the heart and worsening of symptoms. These triggers can, in part, be suppressed by the use of an agent such as morphine sulfate, which acts both as an anxiolytic and a vasodilator. Furosemide (Lasix) is the diuretic of choice, not only for its diuretic effect but also for its immediate vasodilatory action on bronchial vasculature. Admitting these patients to the hospital allows for closer maintenance of homeostasis in their fluid balances and evaluation of any underlying condition that may have precipitated the CHF. Other medications, including angiotensin-converting enzyme inhibitors (ACEIs) or angiotensin receptor blockers (ARBs) and β-blockers, help to control heart failure symptoms by decreasing preload and afterload, and reducing cardiac remodeling.

APPROACH TO:
Congestive Heart Failure

DEFINITIONS

CONGESTIVE HEART FAILURE: Impairment of the ventricle's ability to fill with or eject blood which results in inadequate circulation of blood to meet metabolic needs, characterized by dyspnea, fatigue, and fluid retention

FRAMINGHAM HEART STUDY: Large, prospective cohort study of the epidemiologic factors associated with cardiovascular diseases

CLINICAL APPROACH

CHF can be subdivided into systolic or diastolic dysfunction and right- or left-sided heart failure, all of which can coexist. Systolic dysfunction exists when there is a dilated ventricle with impaired contractility and possibly concomitant valvular disease. Diastolic dysfunction occurs with normal or intact left ventricular ejection fraction (LVEF) but impaired ventricular relaxation and filling, often associated with left ventricular hypertrophy and stiffness, systemic hypertension, or valvular disease. Left heart failure is a syndrome primarily characterized by pulmonary congestion or edema. Right heart failure is a syndrome usually caused by left heart failure. It is characterized by right ventricular (RV) systolic dysfunction accompanied by RV dilatation and tricuspid regurgitation, which causes tissue congestion, including peripheral edema, ascites, and abdominal organ engorgement.

Etiologies

The most common cause of heart failure in the developed world is coronary artery disease, estimated to account for approximately two-thirds of all cases of CHF. Diabetes also plays a large role, and patients with diabetes are twice as likely to develop CHF as those without. Uncontrolled hypertension and valvular disease have become less common primary culprits but are still significant precipitating factors. The most common valvular cause of heart failure in the developed world is senile degeneration of the aortic valve. In undeveloped countries, valve disease secondary to rheumatic fever is more common. Other important risk factors are smoking, sedentary lifestyle, obesity, and lower socioeconomic status. Table 27–1 describes major categories of heart failure with associated disease processes.

Table 27–1 • ETIOLOGIES OF HEART FAILURE

Systolic Heart Failure (Ejection Fraction <40%)

Coronary artery disease	Nonischemic dilated cardiomyopathy
Myocardial infarction[a]	Familial/genetic disorders
Myocardial ischemia[a]	Infiltrative disorders[a]
Chronic pressure overload	Toxic/drug-induced damage
Hypertension[a]	Metabolic disorder[a]
Obstructive valvular disease[a]	Viral
Chronic volume overload	Chagas disease
Regurgitant valvular disease	Disorders of rate and rhythm
Intracardiac (left-to-right) shunting	Chronic bradyarrhythmias
Extracardiac shunting	Chronic tachyarrhythmias

Diastolic Heart Failure (Ejection Fraction >40%–50%)

Pathologic hypertrophy	Restrictive cardiomyopathy
Primary (hypertrophic cardiomyopathies)	Infiltrative disorders (amyloidosis, sarcoidosis)
Secondary (hypertension)	Storage diseases (hemochromatosis)
Aging	Fibrosis
	Endomyocardial disorders

Pulmonary Heart Disease

Cor pulmonale	
Pulmonary vascular disorders	

High-Output States

Metabolic disorders	Excessive blood-flow requirements
Thyrotoxicosis	Systemic arteriovenous shunting
Nutritional disorders (beriberi)	Chronic anemia

[a]Indicates disease process that can lead to diastolic CHF as well.
Reproduced, with permission, from Longo DL, Fauci AS, Kasper DL, et al. Harrison's Principles of Internal Medicine. 18th ed. New York, NY: McGraw-Hill; 2012. Table 234–1.

Epidemiology

In 2013, the American Heart Association estimated there were 5.1 million Americans with heart failure. The Framingham Heart Study found a prevalence of heart failure in men aged 50 to 59 of 8 per 1000, increasing to 66 per 1000 in men over 80. Similar rate increases based on increasing age were seen in women. African Americans have 25% increase higher rates than whites.

Over 1 million hospital admissions in the United States and at least 20% of admissions for patients over age 65 are due to CHF, making it **the most common cause of hospitalization in patients older than 65 years.** Poorer prognosis is seen in patients who are male, older, those with more severe symptoms, coronary artery disease and acute coronary syndrome, hypotension, impaired renal function, hyponatremia, and elevated plasma brain natriuretic peptide (BNP). The most common cause of death is worsening heart failure. Sudden cardiac death, often from a ventricular arrhythmia, may account for up to 30% of all deaths.

Evaluation

Patients presenting with symptoms suggestive of heart failure should be evaluated with a history, physical examination, and focused testing. Diagnosis of heart failure is clinical, and there is no single test that can determine its presence or absence.

The symptoms and signs that occur are unique and characteristic of the alterations to the normal physiologic function of the heart. Signs and symptoms of right-sided heart failure stem from increased pressure in the systemic veins, causing hepatic congestion, venous engorgement, and visceral edema. Symptoms include nausea, vomiting, abdominal distention or bloating, diminished appetite, early satiety, and abdominal pain, particularly in the right upper quadrant (due to hepatic congestion and stretching of the liver capsule). Signs of right-sided heart failure are jugular venous distention, peripheral edema, hepatomegaly, right upper quadrant tenderness, hepatojugular reflux, abdominal ascites, and jaundice.

Left-sided heart failure manifests with elevated pressure in the pulmonary veins, resulting in symptoms of dyspnea on exertion, paroxysmal nocturnal dyspnea, orthopnea, wheezing, tachypnea, and cough. The signs of pulmonary congestion are bilateral pulmonary rales, S_3 gallop rhythm, Cheyne-Stokes respirations (which are associated with low cardiac output), pleural effusion, and pulmonary edema. Pulmonary edema is often the first manifestation of congestive heart failure, but it can also be caused by a variety of noncardiac conditions.

Dyspnea on exertion is the most sensitive symptom for the diagnosis of CHF, but its specificity is much lower. Orthopnea and paroxysmal nocturnal dyspnea are more specific for CHF, but not as sensitive. Symptoms seen in both right- and left-heart failure include weakness, fatigue, nocturia due to increased cardiac preload and decreased renal vasoconstriction in the recumbent position, memory impairment, insomnia, decreased exercise tolerance, headache, stupor, coma, paroxysmal nocturnal dyspnea, and declining functional status. Signs found in both left- and right-heart failure are tachycardia, displaced point of maximal impulse, systolic murmurs (mitral or tricuspid), third heart sound (S_3, ventricular filling gallop) associated with volume overload, fourth heart sound (S_4, atrial gallop) associated with diastolic dysfunction, pulsus alternans, diminished pulse pressure, cyanosis, oliguria, dependent peripheral edema, and cardiac cachexia.

Testing should be designed to confirm CHF (or lead to an alternate diagnosis), identify a cause, and assess the severity of the disease. These initial tests should include blood tests, radiographic studies, electrocardiography, and echocardiography.

Initial blood tests should generally include a complete blood count (CBC), serum electrolytes, magnesium, calcium, renal function tests, urinalysis, hepatic function tests, cardiac enzymes, and BNP. A high white blood cell count can help to identify the presence of an underlying infection, a common triggering event of CHF. Anemia is another common trigger of CHF. In an anemic patient, the oxygen-carrying ability of the blood is reduced so cardiac output must increase to compensate for this. If the anemia is mild, or if the heart is normal, this compensation may occur without producing symptoms; if the anemia is severe or if there is underlying cardiac abnormality (from previous ischemia, hypertension, valvular abnormality, etc), heart failure may occur. Diabetes and hypo- or hyperthyroidism can also precipitate CHF. Testing for concomitant dyslipidemia is also important.

Electrolyte abnormalities are common in the presence of CHF. Neurohumoral responses to a failing heart result in water and sodium retention and potassium excretion. Hyponatremia is a poor prognostic indicator, signifying activation of the renin-aldosterone-angiotensin system. Medications used by patients with chronic heart disease (diuretics, ACEI, ARB, and aldosterone antagonists) also can lead to electrolyte abnormalities. Some electrolyte abnormalities, specifically hypo- or hyperkalemia, hypomagnesemia, and hypocalcemia, can lead to arrhythmias which could incite heart failure or cause significant morbidity in heart failure patients. Increased venous pressure can lead to passive congestion of the liver, resulting in elevated serum transaminases. Severe CHF can lead to jaundice as a consequence of impaired hepatic function caused by congestion.

Serial measurement of cardiac enzymes is necessary to evaluate for the presence of acute myocardial infarction (MI) as the inciting event. Elevated cardiac enzymes that do not reach levels consistent with acute myocardial infarction are seen in about half of patients with systolic heart failure and indicate elevated left ventricular filling pressure due to volume overload.

One of the neurohumoral responses to the presence of a failing ventricle is release of BNP. BNP and its prohormone (pro-BNP) can be used to assist in the diagnosis of CHF as a cause of acute dyspnea. Elevated levels of BNP and pro-BNP are sensitive and specific markers for the diagnosis of CHF. In a dyspneic patient, a level of BNP less than 100 pg/mL essentially excludes a diagnosis of heart failure, and BNP higher than 400 pg/mL indicates high likelihood of heart failure. A pro-BNP level greater than 450 pg/mL in younger patients or 900 pg/mL in older patients also suggests CHF. BNP is not recommended as a screening test nor as a method of monitoring progression of CHF, as the level can be increased by advancing age, renal failure, cardiac ischemia, and pulmonary embolism and can be decreased by acute pulmonary edema, acute mitral regurgitation, and mitral stenosis.

ECG findings in CHF are variable, but can help determine the cause of heart failure. An ECG is useful to evaluate for evidence of acute ischemia or arrhythmia as cause of the CHF and can also reveal the presence of ventricular hypertrophy, often seen in chronic hypertension. Left bundle branch block seen in the setting of heart failure indicates higher 1-year all-cause mortality.

Chest x-ray can help to evaluate for other causes of dyspnea, such as pneumonia, chronic obstructive pulmonary disease, pneumothorax, or lung cancer. A chest x-ray showing cardiomegaly, pulmonary venous congestion, interstitial edema, alveolar edema, or pleural effusion increases the likelihood of CHF in a dyspneic patient. A cardiothoracic ratio greater than 50% indicates systolic dysfunction. **One of the earliest chest x-ray findings in CHF is cephalization of the pulmonary vasculature** (upper lobe pulmonary vein dilation with lower lobe pulmonary vein constriction) which indicates increased preload. As the failure progresses, interstitial pulmonary edema can be seen as perihilar infiltrates, often in a butterfly pattern. Kerley lines, which are spindle-shaped linear opacities in the periphery of the lung bases, appear in later heart failure as well. Pleural effusions can also be found. Effusions are usually bilateral but, if unilateral, are more often seen on the right hemithorax than the left.

Echocardiography is the gold-standard diagnostic modality in the presence of CHF. It can evaluate LVEF, ventricle size, wall thickness, left and right ventricle filling pressures, valve function, and the pericardium, as well as identify regional or global wall motion abnormalities due to ischemic heart disease, and show evidence of cardiomyopathy. It can also find pericardial effusion, tamponade or pericardial constriction. Echocardiography is useful in identifying valvular stenosis or regurgitation, either of which can lead to heart failure. These findings aid in the determination of whether the heart failure is a systolic or diastolic dysfunction, an important distinction in the decision of appropriate treatment.

Some patients may also need cardiac catheterization if coronary artery disease is thought to be a significant contributor to the development of a patient's CHF. Revascularization of coronary lesions causing ischemic heart disease has been shown to improve outcomes in patients with systolic heart failure.

Classification of CHF

CHF severity is characterized by the symptoms a patient has and the degree that the symptoms limit a patient's lifestyle. There are several classification systems in use; two of the most widely used are the New York Heart Association (NYHA) and the American Heart Association (AHA) classifications. Table 27–2 summarizes these systems. The classification of CHF is important in determining the appropriate treatment and prognosis for the patient.

Management of Heart Failure

Prevention is the most important part of managing CHF. The Heart Association classification system helps clinicians identify patients at risk, so that preventive strategies may be implemented early. Aggressive control of hypertension has been shown to reduce incidence of heart failure by up to 50%. Treating patients who have coronary artery disease or who have had a myocardial infarction with ACEI, ARBs, β-blockers, and aldosterone antagonists reduces the risk of progression

Table 27–2 • CLASSIFICATION OF SEVERITY OF CONGESTIVE HEART FAILURE

American Heart Association	New York Heart Association	Limitations	Symptoms
A	—	None	Risk factors
B	I	None with normal activities	Left ventricular dysfunction
B	II	Mild	Fatigue, dyspnea with normal activities
C	III	Moderate	Activities of daily living
D	IV	Severe	At rest

to symptomatic heart failure. Treating dyslipidemia with statin therapy can also reduce incidence of heart failure by 20%.

Controlling other risk factors, such as diabetes mellitus, atherosclerotic vascular disease, and thyroid disease, as well as avoidance of cardiotoxic drugs such as tobacco, alcohol, cocaine, and amphetamines, are important for reducing risk as well.

MANAGING ACUTE CHF

In all cases of acute decompensated CHF, **the initial management imperative is the stabilization of the cardiopulmonary system.** Supplemental oxygen, initially 100% via non-rebreather face mask, should be administered. If necessary, ventilation can be assisted with continuous positive airway pressure (CPAP), bilevel positive airway pressure (BiPAP), or mechanical ventilation. Cardiac and continuous pulse oximetry monitors should be placed and IV access obtained.

The goals of managing an acute exacerbation of CHF are to stabilize hemodynamics, treat reversible underlying conditions contributing to CHF, and to establish an effective regimen for outpatient therapy. About 90% of patients admitted to the hospital with decompensated heart failure are volume overloaded. When volume overload caused by CHF (which frequently causes acute pulmonary edema) is diagnosed, the next step in management is the administration of a loop diuretic. Furosemide is generally the treatment of choice, both for its potent diuretic effect and for its rapid bronchial vasculature vasodilation. Volume overload may also be treated acutely with vasodilators to reduce filling pressures. Nitrates, particularly nitroglycerin when given IV, reduce myocardial oxygen demand by reducing preload and afterload. Nitroglycerin also can rapidly reduce blood pressure and is the treatment of choice in a patient who has CHF and whose blood pressure is elevated. It should be used with caution or avoided in a hypotensive patient.

IV morphine sulfate can be an effective adjunct to therapy. Along with its analgesic and anxiolytic properties, morphine is a venodilator (primary effect) and arterial dilator, resulting in a reduction in preload and an increase in cardiac output. Patients with severely reduced ejection fraction may require short-term use of inotropic agents such as dobutamine or milrinone to improve cardiac output. Vasopressors may also be necessary for hypotension, and dopamine is the preferred agent for CHF patients. Hemodialysis for fluid removal may be required in patients with concomitant end-stage renal disease.

Most patients who present to the emergency department (ED) with symptomatic CHF will require admission to a telemetry unit for treatment and monitoring. To be discharged home directly from the ED, a patient must have had gradual onset of symptoms, rapid resolution of symptoms with treatment, oxygen saturation of greater than 90% on room air, and exclusion of an acute coronary syndrome as the cause of the CHF.

Outpatient Management of Chronic CHF

Patient education is an important aspect of care for all patients with CHF. All patients should be advised about the importance of dietary sodium and fluid restriction. A normal American diet contains 6 to 10 g sodium chloride a day; the American Heart Association, recommends restricting to 1500 mg/d in patients with stage A or B disease because of data correlating the incidence of hypertension and heart failure with sodium intake. Stricter restrictions have been recommended in those with more severe disease, but there is little data to support a specific amount of sodium restriction in patients with stage C or D CHF. Fluid restriction can be considered in patients whose fluid retention is difficult to control. Patients should be warned to avoid nonsteroidal anti-inflammatory medications as these can worsen fluid retention, and reduce the efficacy of diuretics and ACEIs. Overweight and obese patients should be counseled on appropriate caloric restrictions and encouraged to exercise to reduce weight. Exercise training such as cardiac rehabilitation in patients with CHF is associated with improved response to pharmacologic vasodilators, reduced hospitalizations, and improvement in well-being and exercise capacity. The importance of strict management of blood pressure and modification of other cardiac risk factors should be emphasized as well. Obstructive sleep apnea and central sleep apnea are common in patients with systolic heart failure, and treatment with positive airway pressure therapies has been associated with improved ejection fraction and survival.

ACEIs or ARBs should be considered first-line therapy in patients with CHF and reduced left ventricular function. ACEIs and ARBs reduce preload, afterload, improve cardiac output without increasing heart rate, and inhibit tissue renin-angiotensin systems which improves myocardial relaxation and compliance. The result of this is improvement in symptoms and reduction in mortality and hospitalization. Survival is increased by 20% in patients with systolic CHF and with left ventricular systolic dysfunction after MI even without signs or symptoms of CHF. ACEIs or ARBs can also delay the development of symptomatic CHF in asymptomatic patients with a reduced cardiac ejection fraction (AHA stage B or NYHA class I). **Better outcomes are seen at higher doses, so patients should be maintained at the highest tolerable dose.** ACEIs and ARBs are contraindicated in pregnancy, hypotension, hyperkalemia, and bilateral renal artery stenosis, and should be used with caution in patients with renal insufficiency.

The administration of β-blockers, especially in high doses, in the setting of acute CHF, can worsen symptoms; consequently, they should preferentially be started when patients have minimal evidence of fluid retention and few symptoms, and initial doses should be low and titrated up over several weeks. β-Blockers reduce sympathetic tone and the cardiac muscle remodeling associated with chronic heart failure. In combination with ACEIs, β-blockers improve mortality. Contraindications to β-blocker use include symptomatic bradycardia, atrioventricular block in absence of a pacemaker, hypotension, severe peripheral vascular disease, and severe bronchospasm.

Diuretics should be used to reduce volume overload in both the acute and chronic settings. They are most helpful in symptom management, and should be used with ACEI/ARBs and β-blockers for long-term reduction in CHF exacerbations. Loop diuretics (furosemide, bumetanide, torsemide, ethacrynic acid) can be used in all stages of CHF and are useful for pulmonary edema and refractory heart failure. These are preferred because they can increase sodium excretion by 20% to 25% and increase free water excretion. Thiazide diuretics (hydrochlorothiazide, chlorthalidone, others) only increase sodium excretion by 5% to 10% and this effect is reduced in renal insufficiency. Their primary role in management of heart failure is in treatment of hypertension. They can also be used in combination with loop diuretics to potentiate diuresis. Diuretic doses can be adjusted based on daily weight measurements by the patient, and patients should be monitored closely for overdiuresis.

The aldosterone antagonists spironolactone and eplerenone reduce mortality in advanced heart failure, as well as improving symptoms and reducing hospitalizations. Elevated aldosterone levels contribute to sodium and water retention, potassium and magnesium loss, myocardial hypertrophy and fibrosis, and endothelial dysfunction. Aldosterone blockade promotes reversal of these effects. It also functions as a potassium-sparing diuretic and should be considered in NYHA class III and IV heart failure. Patients on this medication must be closely monitored for the development of hyperkalemia, which can become profound and lead to arrhythmia. It should be avoided in patients with renal failure.

Calcium channel blockers, in general, increase mortality in systolic CHF and should be avoided. The exception to this is the dihydropyridine calcium channel blocker amlodipine (Norvasc), which does not increase or decrease mortality, and can be very effective in treating hypertension. Nondihydropyridine calcium channel blockers (diltiazem, verapamil) may be useful in heart failure caused by diastolic dysfunction, as they promote increased cardiac output by lowering heart rate, which allows for more ventricular filling time.

The combination of hydralazine with nitrates has been shown to provide increased survival and decreased hospitalizations when used in combination with ACEIs, β-blockers, and spironolactone in patients with systolic heart failure who self-identified as African American. Digoxin is only indicated to reduce hospital stays in patients with uncontrolled heart failure on appropriate medical therapy or for ventricular rate control in patients with known arrhythmias, such as atrial fibrillation. It can improve symptoms, exercise tolerance, and slightly improve ejection fraction and cardiac output, but it has no mortality benefit, and has a very narrow therapeutic window with significant adverse effects in overdose. Symptoms of digoxin toxicity include nausea, vomiting, headache, somnolence, altered color vision, and arrhythmias. Benefits of digoxin therapy are greatest in patients with NYHA class IV disease, cardiomegaly, and ejection fraction less than 25%.

Approximately, one-third of patients with NYHA class III or IV heart failure and reduced ejection fraction have ECG evidence of abnormal ventricular conduction (ie, prolonged QRS duration), which causes ventricular dyssynchrony. This results in reductions in ventricular filling, left ventricular contractility, paradoxical septal wall motion, and worsening of mitral regurgitation. These patients can be helped by promoting synchronous contraction of both the right and left ventricles using a biventricular pacemaker. This process, also known as **cardiac resynchronization therapy**, has been shown to reduce mortality and hospitalization in patients with symptomatic CHF in spite of maximal medical therapy, as well as improve quality of life, exercise capacity, and LVEF.

Patients with an ejection fraction less than 35%, NYHA class II or III heart failure, and a reasonable life expectancy of at least 1 year are recommended to have an implantable cardioverter-defibrillator (ICD) placed for secondary prevention of sudden cardiac death due to ventricular arrhythmias, especially if the patient has a history of cardiac arrest, ventricular fibrillation, or unstable ventricular tachycardia.

> ## CASE CORRELATION
> - See also Case 20 (Chest Pain).

COMPREHENSION QUESTIONS

27.1 A 57-year-old man who has known New York Heart Association class II heart failure presents to clinic after noting to become dyspneic with significant exertion. On physical examination, his BP is 140/86 mm Hg, pulse 86 beats/min, and respiratory rate 20 breaths/min. A 2/6 pansystolic murmur is best heard at the right sternal border. There is no JVD, but 1+ pretibial and pedal edema are noted. He currently takes an ACEI and aspirin. Which one of the following additional medications has been shown to improve longevity in this situation?

   A. Warfarin (Coumadin)

   B. Digoxin

   C. β-Blocker

   D. Nondihydropyridine calcium channel blocker

   E. Amiodarone (Cordarone)

27.2 A 52-year-old man with a long-standing history of marginally controlled hypertension presents with gradually increasing shortness of breath and reduced exercise tolerance with pain in his calves that causes him to stop walking after one block. His medications include enalapril and metoprolol. His physical examination reveals a blood pressure of 140/90 mm Hg, a respiratory rate of 22 breaths/min, heart rate of 88 beats/min, bibasilar rales, and trace pitting edema. Posterial tibial and dorsalis pedis pulses are 1+. Which of the following diagnostic tests is most appropriate in the further evaluation of this patient?

   A. Cardiac magnetic resonance imaging (MRI)

   B. 12-lead ECG

   C. Spiral computed tomography (CT) of the chest

   D. Two-dimensional echocardiography with Doppler

   E. Posteroanterior and lateral chest radiographs

27.3 A 64-year-old man is noted to have congestive heart failure because of coronary artery disease. Over the past 2 days, he has developed progressive dyspnea and orthopnea. On examination, he is found to be in moderate respiratory distress, has JVD, and rales on pulmonary examination. He is diagnosed with pulmonary edema. Which of the following agents is most appropriate at this time?

A. Hydrochlorothiazide

B. Furosemide

C. Carvedilol

D. Spironolactone

E. Digitalis

27.4 A 70-year-old African-American man with New York Heart Association class III heart failure sees you for follow-up. He has shortness of breath with minimal exertion. The patient is adherent to his medication regimen. His current medications include lisinopril 40 mg twice daily, carvedilol 25 mg twice daily, furosemide 80 mg daily, and spironolactone 25 mg daily. His blood pressure is 100/60 mm Hg, and his pulse rate is 70 beats/min and regular. Physical examination findings include a few scattered bibasilar rales, an S_3 gallop, and no peripheral edema. An ECG reveals a left bundle branch block and echocardiography reveals an ejection fraction of 25%. Which of the following is the best next step for this patient?

A. Increase the furosemide dosage to 80 mg twice daily.

B. Refer for coronary angiography.

C. Increase the lisinopril dosage to 80 mg twice daily.

D. Increase the carvedilol dosage to 50 mg twice daily.

E. Refer for cardiac resynchronization therapy.

ANSWERS

27.1 **C.** β-Blockers are recommended to reduce mortality in symptomatic patients with heart failure. Digoxin is only recommended in patients who are already on maximal medical therapy. Nondihydropyridine calcium channel blockers should be used with caution in patients with heart failure because they can cause peripheral vasodilation, decreased heart rate, decreased cardiac contractility, and decreased cardiac conduction. Anticoagulation with warfarin is not indicated, and amiodarone is used for treatment of arrhythmias.

27.2 **D.** The most useful diagnostic tool for evaluating patients with heart failure is two-dimensional echocardiography with Doppler to assess left ventricular ejection fraction (LVEF), left ventricular size, ventricular compliance, wall thickness, and valve function. It should be performed during the initial evaluation. Chest radiography and 12-lead electrocardiography should be performed in all patients presenting with heart failure, but should not be used as the primary basis for determining which abnormalities are responsible for the heart failure.

27.3 **B.** Furosemide, a loop diuretic, is a first-line agent in CHF exacerbation with pulmonary edema. The other medications listed may be used in the management of CHF, but are not indicated in an acute exacerbation.

27.4 **E.** This patient is already receiving maximal medical therapy. Cardiac resynchronization therapy is recommended for patients in sinus rhythm with an EF less than 35%, QRS greater than 120 ms, and those who remain symptomatic (NYHA III-IV) despite optimal medical therapy.

CLINICAL PEARLS

► The initial hour in the management of a patient with either new-onset CHF or an acute exacerbation is crucial to their outcome.

► Simple measures, such as decreasing cardiac preload by sitting the patient up with their legs on the ground and their arms by their side, maintaining an airway and giving oxygen, and giving sublingual nitroglycerin, can alleviate CHF immediately.

REFERENCES

Dar O, Cowie MR. The epidemiology and diagnosis of heart failure. In: Fuster V, Walsh RA, Harrington RA. eds. *Hurst's the Heart.* 13th ed. New York, NY: McGraw-Hill; 2011.

Francis GS, Tang W, Walsh RA. Pathophysiology of heart failure. In: Fuster V, Walsh RA, Harrington RA. eds. *Hurst's the Heart.* 13th ed. New York, NY: McGraw-Hill; 2011.

King M, Kingery J, Casey B. Diagnosis and evaluation of heart failure. *Am Fam Physician.* 2012 Jun 15;85(12):1161-1168.

King M, Perez O. Heart failure. In: South-Paul JE, Matheny SC, Lewis EL, eds. *Current Diagnosis & Treatment: Family Medicine.* 4th ed. New York, NY: McGraw-Hill; 2015.

Klein L. Heart failure with reduced ejection fraction. In: Crawford MH, ed. *Current Diagnosis & Treatment: Cardiology.* 4th ed. New York, NY: McGraw-Hill; 2014.

Mann DL, Chakinala M. Heart failure: pathophysiology and diagnosis. In: Kasper D, Fauci A, Hauser S, et al., eds. *Harrison's Principles of Internal Medicine.* 19th ed. New York, NY: McGraw-Hill; 2015. Available at: http://accessmedicine.mhmedical.com. Accessed May 25, 2015.

Mehra MR. Heart failure: management. In: Kasper D, Fauci A, Hauser S, et al., eds. *Harrison's Principles of Internal Medicine.* 19th ed. New York, NY: McGraw-Hill; 2015. Available at: http://accessmedicine.mhmedical.com. Accessed May 25, 2015.

Yancy CW, Jessup M, Bozkurt B, et al. 2013 ACCF/AHA guideline for the management of heart failure: a report of the American College of Cardiology Foundation/American Heart Association Task Force on practice guidelines. *Circulation.* 2013 Oct 15;128(16):e240.

A 38-year-old G3P3 divorced executive presents to your clinic for contraceptive advice. She has been in a monogamous relationship with her boyfriend for several months. She denies any drug allergies. She occasionally drinks alcohol and smokes half a pack of cigarettes a day. She mentions that she used to take birth control pills without any problems. All three of her children were born via vaginal delivery without complication. She and her partner are free of sexually transmitted diseases (STDs) based on their recent checkups. She reports that she is tired of using over-the-counter contraceptives because they are inconvenient. She said that her life is very busy because of work. She fears any form of surgery and has not excluded having another child. Her laboratory workup is normal. Her physical examination is normal. She is looking for the "best contraceptive method" for her situation.

▶ What contraceptive options are available to this woman?
▶ Which contraceptives are contraindicated for her?

ANSWERS TO CASE 28:
Family Planning—Contraceptives

Summary: A 38-year-old parous woman presents for counseling regarding her contraceptive options. She is in a monogamous relationship. She reports that she is dissatisfied with using over-the-counter options and that she is not ready for permanent sterilization. She smokes a half-pack of cigarettes daily.

- **Available contraceptive options:** Intrauterine devices (IUDs), progestin implants, injectable progestins, progestin-only oral contraceptives, barrier contraceptives, natural family planning

- **Contraindicated contraceptive options:** Combined estrogen-progesterone contraceptives: oral contraceptive pills, patches, vaginal rings

ANALYSIS
Objectives

1. Know the available methods of contraception.

2. Be aware of contraindications for and of the side effects of contraceptives.

Considerations

Choosing a method of contraception is a personal decision, based on individual preferences, medical history, and lifestyle. In the United States, approximately 50% of pregnancies are unintended and approximately 50% of these pregnancies end in abortion. Approximately 80% of women having unprotected sex will become pregnant within a year. All methods of contraception have a number of risks and benefits of which the patient should be aware, as well as a failure rate, defined as inability to prevent pregnancy over a 1-year period. Sometimes the failure rate is a result of the method and sometimes it is a result of human error. Each method has possible side effects. Some methods require lifestyle modifications. Patients with certain medical conditions cannot use certain types of contraceptives.

There are numerous contraceptive options available and recommendations regarding contraceptive use must be individualized. In the case given, there are several important factors that must be considered. Combined hormonal contraceptives are to be used with caution in women who smoke cigarettes and are not recommended for smokers over the age of 35 because of increased risk of myocardial infarction and stroke. Given the patient's fear of surgery and because she is not certain whether she wants to have more children in the future, surgical sterilization via bilateral tubal ligation or hysteroscopic tubal occlusion or division is not a choice. A vasectomy for the partner, although potentially reversible, should be considered permanent sterilization and not ideal for this patient. Barrier methods are an inconvenience to the patient's busy lifestyle, but still a viable option. Given that both the patient and her boyfriend have no history of STDs and are in a long-term relationship, appropriate methods of contraception for them include IUDs or progestin implants. IUDs can last 3, 5, or 10 years before replacement, depending on the type used, and implants can last 3 years. Both reduce user error associated with pill and barrier contraception. Figure 28–1 is an algorithm that can be used as a guide to approaching family planning options.

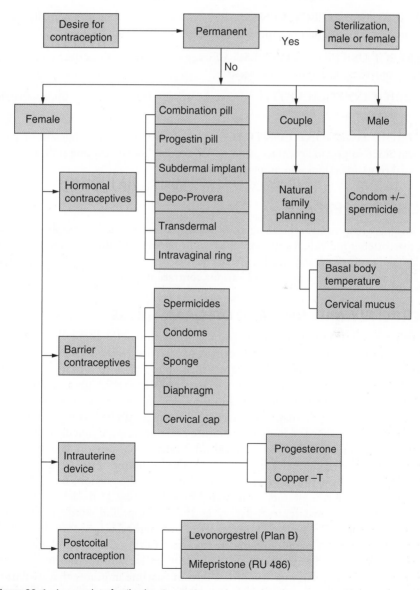

Figure 28–1. Approach to family planning options.

APPROACH TO:
Contraception

DEFINITIONS

INTRAUTERINE CONTRACEPTIVE DEVICE (IUD): Small T-shaped device placed in the endometrial cavity as a method of long-term contraception

TYPICAL USE EFFECTIVENESS: Efficacy of a method as it is actually used, when forgetfulness and improper use can occur

PERFECT USE EFFECTIVENESS: Efficacy of a method in perfect conditions, when consistent and reliable use occur

BARRIER CONTRACEPTIVE: Prevents sperm from entering upper female reproductive tract

STEROID HORMONE CONTRACEPTION: Estrogen plus progestin or progestin alone to provide contraception in various methods, including pills, patches, vaginal rings, injections, and implants

CLINICAL APPROACH

Choosing which contraception agent is best for a patient can be complex. Review of the patient's individual situation, medical problems, and ability to remember to take medication each day are important factors to consider. Table 28–1 summarizes some of the characteristics of various contraceptive agents.

FERTILITY AWARENESS AND OTHER METHODS

Fertility awareness (natural family planning or rhythm method) entails abstinence during the woman's fertile period, or using a barrier method during this time period. Fertility awareness has a failure rate of up to 25% with typical use and 3% to 5% with perfect use. Women with irregular cycles have the highest failure rates. This method is dependent on the ability to identify the approximately 10 days in each menstrual cycle that a woman is fertile, which can be accomplished using calendar calculation, basal body temperature charting, cervical mucus monitoring, or the symptothermal method. The calendar calculation uses the length of past reproductive cycles to predict fertile periods. The beginning of the fertile period is calculated by subtracting 18 days from the shortest of the previous 6 to 12 cycles. The end of the fertile period is calculated by subtracting 11 days from the longest cycle. For a consistent 28-day cycle, the fertile period would occur from days 10 through 17. The basal body temperature method is based on the knowledge that a woman's basal temperature increases during the luteal phase of the reproductive cycle. Temperature must be recorded early in the morning at the same time each day. An increase of 0.4°F from baseline indicates that ovulation has occurred. For this method to be most effective, a woman must either avoid intercourse or use barrier methods from the first day of menses to the third day

Table 28–1 • CONTRACEPTION AGENTS COMPARED INCLUDING BEST-SUITED PATIENTS

Category/Agents	Mechanism	Best Suited for	Disadvantages/ Contraindications
Barrier • Diaphragm • Cervical caps • Condoms (male and female)	Mechanical obstruction to sperm	Avoidance of hormones **Decrease risk of STD (condoms)**	Pelvic organ prolapse Patient discomfort with placing devices on genitals Lack of spontaneity Allergies to material Diaphragm may be associated with more UTIs
Combined hormonal (estrogen and progestin) • Combined oral contraceptives • Contraceptive patch • Vaginal ring	Inhibit ovulation Thicken cervical mucus to inhibit sperm penetration Alters tubal transport Thins endometrium	Iron-deficiency anemia Dysmenorrhea Ovarian cysts Endometriosis OCP—take pill each day **Patch**—less to remember but may cause more nausea **Ring**—less to remember, but may cause vaginal irritation and discharge	Known thrombogenic mutations Active or history of thromboembolic disease Cerebrovascular or coronary artery disease (current or remote) Cigarette smoking (especially over age 35) Uncontrolled hypertension Diabetic retinopathy or nephropathy Peripheral vascular disease Breast or endometrial cancer Unexplained uterine bleeding Migraines with aura Liver tumors (benign or malignant), active liver disease Known or suspected pregnancy Application site reaction (for patches)
Progestin-only oral • Micronor and others	Thickens cervical mucus to inhibit sperm penetration Alters tubal transport Thins endometrium	**Breast-feeding**	Patient needs to remember to take pill at the same time each day

(Continued)

Table 28–1 • CONTRACEPTION AGENTS COMPARED INCLUDING BEST-SUITED PATIENTS (CONTINUED)

Category/Agents	Mechanism	Best Suited for	Disadvantages/ Contraindications
Injectables • Depo-medroxyprogesterone acetate (Depo-Provera, and others)	Inhibits ovulation Thins endometrium Alters cervical mucus to inhibit sperm penetration	Breast-feeding Desires long-term contraception Iron-deficiency anemia Sickle cell disease Epilepsy Dysmenorrhea Ovarian cysts Endometriosis	Depression Osteopenia/osteoporosis—partially reversible with cessation Appetite stimulation leading to weight gain Unexplained uterine bleeding Breast cancer Active or history of thromboembolic disease Cerebrovascular disease Liver tumors (benign or malignant), active liver disease Known or suspected pregnancy
Implants (subdermal in arm) • Etonogestrel (Implanon, Nexplanon)	Inhibits ovulation Thins endometrium Thickens cervical mucus to inhibit sperm penetration	Breast-feeding Desires long-term, reversible contraception (3 years) Iron-deficiency anemia Dysmenorrhea Ovarian cysts Endometriosis	Active or history of thromboembolic disease (relative contraindication) Liver tumors (benign or malignant), active liver disease Unexplained uterine bleeding Breast cancer Hypersensitivity to any of the components of Nexplanon May lead to irregular vaginal bleeding
IUD • Levonorgestrel secreting (Mirena, and others)	Thickens cervical mucus Thins endometrium	Desires long-term, reversible contraception (3 or 5 years) Stable, mutually monogamous relationship Menorrhagia Dysmenorrhea (*Note:* decreased bleeding)	Current STD or recent PID Unexplained uterine bleeding Untreated cervical or endometrial cancer Breast cancer Anatomic abnormalities or uterine fibroids distorting the uterine cavity

(Continued)

Table 28–1 • CONTRACEPTION AGENTS COMPARED INCLUDING BEST-SUITED PATIENTS (CONTINUED)

Category/Agents	Mechanism	Best Suited for	Disadvantages/ Contraindications
• Copper-T (Paragard)	Inhibits sperm migration and viability Changes transport speed of ovum Damages ovum	Desires long-term, reversible contraception (10 years) Stable, mutually monogamous relationship Contraindication to contraceptive hormones	Current STD Current or PID within the past 2 months Unexplained uterine bleeding Malignant gestational trophoblastic disease Untreated cervical or endometrial cancer Breast cancer Anatomic abnormalities or uterine fibroids distorting the uterine cavity Wilson disease May cause more bleeding or dysmenorrhea
Permanent sterilization • Bilateral tubal occlusion • Bilateral tubal ligation	Mechanical obstruction of tubes	Does not desire more children	Contraindications to procedure or surgery May want children in the future

Abbreviations: OCP, oral contraceptive pill; PID, pelvic inflammatory disease; STD, sexually transmitted disease; UTI, urinary tract infection.

after the temperature increase. The cervical mucus method, also called the Billings ovulation method, depends on a woman recognizing the changes in cervical mucus that indicate ovulation is occurring or has occurred. The symptothermal method combines all three; calendar, basal body temperature, and cervical mucus methods.

Other methods include coitus interruptus, also known as the withdrawal method, postcoital douching, and lactational amenorrhea. Coitus interruptus involves withdrawing the penis before ejaculation and has a 27% typical use failure rate. Postcoital douching is used to flush semen out of the vagina, but sperm have been found within cervical mucus within 90 seconds of ejaculation, so this method is unreliable. Lactational amenorrhea occurs with suppression of ovulation due to breast-feeding. During the first 6 months following delivery, women who are exclusively breast-feeding have mostly anovulatory menstrual cycles, and pregnancy rates have been found to be approximately 1%.

BARRIER METHODS

There are **five barrier methods of contraception:** male condom, female condom, diaphragm, sponge, and cervical cap. In each, the method works by keeping the sperm and egg apart. The main possible side effect is an allergic reaction either to the material of the barrier or the spermicides that should be used with them.

Male Condom

Condoms on the market are made of latex rubber, polyurethane, or sheep intestine. Of these types, **only latex and polyurethane condoms are effective in preventing STDs by providing a good barrier to viruses and bacteria.** Polyurethane condoms have a higher rate of breaking or slipping than latex, and thus higher failure rates, but they can be used by patients with a latex allergy. Each condom can only be used once. Condoms have a typical use failure rate of approximately 15%, with most of the failures a result of improper use. Perfect use failure rate is about 2%. For maximal efficacy, a condom must be used with every coital act, should be in place before contact of the penis with the vagina, withdrawal must occur with the penis still erect, the base of the condom must be held during withdrawal, and an intravaginal spermicide or a condom lubricated with spermicide should be employed. Only water-based lubricants should be used with latex condoms as oil-based lubricants reduce efficacy.

Female Condom

The female condom consists of a lubricated polyurethane sheath with a flexible polyurethane ring on each end. One ring is inserted into the vagina much like a diaphragm, while the other remains outside, partially covering the labia. The female condom may offer some protection against STDs but are not as effective as male latex condoms. The estimated typical use failure rate is estimated at 21% and perfect use at 5%.

Sponge

The contraceptive sponge is made of white polyurethane foam. It is shaped like a small doughnut and contains spermicide. The sponge protects for 12 to 24 hours, regardless of how many times intercourse occurs. It is inserted into the vagina to cover the cervix during and after intercourse. After intercourse, the sponge must be left in place for over 6 hours before it is removed and discarded. It does not require fitting by a health professional and is available without prescription. It is to be used only once and then discarded. The typical use failure rate is 32% in parous women and 16% in nulliparous women, decreased to 20% and 9% in perfect use, respectively. An extremely rare side effect is toxic shock syndrome (TSS).

Diaphragm

The diaphragm is a flexible rubber disk with a rigid rim ranging in size from 2 to 4 inches in diameter. It is designed to cover the cervix during and after intercourse, so that sperm cannot reach the uterus. The diaphragm must be fitted by a health professional and the correct size prescribed to ensure a snug seal with the vaginal wall. Spermicidal jelly or cream must be placed on the cervical side of the diaphragm for it to be effective. If intercourse is repeated, additional spermicide should be added with the diaphragm still in place. A diaphragm may be placed up to 6 hours before intercourse, and **should be left in place for 6 to 24 hours after intercourse.** TSS has also been described with diaphragm use, so a diaphragm should not be left in place for longer than 24 hours. The diaphragm used with spermicide has a failure rate of 6% with perfect use and 18% with typical use.

Cervical Cap

The cervical cap is a dome-shaped silicone cap that fits snugly over the cervix. Like the diaphragm, it is used with a spermicide and must be fitted by a health professional. It is more difficult to insert than the diaphragm, but may be left in place for up to 48 hours. There also appears to be an increased incidence of irregular Papanicolaou (Pap) tests in the first 6 months of using the cap, and TSS is an extremely rare side effect. The cap has a failure rate of about 18%.

Spermicides Used Alone

Spermicides come in many forms (foams, films, creams, gels, suppositories, tablets) and work by forming a physical and chemical barrier to sperm. They should be inserted into the vagina within an hour before intercourse. If intercourse is repeated, more spermicide should be inserted. The only spermicidal agent in use in the United States is nonoxynol-9, which is a surfactant that destroys the sperm cell membrane. The failure rate for spermicides in preventing pregnancy when used alone is 29% with typical use and 18% with perfect use. Spermicides are available without a prescription. When **spermicides are used with a condom, the failure rate is comparable to that of oral contraceptives** and is much better than for either spermicides or condoms used alone.

HORMONAL CONTRACEPTION

Hormonal contraception involves ways of delivering estrogen and progesterone. Hormones temporarily interact with the body's reproductive cycle and have the potential for rare but serious side effects. When properly used, hormonal methods are extremely effective.

Oral Contraceptives

There are **two types of oral contraceptive pills (OCPs)**: combination pills, which contain both estrogen and a progestin (a natural or synthetic progesterone), and progestin-only pills (POPs) (commonly known as the "minipill).

Combination pills are the most commonly used contraceptive method. The combination pill suppresses ovulation through inhibition of the hypothalamic-pituitary-ovarian axis, alters the cervical mucus, retards sperm entry, and discourages ovum implantation by creating an unfavorable endometrium. **Combination oral contraceptives offer significant protection against ovarian cancer, endometrial cancer, iron-deficiency anemia from menstrual blood loss, pelvic inflammatory disease (PID), and fibrocystic breast disease.** Women who take combination pills have a lower risk of functional ovarian cysts. The POP reduces cervical mucus and causes it to thicken. The mucus thickening prevents the sperm from reaching the egg and keeps the uterine lining from thickening, which prevents the fertilized egg from implanting in the uterus. The POP is ideal for breast-feeding mothers because it does not interfere with milk production as combination OCPs do. When taken as directed, the failure rate for the POP is 1% to 3%; the failure rate of the combination pill is 1% to 2%. Typical use of OCPs has a failure rate of 8% to 10%.

Women over the age of 35 who smoke cigarettes and women with certain medical conditions should not take the combined OCP. Table 28–2 lists the absolute

Table 28-2 • CONTRAINDICATIONS TO COMBINED HORMONAL CONTRACEPTION

Absolute Contraindications	Relative Contraindications
Previous thromboembolic event	Severe vascular headache (classic migraine, cluster)
Cerebral vascular disease	Severe hypertension (if younger than 35-40 years and in good medical control, can elect OCP)
Coronary occlusion	Diabetes mellitus (prevention of pregnancy outweighs the risk of complicating vascular disease in a diabetic who is younger than 35-40 years)
Impaired liver function	Gallbladder disease (may exacerbate emergence of symptoms when gallstones are present)
Known or suspected breast cancer	Obstructive jaundice in pregnancy
Smokers (>15 cigarettes/day) older than 35 years	Epilepsy (antiepileptic drugs may decrease effectiveness of OCPs)
Congenital hyperlipidemia	Morbid obesity

and relative contraindications to taking the combined OCP. Minor side effects, which usually subside after a few months of usage, include nausea, headaches, breast swelling, fluid retention, weight gain, irregular bleeding, and depression.

When starting an OCP, ideally a patient should take the first pill on the first day of the start of menses. Women may also choose to start on the Sunday after the start of their menses for convenience. A quick-start method has also been proposed, in which patients start taking the pills as soon as they obtain the prescription (if pregnancy is unlikely), which improves compliance. Both Sunday-start and quick-start methods require an additional backup method to be used for the first week. Postpartum, non–breast-feeding women should start the OCP during the fourth week after delivery. Breast-feeding women should start the minipill during the sixth week after delivery. OCPs can be started the day after an induced or spontaneous abortion. **If a pill is missed, it should be taken as soon as possible and the next dose should be taken as usual.** If two or more pills are missed, the patient should be directed to the package insert for instructions and additional backup contraception should be used for at least 7 days following resumption.

The effectiveness of OCPs may be reduced by a few other medications, including some antibiotics, barbiturates, and antifungal medications.

Transdermal Contraceptive

A transdermal contraceptive patch (Ortho Evra and others) is a combined hormone patch containing norelgestromin and ethinyl estradiol. The treatment regimen for each cycle is three consecutive 7-day patches followed by one patch-free week, so that withdrawal bleeding can occur. It can be started in a similar fashion to combined OCPs: on the first day of the menstrual cycle, the first Sunday after the menstrual cycle, or the day the prescription is filled. If the Sunday-start or quick-start methods are used, a backup method of contraception is needed for 7 days. The patch may be placed on the buttocks, lower abdomen, upper outer arm, and upper torso, except for the breasts. If a patch becomes detached, it should be replaced as soon as possible. If the patch is detached for more than 24 hours, it should be replaced and a backup method of contraception used for the next 7 days. **The patch's efficacy and side effects are comparable to that of combined OCPs,** although there may be an increased risk of vascular thrombosis with use of the patch. Women who weigh more than 90 kg may be at increased risk of pregnancy with patch use.

Intravaginal Ring Contraceptive

NuvaRing is a flexible, transparent ring about 5 cm in diameter that delivers etonogestrel and ethinyl estradiol. **A woman inserts the NuvaRing herself, wears it for 3 weeks, then removes and discards the device.** After one ring-free week, during which withdrawal bleeding occurs, a new ring is inserted. It does not need to be fitted by a health professional, and does not need to be removed during intercourse. If a patient or her partner experience problems with the ring during intercourse, it may be removed, but should be replaced within 3 hours. If it is out for more than 3 hours, ovulation may occur. The manufacturer recommends using backup birth control for the first 7 days after placement if not switching from another hormonal contraceptive. Rarely, NuvaRing can slip out of the vagina, and it is recommended to check the position of the ring before and after intercourse. NuvaRing may not be appropriate for women with conditions that increase likelihood of ring expulsion, such as vaginal stenosis, cervical prolapse, cystocele, or rectocele. The efficacy and most side effects of NuvaRing are similar to those of combined OCPs, although vaginitis, discomfort, and foreign body sensation are also commonly reported.

Medroxyprogesterone Injection

Medroxyprogesterone acetate (Depo-Provera, Depo-subQ Provera 104) is an injectable form of a progestin. Medroxyprogesterone acetate has a failure rate of only 0.3% with perfect use, or 3% with typical use. **Each injection provides contraceptive protection for 13 weeks, but can last for up to 4 months.** It is injected every 3 months (90 days) into the gluteus or deltoid muscle. The first dose should be given within 5 days of the onset of menses, so that no backup contraception is needed. Its side effects include irregular menses, weight gain, and injection site reactions. Irregular bleeding and spotting is more significant during the first few months and then is followed by periods of amenorrhea. About half of women develop amenorrhea after a year of medroxyprogesterone acetate use. There may be a prolonged period of time prior to return of fertility after discontinuing Depo-Provera, up to 18 months in a small proportion of women.

Etonogestrel Implant

Contraceptive implants, Implanon and Nexplanon, are inserted subdermally in an in-office minor surgical procedure, and may be removed with another minor procedure. Placement should be timed during the menstrual cycle or during the hormone-free week if using a combined hormonal contraceptive method. The implant contains etonogestrel, the active metabolite of desogestrel, and is effective for 3 years. At the end of 3 years, when the device is removed, a new device may be placed in the same site. The failure rate is less than 1% for women who weigh less than 70 kg.

The potential side effects of the implant include irregular menstrual bleeding, which is the most common reason for discontinuation, headaches, depression, acne, breast tenderness, abdominal pain, and weight gain.

INTRAUTERINE DEVICES

IUDs are small, plastic, flexible devices that are inserted into the uterus through the cervix by a trained physician. **Three IUDs are presently marketed in the United States:** ParaGard T380A, which is a T-shaped plastic device partially covered by copper that is effective for 10 years, Mirena, which is also a T-shaped plastic device, but contains levonorgestrel (a progestin) released over a 5-year period, and Skyla, which is essentially a smaller version of Mirena that releases slightly less levonorgestrel and lasts for 3 years. All are very effective; the copper-T IUD has a 0.6% to 0.8% failure rate, the Mirena has a failure rate of 0.2%, and Sklya has a failure rate of 0.9%. An IUD alters the uterine and tubal fluids, particularly in the case of copper-bearing IUDs, inhibiting the transport of sperm through the cervical mucus and uterus. Progesterone-containing IUDs also thin the uterine lining. Timing of placement should occur during the menstrual cycle and more specifically during the first 7 days of the menstrual cycle for levonorgestrel-containing IUDs.

Manufacturer contraindications for IUD include current or suspected pregnancy; current or recent acute PID or mucopurulent cervicitis; postpartum endometritis or infected abortion in the past 3 months; anatomically distorted uterine cavity, known or suspected uterine or cervical malignancy; unexplained uterine bleeding; and IUD already in place. Copper IUD is also contraindicated in Wilson disease. Levonorgestrel IUDs are also contraindicated in acute liver disease or liver tumor (benign or malignant); breast cancer; and prior ectopic pregnancy. A history of STDs is not a contraindication to IUD placement, but if a woman has a known STD, it is recommended to delay insertion for 3 months following resolution of the infection. Levonorgestrel IUDs may actually reduce the risk of PID by thickening cervical mucus and thinning the endometrium, but caution should be used in patients who are at high risk for PID, and women with multiple sex partners should be counseled to use condoms in conjunction with IUD to reduce risk of contracting an infection.

Side effects include irregular bleeding patterns during the first few months of use, headache, nausea, hair loss, acne, depression, decreased libido, ovarian cysts, and mastalgia. Many patients will become amenorrheic or oligomenorrheic with a levonorgestrel IUD in place, so it can be used to treat patients with menorrhagia. The copper IUD may actually cause heavy, irregular bleeding. Women may also experience some short-term side effects such as cramping and dizziness at the time of insertion; bleeding, cramps, and backache may continue for a few days after the insertion. Complications include expulsion, perforation of the uterus, and ectopic pregnancy. Approximately, 5% of women expel their IUD within the first year. The patient should check that the strings are palpable once a month, and if she cannot find the strings, she should see a health-care provider. The absolute rate of ectopic pregnancy is reduced with the IUD because of its high contraceptive efficacy. However, when accidental pregnancy does occur, there is increased likelihood of ectopic pregnancy. Adolescence and nulliparity are not contraindications.

SURGICAL STERILIZATION

Tubal ligation seals a woman's fallopian tubes so that an egg cannot travel to the uterus. Hysteroscopic tubal obstruction through the placement of sterilization devices in the fallopian tubes is also available. Two types are Food and Drug Administration (FDA) approved: the micro-insert device (Essure) and the polymer matrix system (Adiana). Vasectomy involves closing off a man's vas deferens so that sperm will not be carried to the penis. Vasectomy is a minor surgical procedure, most often performed in a doctor's office under local anesthesia. Hysteroscopic tubal obstruction may be performed with local anesthesia or oral analgesics alone. Tubal ligation is an operating room procedure performed under general anesthesia. Major complications, which are rare in female sterilization, include infection, hemorrhage, and problems associated with the use of general anesthesia. The failure rate is less than 1%. Although there has been some success in reopening the fallopian tubes and the vas deferens, the success rate is low, and **sterilization should be considered irreversible.**

EMERGENCY CONTRACEPTION

All female patients of reproductive age should be made aware of postcoital contraception some of which are available over the counter for adolescent girls of 17 years and older. This knowledge does not increase the likelihood of high-risk behavior. The **Yuzpe method consists of taking high-dose combined OCPs for emergency contraception, and can** decrease the risk of pregnancy by about 75%. This method can be used up to 5 days after unprotected intercourse but is most effective when used within 72 hours. Consider prescribing an antiemetic to be used 1 hour before each dose, as nausea and vomiting are common side effects. Progestin-only emergency contraception is available without a prescription. One or two oral doses of levonorgestrel (Plan B) 0.75 mg, with 12 hours between doses, is more effective than the Yuzpe method, better-tolerated, and can be used up to 5 days after unprotected intercourse. Preven, a convenient emergency contraception kit, includes two doses of medication and a pregnancy test. A single dose of mifepristone (RU-486), a progesterone antagonist, is the most effective emergency contraceptive and has few side effects. A selective progesterone-receptor modulator, known as ulipristal acetate (Ella), is taken in a single dose up to 5 days after unprotected intercourse, and does require a prescription. Placing a copper-containing IUD within 5 days after unprotected sex is the most effective form of emergency contraception, and also provides another 10 years of birth control, but should be avoided in those at risk for STDs, ectopic pregnancy, or if long-term contraception is not desired.

CASE CORRELATION

- See also Cases 4 (Prenatal Care), 16 (Labor and Delivery), and 26 (Postpartum Care).

COMPREHENSION QUESTIONS

28.1   While working in the clinic of the county jail you see a G5P2032 for a well-woman examination. She openly tells you that she was arrested for a history of prostitution. On arrest, she was found to be HIV positive. She is to be released next week and would like contraception. Which of the following agents is most appropriate for this patient?

A.   Oral contraceptive agent

B.   Depot medroxyprogesterone

C.   Intrauterine contraceptive device

D.   Condoms

E.   Cervical cap

28.2   An 18-year-old woman reported having intercourse with her boyfriend 20 hours ago. She was concerned because the condom broke. She used no other form of contraception. The patient reported a history of regular periods since age 14 of heavy flow that usually lasts for longer than 7 days. She is 5 ft 8 in tall and weighs 165 lb. She plays as a forward on her high school basketball team and is worried about becoming pregnant. Which of the following is the most appropriate method of "emergency contraception"?

A.   Yuzpe method

B.   Plan B method

C.   Insertion of a copper IUD

D.   Intramuscular methotrexate

28.3   A 16-year-old adolescent girl presents to your clinic for a well-child check. She has been having regular periods for over 2 years, does not drink or smoke, gets straight As on her report cards, and is in the 75% for height and weight. She is Tanner Stage 5 for both breast and pubic hair development. During your interview, she reveals that she is sexually active and not using contraception. If she continues to have unprotected intercourse, what is the likelihood that she will become pregnant over the course of the next year?

A.   20%

B.   40%

C.   80%

D.   100%

28.4 A 36-year-old woman is seeking contraception. She has delivered her baby 8 weeks ago and is breast-feeding. She undergoes a history and physical examination, and is counseled regarding the various options. She is healthy, drinks an occasional glass of wine per month, does not smoke, and plans to have another child in a year or two. Her blood pressure is 114/70 mm Hg. The patient would like to initiate birth control at this visit. Which method is the most appropriate in her case?

A. Transcervical sterilization (Essure)

B. Natural family planning

C. The minipill

D. Combination oral contraception pills

E. Coitus interruptus

ANSWERS

28.1 **D.** Protection from STDs for this patient, and prevention from transmitting HIV to her future partners is of utmost concern. Condoms are the most effective agents to prevent the transmission of STD. Cervical cap although also a barrier method has high rates of STD transmission. IUDs can be used in selected nulliparous women and in women who desire future fertility. History of STD is not an absolute contraindication to IUD use, but with this patient's high-risk behavior, an IUD should probably be avoided. Oral contraceptives and depot medroxyprogesterone decrease the risk of PID by thickening the cervical mucus but do not provide any protection from STDs.

28.2 **B.** Emergency contraception may include combination hormonal therapy, ideally used within 72 hours but can cause significant nausea and vomiting. Plan B is levonorgestrel and is more effective than the combined OCPs for postcoital contraception without the prominent side effect of nausea. Placing a copper IUD can cause heavy and irregular vaginal bleeding, and would not be a good choice for a patient who already experiences these symptoms. IM methotrexate is not used for emergency contraception.

28.3 **C.** Eighty percent of women having unprotected intercourse will be pregnant in 1 year.

28.4 **C.** The progestin-only pill "minipill" is the most effective form of birth control in the postpartum period for women desiring to breast-feed. Natural family planning and coitus interruptus (withdrawal method) have high rates of user error leading to failure. Essure is a permanent method of birth control that causes occlusion of the fallopian tubes. Combination OCPs can affect a woman's milk supply and have varying safety in lactation.

CLINICAL PEARLS

▶ The male latex condom remains the best shield against HIV and other STDs.

▶ Barrier methods, which work by keeping the sperm and egg apart, usually have only minor side effects.

▶ Combination oral contraceptives offer protection against ovarian cancer, endometrial cancer, iron-deficiency anemia, PID, and fibrocystic breast disease.

▶ Methods of hormonal contraception, when used properly, are extremely effective.

▶ Noncontraceptive benefits of combination oral contraceptives include decreased incidence of benign breast disease, relief from menstrual disorders (dysmenorrhea and menorrhagia), reduced risk of uterine leiomyomata, protection against ovarian cysts, reduction of acne, improvement of bone mineral density, and a reduced risk of colorectal cancer.

▶ Intrauterine and implantable contraceptives are also extremely effective and reduce the contribution of user error to the failure rate.

▶ Surgical sterilization must be considered permanent. Vasectomy is considered safer than tubal ligation.

REFERENCES

Bonnema RA, McNamara MC, Spencer AL. Contraception choices in women with underlying medical conditions. *Am Fam Physician*. 2010;82(6):621-628.

Brunsell SC. Contraception. In: South-Paul JE, Matheny SC, Lewis EL, eds. *Current Diagnosis & Treatment: Family Medicine*. 4th ed. New York, NY: McGraw-Hill; 2015.

Burkman RT, Brzezinski A. Contraception and family planning. In: DeCherney AH, Nathan L, Laufer N, Roman AS, eds. *Current Diagnosis & Treatment: Obstetrics & Gynecology*. 11th ed. New York, NY: McGraw-Hill; 2013.

Cunningham F, Leveno KJ, Bloom SL, et al. In: Cunningham F, Leveno KJ, Bloom SL, et al., eds. *Williams Obstetrics*. 24th ed. New York, NY: McGraw-Hill; 2013.

Esherick JS, Clark DS, Slater ED. Disease management. In: Esherick JS, Clark DS, Slater ED, eds. *Current Practice Guidelines in Primary Care 2015*. New York, NY: McGraw-Hill; 2014.

Hardeman J, Weiss BD. Intrauterine devices: an update. *Am Fam Physician*. 2014 Mar 15;89(6): 445-450.

Hoffman BL, Schorge JO, Schaffer JI, et al. Contraception and sterilization. In: Hoffman BL, Schorge JO, Schaffer JI, et al., eds. *Williams Gynecology*. 2nd ed. New York, NY: McGraw-Hill; 2012.

Smoley BA, Robinson CM. Natural family planning. *Am Fam Physician*. 2012 Nov 15;86(10):924-928.

Wieslander CK, Wong KS. Therapeutic gynecologic procedures. In: DeCherney AH, Nathan L, Laufer N, Roman AS, eds. *Current Diagnosis & Treatment: Obstetrics & Gynecology*. 11th ed. New York, NY: McGraw-Hill; 2013.

A 16-year-old adolescent girl presents for a routine well examination. She is a junior in high school and has no significant medical history. She plays on the school softball team and has a preparticipation clearance form for you to complete. She is accompanied by her mother who wants to know if her daughter should start having routine gynecologic examinations as part of her routine checkup. She states that the patient's last tetanus shot was at the age of 5. She received all of the routine childhood immunizations, including a complete hepatitis B series, and had chickenpox when she was 6 years old. The mother reports that there are no medical problems in the immediate family, but that one of the patient's cousins died at the age of 21 of a sudden cardiac death. When interviewed without the mother in the room, the patient reports to you that she is generally happy, she gets As and Bs in school, and has an active social life. She denies ever being involved in sexual activity, or tobacco or drug use. She says that she will have a "drink or two" at a party with her friends. On examination, her vital signs are normal. Examination of her head and neck, lungs, abdomen, skin, and musculoskeletal and nervous systems are normal. On cardiac auscultation, you hear a 2/6 systolic murmur that gets louder when you have her Valsalva. Peripheral pulses are strong and symmetric; there is good capillary refill and no sign of cyanosis.

► What immunizations should be recommended at this visit?
► At what age is it recommended to start routine Papanicolaou (Pap) smear screening?
► What is the most common cause of sudden cardiac death in young athletes?

ANSWERS TO CASE 29:

Adolescent Health Maintenance

Summary: A healthy 16-year-old adolescent girl presents for a routine checkup and sports preparticipation examination. She is noted incidentally to have a heart murmur.

- **Recommended immunizations:** Tetanus-diphtheria-acellular pertussis (Tdap) booster, meningococcal vaccination, and catch up immunization for the human papillomavirus (HPV) vaccine series as well.

- **Recommended age to start routine Pap smears:** The American College of Obstetrics and Gynecology (ACOG) recommends that initial Pap smears are conducted at age 21. Paps are not indicated at ages younger than 21 regardless of sexual activity or pregnancy.

- **Most common cause of sudden cardiac death in young athletes:** Hypertrophic cardiomyopathy (HCM).

ANALYSIS

Objectives

1. Be familiar with evidence- and expert-based prevention guidelines for adolescents, including the Guidelines for Adolescent Preventive Services (GAPS) for screening examinations and counseling in adolescents.

2. Know the immunizations routinely recommended for adolescents and teenagers.

3. Know the components of and the rationale for performing sports preparticipation examinations.

Considerations

This is a healthy adolescent girl who comes in for a sports preparticipation physical examination. Required sports examinations provide an excellent opportunity for recommended health maintenance such as immunizations, screenings, risk reduction counseling, and general health education. Her history is unremarkable, and she has a 2/6 systolic murmur which increases with Valsalva. The history is the most important component to the sports physical examination. The focus should be on conditions that can lead to sudden cardiac death, which are usually cardiovascular, most commonly hypertrophic cardiomyopathy. Marfan syndrome is associated with aortic root dilation or dissection, hence stigmata of Marfan and family history is also important. The hallmark physical examination finding in HCM is a systolic murmur that decreases in intensity with the athlete in the supine position (increased ventricular filling, decreased obstruction). This contrasts with functional outflow murmurs common in athletes that *increase* in intensity upon lying down. The intensity of the HCM murmur increases with the Valsalva maneuver (decreased ventricular filling, increased obstruction). Any athlete who has a systolic murmur with an intensity of 3/6 or greater; a diastolic, holosystolic, or continuous murmur; or any other murmur that the examiner finds suspicious should be held from participation and referred to a cardiologist for evaluation. Most athletes with HCM are, however, asymptomatic. The individual in this case has only a grade 2/6 murmur, but it is worrisome that it increases in intensity with Valsalva. Most murmurs will decrease in intensity and duration with Valsalva. For this reason, this patient may benefit from referral to cardiology.

APPROACH TO:
Adolescent Health

DEFINITIONS

GUIDELINES FOR ADOLESCENT PREVENTIVE SERVICES: A series of expert- and evidence-based recommendations from the American Medical Association (AMA) regarding the delivery of health services, promotion of well-being, screening for common conditions, and provision of immunizations for adolescents and young adults between the ages of 11 and 21 that is the framework for most adolescent preventive services guidelines.

HPV VACCINE: Immunizations against two, four, or nine high-risk strains of HPV are available. All three are recommended for adolescent girls and young women, ages 9 to 26. The four- and nine-strain HPV vaccines are recommended for males aged 9 to 26 to prevent anal cancer and genital warts. All three vaccines are a series of three injections over 6 months have been shown to be efficacious at reducing the incidence of genital warts and cervical cancer associated with the particular strains of HPV that are included in the vaccine.

CLINICAL APPROACH

Adolescence is a time of physical, emotional, and psychosocial changes. It is also a time of experimentation and, frequently, risk taking. Fortunately, adolescence is also a time of relatively good health for most. However, the choices made during adolescence can affect both the short- and long-term health of the patient. Addressing the unique health-care needs of adolescents can be difficult, as they may be more likely to present to the physician for acute illness than for health maintenance. For this reason, physicians should take the opportunity to consider age-appropriate health maintenance at each encounter with an adolescent and young adult.

Numerous issues can serve as barriers to providing effective care to adolescent patients; one of these is confidentiality. Many adolescents believe that physicians share any information provided with the parent. Consequently, they may not volunteer information, such as sexual activity or use of tobacco, alcohol, and drugs. One commonly used technique to address this is to take a history with the parent in the room, to allow the parent to present any concerns, then interview the patient alone, to allow the patient to speak confidentially with the doctor. **Physicians who** treat adolescent patients should have policies in place to ensure doctor-patient confidentiality while balancing the parent's right to be involved with the child's care. These policies should be discussed with and agreed to by the patient and parent in advance, so as to promote an honest, trusting, and therapeutic relationship.

The AMA has published in 1994 *GAPS* a series of recommendations regarding the delivery of health services, promotion of well-being, screening for common conditions, and provision of immunizations for adolescents and young adults between the ages of 11 and 21. These services are intended to be delivered as part of a series of annual health-care visits that address biomedical and psychosocial aspects of health and emphasize preventive services. Annual visits include counseling of parents and guardians on adolescent health needs and risks in setting of rapid changes and increasing independence. These visits should include at least three complete physical examinations, one in early adolescence (age 11-14), one in middle adolescence (age 15-17), and one in late adolescence (age 18-21).

Other commonly cited guidelines for preventive services in adolescents include the United States Preventive Services Taskforce (USPSTF), American Academy of Pediatrics (AAP), Bright Futures, and the Advisory Committee on Immunization Practices (ACIP). There is good agreement among these guidelines on the following points:

- Following the ACIP guidelines on immunizations in adolescents

- Screening and counseling on prevention of injuries from accidents and violence

- Screening and counseling on prevention of cardiovascular disease (tobacco, obesity, hypertension, and cholesterol)

- Screening and counseling to reduce behavioral risk factors (drugs, alcohol, unsafe sexual practices)

- Promotion of oral and dental health

The **GAPS recommends counseling for both parents and adolescents.** It recommends that physicians provide guidance to parents on normal physical, sexual, and emotional development, signs of physical and emotional problems, parenting behaviors to promote health, and methods to help their child avoid harmful behaviors. Adolescent patients should receive counseling annually on their growth and development, injury prevention, healthy diet, exercise, and avoidance of harmful substances (alcohol, tobacco, drugs, anabolic steroids). Guidance should also emphasize responsible sexual behaviors, including abstinence and contraception, to reduce the risks of sexually transmitted diseases (STDs) and pregnancy.

GAPS recommends the routine screening for several medical, behavioral, and emotional conditions. All adolescents should be screened annually for hypertension, with further evaluation and treatment for those whose blood pressure is above the 90th percentile for their gender and age. All should be screened annually for eating disorders and obesity. All should also be screened for the use of tobacco (both cigarettes and smokeless tobacco), alcohol, and other substances of abuse. Routine drug toxicology screening, however, is not recommended. Lipid screening is recommended for those at above-average risk based on a personal history of comorbid conditions or a family history of hyperlipidemia, coronary artery disease, or other vascular diseases. Tuberculosis (TB) testing should be performed in those at high risk. These risks include having lived (or living) in a homeless shelter or in an area with a high prevalence of TB, having been (or being) incarcerated, having been exposed to active TB, and working in a health-care setting.

All adolescents should be asked about sexual behaviors, including sexual orientation, use of contraception, number of sexual partners, and history of pregnancy or STDs. **Sexually active, symptomatic, and high-risk females should be screened for gonorrhea and *Chlamydia* by urine nucleic acid amplification.** Cervical cancer screening should also be performed at 21 years, regardless of sexual activity. The 2012 ACOG screening guidelines state that screening for cervical cancer with Pap smears should begin at age 21. **Symptomatic and high-risk sexually active males can be screened for presumptive gonorrhea and *Chlamydia* infections by urine nucleic acid amplification.** The Centers for Disease Control and Prevention (CDC) recommends that all adolescents be screened for HIV. The USPSTF recommends HIV confidential screening in adolescent males and females with high-risk behaviors.

Other recommendations include screening all adolescents annually for depression and risk of suicide, with appropriate management or referral of those in need. All should also be questioned annually about emotional, physical, or sexual abuse. Every state mandates the reporting of suspected abuse of minors to the designated child welfare agency or child protective service. Difficulties at school or with learning should also be evaluated annually, with subsequent management to be coordinated with the school and parent/guardian.

The adolescent health visit is also a time to ensure that the patient is appropriately immunized against preventable infections. In those who have received the recommended primary series, a tetanus-diphtheria (Td) booster is recommended at ages 11 to 12 and then, every 10 years thereafter. Because of the continued risk for infection with pertussis, a Tdap is recommended in place of one Td booster for adolescents and adults. Varicella vaccine should be offered to those who have not been vaccinated and who do not have a history of chickenpox. A measles-mumps-rubella (MMR) booster should be given if the patient did not receive a booster at ages 4 to 6. The hepatitis B series should be given to any adolescent who has not been previously immunized. Hepatitis A vaccine can be offered to those who live in areas with high infection rates, travel to high-risk areas, have chronic liver disease, or inject IV drugs, and to males who have sex with males. Routine meningococcal vaccination using a conjugate vaccine (MCV) is recommended at ages 11 to 12. If not previously vaccinated, vaccination before high school is advised. At age 16, patients should receive a meningococcal booster or before going into college dorms or the military barracks if only one dose given before age 16. Vaccination is also recommended for travelers to endemic areas, or the functionally/anatomically asplenic.

Three vaccines (Gardasil, Gardasil 9, and Cervarix) against high-risk strains of HPV are available. All three are recommended for adolescent girls and young women. Gardasil and Gardasil 9 are indicated for males aged 9 to 26 years. These vaccines are a series of three injections over 6 months that have been shown to be efficacious at reducing the incidence of cervical cancer associated with the particular strains of HPV that are included in the vaccine. The Gardasil vaccines have also been shown to effectively reduce the incidence of genital warts. It is preferred to provide HPV vaccination prior to the onset of sexual activity, so the series can be started in children as young as 9 years old, but it is routinely recommended for the ages of 11 to 12. It is also recommended for females and males aged 13 to 26 who have not completed the vaccine series. The HPV vaccine is also useful for those who have started sexual activity, as it may protect against strains of HPV to which the patient has not been exposed.

SPORTS PREPARTICIPATION EXAMINATION

A common reason for healthy adolescents to present to primary care physicians is for a preparticipation examination as a requirement to play a sport in school. The goal of these examinations is to attempt to identify conditions that may place a young athlete at risk during athletic participation. These conditions are primarily cardiac and orthopedic, but are not limited to these systems. **A preparticipation examination allows the physician to provide the comprehensive health maintenance, including counseling, anticipatory guidance, screening, and vaccination, recommended in the GAPS.** These encounters also serve to meet legal and insurance requirements of the school or school system.

The rate of sudden cardiac death in athletes is very low. Congenital cardiac anomalies are the most common etiology, with hypertrophic cardiomyopathy accounting for about one-third and anomalous coronary arteries for about one-fifth of cardiac anomalies. The **history is the most important tool in screening for these abnormalities.** All adolescents and their parents should be asked about personal history of exertional chest pain, dyspnea, syncope, history of heart murmurs, and family history of hypertrophic cardiomyopathy, other congenital cardiac abnormalities, or premature cardiac deaths. Other important historical information includes history of asthma or other pulmonary disorders, orthopedic injuries, heat-related illness, and absence of one of a paired organ (eg, single kidney, testicle, ovary, etc).

It is important to screen for eating disorders, as well as for a desire to change body weight, either for body image or for athletic purposes (eg, "weight cutting" for wrestlers). Eating disorders are more common in female than male athletes. Female patients should be questioned about menstrual irregularities, as amenorrhea could signal anorexia and amenorrheic female athletes could be at risk for osteoporosis.

The examination should be thorough, but several aspects should be emphasized. Blood pressure should be measured and compared with age-and gender-appropriate norms. General appearance, specifically looking for signs of Marfan syndrome, should be noted. These signs, which include arachnodactyly, an arm span greater than height, pectus excavatum, tall-thin habitus, high-arched palate, and ocular lens subluxations, should prompt further evaluation, as persons with Marfan can have aortic abnormalities that predispose to rupture during sports. Auscultation of the heart should be performed, at minimum, in both the laying and standing positions. **The murmur of hypertrophic cardiomyopathy, while not always present, is best heard along the left sternal border and accentuates with activities that decrease cardiac preload and end-diastolic volume of the left ventricle.** Therefore, standing or straining with a Valsalva maneuver would increase the murmur; conversely, squatting would be expected to decrease the murmur. **Any adolescent with stigmata of Marfan syndrome, a murmur suggestive of hypertrophic cardiomyopathy, with a grade 3/6 or louder systolic murmur, or any diastolic murmur should be evaluated by a cardiologist prior to clearance for athletic participation.**

No specific tests are recommended for universal screening of all athletes, although specific tests may be indicated based on history or physical examination findings. Echocardiography is the study of choice for the diagnosis of hypertrophic cardiomyopathy.

Participation in athletics or exercise should be encouraged. **Absolute contraindications to all athletic participation are rare;** more commonly, clearance to participate may be delayed for further evaluation of a suspected condition, rehabilitation of an injury, or recovery from an acute illness. In almost all cases, an adolescent should be able to find some athletic pursuit in which he/she may participate.

CASE CORRELATION

- See also Cases 1 (Health Maintenance, Adult Male), 11 (Health Maintenance, Adult Female), and 18 (Health Maintenance, Geriatric).

COMPREHENSION QUESTIONS

29.1 A high school student is being seen for a sports preparticipation examination. Which of the following should prompt a referral to a cardiologist prior to clearance to participate in high school sports?

    A. Grade 2/6 systolic murmur in an asymptomatic 16-year-old adolescent girl

    B. Grade 1/6 diastolic murmur heard at the apex in a 17-year-old adolescent girl

    C. Grade 2/6 systolic murmur in a 17-year-old adolescent boy that is heard while lying down and that gets softer when standing

    D. An asymptomatic 16-year-old whose grandfather died of a heart attack at age 72

29.2 A 15-year-old adolescent girl is brought in by her mother for a wellness clearance for sports participation at school. She would also like to discuss the addition of birth control. When the mother leaves the room, you learn that the girl is not sexually active but wants to start oral contraceptive pills (OCPs) because she has heard they help with acne and her friends have seen improvement. She does not drink alcohol or smoke and is in honors classes in the ninth grade. She plays on the junior varsity softball team and eats most days in the school cafeteria. Which of the following is recommended routinely in the GAPS and should be performed at this time?

A. Annual complete physical examinations between the ages of 11 and 21

B. Periodic screening for drug use with a urine drug toxicology test

C. Cholesterol testing

D. Annual screening for hypertension

29.3 A 17-year-old adolescent boy reports that he has been sexually active with two female partners in the past year. He has used condoms "sometimes, but not always." He is asymptomatic and has a normal physical examination. Which of the following tests would be recommended to screen him for gonorrhea and *Chlamydia*?

A. Urethral swab.

B. Serum antibodies to *Neisseria gonorrhoeae* and *Chlamydia trachomatis*.

C. Urine for nucleic acid amplification.

D. No screening is recommended.

ANSWERS

29.1 **B.** Any patient with a diastolic murmur, grade 3/6 or louder systolic murmur, murmur suggestive of hypertrophic cardiomyopathy, or signs of Marfan syndrome should be evaluated by a cardiologist prior to clearance to participate in athletics. The murmur of hypertrophic cardiomyopathy typically gets louder with maneuvers that reduce preload, such as the Valsalva maneuver or when standing.

29.2 **D.** GAPS recommends annual screening for hypertension by blood pressure measurement in all adolescents. Complete physical examinations are advised routinely, once during early adolescence, once in mid adolescence, and once in late adolescence, as well as more often when indicated. Lipid screening should be targeted to those who are at high risk based on personal or family history. Routine toxicology screening is not recommended.

29.3 **C.** Urine for nucleic acid amplification is recommended as screening for presumptive gonorrhea or *Chlamydia* in sexually active males. A urethral swab is only appropriate for diagnostic testing in a male who has a urethral discharge.

CLINICAL PEARLS

▶ Adolescents tend to see physicians irregularly. Take the time at each visit, no matter what the reason for the visit, to review health maintenance issues.

▶ Unvaccinated adolescents and teens should be offered vaccination opportunistically and routinely.

▶ True contraindications to participation in all sports are rare. Almost everyone should be able to participate in some form of athletic activity.

REFERENCES

American Medical Association. *Guidelines for Adolescent Preventive Services (GAPS): Recommendations Monograph.* Chicago, IL: American Medical Association; 1997.

Broder KR, Cortese MM, Iskander JK. Advisory Committee on Immunizations Practices (ACIP). Preventing tetanus, diphtheria and pertussis among adolescents: use of tetanus toxoid, reduced diphtheria toxoid and acellular pertussis vaccines. *MMWR Morb Mortal Wkly Rep.* 2006 March 24;55:1-34.

Centers for Disease Control and Prevention (CDC). FDA licensure of quadrivalent human papillomavirus vaccine (HPV4, Gardasil) for use in males and guidance from the Advisory Committee on Immunization Practices (ACIP). *MMWR Morb Mortal Wkly Rep.* 2010;59(20):630-632.

Centers for Disease Control and Prevention (CDC). Prevention and control of meningococcal disease: recommendations of the Advisory Committee on Immunization Practices (ACIP). *MMWR Morb Mortal Wkly Rep.* 2013;62(RR-02):1-22.

Giese EA, O'Connor FG, Brennan FH, Depenbrock PJ, Oriscello RG. The athletic preparticipation evaluation: cardiovascular assessment. *Am Fam Physician.* 2007;75(7):1008-1014.

Ham P, Allen C. Adolescent health screening and counseling. *Am Fam Physician.* 2012 Dec 15;86(12):1109-1116.

Marrazzo JM, Holmes KK. Sexually transmitted infections: overview and clinical approach. In: Kasper D, Fauci A, Hauser S, et al., eds. *Harrison's Principles of Internal Medicine.* 19th ed. New York, NY: McGraw-Hill; 2015. Available at: http://accessmedicine.mhmedical.com. Accessed May 25, 2015.

Womack J. Give your sports physicals a performance boost. *J Fam Pract.* 2010;59(8):437-444.

A 47-year-old African-American man presents to your office for a follow-up visit. He was seen 3 weeks ago for an upper respiratory infection and noted incidentally to have a blood pressure of 164/98 mm Hg. He vaguely remembered being told in the past that his blood pressure was "borderline." He feels fine, has no complaints, and his review of systems is entirely negative. He does not smoke cigarettes, drinks "a couple of beers on the weekends," and does not exercise regularly. He has a sedentary job. His father died of a stroke at the age of 69. His mother is alive and in good health at the age of 72. He has two siblings and is not aware of any chronic medical issues that they have. In the office today, his blood pressure is 156/96 mm Hg in his left arm and 152/98 mm Hg in the right arm. He is afebrile, his pulse is 78 beats/min, respiratory rate 14 breaths/min, he is 70-in tall, and weighs 210 lb. A general physical examination is normal.

▶ What diagnosis (or diagnoses) can you make today?
▶ What further evaluation needs to be performed?
▶ What nonpharmacologic intervention(s) may be beneficial?
▶ What is the recommended initial medication management?

ANSWERS TO CASE 30:

Hypertension

Summary: A 47-year-old man is found to have an elevated blood pressure reading when seen for an unrelated problem visit. On follow-up, his blood pressure remains elevated. He is obese and leads a sedentary lifestyle, but does not have other high risks based on his personal or family history.

- **Diagnoses:** Hypertension and obesity

- **Necessary further evaluation:** Blood glucose; serum potassium, fasting cholesterol panel, estimated glomerular filtration rate (GFR), creatinine, and calcium levels; hematocrit; urinalysis; electrocardiogram (ECG)

- **Nonpharmacologic interventions:** Dietary Approaches to Stop Hypertension (DASH) diet; alcohol limitation to no more than two drinks per day; increased physical activity; weight reduction

- **Recommended initial medication:** Thiazide diuretic or calcium channel blocker

ANALYSIS

Objectives

1. Know the diagnostic criteria for hypertension.

2. Learn the recommended initial evaluation of persons found with an elevated blood pressure.

3. Know the medication and lifestyle modifications that can help to control blood pressure.

4. Learn the complications and risks of uncontrolled hypertension.

Considerations

The patient presented here is typical of one seen every day in primary care offices and represents the most common presentation of hypertension. Most hypertensive patients do not have any symptoms of their disease. They are typically seen for another reason and noted to have a high blood pressure reading. Untreated hypertension significantly raises an individual's risk of myocardial infarction, cerebrovascular accidents, and renal failure, among other conditions. **The risk of cardiovascular disease doubles with each increase in blood pressure of 20/10 mm Hg above 115/75 mm Hg.** Because of the high prevalence of the problem, the lack of symptoms, and the demonstrated efficacy of treatment in reducing the risk of complications, the United States Preventive Services Task Force (USPSTF) recommends screening every adult patient for hypertension by measuring their blood pressure. The appropriate screening interval is not clearly defined, but most practitioners will check the blood pressure of every adult patient at every office visit.

APPROACH TO:
Hypertension

DEFINITIONS

JNC 8: The eighth report of the Joint National Committee on Prevention, Detection, Evaluation and Treatment of High Blood Pressure. A comprehensive, evidence-based review of the diagnosis, evaluation, and management of hypertension published in 2013.

CLINICAL APPROACH

Hypertension is the most common primary diagnosis at physician office visits in the United States each year. **Approximately 50 million Americans have hypertension and approximately 30% are unaware of their problem.** The prevalence is higher in African Americans and in older patients. National Health and Nutritional Examination Surveys (NHANES) data suggest that hypertension is responsible for approximately one-third of heart attacks, one-half of heart failure, and one-fourth of premature deaths. Most patients with end-stage kidney disease are hypertensive. Hypertensive nephrosclerosis is responsible for approximately one-fourth of end-stage kidney disease. **The risk of complications is directly related to the elevation of the blood pressure—the higher the blood pressure, the higher the risk.**

Elevated systolic blood pressure is a greater risk for cardiovascular disease complications than elevated diastolic pressure. Control of systolic blood pressure tends to be more difficult to achieve, and when it is achieved, the diastolic blood pressure usually comes under control as well. The goal of treatment is to get the blood pressure to less than 140/90 in adults up to age 59 and 150/90 mm Hg in patients over age 60. For persons with diabetes or kidney disease, the goal is to achieve a blood pressure of less than 140/90 mm Hg.

Diagnosis and Workup

The diagnosis of hypertension relies on accurate measurement of blood pressure. The appropriate technique is to allow the patient to sit quietly in a chair (not on the examination table) with a supported back and feet on the floor for 5 minutes prior to making the measurement. The blood pressure should be measured at least twice, using a calibrated sphygmomanometer and an appropriately sized cuff for the patient. The blood pressure cuff should encircle at least 80% of the patient's arm; a cuff that is too small can result in a falsely elevated reading.

The diagnosis of hypertension is made based on the average of two properly taken blood pressure measurements at two or more office visits. The JNC 8 did away with the classification of prehypertension, stages 1 and 2 hypertension in order to focus in on when pharmacologic therapy should be started.

When hypertension is diagnosed, an evaluation consisting of a history, physical examination, and focused diagnostic studies should be performed, with the goals of assessing overall cardiovascular risks, identification of possibly secondary causes of hypertension, and determination of the presence of any end-organ damage.

Secondary causes that should be considered include coarctation of the aorta, renovascular and renal disease, Cushing disease, hyperthyroidism, hyperparathyroidism, hyperaldosteronism, pheochromocytoma, and obstructive sleep apnea. Historical information should include personal and family medical histories, an assessment of diet and activity levels, and specific questioning regarding tobacco, alcohol, recreational drug, and medication (both prescription and nonprescription) use. Patients should be questioned about cardiovascular, cerebrovascular, and peripheral arterial disease symptoms.

Along with blood pressure in both arms, examination should include all other vital signs and a measurement of body mass index. Other specific components of the examination should include a funduscopic examination for signs of retinopathy, oropharynx, and neck for signs of obstructive sleep apnea, palpation of the thyroid, auscultation for carotid, femoral, and renal bruits, palpation of peripheral pulses, abdominal palpation for signs of organomegaly or aortic aneurysm, and a complete cardiopulmonary examination.

Initial testing should include measurement of serum potassium, creatinine (with glomerular filtration rate calculation), and calcium, blood glucose, fasting lipids, and hematocrit. A urinalysis should be done to look for proteinuria or cellular components suggestive of renal disease. An ECG should be performed to evaluate for changes consistent with coronary artery disease and to screen for left ventricular hypertrophy (LVH).

Nonpharmacologic Management

Once the diagnosis of hypertension is made, patients should be advised of specific lifestyle modifications that can both reduce their blood pressure and reduce their overall cardiac risk factors. These should include efforts to lose weight if overweight or obese, increase physical activity, and reduce consumption of alcohol. Men should consume no more than two alcoholic beverages a day and women no more than one. Any smoker should be counseled to quit.

A high-potassium and high-calcium diet, the DASH diet plan, reduces blood pressure in an amount comparable to single-agent drug therapy. An informational brochure detailing the DASH diet is available from the National Heart, Lung, and Blood Institute. Combining the various lifestyle modifications provides additive benefits, and these efforts should continue even when the decision is made to start medications.

Pharmacologic Management

Lowering blood pressure reduces the risk of adverse outcomes such as strokes and heart attacks. In the primary treatment of hypertension in African-American patients, thiazide diuretics or calcium channel blockers are the recommended first-line therapy. In non–African-American patients, according to the JNC 8, the first-line pharmacologic treatment can be diuretics, calcium channel blocker, angiotensin-converting enzyme (ACE) inhibitor, or angiotensin receptor blocker (ARB) with a goal of less than 140/90 in those under 60 years and less than 150/90 if 60 years or older. Patients with hypertension who are inadequately controlled with nonpharmacologic interventions alone should be started the agents described earlier unless there

Table 30–1 • JNC 8 RECOMMENDATIONS FOR STARTING SPECIFIC CLASSES OF ANTIHYPERTENSIVE MEDICATION

Indication	Class of Medication
African-American patients	Calcium channel blocker Thiazide diuretic
Nonblack patients younger than 60 years	Angiotensin-converting enzyme inhibitor Angiotensin receptor blocker Thiazide diuretics Calcium channel blockers
Nonblack patients 60 years or older	Calcium channel blocker Thiazide diuretic Angiotensin-converting enzyme inhibitor Angiotensin receptor blocker
Patients with chronic kidney disease	Angiotensin-converting enzyme inhibitor Angiotensin receptor blocker initial or add on for goal of <140/90
History coronary artery disease	β-Blocker (especially if reduced systolic function) Angiotensin-converting enzyme inhibitor Angiotensin receptor blocker
Diabetes mellitus without kidney disease	Nonblack: Angiotensin-converting enzyme inhibitor Angiotensin receptor blocker Thiazide diuretic Calcium channel blocker patients Black: Thiazide diuretics Calcium channel blockers
Patients with heart failure	Angiotensin-converting enzyme inhibitor Angiotensin receptor blocker β-Blocker Spironolactone (Aldactone)
Prevention of recurrent cerebrovascular accident	Angiotensin-converting enzyme inhibitor Angiotensin receptor blocker Calcium channel blockers Thiazide diuretics

is a compelling reason to start another class of medication (Table 30–1). The goal of therapy is to attain and maintain goal blood pressure. If goal blood pressure is not reached with one agent after 1 month, then the physician can either increase the dose of the initial agent or add a second drug.

CASE CORRELATION

- See Case 20 (Chest Pain).

COMPREHENSION QUESTIONS

30.1 A 62-year-old woman presents for a routine physical examination. She is asymptomatic and is not taking any medications. Her blood pressure is found to be 145/85 mm Hg on two readings and her body mass index (BMI) is 29. Review of her chart reveals that her blood pressure was 143/84 mm Hg on a visit 4 months ago for a urinary tract infection. Which of the following is the most accurate statement regarding her blood pressure?

A. Her blood pressure is normal and she is at average risk for developing hypertension.

B. She is at risk for needing pharmacologic treatment for hypertension.

C. She has hypertension and should be started on a thiazide diuretic.

D. She has hypertension and should be started on multidrug therapy.

30.2 A 66-year-old Caucasian woman has an average blood pressure of 155/70 mm Hg despite appropriate lifestyle modification efforts. Her only other medical problems are osteopenia, kidney stones, and mild depression. Her last lipid panel revealed a total cholesterol of 160 mg/dL, high-density lipoprotein (HDL) 40 mg/dL, and low-density lipoprotein (LDL) 90 mg/dL. Which of the following would be the most appropriate treatment at this time?

A. Lisinopril (Prinivil, Zestril)

B. Propranolol (Inderal)

C. Amlodipine (Norvasc)

D. Chlorthalidone

E. Losartan (Cozaar)

30.3 A 48-year-old type 2 Caucasian diabetic man has had persistent blood pressure readings of 150/95 mm Hg for the past 6 months. Current medications include glyburide and metformin. His last HbA_{1c} was 7.9% and the patient has a BMI of 24. On physical examination, position sense is intact but a peripheral neuropathy is detected in a stocking and glove pattern. Vibratory sensation is decreased bilaterally on both lower extremities. Eye examination shows mild papilledema but no cotton wool spots. When questioned, he says that he still occasionally sneaks a cookie after dinner and drinks alcohol nightly. Which of the following is the most appropriate treatment for him?

A. DASH diet and recheck blood pressure in 3 months

B. Thiazide diuretic alone

C. Angiotensin-converting enzyme inhibitor alone

D. Combination of angiotensin-converting enzyme inhibitor and thiazide diuretic

30.4 At a routine checkup, a 6-year-old boy is found to have a blood pressure of 150/90 mm Hg. Repeated blood pressure readings are consistently elevated. The child was delivered at 36 weeks by normal spontaneous vaginal delivery with no complications. All major milestones were met on time and he currently is enrolled in first grade. The child has been healthy up until this point. Which of the following is the most appropriate diagnosis and therapeutic step?

A. The child has essential hypertension and should be started on the DASH diet.

B. The child most likely has hyperthyroidism and should be started on a β-blocker while thyroid studies are performed.

C. The child most likely has renal parenchymal disease and should have a urinalysis and renal ultrasound ordered.

D. The child most likely has "white coat" hypertension and the readings should be ignored if there is no family history of hypertension.

E. The child most likely has a pheochromocytoma and should start a 24-hour urine collection for metanephrines.

ANSWERS

30.1 **B.** This patient's blood pressure falls within the definition of hypertension but outside the need for immediate pharmacologic intervention. She would benefit from the institution of lifestyle modifications to try to reduce her risk of progression.

30.2 **D.** In the JNC 8 guidelines, calcium channel blockers, thiazides, ARBs, and ACE inhibitors are first line in nonblack patients over age 60. In this case, β-blockers may worsen the depression. Thiazide diuretics may improve osteoporosis, and reduce hypercalciuria which can reduce nephrolithiasis.

30.3 **C.** This patient's blood pressure goal is less than 140/90 mm Hg. He is above this goal, so an ACE inhibitor or ARB is first-line therapy regardless of BMI or HbA_{1c}. The dose of the medication can be maximized if blood pressure is not controlled after 1 month, or another agent can be added.

30.4 **C.** Essential hypertension is rarely found in children less than 10 years of age and should be a diagnosis of exclusion. The most common cause of hypertension is renal parenchymal disease, and a urinalysis, urine culture, and renal ultrasonography should be ordered for all children presenting with hypertension.

CLINICAL PEARLS

▶ Check every adult patient's blood pressure at every office visit.

▶ Thiazide diuretics or calcium channel blockers should be the first-line drug treatment in African-American patients with hypertension.

▶ Diuretics, calcium channel blockers, ACE inhibitors, or ARBs are the first line for non–African-American patients less than age 60. Choice of first-line medication can be tailored to mitigate other comorbidities.

▶ All patients with chronic kidney disease should have ACE inhibitors or ARBS as first line or add-on treatment.

▶ All patients with hypertension are at risk for cardiovascular and cerebro-vascular disease. Be sure to address their other significant risks for these diseases, including lipids, smoking, diabetes, and obesity.

REFERENCES

James PA, Oparil S, Carter BL, et al. Evidence-based guideline for the management of high blood pressure in adults: report from the panel members appointed to the Eighth Joint National Committee (JNC 8). *JAMA.* 2014;311(5):507-520.

Kotchen TA. Hypertensive vascular disease. In: Kasper D, Fauci A, Hauser S, et al., eds. *Harrison's Principles of Internal Medicine.* 19th ed. New York, NY: McGraw-Hill; 2015. Available at: http://accessmedicine.mhmedical.com. Accessed May 25, 2015

Langan, R, Jones, K. Common questions about the initial management of hypertension. *Am Fam Physician.* 2015;91(3):172-177.

Riley M, Bluhm B. High blood pressure in children and adolescents. *Am Fam Physician.* 2012;85(7):693-700.

The mother of a 12-month-old male infant calls you at midnight stating that her son has been crying incessantly for the last 6 hours. His bouts of crying last for about 20 minutes, then completely disappear for 15 minutes at a time. Since early afternoon, the child has not been eating much and he has started to vomit the small amounts of juice and milk he had ingested. She decided to call you because the vomitus is now green and the bouts of crying seem to be getting worse.

In the emergency room (ER), you recall that the patient does not have any past medical history, was born at term without complications, and is up-to-date on immunizations. On examination, his temperature is 100°F (37.7°C), his respiration rate is 40 breaths/min, his pulse is 155 beats/min, his blood pressure is 109/60 mm Hg, and his weight is 22 lb. He cries inconsolably for 15 minutes, drawing his legs up to his chest, and then becomes quiet. You notice he still produces tears, and his mucosae are moist. Heart and lung examinations are normal; abdominal examination reveals markedly decreased bowel sounds with generalized tenderness to palpation. You feel a sausage-like mass in the right side of the abdomen. His diaper holds some amount of bloody stool mixed with mucus. The rest of the examination is normal.

▶ What is the most likely diagnosis?
▶ What is the next diagnostic step?
▶ What are the possible complications?

ANSWERS TO CASE 31:
Abdominal Pain and Vomiting in a Child

Summary: This is a 12-month-old infant who had the sudden onset of intermittent crying with vomiting that later became bilious. As the day progressed, his bouts of pain became more severe, each lasting about 20 minutes. On examination, the infant does not yet reveal signs of hypovolemia, sepsis, or shock. On palpation of the abdomen, there is generalized tenderness and a sausage-like mass on the right side. Even though not mentioned by the parent, there is a small amount of bloody-mucous stool that is best described as "currant jelly." This patient has an intussusception that has progressed to an obstruction, and is at risk for perforation with ensuing shock and sepsis.

- **Most likely diagnosis:** Intestinal obstruction caused by intussusception

- **Next diagnostic step:** Abdominal plain x-rays to rule out perforation

- **Possible complications:** If perforation occurs, rapid deterioration as a consequence of shock/sepsis

ANALYSIS

Objectives

1. Become familiar with the most likely causes of intestinal obstruction in the pediatric population.

2. Learn to differentiate between life-threatening abdominal emergencies and urgent conditions.

3. Have a diagnostic approach to the pediatric patient presenting with abdominal pain and vomiting.

Considerations

This 12-month-old infant initially presented with vomiting and intermittent abdominal pain. His vomitus was initially the gastric contents of what he had ingested, but later became bilious, which is suggestive of intestinal obstruction. The description of his abdominal pain tends to reveal the pathophysiologic nature of intussusception. The intermittency and "pain-free" intervals correlate with the gradual and slow telescoping of the intussusceptum (proximal or leading part of the intestine) into the intussuscipiens (distal or receiving end of the intestine). As the "telescoping" progresses, the portions of bowel that are trapped within the lumen of the intestine become edematous, which will ultimately lead to obstruction, ischemia, and perforation of the bowel wall. The sausage-shaped mass felt on examination will not be present in all cases. It represents the portions of bowel that are involved and have become edematous. "Currant jelly" stools are basically a mixture of blood and mucus that has sloughed from the affected bowel wall. This is not present in all cases.

Malrotation with volvulus will also present with a clinical picture of obstruction, and it may be difficult to differentiate among the two solely on clinical findings. Another common condition that may reveal a palpable mass is that of pyloric stenosis, with an olive-shaped mass sometimes palpable in the right upper quadrant. However, pyloric stenosis presents in younger patients and does not involve bouts of severe pain. It is most common in firstborn male children and presents with projectile vomiting.

Before proceeding to diagnostics, the patient should be stabilized with IV fluid hydration and surgery consultation should not be delayed. A nasogastric tube may need to be placed if obstruction is suspected. A plain film of the abdomen is done to rule out perforation. If perforation has occurred, surgical intervention is required. If no perforation is evidenced, an ultrasound of the abdomen may reveal a "coiled spring" lesion, which reflects layers of intestine within the lumen of a different portion of intestine. However, a barium enema will be both diagnostic and therapeutic in the case of intussusception. Although barium is widely used, a water-soluble contrast is preferred if perforation is suspected, because it will not be as irritating to the peritoneum. The therapeutic value of the enema is a result of the constant application of hydrostatic pressure on the intussusceptum, mechanically forcing it to telescope back. Air reduction may also be achieved. This method requires fluoroscopic visualization of bowel-gas patterns until reduction of the intussusceptum is seen. Barium or air reduction is effective in 75% to 90% of cases, after which a 12- to 24-hour observation period is needed until bowel function is adequate and a bowel movement has been produced. The risk of recurrence in this patient with idiopathic intussusception is approximately 10%.

APPROACH TO:
Pediatric Abdominal Pain with Vomiting

DEFINITIONS

INTUSSUCEPTION: A telescoping of the intestine within itself leading to abdominal pain, fever, vomiting, and ultimately bowel necrosis if not resolved

HYPERTROPHIC PYLORIC STENOSIS: Condition of hypertrophy of the pylorus leading to gastric outlet obstruction, commonly manifesting in infants at about 1 month

MALROTATION WITH VOLVULUS: Condition where the small bowel twists around the superior mesenteric artery resulting in vascular compromise to large portions of the midgut, commonly before 1 month

CLINICAL APPROACH

The most important aspect of a diagnostic approach in these cases is to be able to rapidly determine whether or not the condition is an emergency. Although the case presented is that of the most common abdominal emergency among the pediatric population, it is by no means the most common cause of intestinal obstruction.

Among the diagnoses that have to be entertained are hypertrophic pyloric stenosis, malrotation with volvulus/obstruction, foreign-body ingestion, and poisoning.

Etiologies

As described, intussusception will present with intermittent, severe abdominal pain, associated with vomiting that becomes bilious as obstruction sets in. The finding of an elongated mass along the right abdomen is very suggestive of this diagnosis. The location of the mass is because most idiopathic intussusceptions occur at the ileocecal junction. They may be entirely in the jejunum, between the jejunum and ileum, or entirely colonic. "Currant jelly stool" is most often used to describe the finding in this condition and it correlates with the ongoing bowel ischemia as the intussusception and edema progress.

Hypertrophic pyloric stenosis is the most common cause of gastrointestinal (GI) obstruction in infants. It occurs in approximately 3 in 1000 live births, with a male-to-female ratio of 4:1. The usual presenting age is 3 to 6 weeks, and is often described as a "hungry baby" with projectile vomiting. Vomiting is nonbilious and occurs immediately after meals. The infant will demand to be refed immediately. On examination, there may be an olive-shaped mass felt in the right upper quadrant, and peristaltic waves may be seen across the upper abdomen moments before emesis occurs. Ultrasonography shows the thickened pyloric muscles that are causing a gastric outlet obstruction. An upper GI contrast study usually reveals an elongated pyloric canal and a "double-track sign," which is explained by two thin tracts of barium that are created by compressed pyloric mucosa. Once the diagnosis is made, surgical referral is indicated as it is the definitive management. Because of the early age and dramatic nature of the symptoms, parents will usually seek help before the infant becomes severely ill from not eating.

Malrotation occurs in about 1 in 500 live births, but becomes symptomatic in only 1 in 6000 live births. Approximately 60% of patients will be younger than 1 month, with approximately 10% presenting after 1 year, even into adulthood. Because it is primarily a defect that occurs during embryogenesis, the mesentery that is formed will have an abnormally narrow base, which allows the small bowel to move more freely than normal. This creates a problem when the intestinal attachment to the mesentery twists around itself, creating a volvulus. Once obstruction occurs, the child will present with bilious vomiting and abdominal pain. If diagnosis is delayed, the involved segments of bowel will eventually become necrotic, leading to fluid losses and sepsis. The diagnostic approach in such cases will depend on the stability of the patient. If the patient is hypovolemic, hypotensive, has GI blood loss, or has signs of peritonitis, quick stabilization with surgical intervention is necessary. However, if the patient is hemodynamically stable, imaging can be performed to confirm a diagnosis. If malrotation is suspected, an upper GI series is the test of choice. In 75% of patients, the diagnosis will be clearly seen. Diagnostic findings on an upper GI are an obviously misplaced duodenum, or a duodenal obstruction with the classic "beak-like" appearance of the contrast medium caused by a volvulus. Surgery is the only treatment. Although different surgical techniques are applied to prevent a recurrence, a volvulus can repeat itself in as many as 8% of patients. Malrotation can go undiagnosed if a patient never experiences symptoms from it, and older children may present with intermittent vomiting, episodes of abdominal pain, failure to thrive, or syndromes of malabsorption.

Foreign bodies also need to be considered with abdominal pain and vomiting in a pediatric patient. **Only 10% of patients that ingest a foreign body will need an intervention** either to relieve an obstruction or to prevent GI complications. Approximately 90% of patients will pass a foreign body spontaneously, and parents need only to check the stool within 24 hours to confirm passage. Sometimes, if an object can be seen on plain radiographs, a repeat x-ray within 24 hours can be done. **Among objects that require immediate intervention are flat disk, or "button," batteries in the esophagus.** These batteries will conduct electricity when both poles are in contact with the esophageal wall, which may lead to perforation. Sharp objects and multiple magnets also need to be removed. As a general rule, any foreign body in the esophagus needs to be removed in less than 24 hours by upper endoscopy. If a sharp or elongated object (>6 cm) has already passed through the stomach and duodenum, daily x-rays should be done to follow the progress of the object. Those that do not advance within 3 days will require surgical intervention for removal.

Poisoning cannot be overlooked in the evaluation of a child with vomiting and abdominal pain. Among the multiple agents most commonly associated with hospital visits are over-the-counter (OTC) analgesic drugs, cold remedies, insecticides, pesticides, personal care products, and fumes. In a child who presents with vomiting and abdominal pain, a cholinergic syndrome is likely. It is characterized by salivation, lacrimation, diarrhea, vomiting, diaphoresis, intestinal cramps, and seizures. Insecticides and nicotine are among the agents that may induce these symptoms. Antihistamines or tricyclic antidepressants produce dry skin, dry mucosae, urinary retention, and decreased bowel sounds (anticholinergic syndrome). Some medications and substances are radiopaque, such as iron tablets, mercury, lithium, tricyclic antidepressants, Play-Doh, and enteric-coated aspirin. Finding the likely agent of poisoning will mostly depend on the history given. Poison control should be consulted for patients where etiology of ingested toxin is known.

Treatment

Surgical intervention will almost always be necessary if an anatomic/mechanical defect of the GI tract is present. Intestinal obstruction puts a patient at risk for perforation, which further deteriorates a patient's condition. A nasogastric tube is recommended in cases where obstruction has set in and the patient is ill. Careful monitoring of the patient's fluid status is required because of the likelihood of third spacing into ischemic bowel and decreased oral intake.

CASE CORRELATION

- See Case 10 (Acute Diarrhea).

COMPREHENSION QUESTIONS

Match the following etiologies (A-F) to the clinical vignette (31.1-31.6):

A. Malrotation with intermittent volvulus

B. Intussusception

C. Insecticide ingestion

D. Esophageal foreign body

E. Pyloric stenosis

F. Volvulus

31.1 A 6-year-old boy left alone for 10 hours, now with hematemesis and pneumo-mediastinum on chest x-ray.

31.2 A 3-week-old male infant with 2 days of projectile, nonbilious vomiting, and constant feeding.

31.3 A 7-year-old boy with three episodes of severe abdominal pain and vomiting in the last month, previously diagnosed with failure to thrive.

31.4 An 8-month-old female infant with bilious vomiting, constant abdominal pain for 12 hours, and upper GI study showing beak-like appearance of contrast.

31.5 An 11-month-old male infant with intermittent bouts of crying and nonbilious vomiting, with a history of Meckel diverticulum. A small, elongated mass is felt on right side of his abdomen.

31.6 A 4-year-old girl with profuse vomiting, sweating, lacrimation, and diarrhea, who seizes in the emergency room.

ANSWERS

31.1 **D.** The presence of blood in the vomitus and a pneumomediastinum point to an esophageal perforation, most likely from a foreign body in the esophagus.

31.2 **E.** The young age and presence of projectile, nonbilious vomiting after feeding are the keys to this diagnosis. The diagnosis of pyloric stenosis is much more common in males than females.

31.3 **A.** This is the presentation of a malrotation that did not cause enough symptoms at a younger age to lead to a diagnosis.

31.4 **F.** An infant with bilious vomiting and abdominal pain has a volvulus until proven otherwise. The upper GI study is diagnostic of this condition.

31.5 **B.** The intermittent nature of the symptoms and the palpable mass are highly suggestive of intussusception.

31.6 **C.** These symptoms are characteristic of a cholinergic syndrome, possibly caused by insecticide or nicotine poisoning.

CLINICAL PEARLS

▶ Most foreign body ingestions by children will pass spontaneously, but button batteries, sharp objects, and multiple magnets in the esophagus should be removed endoscopically.

▶ The risk of accidental poisoning with common household products and over-the-counter medications should be a routine part of the anticipatory guidance that occurs in a well-child visit.

▶ When a child appears critically ill, do not delay your resuscitative efforts or surgical consultation while you wait for laboratory tests and x-ray results.

REFERENCES

Egan JC, Aiken JJ, Rudolph C. Acute abdominal pain. In: Rudolph C, Rudolph A, eds. *Rudolph's Pediatrics.* New York, NY: McGraw Hill; 2011:1375-1376.

Feltis BA, Schmeling DJ. Intussusception. In: Ziegler M, Azizkhan RG, eds. *Operative Pediatric Surgery.* New York, NY: McGraw-Hill; 2014:592-596.

Hoffenberg E, Brumbaugh D, Furuta GT, et al. Gastrointestinal tract. In: Hay WW Jr., Levin MJ, Deterding RR, Abzug MJ, eds. *Current Diagnosis & Treatment: Pediatrics.* 22nd ed. New York, NY: McGraw-Hill Education; 2013. Available at: http://accessmedicine.mhmedical.com. Accessed May 25, 2015.

An 83-year-old woman is brought to the clinic by her husband who was concerned with his wife's memory problems. He first noticed some memory decline a few years ago, but the onset was subtle and did not interfere with her day-to-day activities. Mainly, she has some difficulty remembering details, is repeating things, and is being forgetful. The patient's family noticed her gradually increasing memory problems, particularly over the past year. She is unable to remember her appointments and relies heavily on written notes and appointment books. Recently, she got lost while driving and was found by her family 10 hours later. She was unable to use her cell phone and was unsure about her home address and phone number. She has also become more reclusive. She does not enjoy her church activities anymore and prefers to stay at home most of the time. She does not want to cook, and she is less attentive to her housework. The patient says that she has always been forgetful. Her medical history is significant for well-controlled hypertension and a history of mastectomy secondary to breast cancer diagnosed 20 years ago. She has no significant history of tobacco or alcohol use. She is independent with all activities of daily living, but needs assistance with medication administration, banking, and transportation. She is up-to-date with her health maintenance and immunization. Her vital signs and general physical examination are normal.

- ▶ What is the most likely diagnosis?
- ▶ What office testing can help to determine a diagnosis?
- ▶ What laboratory testing and imaging studies are indicated at this time?

ANSWERS TO CASE 32:

Dementia

Summary: An 83-year-old woman is noted by her family to have increasing memory difficulties at home. She is forgetful, repeats questions, and does not remember conversations. She had the very significant episode of getting lost in her home town. She is seemingly unaware that there is a problem that is slowly and progressively worsening.

- **Most likely diagnosis:** Dementia of Alzheimer type.

- **Office-based testing that may be beneficial:** Folstein Mini Mental Status Examination (MMSE) is the most widely used instrument. Others available include the Clock Test, the Short Portable Mental Status Questionnaire, the Mini-Cog Test, and the Montreal Cognitive Assessment (MoCa). In addition, a screening test for depression should be performed.

- **Laboratory testing and imaging studies:** Blood count, electrolytes, glucose, calcium, liver function tests, folate, vitamin B_{12}, thyroid-stimulating hormone (TSH), and erythrocyte sedimentation rate. Consider syphilis screening if there is a risk factor or evidence of prior infection, or if patient lives in an area of high incidence. Noncontrast head computed tomography (CT) scan or magnetic resonance imaging (MRI).

ANALYSIS

Objectives

1. Develop a differential diagnosis for dementia.

2. Learn how to appropriately evaluate a complaint of memory loss.

3. Learn about treatment of Alzheimer dementia, the most common specific diagnosis of dementia.

Considerations

This 83-year-old woman is noted by her family to have progressive decrease in cognitive function. She is forgetful, gets lost easily, and this has been slowly but steadily worsening. The most likely diagnosis is dementia; however, other conditions should be considered in the differential diagnosis such as medications, stroke, thyroid disorders, chronic syphilis, or other metabolic conditions. Depression can also present as dementia at times. The workup for this patient includes a careful history and physical examination, imaging of the brain, and selective laboratory tests such as TSH, vitamin B_{12} level, complete blood count (CBC), and comprehensive metabolic panel. Screening for syphilis should also be considered.

APPROACH TO:
Dementia

DEFINITIONS

EXECUTIVE FUNCTIONS: High-level cognitive abilities that control other, more basic, abilities. Executive functions include the ability to start and stop behaviors, alter behaviors to fit circumstances, and adapt behaviors to new situations.

CLINICAL APPROACH

The essential features of the diagnosis of dementia are memory loss and impairment of executive function. Dementia is a clinical diagnosis that can go unrecognized until it is in an advanced stage. Patients rarely report memory loss; the informants are usually their family members. However, relatives may fail to recognize signs and symptoms of dementia because many have a tendency to think that memory loss can be a part of normal aging. Studies of aging have shown that nonverbal creative thinking and new problem-solving strategies may decline with age, but information, skills learned with experience, and memory retention remain intact.

Clinicians should assess cognitive function whenever cognitive impairment or deterioration is suspected. These concerns may be based on direct observation, patient report, or concerns raised by family members, friends, or caretakers. Patients with dementia may have difficulty with one or more of the following:

- Learning and retaining new information (rely on lists, calendars)

- Handling complex tasks (banking, bills, payments)

- Reasoning (adapting to unexpected situations, unfamiliar environment)

- Spatial ability and orientation (getting lost driving, walking)

- Language (word finding, repetition, confabulation)

- Behavior (agitation, confusion, paranoia)

The evaluation of a patient with suspected dementia should include a mental status examination. The **Folstein MMSE** is the most widely used tool in the screening for dementia. The sensitivity of the MMSE for dementia is as high as 87% and the specificity is as high as 82%. The interpretation of the score depends on the patient's education level. It is most accurate in those with at least a high school education.

Another valuable test that can be used in a busy primary care setting is the **Clock Test**. The patient is asked to draw a clock with a specific time. The patient must then accurately draw the clock face with the "big hand" and "small hand" in the correct positions. It is quick, easy to administer, and evaluates executive function in multiple cognitive domains. Other brief cognitive screening tests, such as the Short Portable Mental Status Questionnaire, modified MMSE, MoCA, and Mini-Cog (three-item recall combined with clock drawing) can be used in the primary care setting.

Table 32–1 • CRITERIA FOR PROBABLE ALZHEIMER DISEASE

Dementia confirmed by clinical and neuropsychological examination
Problems in at least two areas of mental functioning
Progressive worsening of memory and mental functioning
No disturbances of consciousness
Symptoms beginning between ages 40 and 90, usually after age 65
No other disorder that could cause the dementia

Data from www.ninds.nih.gov.

In the evaluation of dementia, it is necessary to get information from people who know the patient well. Useful information can be obtained from informant-based functional tests, such as the functional activities questionnaire (FAQ), the instrumental activities of daily living (IADL), and caregiver burden assessments. This information can be important for physicians and families in making plans for long-term care. See Case 18 (Geriatric Health Maintenance) for more on functional assessment.

ALZHEIMER DISEASE

Alzheimer disease is the most common cause of dementia. Although a definitive diagnosis can only be made by the presence of neuritic plaques and neurofibrillary tangles detected on autopsy, clinical diagnostic criteria have been developed (Table 32–1). **Common diagnostic criteria include the gradual onset and progression of cognitive dysfunction in more than one area of mental functioning that is not caused by another disorder.**

The initial evaluation includes a detailed history, from both the patient and another informant (usually a spouse, child, or other close contact) and complete physical and neurologic examinations to evaluate for any focal neurologic deficit that may be suggestive of a focal neurologic lesion. **A validated test, such as the MMSE, should be used to confirm the presence of dementia.** The results of this test can also be used to follow the clinical course, as a reduction in score over time is consistent with worsening dementia.

A focused evaluation to rule out other causes of dementia must be performed as well. The physical examination should focus on neurologic deficits consistent with prior strokes, signs of Parkinson disease (eg, cogwheel rigidity and/or tremors), gait abnormalities or slowing, and eye movements. Patients with Alzheimer disease generally have no motor deficits at presentation.

Depression in the elderly can present with symptoms of memory disturbance. This is known as "pseudodementia." As depression is common and treatable, a screening test for depression should be performed when dementia is evaluated. Similarly, hypothyroidism and vitamin B_{12} deficiency are common and treatable conditions that can cause cognitive problems. TSH and vitamin B_{12} levels should be performed as a routine part of the workup. Neurosyphilis could present in this fashion, but is such an uncommon diagnosis that routine screening would not be recommended. Evaluation for neurosyphilis would be warranted if there were identified high-risk factors, history of the disease, or if the patient lived in an area with a high

Table 32–2 • MEDICATIONS USED IN THE TREATMENT OF ALZHEIMER DEMENTIA

Cholinesterase Inhibitors	Indications	Side Effects/Comments
Donepezil (Aricept)	Mild-moderate Alzheimer dementia	Common: nausea, vomiting, diarrhea, dizziness, headaches
Galantamine (Razadyne)	Mild-moderate Alzheimer dementia	Severe: arrhythmias, dementia bradycardia, urinary obstruction
Rivastigmine (Exelon)	Mild-moderate Alzheimer dementia	
N-methyl-D-aspartate (NMDA) antagonist Memantine (Namenda)	Moderate-severe Alzheimer dementia	Side-effect profile comparable to placebo; can be used in combination with cholinesterase inhibitors

prevalence of syphilis. Neuroimaging with either a noncontrast CT scan or an MRI of the brain is recommended to rule out other confounding diagnoses. Other testing, such as positron emission tomography (PET), genetic testing, and spinal fluid analysis are not routinely recommended. Referral to neurology is appropriate when diagnosis is uncertain.

When the diagnosis of Alzheimer disease is made, a comprehensive care plan should be initiated. **The management of Alzheimer disease must be directed both at the patient and at the patient's family or caregivers.** The goals of therapy are to maximize the cognition, delay functional decline, and prevent or improve the behavioral disturbances.

Table 32–2 lists the medications that are primarily used in the treatment of Alzheimer disease. Family members should understand that the **medications may delay the progression of the disease but may not reverse any decline that has already occurred.** For that reason, the medications may be more beneficial if started earlier in the course of the disease.

Antipsychotic medications have also been used to control hallucinations and agitation in patients with Alzheimer disease. However, this is an "off-label" use of medication and data show a higher death rate associated with the use of the newer antipsychotics. The Food and Drug Administration (FDA) has placed a black box warning against the use of typical and atypical antipsychotic medications for dementia-related psychosis due to the increased risk of deaths. Herbal medications such as Ginkgo biloba and huperzine A have inconsistent evidence for efficacy, but appear to be safe alternatives. These should not be used with prescription medications due to potential interactions.

Behavioral interventions also may be beneficial. These can include scheduled toileting in an effort to reduce episodes of incontinence, writing reminder notes, keeping familiar objects around, providing adequate lighting, and making duplicates of important objects (eg, keys) in case they get lost. Caregivers also need support and may benefit from appropriate training, support groups, and periodic respite care.

Unfortunately, even with the best of care, Alzheimer disease is relentless and progressive. Families may have significant difficulties and conflicts regarding issues surrounding end-of-life care and placement in assisted living or nursing homes. Resources such as local chapters of the Alzheimer Association (www.alz.org) may provide valuable services, information, and support.

VASCULAR DEMENTIA

Vascular dementia, or multi-infarct dementia, is the second most common cause of dementia. In vascular dementia, there is neuronal loss as a consequence of one or more strokes. The **symptoms are related to the amount and location of the neuronal loss.** Vascular dementia can exist along with Alzheimer disease or other causes of dementia, resulting in a mixed-dementia syndrome. Unlike Alzheimer disease, which is a gradually progressive process, **vascular dementia often has a sudden onset and progresses in a stepwise fashion.** Patients tend to function at a certain level and then show an acute deterioration when the initial, or subsequent, infarcts occur. The risk factors include those for cerebrovascular disease (hypertension, tobacco use, diabetes, etc). There are no controlled trials showing medication effectiveness in vascular dementia, so the treatment is aimed at reducing the risk of further neurologic damage.

LEWY BODY DEMENTIA

Lewy body dementia is the third most common form of dementia. This dementia presents early on with **vivid hallucinations, fluctuation in cognition, and often parkinsonian extrapyramidal signs and postural instability.** Tremor is less apparent and levodopa is not very effective in these patients. Daytime drowsiness and sleeping, staring into space for prolonged periods of time, and episodes of disorganized speech can further distinguish Lewy body dementia from Alzheimer disease. Therapies are similar as those for Alzheimer disease.

FRONTOTEMPORAL LOBE DEMENTIA

Frontotemporal lobe dementia is the fourth most common form of dementia and due to the behavioral disturbances associated with this, dementia can be very distressing for the patient's family. In this form of dementia, patient's personalities can significantly change, becoming antisocial or disinhibited from social norms with poor impulse control. Patients can develop apathy, emotional blunting, and perseveration behaviors including echolalia, and stereotypical behaviors such as toe tapping and repetitive motor activity. There are little pharmacologic therapies with significant evidence for efficacy. Counseling and support of the family can mitigate the stress of caring for these patients.

OTHER ILLNESSES ASSOCIATED WITH DEMENTIA

Numerous other conditions may present with dementia or have dementia as a prominent symptom. **Parkinson disease** commonly has an associated dementia, especially as the overall disease advances. **Huntington disease** is an autosomal dominant disorder that presents with progressive dementia, depression, and choreiform movements. Dementia can be a complication of **chronic alcohol abuse,** reinforcing the need for a complete history of substance use. Potentially reversible forms of dementia include **normal pressure hydrocephalus** (the triad of dementia, gait disturbance, and urinary incontinence), **chronic subdural hematoma,** and **depression.** Many **prescription and over-the-counter medications** can cause memory disturbances. Chief among these are anticholinergic medications, sedatives (benzodiazepines), sleeping pills, and narcotic pain medications. As noted previously, hypothyroidism, vitamin B_{12} deficiency, and neurosyphilis may present as dementing illnesses. **Metabolic abnormalities,** such as hyponatremia or abnormal calcium levels, and other infections, such as **AIDS,** can also cause dementia.

DELIRIUM

Delirium is an **acute change in mental status that is characterized by fluctuations in levels of consciousness.** It is usually caused by an acute medical illness, the use of a medication, or the withdrawal from a drug or alcohol. Delirium affects 10% to 30% of hospitalized patients, with a higher incidence in the elderly, in those with an underlying dementia, and in those with multiple underlying medical conditions. **The treatment of delirium is treatment of the condition that precipitated it.** Delirium is often reversible if the underlying cause can be found and aggressively managed. Patients with delirium have significantly longer hospital stays and increased mortality rates.

CASE CORRELATION

- See Case 25 (Major Depression).

COMPREHENSION QUESTIONS

32.1 A 63-year-old man is brought in by his family because of memory loss. They have noted a worsening of his symptoms over several months. They also report that he has had multiple falls, hitting his head on one occasion, and has had frequent urinary incontinence. On examination, a gait apraxia is noted. Which of the following is the most likely diagnosis?

A. Alzheimer disease

B. Normal pressure hydrocephalus

C. Dementia with Lewy bodies

D. Delirium

32.2 An 82-year-old woman is admitted to the hospital for altered mental status. Her family says that she has been confused and falling asleep frequently and that she has been hallucinating—talking to people who are not in the room. They report that prior to this illness, she was independent and "sharp as a tack." On urine analysis, she is found to have a urinary tract infection (UTI). Which of the following is the most appropriate treatment?

A. Start rivastigmine (Exelon) for worsening of Alzheimer dementia.

B. Start an alerting agent such as modafinil (Provigil) for symptomatic treatment of her hypersomnia.

C. Start an antibiotic for treatment of her infection and optimize management of any other medical conditions.

D. Give her a dose of ziprasidone (Geodon) for her hallucinations.

32.3 A 77-year-old man is brought to your office by his wife, who states that he has been having mental difficulties in recent months, such as not being able to balance their checkbook or plan for his annual visit with the accountant. She also tells you that he has reported seeing animals in the room with him that he can describe vividly. He takes frequent naps and stares blankly for long periods of time. He seems almost normal at times, but randomly appears very confused at other times. He has also been dreaming a lot and has fallen down more than once recently. He currently takes aspirin, 81 mg/d. On examination, the patient walks slowly with a stooped posture and almost falls when turning around. He has only minimal facial expressiveness. No tremor is noted and the remainder of the examination is normal. He is able to recall three words out of three, but clock drawing is abnormal. Laboratory studies are normal and a CT of the brain shows changes of aging. What type of dementia does this patient most likely have?

A. Dementia with Lewy bodies

B. Alzheimer disease

C. Frontotemporal dementia

D. Vascular dementia

E. Dementia of Parkinson disease

32.4 A 66-year-old woman is brought in by her family because of difficulty with memory and disorientation that has worsened over the past 6 months. A careful history and physical examination is performed. Which of the following tests is most appropriate in this patient?

A. Head CT or MRI

B. Lumbar puncture

C. Rapid plasma reagin (RPR)

D. Electroencephalogram (EEG)

ANSWERS

32.1 **B.** Normal pressure hydrocephalus classically causes dementia, incontinence, and gait disturbance. All of the other listed conditions may cause memory disturbance, but the constellation of these three symptoms is most consistent with normal pressure hydrocephalus.

32.2 **C.** This scenario is one that is commonly seen in elderly patients and is consistent with delirium. The patient is elderly and has an infection, causing both an acute change in her mental status and a fluctuating level of consciousness. The treatment is to treat the underlying infection and any associated medical conditions.

32.3 **A.** This patient has dementia with Lewy bodies, which is the third most common type after Alzheimer disease and vascular dementia. He demonstrates typical signs and symptoms, including well-formed hallucinations, vivid dreams, fluctuating cognition, sleep disorder with periods of daytime sleeping, frequent falls, deficits in visuospatial ability (abnormal clock drawing), and rapid eye movement (REM) sleep disorder (vivid dreams). In Alzheimer disease, the predominant early symptom is memory impairment without the other symptoms found in this patient. In dementia of Parkinson disease, extrapyramidal symptoms such as tremor, bradykinesia, and rigidity precede the onset of memory impairment by more than 1 year. Frontotemporal dementia presents with behavioral changes, including disinhibition, or language problems such as aphasia.

32.4 **A.** A noncontrast head CT or MRI is recommended by the American Academy of Neurology for the routine evaluation of dementia. All of the other tests may be appropriate if there is a finding on the history or examination that calls for further testing (an exposure to syphilis, episodes suggestive of seizures, or symptoms of normal pressure hydrocephalus for which a spinal tap may be performed).

CLINICAL PEARLS

▶ The presentation of acutely altered mental status (delirium) should prompt an aggressive workup for an underlying cause, as treatment may result in correction of the mental status.

▶ Alzheimer disease is a disease of the family, not just the individual. It is critical to treat the patient while giving support to the caregivers.

REFERENCES

Alzheimer's Association website: www.alz.org. Accessed November 7, 2015.

American Geriatric Society website: www.americangeriatrics.org. Accessed November 7, 2015.

Cardarelli R, Kertesz A, Knebl JA. Frontotemporal dementia: a review for primary care physicians. *Am Fam Physician*. 2010 Dec 1;82(11):1372-1377.

Neef D, Walling AD. Dementia with Lewy bodies: an emerging disease. *Am Fam Physician*. 2006;73(7):1223-1230.

Seeley WW, Miller BL. Dementia. In: Kasper D, Fauci A, Hauser S, et al., eds. *Harrison's Principles of Internal Medicine*. 19th ed. New York, NY: McGraw-Hill; 2015. Available at: http://accessmedicine.mhmedical.com. Accessed May 25, 2015.

Simmons BB, Hartmann B, Dejoseph D. Evaluation of suspected dementia. *Am Fam Physician*. 2011 Oct 15;84(8):895-902.

A 20-year-old woman comes to clinic for an annual physical examination. She has no complaints. She has no significant medical or surgical history. She is currently taking oral contraceptive pills because of her irregular menstrual cycles. She attained menarche at age 13 and has had irregular cycles since. She has never been sexually active. Her family history is positive for hypertension and obesity in both her parents. On examination, her blood pressure (BP) is 120/85 mm Hg, her pulse is 78 beats/min, and her respiratory rate is 14 breaths/min. Her weight is 188 lb, and she is 63-in tall. Her physical examination is unremarkable except for a brownish/black, velvety thickening of the skin on the back of her neck, hirsutism, and abdominal obesity.

▶ What are the clinical issues that need to be addressed during this preventive visit?
▶ What is your next step in the evaluation of this patient?
▶ What are the therapeutic options available for this patient?

ANSWERS TO CASE 33:
Obesity

Summary: A 20-year-old obese woman presents for a routine examination. Along with her abdominal obesity, she has irregular menstrual cycles, acanthosis nigricans, and hirsutism.

- **Clinical issues to address:** Obesity and possible polycystic ovarian disease.

- **Next steps in evaluation:** Calculate a body mass index (BMI), measure waist circumference, repeat blood pressure. Order laboratory tests to measure fasting glucose, lipids, thyroid-stimulating hormone (TSH), and liver enzymes.

- **Therapeutic options:** Assess her interest in losing weight. If she is interested, collaborate with the patient to devise weight-loss goals and advise on diet and physical activity to achieve these goals. If she is not interested, advise on the health benefits of weight loss and address other risk factors. In either case, arrange follow-up. At subsequent visits, you can consider adding pharmacotherapy as an adjunct to diet and exercise.

ANALYSIS

Objectives

1. Understand the etiology and pathogenesis of obesity.

2. Know other comorbid conditions associated with obesity.

3. Learn the diagnostic criteria for obesity and the metabolic syndrome.

4. Understand the therapeutic options available for the management of obesity.

Considerations

Obesity is a chronic and stigmatizing disease that begins early in life. Increased caloric intake, decreased physical exertion, and genetic predisposition are common causes of obesity. Routine physical examination visits serve as a good platform to address issues related to obesity and its associated comorbid conditions. This visit should be taken as an opportunity to address obesity, metabolic risk, and its management.

In this case, this patient's weight is 188 lb, and she is 63-in tall; thus, her BMI is 33.5 kg/m². Further measurements included a waist circumference of 36 in and a repeat blood pressure of 125/85 mm Hg. Her laboratory test results included total cholesterol of 202 mg/dL, high-density lipoprotein (HDL) cholesterol of 35 mg/dL, low-density lipoprotein (LDL) cholesterol of 120 mg/dL, and triglycerides of 172 mg/dL. Her fasting glucose was 104 mg/dL, and she had normal renal and liver function tests.

Increased body weight is a major risk factor for the development of disease and for premature death. The metabolic syndrome is an important risk factor for subsequent development of type 2 diabetes and cardiovascular disease (CVD). The metabolic syndrome presents in 5% of the population at normal weight, 22% of those who were overweight, and 60% of those who were obese. She has metabolic syndrome based on her abdominal circumference, increased triglycerides, low HDL, and mildly elevated LDL cholesterol levels. She may also need further investigation for the presence of polycystic ovarian syndrome (PCOS) because of her obesity, hirsutism, and history of irregular cycles. PCOS should be a consideration in patients with chronic anovulation, ovarian cysts, and evidence of hyperandrogenism. Both the metabolic syndrome and PCOS are very closely associated with obesity and insulin resistance.

Based on the provided information, in this situation, the key clinical implication of these diagnoses is identification of a patient needing aggressive lifestyle modification focused on weight reduction and increased physical activity.

APPROACH TO:
Obesity

DEFINITIONS

BODY MASS INDEX: A measurement of the relative composition of lean body mass and body fat, calculated as (weight in kilograms)/(height in meters)^2.

METABOLIC SYNDROME (syndrome X, insulin resistance syndrome): A constellation of metabolic abnormalities that confer increased risk of cardiovascular disease and diabetes mellitus. Major features include central obesity, hypertriglyceridemia, low HDL cholesterol, hyperglycemia, and hypertension.

OVERWEIGHT: Defined as BMI greater than or equal to 25 kg/m^2, the point at which all-cause, metabolic, cancer, and cardiovascular morbidity begins to rise.

OBESITY: A state of excess adipose tissue mass. Defined by most authorities as BMI greater than or equal to 30 kg/m^2. **Morbid obesity** is defined as a BMI greater than or equal to 40 kg/m^2. **Super obesity** is defined as a BMI greater than or equal to 50 kg/m^2.

SATIATION: Level of fullness during a meal.

SATIETY: Level of hunger after a meal.

CLINICAL APPROACH

Obesity is a chronic and easily diagnosed disease that is associated with life-threatening morbidity and mortality. Data from the National Health and Nutrition Examination Surveys (NHANES) show that in 2011 to 2012, 16.9% of 2- to 19-year-olds and 35.1% of adults aged 20 or older were obese. Overall, there was no significant change from 2003 to 2004 through 2011 to 2012 in obesity in 2- to 19-year-olds, or obesity in adults.

Table 33–1 • NCEP-ATP III CRITERIA FOR METABOLIC SYNDROME	
Three of more of the following:	
Waist circumference	Waist circumference >102 cm (M), >88 cm (F)
Hypertriglyceridemia	Triglycerides ≥150 mg/dL or specific medication
Low HDL cholesterol	HDL cholesterol <40 mg/dL if male or <50 mg/dL if female or specific medication
Hypertension	Blood pressure ≥130 mm Hg systolic or ≥85 mm Hg diastolic or specific medication
Fasting plasma glucose	Fasting plasma glucose ≥100 mg/dL or specific medication or previously diagnosed type 2 diabetes

Metabolic Syndrome

Current minimum estimates are that the prevalence of metabolic syndrome in the United States is at least 34.5% using the Adult Treatment Panel (ATP) III criteria (Table 33–1). The metabolic syndrome is an important risk factor for subsequent development of type 2 diabetes and cardiovascular disease. Thus, the key clinical implication of a diagnosis of metabolic syndrome is identification of a patient needing aggressive lifestyle modification focused on weight reduction and increased physical activity.

Diagnostic Tools

BMI is used as a measure of weight status and aid to predict risk of disease as it generally correlates well as an estimate of total body fat. However, **BMI is not as accurate a measure of overweight/obesity in patients with heart failure, pregnant women, body builders, professional athletes, elderly patients, and certain ethnic groups.** Moreover, abdominal obesity is associated with increased risk for hypertension, heart disease, dyslipidemia, and diabetes. Additional measurements, like waist circumference, and waist-to-hip ratio, need to be used to accurately identify the population at risk. Direct measurement of percentage of body fat may also provide additional information. Table 33–2 lists the classification of overweight/obesity based on BMI.

Table 33–2 • DEFINITION OF OBESITY BASED ON BMI	BMI (kg/m²)	Obesity Class
Underweight	<18.5	
Normal	18.5-24.9	
Overweight	25.0-29.9	
Obesity	30.0-34.9	I
	35.0-39.9	II
Extreme obesity (also called morbid, or severe, obesity)	>40	III
Super obesity	>50	III

Along with the measurements mentioned earlier, a health history, physical examination, and **focused laboratory workup** should be performed to look for complications and comorbid conditions. Any previous weight-loss efforts, recent smoking cessation, daily physical activity levels, and eating habits should be assessed to identify factors that might be contributing to weight gain and obesity. A **fasting glucose and glycosylated hemoglobin** level should be measured to evaluate for diabetes mellitus and impaired glucose tolerance. The presence of acanthosis nigricans—a velvety, hyperpigmented thickening of the skin commonly found on the neck and axillary regions—may also be a sign of insulin resistance. **Fasting lipids** should also be measured, both to evaluate for the presence of metabolic syndrome and for the assessment of the patient's risk for cardiovascular disease. **TSH** should be measured to screen for hypothyroidism. **Liver enzymes** should be requested, as abnormal results may indicate the development of a fatty liver.

Pathogenesis

Energy balance is the relationship of energy intake to energy expenditure. When more energy is expended than taken in, weight loss ensues. When the intake of energy exceeds the amount expended, weight gain occurs. In all persons, **obesity is caused by ingesting more energy relative to the amount of energy expended.** Energy balance is affected by genetic, physiologic, and environmental factors.

It has been **estimated that genetic background can explain 40% or more of the variance in body mass in humans.** The genetic component is complex and involves the interaction of multiple genes. However, the marked increase in obesity cannot be completely attributed to genetics. Social factors such as lower education level, lower socioeconomic class, and diet composition are all associated with high risk of obesity. Likewise, physiologic factors such as various gut hormones, level of spontaneous physical activity (fidgeting), and age-related decline in energy expenditure are key determinants in regulation of food intake and energy expenditure. An **increase in energy consumption with a decrease in physical activity is thought to be the main contributor to the current obesity epidemic.** Among numerous issues, the availability of convenience foods and the increase in palatability and serving size, compounded with industrialization leading to a sedentary lifestyle, has led to an altered energy balance.

Health Hazards Associated With Obesity

Obesity is a risk factor for the development of diabetes and cardiovascular disease. It is a risk factor for numerous other medical conditions (Table 33–3). In general, greater BMI is associated with more health complications and grade II or higher obesity is associated with greater risk of mortality. Also, the more complications that develop, the more difficult it becomes to manage the underlying obesity. For example, a person with degenerative arthritis and heart disease may have significant symptoms during exercise, impairing his or her ability to expend more energy in an effort to lose weight.

Treatment

Treatment of obesity should begin in patients with a BMI greater than 25 or who have visceral obesity, documented by increased waist circumference greater

Table 33–3 • COMMON MEDICAL COMPLICATIONS OF OBESITY
Cardiovascular disease
Cerebrovascular disease
Cholelithiasis
Chronic kidney disease
Degenerative joint disease
Eating disorders
Nonalcoholic fatty liver disease/nonalcoholic steatohepatitis
Hyperlipidemia
Hypertension
Infertility/reduced fertility
Malignancies
Menstrual cycle irregularities
Mood disorders
Polycystic ovary syndrome
Psychosocial dysfunction
Sleep apnea
Type 2 diabetes mellitus

than 40 in men and greater than 35 in women or a waist-to-hip ratio greater than 0.9 in men and greater than 0.85 in women. Weight loss of as little as 5 lb reduces the risk of developing comorbid conditions. Developing a **treatment plan** for obesity is complex and should use a **combination of dietary restrictions, increased physical activity, and behavior therapy** as a gold standard.

Dietary intervention is the cornerstone of weight-loss therapy. Most diets work in two principal dimensions: energy content and nutrient composition. The National Heart, Lung, and Blood Institute (NHLBI) recommend initiating treatment with a calorie deficit of 500 to 1000 kcal/d compared with the patient's habitual diet. This reduction produces a weight loss of 1 to 2 lb/wk (0.45 to 0.91 kg/wk). **Loss of more than 5% of initial body weight can improve CVD risk.** There are different kinds of specific dietary modifications recommended, but they all work based on calorie restriction. The selection of a diet should be based on patient preferences to promote optimal dietary adherence, a key determinant of weight loss irrespective of the type and nutrient composition of the diet. In addition, calorie restriction should not compromise the nutrient content of the diet; patients should still aim for a balanced meal.

The addition of exercise training to a diet program can add to the weight loss. However, **physical activity alone is not an effective method for achieving weight loss.** Although increasing physical activity is not effective for weight loss when used alone, physical activity is very important for long-term weight management and cardiovascular health benefits. Physical activity can improve insulin sensitivity and glycemic control, decrease abdominal fat, and reduce cardiovascular risk. Patients should engage in moderate to vigorous physical activity for at least 30 min/d, 5 to 7 d/wk, both to maintain weight loss and for the independent health benefits of exercising.

The purpose of behavior modification therapy is to help patients identify and make long-term changes in their eating and physical activity habits that contribute to obesity. The targets of behavior modification are avoiding triggers, maintaining dietary diaries, using portion-controlled plates, slowing rate of eating to enhance satiation, avoidance of high-risk situations, increasing physical activity, and breaking repetitive behaviors, such as watching TV while eating.

Pharmacotherapy

Table 33–4 lists the medications commonly used in the treatment of obesity. Pharmacologic therapy may be offered to those with a BMI greater than 30, or

Table 33–4 • MEDICATIONS USED IN THE TREATMENT OF OBESITY		
Drug Name (Trade Name)	**Mechanism of Action**	**Notes**
Bupropion-naltrexone (Contrave)	Antidepressant and opioid antagonist	Not recommended as first line. Can be used in obese smokers that want to quit. Full cardiovascular effects are unknown, but this should not be used with uncontrolled hypertension. Warn about suicidal ideation in young adults.
Dextroamphetamine (Dexedrine, Dextrostat)	Sympathomimetic (increased norepinephrine release)	All: Numerous drug interactions; stimulant side effects include insomnia, agitation, tachycardia, hypertension; additive effects with other stimulants (caffeine, cold medications, etc); can be addicting; avoid with monoamine oxidase (MAO) inhibitors; all indicated for short-term (generally interpreted as up to 12 weeks) use only
Phendimetrazine (Bontril)	Sympathomimetic (increased norepinephrine release)	
Diethylpropion (Tenuate)	Sympathomimetic (increased norepinephrine release)	
Phentermine (Fastin, Pro-Fast, Ionamin, Adipex-P)	Sympathomimetic (increased norepinephrine release)	
Phentermine-topiramate (Qsymia)	Sympathomimetic (increased norepinephrine release) and anticonvulsant	Significant side effects of topiramate include paresthesias, somnolence, and difficulty concentrating. Topiramate has also been associated with metabolic acidosis.
Lorcaserin (Belviq)	Serotonin receptor agonist	Selective serotonin 2C receptor agonist, which decreases cardiac side effect of nonselective serotonin agonists.
Orlistat (Xenical, Alli)	Selective inhibitor of pancreatic lipase, results in reduced intestinal digestion of fat and increased fecal fat excretion	Recommended as first-line pharmacotherapy along with behavioral and dietary changes. GI side effects common: diarrhea, fecal incontinence, bloating, cramps, gas, oily stools; must follow low-fat diet to reduce side effects; may give vitamin supplements for decreased absorption of fat-soluble vitamins (A, D, E) and β-carotene; indicated for short- or long-term use

BMI of 27 to 30 with comorbid conditions. Orlistat, lorcaserin, and phentermine/topiramate are US Food and Drug Administration (FDA) approved for long-term weight-loss management. All of these approved medications have generally been found to have modest weight loss over placebo and often are limited in efficacy due to side effects and/or cost.

With the exception of orlistat, which inhibits the absorption of dietary fat, all medications approved for obesity act as anorexiants. Anorexiant medications increase satiation, satiety, or both, by affecting the monoamine system in the hypothalamus. Increasing satiation results in a reduction in the amount of food eaten, whereas increasing satiety reduces the frequency of eating. The FDA-approved medications, which should be used as adjuncts to diet, exercise, and behavioral treatments, are generally recommended to be used short term. Their use should be tapered off after prolonged use or if there is lack of efficacy. Metformin and exenatide, medications approved for treatment of type 2 diabetes mellitus, may be a useful adjunct for weight loss in patients with comorbid obesity. Metformin can also help with weight loss in patients with polycystic ovary syndrome.

Many previously approved medications for weight loss have been removed from the market due to significant risks greater than benefits. Over-the-counter weight-loss medications and supplements have similar risk-benefit profiles or have limited research for safety and efficacy.

Bariatric Surgery

Patients with a **BMI greater than 40 who have failed diet and exercise (with or without drug therapy), or greater than 35 with serious comorbid conditions, are potential candidates for surgical treatment of obesity.** Weight-loss surgeries fall into one of two categories: restrictive and restrictive-malabsorptive. Restrictive surgeries, such as laparoscopic adjustable gastric banding, limit the amount of food the stomach can hold and slow the rate of gastric emptying. Restrictive-malabsorptive bypass procedures, such as the Roux-en-Y gastric bypass, combine the elements of gastric restriction and selective malabsorption.

The two most common surgeries done are Roux-en-Y gastric bypass and laparoscopic adjustable gastric banding, or "lap banding." The Rouex-en-Y procedure involves the construction of a small (10-30 mL) gastric pouch that empties into a segment of jejunum. With the small pouch and the small outlet to limit caloric intake, the Rouex-en-Y is mostly a restrictive procedure with some degree of associated malabsorption. Surgical mortality rate from bariatric surgery is generally less than 1% but varies with the procedure, patient's age and comorbid conditions, and experience of the surgical team. The most common surgical complications include stomal stenosis or marginal ulcers (occurring in 5%-15% of patients) that present as prolonged nausea and vomiting after eating or inability to advance the diet to solid foods.

In lap banding, an adjustable silicone gastric band is laparoscopically placed around the upper stomach just distal to the gastroesophageal junction. The band has a balloon connected to a subcutaneously implanted port, which can be inflated or deflated to reduce the circumference of the band. Complications of the banding procedure are less common and less severe than in gastric bypass, but the long-term weight loss may also be less. The adjustable band allows for the flexibility of addressing various nutritional demands after the surgery. For example, the band can be adjusted to have the stoma widened to accommodate a greater demand for caloric and fluid intake when a patient becomes pregnant.

COMPREHENSION QUESTIONS

33.1 A 15-year-old adolescent boy is brought into the clinic by his mother. He has been experiencing chest pain, shortness of breath, and is having increased episodes of asthma exacerbation. He is 5 ft 10 in in height and weighs 399 lb. An ECG in the office shows a normal sinus rhythm. He is unable to participate in school athletics due to his weight and has little physical activity after school. He has friends, but has some esteem issues because of being so large. He often finds it hard to find current trendy clothes in his size, but says it's ok because he is not the largest person at his school. His mother, who is also morbidly obese, is worried that he will have a heart attack and wants him to lose weight. Which of the following patients has the best evidence to be a candidate for bariatric surgery as initial treatment for obesity?

A. A man with a BMI of 32 and arthritis of the knees.

B. A woman with a BMI of 33 and type 2 diabetes.

C. A woman with a BMI of 42 but no identifiable complications.

D. Any obese patient who desires bariatric surgery should have it offered.

33.2 A patient you have been seeing for 10 years recently lost his health insurance because his BMI is too high. He was born with achondroplasia and is 4 ft 8 in in height and weighs 192 lb. He has been in good health and takes no medications. On examination, his BP is 122/76 mm Hg, pulse 56 beats/min, and respiratory rate 16 breaths/min. For which of the following patients is a BMI measurement most likely to be an accurate assessment of obesity?

A. A bodybuilder with a BMI of 38

B. A pregnant woman with a BMI of 31 in her 37th week of gestation

C. A man with congestive heart failure, pitting edema, and a BMI of 30

D. A hypertensive woman with a BMI of 32

33.3 A 34-year-old Hispanic woman comes to clinic to discuss weight management. She is currently 5-ft 2-in tall and weighs 265 lb. She says she always had a hard time managing her weight as a child, but let things get out of control when she was living on her own in college. She has had two children in the past 5 years. She gained 50 lb with the first child and lost 30 lb. With the second child she gained 35 lb and lost 10 lb. She has tried many fad diets where she initially loses weight but eventually gains it back. She exercises some but is limited by osteoarthritis of the knees. She has thought about gastric bypass but is fearful of undergoing a surgical procedure. Which of the following medications may be used for the long-term management of obesity?

A. Orlistat

B. Phendimetrazine

C. Dextroamphetamine

D. Phentermine

ANSWERS

33.1 **C.** Bariatric surgery can be effective but carries significant risks. The best evidence is for people with a BMI of greater than 40 who have failed diet and exercise (with or without drug therapy) or with a BMI of greater than 35 and obesity-related complications. Grade 1 obesity with diabetes mellitus or significant medical conditions related can be considered for bariatric surgery, but the evidence of benefit over risk is less robust.

33.2 **D.** A BMI reading will not accurately assess the ratio of lean body mass to body fat in highly muscled persons (weightlifters, athletes), persons with decreased muscle mass (elderly), in pregnant women, and in symptomatic congestive heart failure.

33.3 **A.** Orlistat is indicated for the long-term treatment of obesity. All of the pure stimulant medications should be for short-term use only.

CLINICAL PEARLS

▶ Obesity is a chronic disease that is reaching epidemic status in the United States and worldwide.

▶ BMI is a common tool used to grade obesity, but in certain cases it may be inadequate.

▶ Obesity treatment should always include dietary restriction, increased activity, and behavioral modifications.

▶ Even 5% to 15% weight loss can significantly reduce the complications associated with obesity.

REFERENCES

Bray GA. *Contemporary Diagnosis and Management of Obesity and the Metabolic Syndrome.* 4th ed. Newton, PA: Handbooks in Healthcare; 2011.

Centers for Disease Control and Prevention (CDC). Available at: www.cdc.gov/obesity. Accessed November 7, 2015.

Dyson PA. The therapeutics of lifestyle management on obesity. *Diabetes Obes Metab.* 2010;12(11): 941-946.

Flier JS, Maratos-Flier E. Biology of obesity. In: Kasper D, Fauci A, Hauser S, et al., eds. *Harrison's Principles of Internal Medicine.* 19th ed. New York, NY: McGraw-Hill; 2015. Available at: http://accessmedicine.mhmedical.com. Accessed May 25, 2015.

Grundy SM, Smith SC, Jr. Metabolic syndrome, obesity, and diet. In: Fuster V, Walsh RA, Harrington RA, eds. *Hurst's the Heart.* 13th ed. New York, NY: McGraw-Hill; 2011.

Moyer VA. U.S. Preventive Services Task Force. Screening for and management of obesity in adults: U.S. Preventive Services Task Force recommendation statement. *Ann Intern Med.* 2012 Sep 4;157(5):373-378.

Ogden CL, Carroll MD, Kit BK, Flegal KM. Prevalence of childhood and adult obesity in the United States, 2011-2012. *JAMA.* 2014;311(8):806-814.

A 33-year-old woman presents with a complaint of headaches. She has had headaches since she was a teenager, but they have become more debilitating recently. The episodes occur once or twice each month and last for up to 2 days. The pain begins in the right temple or at the back of the right eye and spreads to the entire scalp over a few hours. She describes the pain as a sharp, throbbing sensation that gradually worsens and is associated with severe nausea. Several factors aggravate the pain, including loud noises and movement. She has taken several over-the-counter medications for the pain, but the only thing that works is going to sleep in a quiet, darkened room. A thorough history reveals that her mother suffers from migraine headaches. Her vital signs, general physical examination, and a thorough neurologic examination are all within normal limits.

▶ What is the most likely diagnosis?
▶ What imaging study is most appropriate at this time?
▶ What are the most appropriate therapeutic options?

ANSWERS TO CASE 34:
Migraine Headache

Summary: A 33-year-old woman presents with headaches that are throbbing and over her right eye. Her headaches have occurred since she was a teenager and have progressively worsened. She has not found relief from over-the-counter preparations.

- **Most likely diagnosis:** Migraine without aura.

- **Most appropriate imaging study:** No imaging is indicated at this time as there are no "red flag" symptoms or signs.

- **Most appropriate therapy:** A "triptan" medication given in a means that does not have to be swallowed (eg, subcutaneous, intranasal, or orally dissolving tablet).

ANALYSIS

Objectives

1. Know the differential diagnosis of chronic headache.

2. Learn the "red flag" symptoms and signs that should prompt rapid, specific diagnostic and treatment interventions.

3. Know how to manage common headache syndromes.

Considerations

The patient described in the case has symptoms that are very characteristic of classic migraines without aura. Her headaches are unilateral, throbbing in nature, and have been progressively worsening. Migraine headaches are the most common headaches of vascular origin and the second most common cause of headaches overall. Migraines are a member of a group of primary headache syndromes differentiated by their associated features. Migraines typically cause recurrent episodes of headache, nausea, and vomiting. They can also be associated with other neurologic symptoms such as photophobia, light-headedness, paresthesias, vertigo, and visual disturbances. In the patient described in this case, the history and lack of physical findings can reasonably lead to the diagnosis of migraine headaches without aura ("common migraine"), the most frequently occurring form. Other classifications of migraines include migraine with aura ("classic migraine"), ophthalmoplegic migraine, retinal migraine, and childhood periodic syndromes that may be precursors to or associated with migraines. During the evaluation of this patient, the focus should be on determining the etiology of the headache, assessing for any red flags (Table 34–1) that may indicate worse pathologic causes, identifying triggers, and therapy for the condition.

According to the International Headache Society, symptoms diagnostic of migraine headache (Table 34–2) include moderate to severe headache with a pulsating quality; unilateral location; nausea and/or vomiting; photophobia;

Table 34–1 • "RED FLAG" SYMPTOMS AND SIGNS IN THE EVALUATION OF HEADACHES

Red Flag	Differential Diagnosis	Workup Studies
Sudden-onset maximum severity "worst headache" or new and different headache	Subarachnoid hemorrhage, pituitary apoplexy, hemorrhage into a mass lesion or vascular malformation, mass lesion	Neuroimaging first; lumbar puncture if neuroimaging negative
Headaches increasing in severity and frequency, brought on by Valsalva or physical exertion	Mass lesion, subdural hematoma, medication overuse	Neuroimaging, drug screen
Headache beginning after age 50; especially if jaw pain on chewing (jaw claudication)	Temporal arteritis, mass lesion	Neuroimaging, erythrocyte sedimentation rate level
New-onset headache in patient with risk factors for HIV infection or cancer	Meningitis, brain abscess (including toxoplasmosis), metastasis	Neuroimaging first; lumbar puncture if neuroimaging negative
Headache with signs of systemic illness (fever, stiff neck, rash)	Meningitis, encephalitis, Lyme disease, systemic infection, collagen vascular disease	Neuroimaging, lumbar puncture, serology
Focal neurologic signs or symptoms of disease (other than typical aura)	Mass lesion, vascular malformation, stroke, collagen vascular disease	Neuroimaging, collagen vascular evaluation (including antiphospholipid antibodies)
Papilledema	Mass lesion, pseudotumor cerebri, meningitis	Neuroimaging, lumbar puncture
Headache subsequent to head trauma	Intracranial hemorrhage, subdural hematoma, epidural hematoma, posttraumatic headache	Neuroimaging of brain, skull, and cervical spine

Data from South-Paul JE, Matheny SC, Lewis EL, et al. Current Diagnosis and Treatment in Family Medicine. *New York, NY: McGraw-Hill; 2004:330.*

phonophobia; worsening with activity; multiple attacks lasting for 4 hours to 3 days; and absence of history or physical examination findings that would make it likely that the headache is the result of another cause. Common triggers of migraine headaches include menses, fatigue, hunger, and stress.

Table 34–2 • SIMPLIFIED DIAGNOSTIC CRITERIA FOR MIGRAINE

Repeated attacks of headache lasting 4-72 h in patients with a normal physical examination, no other reasonable cause for the headache, and:

At Least 2 of the Following Features:	Plus at Least 1 of the Following Features:
Unilateral pain	Nausea/vomiting
Throbbing pain	Photophobia and phonophobia
Aggravation by movement	
Moderate or severe intensity	

Adapted from the International Headache Society Classification (Headache Classification Committee of the International Headache Society, 2004).

APPROACH TO:
Migraine Headaches

DEFINITIONS

PRIMARY HEADACHE SYNDROME: Headaches in which headache and associated features occur in the absence of any exogenous cause. The most common are migraine, tension-type headache, and cluster headache.

MIGRAINE HEADACHES: Vascular headaches typically throbbing unilateral in character, and may be present with or without an aura. There is a high female predominance.

TENSION HEADACHE: The most common primary headache syndrome, typically presenting with pericranial muscle tenderness and a description of a bilateral band-like distribution of the pain.

CLUSTER HEADACHE: Unilateral headaches that may have a high male predominance, can be located in the orbital, supraorbital, or temporal region. It is generally described as a deep, excruciating pain lasting from 15 minutes to 3 hours. These headaches are usually episodic; however, a small subset may have chronic headaches.

CHRONIC DAILY HEADACHE: Experiencing headache on 15 days or more per month. Chronic daily headache (CDH) is not a single entity; it can encompass a number of headache syndromes, including chronic tension headaches, migraines, infection, inflammation, trauma, and medication overuse.

CLINICAL APPROACH

Headaches are an extremely common complaint in primary care, urgent care, and emergency settings. The vast majority of adults have at least one headache each year, although most do not present for medical care. **The role of the practitioner is to attempt to accurately diagnose the cause of the headache, rule out secondary causes of headaches ("red flags") that may signify a serious underlying pathology, provide appropriate acute management, and assist with headache prevention when needed.** It is important that each individual headache be evaluated in the context of patient's prior headaches. The clinician should remain alert to the possibility of a secondary cause for the headache. Migraine headaches do not preclude the presence of underlying pathology.

The medical history in a patient with headaches should focus on several important areas. The quality and characteristics of the headache and its specific location and radiation should be identified. The presence of associated symptoms, especially neurologic symptoms that may suggest the presence of a focal neurologic lesion or increased intracranial pressure, must be documented. The age at which the patient first developed the headaches, the frequency and duration of the headaches, and the amount of disability and distress that is caused to the patient should be explored. It is also important to note what the patient has done to try to treat the headaches in the past, including as much detail as possible regarding medication usage (both prescription and over-the-counter [OTC]). Determining functional limitations during headaches and categorization of the migraine severity level should also be determined as it will affect the choice of treatment:

Mild: Patient is aware of a headache but able to continue daily routine.

Moderate: The headache inhibits daily activities but is not incapacitating.

Severe: The headache is incapacitating.

Status: A severe headache that has lasted more than 72 hours.

Clinicians should stratify treatment based on severity rather than using stepped care.

The examination should include both a general and a detailed neurologic examination. A funduscopic examination revealing papilledema may be supportive of the presence of increased intracranial pressure. **Identifying a focal neurologic deficit increases the likelihood of finding a significant central nervous system (CNS) pathology as the cause of the headache.**

A patient with symptoms and signs consistent with migraine and who does not have any "red flag" findings (see Table 34–1) does not require any further testing prior to instituting treatment. Neuroimaging should be performed if there is an unexplained neurologic abnormality on examination or if the headache syndrome is not typical of either migraines or some other primary headache disorder. The **presence of rapidly increasing headache frequency or a history of either lack of coordination, focal neurologic symptom, or headache awakening the patient from sleep raises the likelihood of finding an abnormality on an imaging test.** Magnetic resonance imaging (MRI) may be more sensitive than computed tomography (CT) scanning for the identification of abnormalities, but it may not be more sensitive at identifying *significant* abnormalities. CT scanning would be initial imaging for "thunderclap" headaches where intracranial bleeds are considered. Other testing (eg, blood tests, electroencephalogram [EEG]) should only be performed for diagnostic purposes if there is a suspicion based on the history or physical examination.

The treatment of headache is best individualized based on a thorough history, physical examination, and the interpretation of any additional study results. Migraines can often be managed to some degree by a variety of nonpharmacologic approaches. Nonpharmacologic treatment can include patient education, bed rest in a dark room, and removal of known triggers. Most patients benefit from simple avoidance of specific headache triggers. Lifestyle modifications may be helpful. These could include diet changes, regular exercise, regular sleep patterns, avoidance of excess caffeine and alcohol, and avoidance of acute changes in stress levels. Migraine patients do not encounter more stress or triggers than the general population; however, they may have overresponsiveness to these triggers. Some techniques to manage stress may include yoga, meditation, hypnosis, and conditioning techniques such as biofeedback. Other nonpharmacologic treatments which may be effective in some patients include cold applications, constant temporal artery pressure, acupuncture, and hyperbaric oxygen.

The US Headache Consortium lists the following general management guidelines for the treatment of migraine headaches:

- Educate migraine patients about their condition and its treatment, and to participate in their own management.

- Use migraine-specific agents (eg, triptans, dihydroergotamine, ergotamine) in patients with more severe migraines, and in those whose headaches respond poorly to treatment with nonsteroidal anti-inflammatory drugs (NSAIDs) or combination analgesics, such as aspirin plus acetaminophen plus caffeine.

- Select a nonoral route of administration for patients whose migraines present early with nausea or vomiting as a significant component of the symptom complex.

- Consider using a self-administered rescue medication for patients with severe migraine who do not respond well to other treatments.

- Guard against medication-overuse or rebound headaches. Patients who require acute treatment on two or more occasions per week should probably be on prophylactic treatment.

The goal of therapy in migraine prophylaxis is a reduction in the severity and frequency of headache by 50% or more. Options for pharmacologic treatment and prophylaxis of migraines are listed in Tables 34–3 and 34–4, respectively.

OTHER HEADACHE SYNDROMES

Tension-Type Headache

Tension headache is the most prevalent form of primary headache disorder, typically presenting with pericranial muscle tenderness and a description of a bilateral band-like distribution of the pain. Headaches can last from 30 minutes to 7 days and there is no aggravation by walking stairs or similar routine physical activity. There is no associated nausea or vomiting. Both photophobia and phonophobia are absent, or one, but not the other, is present. They can be either episodic (<180 d/y) or chronic (>180 d/y).

Initial medical therapy of episodic tension-type headache includes aspirin, acetaminophen, and NSAIDs. Combination analgesics containing caffeine are second-line options. Measures to minimize risk of medication-overuse headaches include limiting use of drugs to treat acute headache to 2 to 3 d/wk, avoiding opioids and sedative hypnotics, and monitoring medication intake.

The general management principles for the treatment of migraine headaches can also be applied to the treatment of chronic tension-type headaches. In frequent headache sufferers, the combination of antidepressant medications and stress management therapy reduces headache activity significantly. Other prophylactic treatments of chronic tension-type headaches include electromyography (EMG) biofeedback, acupuncture, cognitive behavioral therapy, and relaxation training. Pharmacologic therapies for prophylaxis include amitriptyline as a first line, mirtazapine, venlafaxine, calcium channel blockers, and β-blockers.

Cluster Headache

Cluster headache is strictly unilateral in location and can be located in the orbital, supraorbital, or temporal region. It is generally described as a deep, excruciating

Table 34–3 • TREATMENT OF ACUTE MIGRAINE

Drug	Trade Name	Dosage
Simple Analgesics		
Acetaminophen, aspirin, caffeine	Excedrin Migraine	Two tablets or caplets q6h (max 8 per day)
NSAIDs		
Naproxen	Aleve, Anaprox, generic	220-550 mg PO BID
Ibuprofen	Advil, Motrin, Nuprin, generic	400 mg PO q3-4h
Tolfenamic acid	Clotam Rapid	200 mg PO; may repeat ×1 after 1-2 h
Diclofenac potassium	Cambia	50 mg PO (powder packet mixed with water)
5-HT$_1$ Receptor Agonists		
Oral		
Ergotamine 1 mg, caffeine 100 mg	Cafergot	One or two tablets at onset, then one tablet q½h (max 6 per day, 10 per week)
Naratriptan	Amerge	2.5-mg tablet at onset; may repeat once after 4 h
Rizatriptan	Maxalt Maxalt-MLT	5-10-mg tablet at onset; may repeat after 2 h (max 30 mg/d)
Sumatriptan	Imitrex	50-100-mg tablet at onset; may repeat after 2 h (max 200 mg/d)
Frovatriptan	Frova	2.5-mg tablet at onset; may repeat after 2 h (max 5 mg/d)
Almotriptan	Axert	12.5-mg tablet at onset; may repeat after 2 h (max 25 mg/d)
Eletriptan	Relpax	40 or 80 mg
Zolmitriptan	Zomig Zomig Rapimelt	2.5-mg tablet at onset; may repeat after 2 h (max 10 mg/d)
Nasal		
Dihydroergotamine	Migranal Nasal Spray	Prior to nasal spray, the pump must be primed 4 times; 1 spray (0.5 mg) is administered, followed in 15 min by a second spray
Sumatriptan	Imitrex Nasal Spray	5-20 mg intranasal spray as 4 sprays of 5 mg or a single 20-mg spray (may repeat once after 2 h, not to exceed a dose of 40 mg/d)
Zolmitriptan	Zomig	5-mg intranasal spray as one spray (may repeat once after 2 h, not to exceed a dose of 10 mg/d)

(Continued)

Table 34–3 • TREATMENT OF ACUTE MIGRAINE (CONTINUED)

Drug	Trade Name	Dosage
Parenteral		
Dihydroergotamine	DHE-45	1 mg IV, IM, or SC at onset and q1h (max 3 mg/d, 6 mg per week)
Sumatriptan	Imitrex Injection Alsuma Sumavel DosePro	6 mg SC at onset (may repeat once after 1 h for max of 2 doses in 24 h)
Dopamine Receptor Antagonists		
Oral		
Metoclopramide	Reglan,[a] generic[a]	5-10 mg/d
Prochlorperazine	Compazine,[a] generic[a]	1-25 mg/d
Parenteral		
Chlorpromazine	Generic[a]	0.1 mg/kg IV at 2 mg/min; max 35 mg/d
Metoclopramide	Reglan,[a] generic	10 mg IV
Prochlorperazine	Compazine,[a] generic[a]	10 mg IV
Other		
Oral		
Acetaminophen, 325 mg, *plus* dichloralphenazone, 100 mg, *plus* isometheptene, 65 mg	Midrin, generic	Two capsules at onset followed by 1 capsule q1h (max 5 capsules)
Nasal		
Butorphanol	Generic	1 mg (1 spray in 1 nostril), may repeat if necessary in 1-2 h
Parenteral		
Opioids	Generic[a]	Multiple preparations and dosages

[a]Not all drugs are specifically indicated by the FDA for migraine. Local regulations and guidelines should be consulted.
Note: Antiemetics (eg, domperidone 10 mg or ondansetron 4 or 8 mg) or prokinetics (eg, metoclopramide 10 mg) are sometimes useful adjuncts.
Abbreviations: 5-HT, 5-hydroxytryptamine; NSAIDs, nonsteroidal anti-inflammatory drugs.
Reproduced, with permission, from Kasper D, Fauci A, Hauser S, et al. Harrison's Principles of Internal Medicine. 19th ed. New York, NY: McGraw-Hill Education; 2015. Table 447–4.

pain lasting from 15 minutes to 3 hours. The frequency can vary from one every other day to eight attacks per day. Cluster headaches are associated with ipsilateral autonomic signs and symptoms, and have a much greater prevalence in men. Compared to migraine sufferers who often desire sleep and a quiet, dark environment during their headache, individuals with cluster headache pace around, unable to find a comfortable position. The first-line treatment of cluster headache includes 100% oxygen at 6 L/min, and triptans. Second-line treatment for acute attacks includes intranasal lidocaine, dihydroergotamine, prednisone, octreotide, and somatostatin. Verapamil, lithium, melatonin, antiepileptics, and prednisone may

Table 34–4 • PREVENTIVE TREATMENTS IN MIGRAINE[a]		
Drug	**Dose**	**Selected Side Effects**
Pizotifen[b]	0.5-2 mg qd	Weight gain Drowsiness

β-Blocker
  Propranolol
  Metoprolol
	
	40-120 mg BID
	25-100 mg BID
		
		Reduced energy
		Tiredness
		Postural symptoms
		Contraindicated in asthma

Antidepressants
  Amitriptyline
  Dosulepin
  Nortriptyline
 	
  Venlafaxine
	
	10-75 mg at night
	25-75 mg at night
	25-75 mg at night
	
	75-150 mg/d
		
		Drowsiness
		
		Note: Some patients may only need a total dose of 10 mg, although generally 1-1.5 mg/kg body weight is required

Anticonvulsants
  Topiramate
 	
  Valproate
	
	25-200 mg/d
	
	400-600 mg BID
		
		Paresthesias
		Cognitive symptoms
		Weight loss
		Glaucoma
		Caution with nephrolithiasis
		Drowsiness
		Weight gain
		Tremor
		Hair loss
		Fetal abnormalities
		Hematologic or liver abnormalities

Serotonergic drugs Methysergide[c]	 1-4 mg qd	 Drowsiness Leg cramps Hair loss Retroperitoneal fibrosis (1-mo drug holiday is required every 6 mo)

Other classes
  Flunarizine[b]
 	
  Candesartan
	
	5-15 mg qd
	
	16 mg daily
		
		Drowsiness
		Weight gain
		Depression
		Parkinsonism
		Dizziness

Chronic migraine Onabotulinum toxin type A	 155 U	 Loss of brow furrow

(Continued)

Table 34–4 • PREVENTIVE TREATMENTS IN MIGRAINE[a] (CONTINUED)		
Drug	Dose	Selected Side Effects
No convincing evidence from controlled trials		
Verapamil		
Controlled trials demonstrate *no effect*		
Nimodipine Clonidine Selective serotonin reuptake inhibitors: fluoxetine		

[a]Commonly used preventives are listed with typical doses and common side effects. Not all listed medicines are approved by the US Food and Drug Administration; local regulations and guidelines should be consulted.
[b]Not available in the United States.
[c]Not currently available worldwide.
Reproduced, with permission, from Kasper D, Fauci A, Hauser S, et al. Harrison's Principles of Internal Medicine. 19th ed. New York, NY: McGraw-Hill Education; 2015. Table 447–6.

be used for prophylactic treatment. Because of side effects related to chronic use, ergotamine and prednisone need to be used with caution.

Chronic Medical Conditions

Patients with certain underlying medical conditions have a greater incidence of having an organic cause of their headache. Patients with cancer may develop headaches as a consequence of metastases. Someone with uncontrolled hypertension (with diastolic pressures >110 mm Hg) may present with the chief complaint of headache. Patients with HIV infection or AIDS may present with central nervous system metastases, lymphoma, toxoplasmosis, or meningitis as the cause of their headache. It is always important to evaluate each headache in context and consider secondary causes.

Medication-Related Headache

Numerous medications have headache as a reported adverse effect. Medication-overuse headache (formerly drug-induced or "rebound" headache) may occur following frequent use of any analgesic or headache medication. This includes both nonprescription (eg, acetaminophen, NSAIDs) and prescription medications. Caffeine use, whether as a component of an analgesic or a beverage, is another culprit in this category. The duration and severity of the withdrawal headache following discontinuation of the medication vary depending on the medication(s) involved. Any contributing, underlying psychological conditions that may lead to medication overuse may make discontinuation of the medication difficult and should be addressed.

COMPREHENSION QUESTIONS

34.1 A 28-year-old man presents for evaluation of headaches. He has had several episodes of unilateral throbbing headaches that last 8 to 12 hours. When they occur, he gets nauseated and just wants to go to bed. Usually they are relieved after he lays down in a dark, quiet room for the remainder of the day. He is missing significant work time due to the headaches. He has a normal examination today. Which of the following statements is accurate regarding this situation?

A. He needs a CT scan of his head to evaluate for the cause of his headache.

B. When he gets his next headache, he should breathe in 100% oxygen and use a triptan medication.

C. If he has not already done so, he should use aspirin 650 mg orally every 4 hours as needed and take a stress-management class.

D. An injectable or nasal spray triptan is most appropriate.

34.2 A 52-year-old woman presents to the office for an acute visit complaining of 2 hours of headache. She says that it came on suddenly with no account of trauma and is the worst headache she has ever had. She has had migraines since she was an early adult. The pain is described as "stabbing" and is more severe on the left side. She takes no medications and recently stopped taking oral contraceptive pills after going through menopause. Her blood pressure is elevated at 145/95 mm Hg, but otherwise she has no focal neurologic abnormalities on examination. She is alert and oriented to person, place, time, and situation. Which of the following is the most appropriate management at this time?

A. Prescribe a triptan medication.

B. Schedule a noncontrast head CT scan for tomorrow morning.

C. Call 911 and transfer the patient to the nearest emergency room.

D. Prescribe an antihypertensive medication and follow up in 2 weeks.

34.3 A 43-year-old man presents with headaches that he has had daily for several months. Every morning at work, usually between 9 and 10 AM, he has to take 650 mg of acetaminophen to relieve the headache. This has been going on for the past 3 months and he is at the point of looking for a new job, as he thinks that job stress is the cause of his symptoms. His examination is normal. Which of the following is the most appropriate advice for him?

A. Continue with the as-needed acetaminophen and find a less-stressful career.

B. He should start an antidepressant for headache prophylaxis.

C. His headaches are most likely to improve if he stops taking the acetaminophen.

D. A triptan is a more appropriate treatment for him.

ANSWERS

34.1 D. This patient gives a history very consistent with common migraine headaches. There are no red flags found on history or examination, so no further testing is necessary at this point. As he has significant nausea, he may benefit from nonoral medication. A triptan delivered by injection or nasal spray is a reasonable starting point for him.

34.2 C. The acute onset of the most severe headache in a patient's life is concerning for the presence of a subarachnoid hemorrhage. This is a medical emergency. This patient should be transported by emergency medical services to the nearest emergency facility for stabilization and management.

34.3 C. This situation is typical of a medication-related headache. While finding a new, less-stressful job may be beneficial, the problem will not resolve until he discontinues the daily use of his over-the-counter analgesic.

CLINICAL PEARLS

▶ Migraine headaches can occur in children and adolescents, as well as adults.

▶ Most patients presenting for the evaluation of headaches do not need diagnostic testing beyond the history and physical. However, the presence of focal neurologic deficits or other red flag symptoms/signs should prompt an immediate workup or referral.

REFERENCES

Beithon J, Gallenberg M, Johnson K, et al. Institute for Clinical Systems Improvement: diagnosis and treatment of headache. Available at: http://bit.ly/Headache0113. Updated January 2013. Accessed April 19, 2015.

Goadsby PJ, Raskin NH. Migraine and other primary headache disorders. In: Kasper D, Fauci A, Hauser S, et al., eds. *Harrison's Principles of Internal Medicine*. 19th ed. New York, NY: McGraw-Hill; 2015. Available at: http://accessmedicine.mhmedical.com. Accessed May 25, 2015.

Headache Classification Committee of the International Headache Society. *The International Classification of Headache Disorders*. 3rd ed. (beta version). *Cephalgia*. 33(9):629-808.

Migraine in Adults. In Dynamed [database online]. EBSCO Information Services. Available at: http://search.ebscohost.com/login.aspx?direct=true&site=DynaMed&id=114718. Updated July 25, 2014. Accessed February 15, 2015.

Silberstein SD, Holland S, Freitag F, et al. Evidence-based guideline update: pharmacologic treatment for episodic migraine prevention in adults. *Neurology*. 2012;78:1337-1345.

A 56-year-old white man comes in for a routine health maintenance visit. He is new to your practice and has no specific complaints today. He has hypertension for which he takes hydrochlorothiazide. He has no other significant medical history. He does not smoke cigarettes, occasionally drinks alcohol, and does not exercise. His father died of a heart attack at age 60 and his mother died of cancer at age 72. He has two younger sisters who are in good health. On examination, his blood pressure is 130/80 mm Hg and his pulse is 75 beats/min. He is 6-ft tall and weighs 200 lb. His complete physical examination is normal. You order a fasting lipid panel, which subsequently returns with the following results: total cholesterol 242 mg/dL; triglycerides 138 mg/dL; high-density lipoprotein (HDL) cholesterol 48 mg/dL; and low-density lipoprotein (LDL) cholesterol 155 mg/dL.

▶ What are the indications for statin therapy?
▶ What other laboratory testing is indicated at this time?
▶ What is the recommended management at this point?

ANSWERS TO CASE 35:
Hyperlipidemia

Summary: A 56-year-old white man with well-controlled hypertension is found to have elevated cholesterol on a screening blood test as part of a physical examination. He has no known history of coronary artery disease or of any coronary artery disease risk equivalent.

- **Recommendations for statin treatment:** American College of Cardiology/ American Heart Association (ACC/AHA) and National Institute for Clinical Evidence (NICE) guidelines recommend treatment with statins based on calculated risk using validated prediction rules.

- **Further testing at this time:** Blood glucose, creatinine, liver function tests, thyroid-stimulating hormone (TSH).

- **Initial management of his elevated cholesterol:** Therapeutic lifestyle changes (TLCs) with consideration for implementation of statin therapy.

ANALYSIS

Objectives

1. Know the risk factors for cardiovascular disease (CVD).

2. Know the new ACC/AHA and NICE recommendations for prevention of CVD.

3. Know the previous Adult Treatment Panel (ATP) III guidelines for the diagnosis, evaluation, and management of hyperlipidemia.

4. Be able to counsel patients on therapeutic lifestyle changes to lower their cholesterol levels.

Considerations

This case illustrates a 56-year-old white man with well-controlled hypertension and total cholesterol 242 mg/dL; triglycerides 138 mg/dL; HDL cholesterol 48 mg/dL; and LDL cholesterol 155 mg/dL. Based on the pooled cohort risk equation, his 10-year risk of atherosclerotic cardiovascular disease is 9.3% (based on his age, race, nonsmoking status, controlled hypertension, total cholesterol, and HDL level). Whether medication for cholesterol levels is initiated at this time is based on which of the current recommendations you follow; however, any medication regimen should be accompanied by therapeutic lifestyle changes such as weight loss, exercise, and diet.

APPROACH TO:
High Cholesterol

DEFINITIONS

ACC/AHA: American College of Cardiology and American Heart Association, which made joint recommendations for cholesterol management based on risk assessment in 2013.

ATP III: The third report of the National Cholesterol Education Program Expert Panel on the Detection, Evaluation, and Treatment of High Blood Cholesterol in Adults, released in 2002.

HDL CHOLESTEROL: High-density lipoprotein cholesterol.

LDL CHOLESTEROL: Low-density lipoprotein cholesterol.

NICE: National Institute for Clinical Excellence based in the United Kingdom, which made recommendations for cholesterol management based on risk assessment.

STATIN: Medication in the β-hydroxy-β-methylglutaryl-coenzyme A (HMG-CoA)–reductase inhibitor class. These are the most widely used medications for lowering LDL cholesterol.

CLINICAL APPROACH

Treatment recommendations for high cholesterol are evolving. Previous recommendations were based on the third report of the National Cholesterol Education Program Expert Panel on the Detection, Evaluation, and Treatment of High Blood Cholesterol in Adults, otherwise known as ATP III, released in 2002. New recommendations developed in 2013 by the ACC/ AHA and also recommendations by the NICE developed in the United Kingdom are different from the ATP III and vary in their recommendations from each other. Both new recommendations use risk assessment tools in order to determine if an individual should be treated with a cholesterol medication. The American Academy of Family Physicians (AAFP) later released its qualifications to the new guidelines. Like many changing areas of medicine, the current guidelines for treatment of high cholesterol are actively changing and providers have the opportunity to decide which recommendations to use in collaboration with patients on joint decision making. We will provide the guidelines for comparison and the AAFP qualifications to the new guidelines.

It is important to remember that cholesterol is not a disease. High cholesterol is a risk factor for coronary heart disease (CHD). As such, **an individual's cholesterol levels must be interpreted in the context of their overall risks for CHD.** The recommended intensity of the statin medication should be proportionate to their risk of CHD: the higher one's risk, the higher the intensity of the statin therapy. It is also important to note that for patients that do not tolerate high-intensity statins, using a lower-intensity statin would still provide some cardiovascular benefit, if the lower-intensity statin can be tolerated.

As mentioned earlier, the ATP III guidelines focused on risk factors to determine treatment and there were set goals for LDL levels to guide treatment. New recommendations no longer recommend treating to a goal LDL and use risk assessment scores in order to determine who should be treated with statin therapy. The classification and management guidelines for ATP III are seen in Table 35–1.

The ACC and AHA have developed guidelines for selecting patients for statin therapy. Statin therapy is recommended in all patients with known cardiovascular disease or LDL greater than 190 mg/dL. Statin therapy has been recommended for four additional groups of adults greater than or equal to 21 years:

- Patients less than or equal to **75 years with clinical CVD**

- Patients with LDL cholesterol greater than or equal to **190 mg/dL**

Table 35–1 • ATP III CLASSIFICATION OF LIPID LEVELS AND MANAGEMENT GUIDELINES

Cholesterol Level Classification

LDL Cholesterol (mg/dL)

<100	Optimal
100-129	Near optimal/above optimal
130-159	Borderline high
160-189	High
190 or greater	Very high

Total Cholesterol (mg/dL)

<200	Desirable
200-239	Borderline high
240 or greater	High

HDL Cholesterol (mg/dL)

<40	Low
60 or greater	High

Management Guidelines

Risk Category	LDL Goal	LDL Level to Start Therapeutic Lifestyle Change	LDL Level to Consider Medication
CHD or CHD equivalent	<100	≥100	≥130 (optional for 101-129)
Two or more risks factors	<130	≥130	10-y risk 10%-20% ≥160 10-y risk <10% ≥190
0-1 risk factors	<160	≥160	≥190

Data from ATP III report.

- **Patients aged 40 to 75 with diabetes and LDL cholesterol** greater than or equal to **70 mg/dL**

- **Patients aged 40 to 75 with 10-year CVD risk** greater than or equal to **7.5% and** LDL greater than or equal to **70 mg/dL**

It is reasonable to consider statin therapy after evaluating benefits versus risks in patients with clinical CVD older than 75 years, diabetic patients less than 21 years or greater than 75 years, or with patients whose atherosclerotic CVD (ASCVD) 10-year risk is between 5% and less than 7.5%, and 40 to 75 years with LDL 70 to 189 mg/dL and without diabetes or clinical CVD. Numerous risk calculators are available online. By determining the individual risk, one can then determine the appropriate management for the patient.

The NICE recommendations for the primary prevention of CVD use the QRISK2 risk assessment tool and begin statin therapy for adults with greater than or equal to 10% 10-year risk. Statin therapy should begin with focus on high intensity and low cost. NICE recommends offering atorvastatin 20 mg for primary prevention if 10-year risk greater than or equal to 10% and to people aged 85 or older. Monitor statin therapy with liver function tests at baseline, at 3 months, and at 12 months. If statin is contraindicated or not tolerated, ezetimibe can be offered. For patients with known CHD, treatment should be started with atorvastatin 80 mg. NICE recommends against use of fibrates, nicotinic acid, anion exchange resins, or omega-3 fatty acids for primary or secondary prevention.

The ACC/AHA and NICE recommendations require risk assessment in order to determine the patient's risk of coronary disease and need for lipid-lowering medication. Several risk assessment tools are available including Framingham risk estimation, QRISK and ASSIGN, pooled cohort equations, and coronary artery calcium scoring. NICE recommends QRISK2 and ACC/AHA uses pooled cohort equations, which may overestimate risk. Assessment scores can overestimate or underestimate risk in certain groups, so use of the appropriate assessment tool for the patient is important. There is insufficient data to support one assessment tool over another for predicting cardiovascular risk. Comparison of ACC/AHA and NICE guidelines are provided in Table 35–2.

The AAFP released its clinical practice guideline with endorsement of the AHA/ACC recommendations, with qualifications, in June, 2014. The key recommendations are listed in Table 35–3. The qualifications listed by the AAFP were that the CVD risk assessment tool has not been validated and may overestimate risk and a cutoff of 7.5%, rather than 10%, will significantly increase the number of patients on statins. Also, many of the recommendations were based on expert opinion, although some points were evidence based, and 7 out of 15 members of the guideline panel had conflicts of interest.

Evaluation

When high blood cholesterol is identified, an investigation should be performed to evaluate for **secondary causes of dyslipidemia.** Included among these causes are

Table 35–2 • ACC/AHA AND NICE GUIDELINES FOR TREATING CHOLESTEROL		
ACC/AHA Guidelines		
Risk Category	**Statin Therapy Recommended If**	**Reasonable to Consider Statin Therapy If**
Clinical atherosclerotic cardiovascular disease	Age 20-75	Age >75
LDL-C ≥190 mg/dL	Age ≥21	NA
Diabetes plus LDL-C 70-189 mg/dL	Age 40-75	Age 21-40 or >75
Age 40-75 plus LDL-C 70-189 mg/dL	Estimated 10-y risk of atherosclerotic cardiovascular disease ≥7.5%	Estimated 10-y risk of atherosclerotic cardiovascular disease 5% to <7.5%
Age 40-75 plus LDL-C 70-189 mg/dL	Estimated 10-y risk of atherosclerotic cardiovascular disease ≥7.5%	Estimated 10-y risk of atherosclerotic cardiovascular disease 5% to <7.5%
NICE Guidelines		
Risk Category	**Drug Recommendations**	
Existing cardiovascular disease (secondary prevention)	Atorvastatin 80 mg/d for all adults with cardiovascular disease Do not delay statin treatment in patients with acute coronary syndrome	
10-y cardiovascular disease risk >10%	Atorvastatin 20 mg/d	
10-y cardiovascular disease risk <10%	Optimize all other modifiable cardiovascular risk factors Statin not recommended	

Abbreviations: ACC/AHA, American College of Cardiology/American Heart Association; LDL-C, low-density lipoprotein C; NICE, National Institute for Health and Clinical Excellence.
Data from Dynamed, NICE, and ACC/AHA guidelines.

diabetes, hypothyroidism, obstructive liver disease, and chronic renal failure. Consequently, a reasonable laboratory workup includes fasting blood glucose, TSH, liver enzymes, and a creatinine level. Certain medications, including progestins, anabolic steroids, and corticosteroids, also can result in elevated cholesterol. Consideration should be given to changing or discontinuing these when possible.

Management

TLCs are the cornerstone of all treatments for hyperlipidemia. All patients should be educated on healthier living, including dietary modifications, increased physical activity, and smoking cessation. Weight reduction should be encouraged.

Specific dietary recommendations include limiting trans-fatty acid intake to less than 1% of total calories, limiting saturated fats to less than 7% of total calories, replacing saturated fats with polyunsaturated fats, and have a total intake of less than 200 mg/d of cholesterol. Total dietary fat should be kept to no more than

Table 35-3 • AAFP CLINICAL PRACTICE GUIDELINES KEY
RECOMMENDATIONS FOR CHOLESTEROL MANAGEMENT

Individuals with LDL-C ≥190 mg/dL or triglycerides ≥500 mg/dL should be evaluated for secondary causes of hyperlipidemia.

Adults ≥21 y with a primary LDL-C ≥190 mg/dL should be treated with high-intensity statin therapy unless contraindicated.

Adults 40-75 y with an LDL-C 70-189 mg/dL without clinical ASCVD or diabetes and an estimated 10-y ASCVD risk ≥7.5% should be treated with moderate- to high-intensity statin therapy.

Adults 40-75 y with diabetes mellitus and an LDL-C 70-189 mg/dL should be treated with moderate-intensity statin therapy.

Individuals ≤75 y who have clinical ASCVD should be treated with high-intensity statin therapy unless contraindicated.

There is not enough evidence to recommend for or against treating blood cholesterol to target levels.

There is not enough evidence to recommend the use of nonstatin medication combined with statin therapy to further reduce ASCVD events.

Abbreviations: ASCVD, atherosclerotic cardiovascular disease; LDL-C, low-density lipoprotein C.
Data from AAFP Clinical Practice Guideline on Cholesterol.

35% of total calories, with less than 10% polyunsaturated fat. AHA diet and life-style modifications include balancing calorie intake and physical activity to achieve or maintain healthy body weight, consuming a diet rich in vegetables and fruits and choose whole-grain, high-fiber foods, consume fish, especially oily fish, at least twice a week, minimize added sugars and sugary beverages, choose low-salt foods, and consume alcohol in moderation. The addition of dietary soluble fiber and plant stanols/sterols can be beneficial as well. Soluble fiber 10 to 25 g and of plant stanols/sterols 2 g can be added to reduce CVD and CHD risk. Referral to a dietician may be helpful as well. When TLC is instituted, regular follow-up must be arranged.

Pharmacotherapy may be considered in patients with ASCVD risk greater than 7.5% for ACC/AHA and 10% for NICE. **TLC should continue to be reinforced and encouraged even when starting medications.** In someone with known CHD, statin therapy is recommended in all guidelines. **The first-line pharmacotherapy for LDL cholesterol reduction is a statin.** Statins not only reduce LDL cholesterol but also reduce the rates of coronary events, strokes, cardiac death, and all-cause mortality. Ezetimibe is recommended as the second therapy for patient who cannot tolerate any level of statin or have contraindications. A list of medications available for treatment of hyperlipidemia is included on Table 35-4.

Cholesterol treatment is an example where new recommendations can create controversy in the management of chronic disease. The recommendations for evaluation, treatment, and ongoing management of high cholesterol have changed significantly over recent years with a focus on risk assessment. New development of treatments will also lend to ongoing changes in the new future.

Table 35–4 • MEDICATIONS USED TO LOWER CHOLESTEROL

Drug Class/ Medication	Effects	Side Effects	Contraindications
Statin • Lovastatin • Pravastatin • Fluvastatin • Atorvastatin • Rosuvastatin • Simvastatin	LDL ↓18%-55%; HDL ↑5%-15%; triglycerides (TG) ↓7%-30%	Myopathy, myalgia, increased liver enzymes	Active or chronic liver disease; relative contraindication with cytochrome P-450 inhibitors, cyclo- sporine, macrolides, antifungals
Bile acid sequestrants • Cholestyramine • Colestipol • Colesevelam	LDL ↓15%-30%; HDL ↑3%-5%; TG no change; or increase	GI distress, constipation, decreased absorption of other meds	Dysbetalipoprotein- emia; TG >400
Nicotinic acids • Immediate-release, sustained-release, or extended-release nicotinic acid	LDL ↓5%-25%; HDL ↑15%-35%; TG ↓20%-50%	Flushing, hyperglycemia, hyperuricemia, upper GI distress, hepatotoxicity	Absolute: chronic liver disease, severe gout Relative: diabetes, hyperuricemia, peptic ulcer disease
Fibric acids • Gemfibrozil • Fenofibrate	LDL ↓5%-20%; HDL ↑10%-20%; TG ↓20%-50%	Dyspepsia, gallstones, myopathy, unexplained non-CHD deaths in WHO study	Severe renal disease, severe hepatic disease
Cholesterol absorption • blocker • Ezetimibe	LDL ↓13%-25%; HDL ↑3%-5%;TG ↓5%-14%	Abdominal pain, diarrhea	Hepatic insufficiency/ active liver disease
Monoclonal antibody, • PCSK9 inhibitors • Evolocumab • Alirocumab	LDL ↓50% 82.3% LDL <70	Nasopharyngitis, upper respiratory tract infection, influenza, back pain	Pending approval by the FDA

Data from ATP III report, ezetimibe product information, and Sullivan, Olsson AG, Scott R, et al.

CASE CORRELATION

- See Cases 20 (Chest Pain) and 30 (Hypertension).

COMPREHENSION QUESTIONS

35.1 A 62-year-old smoker with a known history of CHD presents for establishment of care. He has normal blood pressure. His LDL cholesterol is 105 mg/dL, HDL cholesterol is 28 mg/dL, and total cholesterol is 170 mg/dL. According to the NICE guidelines, what medication therapy should be initiated at this time?

A. Ezetimibe

B. Atorvastatin

C. Niacin

D. Gemfibrozil

35.2 A 55-year-old woman presents to your office for follow-up. She was discharged from the hospital 1 week ago following a heart attack. She has quit smoking since then and vows to stay off cigarettes forever. Her lipid levels are total cholesterol 240 mg/dL, HDL 50 mg/dL, LDL 150 mg/dL, and triglycerides 150 mg/dL. Which of the following is the most appropriate management at this time?

A. Institute therapeutic lifestyle changes alone.

B. Institute therapeutic lifestyle changes and start on a statin.

C. Start on a statin.

D. Institute therapeutic lifestyle changes and start on a statin and nicotinic acid.

35.3 A 48-year-old man with no significant medical history and no symptoms is found to have elevated cholesterol at a health screening. Which of the following tests is part of the routine evaluation of this problem?

A. ECG

B. Stress test

C. Complete blood count (CBC)

D. Thyroid-stimulating hormone

ANSWERS

35.1 **B.** This patient has known CHD and should be started on statin therapy.

35.2 **B.** This patient has known CHD, documented by her recent myocardial infarction. All guidelines recommend therapeutic lifestyle changes as an integral part of care. With known CHD, statin therapy is also indicated. ACC/AHA guidelines would recommend high-intensity statin therapy.

35.3 **D.** Hypothyroidism is a potential cause of secondary dyslipidemia. A TSH is a reasonable test to perform in this setting. There is no indication to screen for CHD with an ECG or stress test in this asymptomatic person. Other tests to perform could include fasting blood glucose, liver enzymes, and a measurement of renal function.

CLINICAL PEARLS

▶ Lipid levels must always be interpreted in the context of the individual's overall risk factors for CHD.

▶ Statins have the best data to support improvement in outcomes that are clinically significant, such as heart attacks, strokes, and death. Unless there is a contraindication, a statin should be the first medication used for cholesterol reduction.

▶ Remind patients who are taking lipid-lowering medications that lifestyle modifications are still necessary. Medications are not a substitute for a healthy lifestyle.

REFERENCES

American Academy of Family Physicians Clinical Practice Guideline: Cholesterol. Available at: http://www.aafp.org/patient-care/clinical-recommendations/all/cholesterol.html. Accessed May 12, 2015.

Grundy SM, Cleeman JI, Merz CN, et al. NCEP report: implications of recent clinical trials for the National Cholesterol Education Program Adult Treatment Panel III guidelines. *Circulation.* 2004;110:227-239.

Hypercholesterolemia (2015, April 27). In DynaMed Plus [database online]. EBSCO Information Services. Available at: http://dynamed.com/. Accessed May 12, 2015.

National Cholesterol Education Program. The third report of the NCEP Expert Panel on the detection, evaluation and treatment of high blood cholesterol in adults. Item no: 02-5215; 2002.

National Institute for Health and Care Excellence (NICE). Lipid modification: cardiovascular risk assessment and the modification of blood lipids for the primary and secondary prevention of cardiovascular disease. *BMJ.* 2014 Jul 17;349:g4356.

Stone NJ, Robinson JG, Lichtenstein AH, et al. 2013 ACC/AHA guideline on the treatment of blood cholesterol to reduce atherosclerotic cardiovascular risk in adults: a report of the American College of Cardiology/American Heart Association Task Force on Practice Guidelines. *Circulation.* 2014 Jun 24;129(25 suppl 2):S1-S45.

Rader DJ, Hobbs HH. Disorders of lipoprotein metabolism. In: Kasper D, Fauci A, Hauser S, et al., eds. *Harrison's Principles of Internal Medicine.* 19th ed. New York, NY: McGraw-Hill Education; 2015. Available at: http://accessmedicine.mhmedical.com. Accessed May 25, 2015.

Sullivan D, Olsson AG, Scott R, et al. Effect of a monoclonal antibody to PCSK9 on low-density lipoprotein cholesterol levels in statin-intolerant patients: the GAUSS randomized trial. *JAMA.* 2012;308(23):2497-2506.

Van Horn L, McCoin M, Kris-Etherton PM, et al. The evidence for dietary prevention and treatment of cardiovascular disease. *J AM Diet Assoc.* 2008 Feb;108(2):228-331.

A 20-month-old girl, new to your practice, is brought in by her mother because she's been crying and not walking for the past day. Her mother reports that the child is "very clumsy and falls a lot." She says that the little girl may have injured her leg by falling off the sofa because, she repeats, "she really is clumsy and falls a lot." Upon review with the mother, she states that the child has no significant medical history and takes no medications regularly. There are two older children in the family, ages 4 and 6, who are in good health but also are "clumsy and forever hurting themselves." The husband lives in the home. Without any questioning or prompting, the mother states that her husband is "a good man but he's under a lot of stress." You ask the mother to undress the child for an examination and she quickly replies, "Do you really have to undress her? She's very shy." You politely, but firmly, say that you need to examine her and she removes the child's pants. You see that her right knee is visibly swollen and tender to palpation on the medial bony prominences. You also note numerous bruises of the buttocks and posterior thighs, which appear to be of different ages. There are also several small, circular scars on the legs, each about a centimeter in size. "See how clumsy she is?" the mother says, pointing to her bruises. An x-ray of the child's knee shows a corner fracture of the distal femoral metaphysis.

► What is the likely mechanism of this child's injuries?
► What further evaluation is necessary at this time?
► What legal obligation must a physician fulfill in this circumstance?

ANSWERS TO CASE 36:

Family Violence

Summary: A 20-month-old girl is brought to the office for evaluation of crying and not walking. On examination, she is found to have multiple bruises and circular wounds that are suspicious for cigarette burns. Her knee x-ray shows a metaphyseal corner fracture, an injury that is inconsistent with the stated history of "falling off the sofa."

- **Most likely mechanism of injuries:** Inflicted injuries, including leg injury from forceful pulling, bruising from hitting the child's legs, and cigarette burns

- **Further evaluation at this time:** Complete, unclothed physical examination of child (including ophthalmoscopic and neurologic examinations); radiographic skeletal survey

- **Legal obligation of physician:** Report of suspected child abuse to the appropriate child protective services organization

ANALYSIS

Objectives

1. Learn the symptoms and signs suggestive of child maltreatment and abuse.

2. Know the situations in which the risk of family violence increases.

3. Learn some of the medicolegal requirements involved in situations of family violence.

Considerations

Family violence can occur in families of any socioeconomic class and in households of any composition. The term *family violence* **includes child abuse, intimate partner violence (IPV), and elder abuse.** The abuse that occurs can be physical, sexual, emotional, psychologic, or economic. It can take the forms of battering, raping, threatening, intimidating, isolating from friends and family, stealing, and preventing the earning of money, among many others.

In the case presented here, there are several signs of intentionally inflicted injuries to the child. The presence of numerous bruises of varying ages, especially on relatively protected areas such as the buttocks and upper posterior thighs, should raise suspicions. Finding injuries inconsistent with the reported history also can be a clue. Certain types of fractures, such as metaphyseal corner fractures (caused by forceful jerking or twisting of the leg) are usually a result of abuse. The identification of wounds consistent with cigarette burns is highly specific for abuse.

Physicians often find these situations extremely difficult and uncomfortable to deal with. They may feel caught between two partners—both of whom are patients—but who give conflicting stories. They may have concerns about the legal implications of their findings and fear legal actions if they make reports to authorities. They may have frustrations in dealing with a person who will not leave an abusive spouse and may feel ill-trained to deal with many of these situations. By knowing situations in which family violence is more likely to occur, knowing the laws regarding disclosure and reporting, and learning to recognize the signs of family violence, physicians can be better prepared to address these situations when they occur.

APPROACH TO:
Family Violence

DEFINITIONS

CHILD MALTREATMENT: An all-inclusive term covering physical abuse; sexual abuse; emotional abuse; parental substance abuse; physical, nutritional, and emotional neglect; supervisional neglect; and Munchausen syndrome by proxy.

ELDER MISTREATMENT: Intentional or neglectful acts by a caregiver or trusted individual that harm a vulnerable older person.

NEGLECT: Failure to provide the needs required for functioning or for the avoidance of harm.

PHYSICAL ABUSE (BATTERY): Intentional physical actions (eg, biting, kicking, punching) that can cause injury or pain to another person.

CLINICAL APPROACH

Family violence is a pattern of abusive behavior in any relationship in which one individual gains or maintains power or control over another individual. This abuse can take the form of physical violence (battery), sexual violence, intimidation, emotional and psychological abuse, economic control, neglect, threats, and isolation from others. During screening, evaluation, and intervention of cases of domestic and family violence, it is important to consider cultural influences and the unique dynamics of special populations (eg, lesbian, gay, bisexual, transgender, older couples, and immigrant populations).

Intimate Partner Violence

Although IPV is most common to think of this as a man abusing a woman, abuse can occur both in homosexual relationships and in heterosexual relationships with a male victim. It is estimated that 1.5 million women and 834,700 men annually are raped and/or physically assaulted by an intimate partner. **Women are more likely to be injured, sexually assaulted, or murdered by an intimate partner and studies show that women have a one in four lifetime risk of such abuse.**

Abuse can occur in any relationship or in any socioeconomic class. Certain situations increase the likelihood, or escalate the occurrences, of abuse. These situations include changes in family life (such as pregnancy, illnesses, and deaths), economic stresses, and substance abuse. Personal and family histories of abuse also increase the likelihood of family violence. Most women do not disclose abuse to their physicians.

Numerous professional organizations, such as the American Medical Association, the American Academy of Family Physicians, and the American College of Obstetricians and Gynecologists, advocate for the routine screening of women for abuse by direct and nonjudgmental questioning. Numerous tools exist for screening, from simple questioning to more formal inventory tools. The simple question, "Do you feel safe in your home?" has a sensitivity of 8.8% and a specificity of 91.2%, so more formal testing may be necessary in some cases. Since 2013, the United States Preventive Services Task Force (USPSTF) has recommended (B grade) that clinicians regularly screen women of childbearing age for intimate partner violence. It also found insufficient evidence to assess the balance of benefits and harms of screening all elderly or vulnerable adults for abuse and neglect and found insufficient evidence to recommend routine intimate partner violence screening. The USPSTF does recommend that **all clinicians should be alert to physical and behavioral signs and symptoms associated with abuse and neglect and that direct questions about abuse are justifiable** due to high levels of undetected abuse in women and the potential value of helping these patients. Multiple studies have shown that screening does not result in harm to participants. Recommendations regarding interactions with victims of abuse include exhibiting compassionate, nonjudgmental, supportive care in a private, secure environment.

Victims of abuse can present with varied symptoms and signs suggestive of the problem. Direct physical findings can include obvious traumatic injuries, such as contusions, fractures, "black eyes," concussions, and internal bleeding. Genital, anal, or pharyngeal trauma, sexually transmitted diseases (STDs), and unintended pregnancy may be signs of sexual assault. Depression, anxiety, panic, somatoform and posttraumatic stress disorders, and suicide attempts can also result from abusive relationships.

Some signs and symptoms may be less obvious and may require numerous encounters until the finding of family violence is made. Victims of abuse may present to doctors frequently for health complaints or have physical symptoms that cannot otherwise be explained. Delays in treatment for physical injuries may be a sign of IPV. Chronic pain, frequently abdominal or pelvic pain, is commonly a sign of a history of abuse. The development of substance abuse or eating disorders may prompt inquiry into family violence as well. Children of women abused often directly witness the abuse of their mother. Children and adolescents of abused women can exhibit aggression, anxiety, bedwetting, and depression.

When abuse is identified, an initial priority is to assess the safety of the home situation. Direct questioning regarding increasing levels of violence, the presence of weapons in the home, as well as the need for a plan for safety for the victim and others at home (children, elders), is critical. Resources and support, such as shelters, community-based treatment, and advocacy programs, should be provided. It may be helpful to allow the patient to contact a shelter, law enforcement, family members, or friends, while still in the doctor's office. Multidisciplinary interventions, including family, medical, legal, mental health, and law enforcement, are often necessary.

The laws regarding clinician reporting of partner violence vary from state to state. It is important to know the statutes in your locality. Many states do not require contacting legal authorities if the victim of the abuse is a competent adult.

Child Abuse

Approximately 1 million cases of child abuse, with more than 1000 deaths, are reported each year in the United States; the number of unreported cases makes the overall prevalence much higher. Child abuse is the third leading cause of death in children between 1 and 4 years and almost 20% of child homicide victims have contact with health-care professionals within a month of their death. The situations that increase the risk of child abuse are similar to those that increase the likelihood of other family violence. These include parental depression and previous history of abuse, substance abuse, social isolation, and increased stress. Societal factors include dangerous neighborhoods and poor access to recreational resources. Children who are chronically ill or who have physical or developmental disorders may be at even higher risk. Protective factors include family support from community or relatives, parental ability to ask for help, and access to mental health resources. Identification of at-risk families and home visitation interventions has been shown to significantly reduce child abuse. Short- and long-term physical, psychological, and social consequences are often seen in the victims of child abuse.

Certain history and physical examination findings raise the suspicion for child abuse. Several presenting history and behavioral features may be associated with increased risk of maltreatment or abuse (Table 36–1). Injuries that are inconsistent with the stated history or a history that repeatedly changes with questioning should raise the suspicion of abuse. Children who are taken to numerous different physicians or emergency rooms, or who are brought in repeatedly with traumatic injuries, may be victims. Delay in seeking medical care for an injury may also be a clue to abuse. **Any serious injury in a child less than 5 years, especially in the absence of a witnessed event, should be viewed with suspicion.**

Children frequently have bruises, fractures, and other injuries that occur accidentally and it can be difficult to distinguish with certainty whether an injury is

Table 36–1 • CONCERNING FEATURES THAT MAY BE ASSOCIATED WITH CHILD ABUSE
Evolving or absent history about injury
Delay in seeking care for concerning condition
Unusual interactions between child and parent
Overly compliant child with painful medical procedures
Overly affectionate behavior from child to medical staff
Protective of abusing parent
Parental substance abuse or intoxication
Poor self-esteem in parent
History of abuse in parent's childhood
History of domestic abuse
Loss of control of parent triggered by child's behavior

Adapted from Tintinalli's Emergency Medicine: A Comprehensive Study Guide. *7th ed. New York, NY: McGraw-Hill; 2011.*

Table 36–2 • INJURIES SUGGESTIVE OF CHILD ABUSE
Stocking-and-glove burns of the extremities (immersion in scalding water)
Burns of the buttock and groin that spare the intertriginous areas (immersion in scalding water)
Centimeter-sized circular burns (cigarettes)
Multiple bruises of differing ages (most common manifestation of child abuse)
Epiphyseal separations
Multiple fractures and fractures in different stages of healing
Unexplained injury to buttocks, thighs, ears, neck
Bite marks
Bruises in the shape of a hand, belt buckle, or loops of a cord
Retinal hemorrhages ("shaken baby syndrome")
Corner or "bucket-handle" fractures of metaphysis of long bones
Spiral fracture of femur or humerus
Rib fractures, especially posteromedial fractures
Vertebral body fractures and subluxations
Digital fractures
Scapular fractures
Spinous process fractures
Sternal fractures
Complex, bilateral, or wide skull fractures
Injury to external genitalia
Sexually transmitted diseases, genital warts
Circumferential hematoma of anus (forced penetration)

accidental or intentional. However, **certain types of injuries are uncommon as accidents** (Table 36–2). The presence of these injuries is highly suggestive of child abuse. **Neglect is also a form of child abuse.** An injury or illness that occurred because of lack of appropriate supervision may be a sign of neglect. Failure to provide for basic nutritional, health-care, or safety needs may be other forms of neglect.

When an injury suspicious for child abuse is identified, attention should initially focus on treatment and protection from further injury. A complete examination should be performed and all injuries documented with drawings or photographs. An x-ray skeletal survey can be performed to look for evidence of current or previous bony injuries. Skeletal survey is typically recommended for all cases of suspected abuse in children younger than 2 years. Ophthalmologic examination should be performed to look for retinal hemorrhages. Other imaging, such as computed tomography (CT) of the head, nuclear medicine imaging, or positron emission tomography may be indicated depending on patient circumstance. Laboratory studies can be useful in both identifying disorders that might explain observed findings and finding occult or more severe injury not evident on examination. Testing for sexually transmitted illnesses may be necessary as well. The clinical findings, pertinent history, and results of evaluation should be documented carefully and legibly.

All 50 states require reporting of suspected child abuse to child protective services or other appropriate authorities (refer to local laws to determine the appropriate authority). Parents should be informed that a report is going to be made and the process that is likely to occur after the report is made in a neutral nonaccusatory manner that emphasizes your role as an advocate for the child's health and safety. Consideration must also be given to the possibility that there are other victims of abuse in the home (spouse, other children, elders). **Any health-care provider who makes a good-faith report of suspected abuse or neglect is immune from any legal action, even if the investigation reveals that no abuse occurred.** Providers may be held liable for failure to report child abuse.

Elder Abuse

Many types of elder abuse may occur, including physical, sexual, and psychological abuse, neglect, and financial exploitation. The estimated prevalence of elder abuse ranges from 2% to 10% and out of the 1 in 10 elders that may experience abuse, only 1 in 5 are reported. Along with the other risks for domestic violence, several factors unique to the care of elders may play a role. The majority of abusers are family members. Caregiver frustrations and burnout are commonly heard excuses for abuse. Abusers often have histories of mental health problems or substance abuse and have little insight into the fact that they are abusing the patient. Women older than 75 years are statistically the most abused group. **Persons who are older, more cognitively and physically debilitated, and have less access to resources are more likely to be abused or exploited.**

A history of abuse may be difficult to obtain, as the patient may fear worsening of the abuse or may not have the cognitive ability to make an accurate report. If feasible, it is **helpful to interview the patient without the presence of the caregiver.** Screening the caregiver for stress, in private, with referral for community resources may prevent abuse in the elderly. The physical examination, like in child abuse, should carefully document any injuries that are found. Suspicions of dehydration or malnutrition should be confirmed with appropriate laboratory testing, and radiographs should be performed as necessary.

By law, elder abuse should be reported to the appropriate adult protective services, but the reporting requirements vary by state. A multidisciplinary approach involving medical providers, social workers, legal authorities, and families is usually necessary to address the issues involved.

COMPREHENSION QUESTIONS

36.1 A 42-year-old woman presents to your office for evaluation of chronic abdominal pain. She has seen you multiple times for this complaint, but the workup has always been negative. On examination, her abdomen is soft and there are no peritoneal signs. She has no rash, but does have a purpuric lesion lateral to her left orbit. Which of the following is the best next step in management?

    A. Ask the patient about physical abuse and report suspicions to the local police.

    B. Ask the patient about physical abuse and provide information about local support services.

    C. Exclude a bleeding diathesis before inquiring about abuse.

    D. Order an abdominal x-ray.

    E. Refer to psychiatry.

36.2 A 7-month-old male infant presents to the emergency department (ED) with his father after a 1-day history of intractable vomiting. On examination, the child is lethargic. The anterior fontanel is closed. An abdominal x-ray shows a nonspecific bowel gas pattern and incidentally reveals a mid-shaft fracture of the right femur. When confronted about the fracture, the father states that the child climbed onto a chair and jumped off yesterday. Which of the following is the most appropriate next step in management?

A. Outpatient radiographic bone survey

B. Consulting a child abuse specialist

C. Social services consult

D. Disclosing to the parent the intention of contacting child protection services

E. Inpatient noncontrast CT of the head

36.3 Which of the following injuries is most likely to be caused by abuse of a toddler?

A. Three or four bruises on the shins and knees

B. Spiral fracture of the tibia

C. A displaced posterior rib fracture

D. A forehead laceration

36.4 An 80-year-old man who resides in a local nursing home is seen in your office for unexplained scratches on arms, and band-like bruises on wrists and ankles consistent with restraint use. The patient is mildly demented, and appears scared. There is no family to contact. Examination and laboratory results show no medical reason for easy bruising. Which of the following should be your next step?

A. Refer to nursing home social worker.

B. Contact nursing home ombudsmen program.

C. Have the patient observed by nursing home staff.

D. Contact nursing home vice president for nursing care.

E. Send the patient back to the nursing home.

ANSWERS

36.1 **B.** It is appropriate to discuss your concerns in a nonaccusatory, nonjudgmental fashion with your patient. Waiting for her to bring up the subject may result in her suffering further abuse. The reporting of the abuse of competent adults (not elders) is not mandated by law in most states. You should offer assistance, evaluate her safety, and provide her with information regarding available services in the area. There is no reason to exclude a bleeding diathesis before approaching the subject of abuse.

36.2 **E.** This child has injuries consistent with physical abuse. In children less than 1 year, 75% of fractures are due to abuse. Moreover, the shape of a fracture—spiral, transverse, etc—is less important in suspected abuse than the age of the child and location of the fracture. The purported history of fall is inconsistent with the developmental abilities of a 7-month-old infant. The infant has intractable vomiting and is lethargic on examination. These findings are worrisome for neurologic damage. An inpatient evaluation with CT should be ordered to exclude intracranial bleed, since this disorder may lead to irreversible brain damage or even death if not identified quickly and protects the child from further abuse while workup is being completed. Outpatient management with close follow-up and referral to child protective services is appropriate if caregivers are not suspected of being the abusers. While a radiographic bone survey is indicated in all children less than 2 years with suspected abuse, it should be done after excluding more urgent conditions. If you are concerned that the child may be at further risk of abuse and that notifying the parents of your concerns would put the child at immediate danger, it is not necessary to notify the parents of your report to law enforcement or Child Protective Services. However, in most cases, the parents should have the opportunity to discuss these concerns with you. Lastly, the anterior fontanel closes between 4 and 26 months (average 13.8 months). It may bulge in conditions, such as meningitis or intracranial hemorrhage, which increase intracranial pressure.

36.3 **C.** A posterior rib fracture is often the result of grabbing and squeezing the chest violently. It is very suspicious for abuse. A spiral fracture of the tibia is known as a "toddler's fracture" and is a common injury that is often confused with abuse, but not often caused by abuse. Bruises on the anterior and over bony prominences such as the shins, knees, and forehead injuries are common from falls while learning to walk. Well-padded areas that are bruised such as the thigh, buttock, and cheeks increase likelihood of abuse.

36.4 **B.** Clinicians have a legal duty to report possible elder to abuse to adult protective Services in their community. If the patient is living in a nursing care facility, each state has nursing home ombudsmen who can investigate. The ombudsmen program is mandated by the Federal Older Americans Act. If you feel that this patient is in immediate danger, he can be admitted for evaluation of bruising while the ombudsmen and local adult protective services investigate for substandard care or abuse at the nursing care facility.

CLINICAL PEARLS

▶ Suspected child and elder abuse must be reported. Good-faith reports of suspected abuse are a shield to lawsuits; failure to report can result in legal action against the physician.

▶ When seeing a suspected abuse victim, always consider the possibility that there could be other abuse victims in the household.

REFERENCES

Berkowitz C. Child abuse and neglect. In: Tintinalli JE, Stapczynski J, Ma O, et al., eds *Tintinalli's Emergency Medicine: A Comprehensive Study Guide.* 7th ed. New York, NY: McGraw-Hill; 2011.

Cronholm P, Fogarty C, Ambuel B, Harrison S. Intimate partner violence. *Am Fam Physician.* 2011 May 15;83(10):1165-1172.

Eyler AE, Cohen M. Case studies in partner violence. *Am Fam Physician.* 1999;60:2569-2576.

Gibbs LM, Mosqueda L. The importance of reporting mistreatment of the elderly. *Am Fam Physician.* 2007 Mar 1;75(5):628.

Hancock M. Intimate partner violence and abuse. In: Tintinalli JE, Stapczynski J, Ma O, et al., eds. *Tintinalli's Emergency Medicine: A Comprehensive Study Guide.* 7th ed. New York, NY: McGraw-Hill; 2011.

Hoover R, Polson, M. Detecting elder abuse and neglect: assessment and intervention. *Am Fam Physician.* 2014 Mar 15;89(6):453-460.

Kodner C, Wetherton A. Diagnosis and management of physical abuse in children. *Am Fam Physician.* 2013 Nov 15;88(10):669-675.

Krennerich E. Trauma, burns, and common critical care emergencies. In: Engorn B, Flerlage J, eds. *The Johns Hopkins Hospital: The Harriet Lane Handbook: A Manual for Pediatric House Officers.* 20th ed. Philadelphia, PA: Saunders; 2015.

United States Preventive Services Task Force. Intimate partner violence and abuse of elderly and vulnerable adults: screening. January 2013. Available at: www.uspreventativeservicestaskforce.org. Accessed February 21, 2015.

A 12-year-old boy is brought to the physician's office with right thigh pain and a limp. His mother has noticed him limping for the past week or so. He denies any injury to his leg but says that it hurts some when he plays basketball with his friends. He denies back pain, hip pain, or ankle pain. He occasionally gets some pain in the right knee but does not have any swelling or bruising. He has no significant medical history, does not take any medications regularly, and otherwise feels fine. On examination, he is an overweight adolescent. His vital signs and a general physical examination are normal. When you have him walk, he has a prominent limp. You note that he seems to keep his weight on his left leg for a greater proportion of his gait cycle than he does on the right leg. Examination of his back reveals a full range of motion, no tenderness, and no muscle spasm. He gets pain in the right hip when it is passively internally rotated. When the hip is passively flexed, there is a noticeable external rotation. There is no thigh muscle atrophy. His right knee and the remainder of his orthopedic examination are normal.

► What is the most appropriate test to order first for this patient?
► What is the most likely diagnosis?
► What complication could occur if this problem is not diagnosed and treated?

ANSWERS TO CASE 37:
Limping in Children

Summary: An overweight 12-year-old boy presents for evaluation of a limp and thigh pain. There is no history of injury or trauma. He is found to have pain on internal rotation of the hip and his hip externally rotates when passively flexed. He bears weight more on his left leg than his right while walking.

- **Most appropriate test to order:** X-ray of the right hip

- **Most likely diagnosis:** Slipped capital femoral epiphysis

- **Complication for which he is at risk:** Avascular necrosis of the hip

ANALYSIS

Objectives

1. Develop a differential diagnosis of the most likely causes of leg pain and limping in children.

2. Know common causes of leg pain and limping in children of different ages.

3. Know appropriate examination, laboratory, and radiologic evaluation for the limping child.

Considerations

Leg pain is a common complaint in childhood. The **most common causes of leg pain in children are acute trauma** (sprains, strains, contusions) or **overuse injuries.** However, leg pain and limping can be a sign of a more serious, even life-threatening, pathology. Learning an approach to the evaluation and the common diagnoses involved may help in the identification of these problems earlier, when a better outcome is more likely.

To understand a limp, it is first important to understand the normal gait. Gait is composed of two phases: the "swing" and the "stance" phases. The stance phase is the weight-bearing phase and accounts for approximately 60% of the gait cycle. The swing phase is the non–weight-bearing phase, when the foot lifts off the ground and is propelled forward. The **antalgic gait occurs when the stance phase of gait is shortened on the side of pain, usually because of pain during weight bearing.** Antalgic gait is the most common type of limp and is the type of gait described in this case.

There are many causes of limp with pain in children; some of the more common causes may be broadly categorized as being primarily orthopedic, reactive, infectious, rheumatologic, or neoplastic. The prevalence of the specific diagnoses also varies by age. Limp without pain is usually due to congenital orthopedic anomalies or neuromuscular disorders.

In the specific case presented, there are several symptoms and signs that make the diagnosis of slipped capital femoral epiphysis (SCFE) likely. The absence of a specific injury is significant, as SCFE is the most common nontraumatic hip pathology in adolescents. The initial complaint of thigh pain may lead to other considerations, but **hip pathology will frequently present with pain in the groin, thigh, or even the knee.** The patient's age and body habitus are typical for SCFE, which is classically described as occurring most often in overweight adolescent males. Pain with internal rotation of the hip and the finding of external rotation on passive flexion of the affected hip are also suggestive of SCFE.

APPROACH TO:
Limping With Pain in Children

DEFINITIONS

AVASCULAR NECROSIS: Death of living bone tissue caused by disruption of blood flow

DYSPLASIA: Abnormal growth or development

CLINICAL APPROACH

As always, the initial approach should include a good focused history and physical. The clinician should ask questions about recent trauma, onset, and duration of limp, recent illnesses (viral, pharyngitis, rashes, tick bites, diarrhea, urethritis). Past medical history, previous levels of function, and family history of musculoskeletal disorders can help with diagnosis. Associated symptoms like fever, weight loss, anorexia, or pain are especially important. A key characteristic in the evaluation of the child with a limp is assessing whether there is pain or no pain. In an antalgic gait, the cause of the pain may range from the back to the foot (Table 37–1). Therefore, unless there is an obvious source of pain, the examination should include assessment of the back, pelvis, buttock, leg, and foot. In the child who clings to the parent, separating the child from the parent will allow the clinician to observe the child's gait when they walk back to the parent. The child who walks stiffly may be avoiding moving the spine indicating a possible discitis. Those with nonantalgic gait abnormalities (Trendelenburg gait, inability to dorsiflex the foot, locked knees, toe walking) can have congenital, neurologic, or limb length disorders. Inspecting the feet may show clawing of the toes or cavus deformity, which are signs of neuromuscular conditions.

Because hip pathology often presents with vague pain and hip conditions are likely to need emergent treatment, **evaluation of the hip may be the most important part of the examination of a patient in whom the site of pathology is not immediately obvious.** Restricted internal rotation appears to be the most sensitive marker of hip pathology in children, followed by a lack of abduction. Internal rotation of the hip increases the intracapsular pressure within the acetabulum. Pain during a leg roll (supine child with extended hip and knee; one examiner stabilizes the pelvis while another rolls leg internally and externally) and limited internal rotation of less than 30 degrees may indicate infectious or orthopedic hip pathology. The FABER test (*Flexion, ABduction, External Rotation*—the ipsilateral ankle placed

Table 37–1 • COMMON CAUSES OF LIMP WITH PAIN IN CHILDREN

Orthopedic
- Fracture
- Stress fracture
- Pathologic fracture through tumor or cyst
- Sprain/strain/contusion
- Slipped capital femoral epiphysis
- Early Legg-Calvé-Perthes disease

Reactive
- Toxic synovitis
- Transient synovitis following viral infection
- Rheumatic fever

Infectious
- Septic arthritis
- Osteomyelitis
- Cellulitis
- Discitis
- Gonococcal arthritis

Rheumatologic
- Juvenile rheumatoid arthritis
- Systemic lupus erythematosus

Tumor
- Benign tumors (osteoid osteoma, osteoblastoma)
- Ewing sarcoma
- Osteosarcoma

Other
- "Growing pains"

on the contralateral knee and mild downward pressure placed on the ipsilateral knee) can find pathology located in the sacroiliac joint, often seen in rheumatologic disorders. Bone pain or point tenderness can indicate osteomyelitis or malignancy. Limps from overuse injuries of the foot (eg, Sever disease) and knee disorders (eg, Osgood-Schlatter disease) can occur. If there is significant abdominal pain on history or examination, consider an acute abdomen or psoas abscess.

X-rays should be obtained when the differential indicates a likelihood of bony abnormalities. An ultrasound of the hip is more sensitive for an effusion of the hip and can be considered. In nonverbal children, x-rays from hip to feet can find a fracture in a significant minority of children with limp. A complete blood count (CBC) should be drawn if there is concern of an infection, inflammatory arthritis, or malignancy. An erythrocyte sedimentation rate (ESR) and C-reactive protein (CRP) should be considered in evaluating infectious and rheumatologic etiologies. Consider Lyme disease in endemic areas, as this can mimic both infectious and rheumatologic causes of hip disorders. If there was a recent pharyngitis, consider antistreptolysin (ASO) titers. In teens with history of urethritis or febrile diarrhea, consider urine chlamydial antigens or stool cultures for possible Reiter syndrome. Any joint where septic arthritis is considered should have a joint aspiration and evaluation of synovial fluid. Fever greater than 99.5°F and ESR greater than 20 is

Table 37–2 • COMMON ORTHOPEDIC CAUSES OF LIMP WITHOUT PAIN IN CHILDREN
Congential dislocation (developmental dysplasia) of the hip
Spastic hemiplegia (cerebral palsy)
Legg-Calvé-Perthes (subacute and chronic)
Leg-length discrepancy
Proximal focal femoral dysplasia
Congenital short femur
Congenital bowing of the tibia

Data from Hollister JR. Rheumatic diseases. In: Hay WW, Levin MJ, Sondheimer JM, et al, eds. Current Pediatric Diagnosis and Treatment. *15th ed. New York, NY: McGraw-Hill; 2001:734; Leet AI, Skaggs DL. Evaluation of the acutely limping child.* Am Fam Physician. *2000;61: 1011-1018; and Crawford AH. Orthopedics. In: Rudolph CD, Rudolph AM, Hostetter MK, eds.* Rudolph's Pediatrics. *21st ed., New York, NY: McGraw-Hill; 2003: 2419-2458.*

97% sensitive for septic hip joint. Testing of the fluid should include culture for gonorrhea in teens that are sexually active.

The evaluation of limping without pain (Table 37–2) should include measurements for leg length discrepancies (measure umbilicus to medial malleolus) and observation for muscular atrophy or limb deformity. Barlow (hip and knee flexed 90 degrees, hold the knee and attempt to displace the thigh posterior), Ortolani (guided abduction), and Galeazzi (knee height discrepancy when patient lies supine with ankles to buttocks and hips and knees flexed) tests can be used to assess for congenital hip abnormalities and femoral length discrepancies.

Infants and Toddlers

Common causes of limping in children in this age group are septic arthritis, fractures, and complications of congenital hip dysplasia. **Septic arthritis** is usually monoarticular and associated with systemic signs such as fever. In young infants, the symptoms may be less obvious, such as crying, irritability, and poor feeding. Children who are ambulatory (crawlers or walkers) will often refuse to do anything that puts weight on the affected joint because of pain. Infection of a joint causes a septic effusion, which raises the pressure inside of the joint capsule. **Children with a septic hip joint will often lay with their hip flexed, abducted, and externally rotated**, which helps to reduce the pain, and they will have significant pain with any internal rotation or extension of the joint. Children with a septic joint will usually have an elevated white blood cell (WBC) count, ESR, and CRP. Definitive diagnosis comes from joint aspiration. **Any suspected septic joint must be aspirated.** In younger infants (4 months or younger), group B *Streptococcus* and *Staphylococcus aureus* are the most common pathogens involved. In older infants and children under the age of 5, *S aureus* and *Streptococcus pyogenes* are the usual causes. Treatment is urgent surgical irrigation and debridement, along with antibiotics.

Unsuspected **fractures**—either stress fractures or traumatic fractures—can present with pain and limping. Abuse must be suspected if the injury is inconsistent with the history presented, if the history changes with repeated questioning, if the child is said to have performed an act outside of his developmental ability, or if a fracture usually associated with abuse is found (see Case 36). However, the **history**

Table 37–3 • RED FLAGS REQUIRING IMMEDIATE THOROUGH INVESTIGATION IN A CHILD WITH NONTRAUMATIC LIMP
Child <3 years old
Child unable to bear weight
Fever in child with limp
Child with comorbid systemic illness
Child >9 years old with pain or restricted hip movements

Data from Perry DC, Bruce C. Evaluating the child who presents with an acute limp. BMJ. 2010 Aug 20;341:c4250. doi: 10.1136/bmj.c4250.

may not reveal the source of the injury, as a child may fall outside of the view of the parent (see Table 37–3). **A traumatic injury may not result in limping or in complete immobility, but may cause a change in how the child ambulates.** For example, a child who previously walked and now refuses to walk but will crawl, may have an injury of the lower leg or foot.

A **toddler's fracture** is one example of an unsuspected fracture that may present primarily as a limp or a refusal to walk. This fracture is a **spiral fracture of the tibia that results from twisting while the foot is planted.** The diagnosis may be suspected in the setting of an acute limp or change in ambulation, a normal examination of the knee and upper leg, and tenderness of the tibia. It can be confirmed with a plain film x-ray. Undiagnosed **congenital developmental dysplasia of the hip (DDH) may present as a painless limp that is present from the time that the child learns to walk.** All newborns and infants should have their hips examined for instability or dislocation. If undiagnosed, contractures may form that limit movement of the hip. When the child learns to walk, the child will have a painless limp. The diagnosis may be confirmed by x-rays showing abnormal hip alignment. If the problem is found in the first few weeks of life, the child can be treated with splinting of the hip and normal development usually follows. If diagnosed late, the treatment is often surgical.

Young Children

Transient synovitis is a self-limited inflammatory response that is a common cause of hip pain in children. It occurs typically in children ages 3 to 10, is more common in boys than in girls, and **often follows a viral infection.** It is frequently seen as gradually increasing hip pain that results in a limp or refusal to walk. These children have a low-grade or no fever, a normal WBC count, and a normal ESR. On examination, there is pain with internal rotation of the hip and the overall range of motion is limited by pain. X-rays are either normal or show some nonspecific swelling. In a situation where the patient is afebrile, has pain-free rotation of hip greater than 30 degrees, has a normal WBC count, normal ESR, CRP, and short-term follow-up can be assured, the patient can be followed clinically and should improve in a few days. If these conditions are not met and the diagnosis of a septic joint is considered, or if a patient followed expectantly continues to worsen, an aspiration should be done. Kocher criteria are often utilized to assess risk for septic arthritis in children. The four criteria are fever greater than 101.3°F (38.5°C), non–weight-bearing, ESR greater than 40, WBC count greater than 12,000. Zero criteria present equals less than 0.2% risk, one criteria is 3%, two criteria is 40%, three criteria is 93%, and four criteria is almost 100% chance of septic arthritis. **A septic joint will have a purulent aspirate with a WBC count greater than 50,000/μL; transient synovitis will have a yellow/clear aspirate with a lower WBC count (<10,000/μL).**

Legg-Calvé-Perthes (LCP) disease is an **avascular necrosis of the femoral head** that typically occurs in children ages 4 to 8. It is much more common in boys than in girls. Any disruption of blood flow to the femoral capital epiphysis, such as trauma or infection, may cause avascular necrosis. In LCP disease, the etiology of the disruption of blood flow is unknown. Children typically have a gradual onset of hip, thigh, or knee pain, and limping over a few months. Early in the course, x-rays of the hip may appear normal. Later radiographic findings include collapse, flattening, and widening of the femoral head. Bone scans or magnetic resonance imaging (MRI) may be necessary to confirm the diagnosis. The **treatment is usually conservative**, with protection of the joint and efforts to maintain range of motion. Children who develop more severe necrosis or who develop the disease at older ages may have a worse outcome and a higher risk of developing degenerative arthritis.

Adolescents

The capital femoral epiphysis is the growth plate that connects the metaphysis (femoral head) to the diaphysis (shaft of the femur). A **slipped capital femoral epiphysis** is a separation of this growth plate, which results in the femoral head being medially and posteriorly displaced. This may be caused by an acute injury, but more often is not. It is most often seen in overweight adolescent boys and presents as pain in the hip, thigh, or knee along with a limp. Examination reveals **limited internal rotation** and obligate **external rotation when the hip is passively flexed**. Early x-rays may show only widening of the epiphysis; later x-rays can show the slippage of the femoral head in relation to the femoral neck. The treatment is surgical pinning of the femoral head. These patients must be closely followed, as approximately 20% to 50% will develop avascular necrosis and 33% will develop SCFE in the contralateral hip.

Other causes of limb pain are common in adolescents. Sprains, strains, and overuse injuries are the most common cause of limb pain in this population, and are usually readily diagnosed on history and examination (see Case 12). Sexually active adolescents or teens are at risk for sexually transmitted diseases (STDs) and their complications, including gonococcal arthritis. In this population, an appropriate history, sexual history, and review of systems are necessary.

All Ages

Septic arthritis, fractures, neuromuscular disorders, and neoplasms can cause a limp in children of all ages. Night sweats, anorexia, weight loss, and pain that wakens the child at night are suspicious for malignancy. "Growing pains" is a diagnosis of exclusion. It should be considered if the pain is only at night, is bilateral, is not present during the day, and if no other pathology is found.

> ## CASE CORRELATION
> • See also Cases 3 (Joint Pain) and 5 (Well-Child Care).

COMPREHENSION QUESTIONS

37.1 A 6-year-old young boy is brought in for evaluation of a painful hip. He has been limping and not wanting to walk for the past 2 days. He has had no obvious injury. He feels a little better if he is given some ibuprofen. He has not had a fever and does not have any other current symptoms, although he had "the flu" last week. On examination, his vital signs are normal. His right hip has some pain with internal rotation. He walks with a pronounced limp. Which of the following statements is most appropriate?

A. He can be sent home with a prescription for ibuprofen.

B. He should have a CBC and ESR.

C. He should have an aspiration of his hip in the office.

D. If he has a normal x-ray, no further workup is needed.

37.2 An 18-month-old African-American girl is brought into your office because she has been crying and stopped walking today. She will crawl, however. Her mother denies any injury to the child. On examination, she is crying but consolable in her mother's arms. She has bruising and swelling just proximal to the left ankle. An x-ray reveals a spiral fracture of the tibia. Which of the following best describes your advice to the mother of the patient?

A. You are going to report this to child protective services as suspected abuse.

B. You are going to refer the child for a bone biopsy because this is a pathologic fracture that may represent a neoplasm.

C. This is a common fracture resulting from twisting on a planted foot.

D. You should draw blood to evaluate for sickle cell disease, which may cause infarction of the bone.

37.3   A 2-year-old boy is brought in with fever and poor feeding. He started getting sick yesterday and has worsened significantly today. He has had no recent illnesses or injuries, and no known ill contacts. On examination, his temperature is 101°F (38.3°C), is tachycardic, and appears ill. He is lying on his back with his left leg flexed and abducted at the hip. A head, ears, eyes, nose, and throat (HEENT) examination is normal, the heart is tachycardic but regular, and the lungs are clear. The abdomen is nontender and has normal bowel sounds. He screams in pain when you move his left leg from its resting position. Blood work reveals an elevated WBC count of 15,000 mm^3 and an ESR of 45 mm/h (normal: 0-10). An x-ray of his left hip shows a widened joint space but no fractures. Which of the following is your next step at this point?

A.   Oral antibiotic and follow-up in 1 day

B.   MRI of the hip and referral to an orthopedist

C.   Anti-inflammatory medication and close follow-up

D.   Hip joint aspiration

37.4   A 6-year-old boy appears in the office with a 2-month history of slight limp. He has no significant past medical history and takes no medications. He has normal vital signs and is noted to have antalgic gait and decreased range of motion in the left hip (internal rotation more limited). He has mild pain on palpation of the anterior capsule on the left side. X-ray shows fragmentation of the femoral head. Which of the following is the most likely diagnosis?

A.   Toxic synovitis of hip

B.   Avascular necrosis of hip (Legg-Calvé-Perthes)

C.   Slipped capital femoral epiphysis

D.   Femoral shaft fracture

ANSWERS

37.1   **B.** The case presented is suspicious for transient synovitis following a viral illness. A CBC and ESR should be drawn. With a normal CBC and ESR, and if follow-up can be assured, this child could be treated expectantly, given an oral nonsteroidal anti-inflammatory drug (NSAID) with the expectation of a recovery in a few days.

37.2   **C.** The case presented is classic for a toddler's fracture. Spiral fractures of other long bones (femur, humerus) are more suspicious for abuse. Orthopedic referral is appropriate for management, but a bone biopsy or further workup is not necessary at this time.

37.3   **D.** The child in this case has all of the symptoms and signs of a septic hip joint. This situation demands a joint aspiration to confirm the diagnosis. If it is confirmed, he should be promptly referred for urgent surgical management.

37.4 **B.** This child is in the correct gender and age group with signs, symptoms, and radiologic findings associated with Legg-Calvé-Perthes disease. It is often a self-healing disorder. Treatment is focused on limiting pain and avoiding functional loss. Depending on severity and age, treatment may include watchful waiting, physical therapy, casting, and surgery.

CLINICAL PEARLS

▶ Hip pathology may not cause hip pain; it may cause groin, thigh, or knee pain instead.

▶ Because of the high risk of bilateral disease, follow-up in SCFE cases should include examination and x-rays of the unaffected hip until the growth plate closes.

▶ A limp that is nonantalgic usually does not need urgent evaluation.

REFERENCES

Herring JA. The musculoskeletal system. In: Rudolph CD, Rudolph AM, Lister G, et al., eds. *Rudolph's Pediatrics.* 22nd ed. New York, NY: McGraw-Hill; 2011:839-876.

Peck M. Slipped capital femoral epiphysis: diagnosis and management. *Am Fam Physician.* 2010 Aug 1;82(3):258-262.

Perry DC, Bruce C. Evaluating the child who presents with an acute limp. *BMJ.* 2010 Aug 20;341:c4250.

Sawyer JR, Kapoor M. The limping child: a systematic approach to diagnosis. *Am Fam Physician.* 2009 Feb 1;79(3):215-224.

On the third postoperative day following an uneventful open appendectomy under spinal anesthesia, a 70-year-old man with history of hypertension and benign prostatic hyperplasia (BPH) suddenly developed a temperature of 102.5°F (39.1°C) accompanied by chills and vomiting. Just before surgery, a urethral catheter was placed, which was removed 24 hours later, only to be replaced when he was unable to urinate on his own on the second postoperative day. Physical examination is unremarkable except for costovertebral angle tenderness and suprapubic tenderness. He has no abdominal guarding or rebound tenderness.

▶ What is the most likely cause of postoperative fever?
▶ What is the next diagnostic step?
▶ What is the most appropriate treatment at this time?

ANSWERS TO CASE 38:
Postoperative Fever

Summary: A 70-year-old man with history of hypertension and BPH who underwent open appendectomy under spinal anesthesia develops fever, chills, and vomiting on the third postoperative day. Physical examination shows costovertebral tenderness and suprapubic tenderness. He has a urethral catheter in place because of a problem in voiding.

- **Most likely cause of postoperative fever:** Urinary tract infection (UTI) with probable pyelonephritis
- **The next diagnostic step:** Urinalysis (UA) and urine culture
- **Treatment:** Antibiotics

ANALYSIS

Objectives

1. Identify the different causes of postoperative fever based on the timing of onset, nature of surgery, and patient's risk factors.

2. Understand the different clinical presentations that point to the etiology of postoperative fever.

Considerations

This 70-year-old man with history of hypertension and BPH is at high risk for UTI because he recently underwent a pelvic procedure under spinal anesthesia and because he has urinary retention secondary to BPH. In addition, the use of a urethral catheter poses an additional risk for bacterial seeding of the urinary bladder. Suprapubic pain and costovertebral tenderness are physical findings suggestive of UTI, most likely acute pyelonephritis. For those without a urethral catheter, symptoms such as dysuria, urgency, and frequency are common. UTI is high on the list of causes of fever in the third postoperative day, although it could also occur anytime during the postoperative period. Urinalysis may detect presence of bacteriuria, pyuria, nitrites, and leukocyte esterase. Urine culture would determine the type of offending organism, the most common of which are *Escherichia coli*, *Proteus*, *Klebsiella*, *Staphylococcus epidermidis*, *Pseudomonas*, and *Candida*. In this patient, the urethral catheter needs to be changed now and discontinued as soon as he is able to void his own. Symptomatic patients and those who are at high risk for infection are usually treated with appropriate IV antibiotics according to the most likely pathogens. The antibiotics subsequently can be adjusted based on culture results. Blood cultures should be ordered if urosepsis is suspected. Most importantly, it is crucial to address and treat the cause of urinary retention (eg, BPH, kidney stone) to prevent recurrence and avoid complications.

APPROACH TO:
Postoperative Fever

DEFINITIONS

DRUG FEVER: Fever that coincides with the administration of a particular drug and cannot otherwise be explained by clinical and laboratory findings. Resolution of the fever occurs with discontinuation of the suspected drug. Drugs that are usually implicated are β-lactams, sulfa derivatives, anticonvulsants, allopurinol, heparin, and amphotericin B.

MALIGNANT HYPERTHERMIA: A rare autosomal dominant disorder characterized by fever of greater than 104°F (40°C), tachycardia, metabolic acidosis, rhabdomyolysis, and calcium accumulation in skeletal muscle leading to rigidity. This may occur up to 24 hours after exposure to anesthetic agents such as halothane and succinylcholine. Treatment includes discontinuing offending agents and supportive therapy, such as antipyretics, oxygen hyperventilation, cooling blankets, sodium bicarbonate for acidosis, and dantrolene IV.

SURGICAL SITE INFECTION (SSI): A concept introduced by the Centers for Disease Control and Prevention (CDC) and various consensus panels to replace the term surgical wound infection. This refers to any infection that occurs in the site of surgery within 30 days of an operative procedure or within 1 year with implants. SSIs are classified as superficial, deep, or organ/space infections. SSI is a common nosocomial infection.

CLINICAL APPROACH

Fever (defined as >38°C/100.4°F) is the most common postoperative complication, occurring in 50% of major surgery in the immediate postoperative period. **As an integral part of informed consent prior to surgery, patients need to be made aware by the physician of the possibility of experiencing postoperative febrile episodes.** In addition, adequate preoperative evaluation, which includes performing a history and physical examination to identify risk factors, medications, nutritional status, and comorbid conditions, is imperative to avoid possible life-threatening situations during the perioperative period. Preoperative and perioperative strategies can be used to reduce the risk of developing a postoperative fever (Table 38–1). Fortunately, postoperative fever typically resolves spontaneously and most of the time does not necessarily indicate the presence of infection.

The etiology of postoperative fever could be infectious or noninfectious (Tables 38–2 and 38–3). Most postoperative fevers are not infectious, but require a good thorough history and physical to rule infectious causes out. The mnemonic "**5 Ws**" helps in remembering the most common causes of postoperative fever in roughly the order of frequency: **wind** (pneumonia), **water** (UTI), **wound** (SSI), **walking** (deep venous thrombosis [DVT]), and **wonder drugs** (drug fever). When a surgical patient develops fever, the differential diagnosis and investigative methods

Table 38–1 • STRATEGIES TO REDUCE THE RISK OF POSTOPERATIVE FEVER
Preoperative Interventions
• Optimize nutritional status. • Smoking cessation. • Treat any existing active infections. • Optimize management of existing medical conditions (eg, diabetes). • Reduce dosage of immunosuppressive therapies (when indicated).
Perioperative Interventions
• Administer perioperative antibiotics. • Use noninvasive ventilation. • If intubation necessary, use pneumonia prevention protocols. • Remove catheters, IV lines, tubes, and drains as soon as safe. • Change lines after 72-96 h if they are still needed. • DVT prophylaxis using early mobilization, sequential compression devices, subcutaneous heparin, or low-molecular-weight heparin.

Abbreviation: DVT, deep venous thrombosis.

are directed by the timing of the fever, the type of surgery performed, the preexisting clinical conditions, and the presenting symptoms. Comorbid conditions that increase risk for infectious postoperative fevers include increasing age, frailty, smoking, diabetes, and immunosuppression. A thorough physical examination should be initiated, followed by inspection of the surgical site, a review of all medications, and a consideration of hospital-related causes (IV lines and catheters). In the absence of significant risk factors and clear lack of clinical and physical signs of infection, laboratory tests may not be required.

Tissue trauma during surgery stimulates an inflammatory response that leads to release of pyrogenic cytokines (ie, interleukin, tumor necrosis factor, interferons) from the tissues. In general, more extensive surgical procedures are associated with more tissue trauma and a greater degree of fever response. Elevated levels of bacterial endotoxins and exotoxins that are released from the endogenous gut flora of the colon as a result of surgical complications also elicit the same inflammatory response. This reaction leads to elevation of the thermoregulatory set point and production of fever (temperature >100.4°F [38°C]). This explains why suppression of cytokine release by nonsteroidal anti-inflammatory drugs (NSAIDs), steroids, or acetaminophen may alleviate fever and enhance patient comfort.

There are few causes of **fever in the immediate postoperative period**. Medications and blood products are commonly associated with fevers immediately postoperative. A dangerous cause in this period is **malignant hyperthermia**, which is an inherited disorder characterized by markedly elevated temperature, up to 104°F (40°C), typically within 30 minutes after induction of inhalational anesthesia (ie, halothane) or depolarizing muscle relaxant (ie, succinylcholine). Another cause of immediate postoperative fever is **bacteremia**, which occurs more commonly in urologic procedures that involve instrumentation, for example, transurethral resection of the prostate. Gram-negative bacteria are the most common pathogen. Within 30 to 45 minutes, the patient develops chills and temperature that could exceed

Table 38–2 • COMMON CAUSES OF POSTOPERATIVE FEVER

Approximate Onset of Fever	Infectious	Noninfectious
Intraoperative up to 24 h after surgery	Preexisting infection	Surgical trauma
	Bacteremia from urologic procedures	Medications
	Intraperitoneal leak (up to 36 h)	Blood products (at time of transfusion)
	Invasive soft-tissue infection	Malignant hyperthermia
	Toxic shock syndrome	
1 d to 1 wk from surgery	UTI (often with indwelling urethral catheters or following genitourinary procedures)	Acute myocardial infarction
	Pneumonia (eg, ventilator-associated or aspiration)	Alcohol/drug withdrawal
	SSI	Gout
	Catheter-related infection	Pancreatitis
	Preexisting infection	Pulmonary embolism
	Cellulitis	Superficial vein thrombophlebitis (often at IV site)
	Viral upper respiratory tract infection	Benign postoperative fever (diagnosis of exclusion)
1 to 4 wk after surgery	SSI	Medication toxicity
	Pseudomembranous colitis	DVT
	Antibiotic-associated diarrhea (ie, *Clostridium difficile*)	Pulmonary embolism
	Catheter-related infection (ie, central venous catheters)	Thrombophlebitis (particularly in those with impaired mobility)
	Device-related infections	
	Abscess	
>1 mo after surgery	Blood-transfusion viral and parasitic infections (ie, hepatitis, CMV, HIV, toxoplasmosis, *Plasmodium malariae*, babesiosis)	Postpericardiotomy syndrome
	Infective endocarditis	
	Postpericardiotomy syndrome (following cardiac surgery)	
	SSI	
	Device-related infections	
	Vascular graft infection	

Abbreviations: DVT, deep venous thrombosis; SSI, surgical site infection; UTI, urinary tract infection.

Table 38–3 • OTHER CAUSES OF POSTOPERATIVE FEVER WITH VARIABLE TIMING OF ONSET

Infectious	Noninfectious
Abscess	Withdrawal reaction from drugs/alcohol
Sinusitis	Subarachnoid hemorrhage
Otitis media	Bowel infarction
Parotitis	Pancreatitis
Meningitis	Hyperthyroidism/thyroid storm
Acalculous cholecystitis	Dehydration
Osteomyelitis	Acute hepatic necrosis
Bacteremia	Hypoadrenalism/addisonian crisis/acute adrenal insufficiency
Empyema	Neoplastic fever
Fungal sepsis	Suture reaction
Hepatitis	Systemic inflammatory response syndrome (SIRS)
Decubitus ulcers	Pheochromocytoma
Perineal infections	Lymphoma
Peritonitis	Hematoma
Pharyngitis	Seroma
Tracheobronchitis	Myocardial infarction/stroke
	Gout/pseudogout
	Transfusion reaction
	Organ transplant–related infection
	Neuroleptic malignant syndrome

104°F (40°C). Accompanying symptoms such as tachycardia, tachypnea, oliguria, and hypotension are common.

If fever occurs within 36 hours postlaparotomy, there are two important infectious etiologies to keep in mind—**bowel injury with leakage of gastrointestinal contents into the peritoneum** and **invasive soft-tissue wound infection** caused by β-hemolytic streptococci or *Clostridium* species. The former is accompanied by hemodynamic instability. Much less common in this setting is **toxic shock syndrome** caused by *Staphylococcus aureus*.

Within the first 48 to 72 postoperative hours, **atelectasis** (partial collapse of peripheral alveoli) causes 90% of pulmonary complications of surgery, particularly following abdominal and thoracoabdominal procedures. Contrary to popular belief, its close association with early postoperative fever is probably coincidental. The alveolar collapse is compounded by the loss of functional residual capacity in almost all patients and 50% reduction of vital capacity intraoperatively. Chest x-ray may reveal discoid infiltrate and an elevated hemidiaphragm. Although fever is not likely a consideration, hypoxemia, pneumonia, and scarring that can lead to bronchiectasis can be a consequence of atelectasis.

Instructing the patient on deep inspiration and coughing, the use of incentive spirometry, and the provision of adequate pain control can facilitate the opening of the alveoli. Without resolution of atelectasis, **pneumonia** may ensue. Patients who are on mechanical ventilators are at highest risk for pneumonia (ventilator-associated pneumonia). Fever associated with productive cough, pulmonary crackles, worsening oxygenation, elevation of white blood counts (WBCs), positive sputum culture, and new infiltrates in chest x-ray are the usual indicators of pulmonary infection. Postoperative pneumonia is typically polymicrobial. Enterobacteriaceae and *S aureus* or Enterobacteriaceae and streptococci are common bacterial combinations. Appropriate use of broad-spectrum IV antibiotic therapy is the treatment. **Aspiration** as the possible cause of pneumonia should be suspected in the elderly, those who reside in a nursing home, and those with neurologic dysphagia, compromised cough reflex, altered mentation, endotracheal intubation, and gastroesophageal reflux disease (GERD). Antibiotics are typically given following a witnessed aspiration and discontinued after 48 to 72 hours with no development of infiltrates. **Gram-negative coverage is required for aspiration pneumonia**, with the current agents of choice being piperacillin/tazobactam, meropenem, or cefepime with metronidazole. Vancomycin can be considered to cover for methicillin-resistant *S aureus* (MRSA). It is also around this time that **UTI** should be entertained as part of differential diagnosis. Mild UTIs can be treated with similar agents or with a third-generation cephalosporin or fluoroquinolone. For severe cases or if drug-resistant bacteria are suspected, carbapenems are recommended.

The patient with persistent fever 5 to 7 days after surgery needs to have a thorough examination of the operative site to check for signs of infection, which include erythema, pain, local edema, and purulent discharge. **Surgical site infections** (SSIs) have markedly decreased through wide practice of aseptic technique and team-based perioperative management protocols. Patients at high risk of wound infection are those who underwent lengthy surgical procedure, received blood transfusion, are malnourished, are immunosuppressed, and those who have diabetes mellitus. Prophylactic antibiotics should be given within 1 hour before surgery and discontinued within 24 hours after surgery to lower the risk of SSI. Skin site infections may be treated with oxacillin or with vancomycin if MRSA is common in the institution or environment. Deep abdominal infections are often treated with a cephalosporin, such as cefoxitin, or a combination of fluoroquinolone plus metronidazole to cover anaerobic, enterococci, and enteric gram-negative bacilli infections.

Drug fevers are often associated with rash and/or lupus-like syndromes. They also may have renal, liver, lung, joint, or hematologic dysfunction associated with the drug toxicity. The risk of developing drug fever correlates with the number of drugs prescribed. Antimicrobial agents account for roughly one-third of all cases. Common antimicrobial agents associated with drug fever include minocycline, cephalosporins, fluoroquinolones, sulfonamides, and penicillins. Drug fever typically resolves within 72 to 96 hours after the discontinuation of the offending agent.

Purulent drainage and fluctuance indicate the presence of abscess, which requires incision and drainage. When cellulitis is confirmed, treatment with antibiotic is warranted. Gram-positive bacteria, such as *S aureus*, *S epidermidis* (especially with implants or devices), *Streptococcus pyogenes*, and *Enterococcus*, are important pathogens. Fungal etiology should not be ruled out in patients with severe comorbid conditions. On rare occasions, deep abscesses produce fever 10 to 15 days after surgery. A high level of suspicion leads to diagnostic imaging such as computed tomography (CT) scan of the body region most likely to be infected, which depends on the location of the surgery. Interventional radiology specialists could be called upon for radiologically guided drainage of the abscess, which is the definitive treatment. Antibiotics should include coverage for gram-negative enteric bacilli and anaerobes, especially when intra-abdominal or pelvic infections are suspected. Gallium scans may be helpful in finding sites of infection in patients without localizing symptoms and workup.

Intravascular catheter or line-associated infection needs to be entertained when the patient has had IV devices for 3 days or more, even when the site appears clean. Any unnecessary lines should be discontinued, as they are potential sites of infection. The catheter tip is cultured to reveal the offending organism that would direct treatment.

Fever caused by **DVT** usually occurs 1 to 4 weeks postoperatively. Half of the time patients with DVT are asymptomatic. Common complaints are unilateral leg swelling, tenderness, pain, and warmth. The **Homan sign** (pain in the calf on foot dorsiflexion) is demonstrated in some cases. When possible, surgical patients are encouraged to ambulate early; otherwise, subcutaneous heparin or low-molecular-weight heparin are useful prophylactic measures. If the patient is at high risk for bleeding, intermittent pneumatic compression devices can help. Diagnosis is made by duplex ultrasound. Patients who develop **pulmonary embolism** usually have concomitant DVT. The treatment of DVT and pulmonary embolism is initiated with low-molecular-weight heparin or unfractionated heparin, followed by warfarin.

The type of surgery also provides a clue as to the associated risks of fever-associated surgical morbidity. In general, laparoscopic surgery comparatively causes fewer cases of fever than open surgery due to less tissue trauma. Pleural effusion develops in all patients undergoing cardiothoracic surgery and 5% of those patients acquire pneumonia. Particularly unique to abdominal surgery is deep abdominal abscess and pancreatitis. Obstetric and gynecologic surgery could be complicated by postpartum endometritis/deep pelvic abscess, necrotizing fasciitis, and pelvic thrombophlebitis. SSI is the most common infectious cause of fever in orthopedic surgery. Prostatic and perinephric abscess are more commonly seen in urologic procedures. Arterial embolization, or "blue toe" syndrome due to emboli from an infected vascular graft can occur following vascular surgery, especially in grafts involving the groin and the legs. Endovascular aortic aneurysm repair may be complicated by "postimplantation syndrome" characterized by self-limited fever, elevated C-reactive protein (CRP) levels, leukocytosis, and negative blood cultures. Patients undergoing genitourinary procedure are at greater risk of having UTI. Meningitis is a common cause of fever following a neurosurgical procedure. Neurosurgery patients, who are usually immobilized and less aggressively anticoagulated to avoid brain hemorrhage, have the highest incidence of DVT.

COMPREHENSION QUESTIONS

38.1 A 60-year-old man with adenocarcinoma of the colon underwent left hemico-lectomy with primary anastomosis. Thirty hours after surgery, he was found to have a fever of 102°F (38.8°C), blood pressure of 90/60 mm Hg, heart rate of 140 beats/min, respirations of 24 breaths/min, and low urine output. Physical examination showed diffuse abdominal tenderness. The surgical site is clean and Gram stain did not show any organism. Urinalysis was negative and the complete blood count (CBC) showed leukocytosis. Which of the following is the most likely cause of this patient's fever?

A. Pneumonia

B. Intraperitoneal leak from bowel injury

C. Surgical site infection

D. Deep tissue abscess

38.2 An 84-year-old nursing home resident underwent emergency open chole-cystectomy under general anesthesia. She has advanced Parkinson disease, hypertension, and diabetes, and was receiving nutrition via nasogastric tube (NGT). On the second postoperative day, she was noted to be coughing and vomiting. Four days later, she had a temperature of 102°F (38.8°C), heart rate of 90 beats/min, respiratory rate of 25 breaths/min, blood pressure of 120/70 mm Hg, and oxygen saturation of 87% on room air. She had a pro-ductive cough with what the nursing staff describes as "putrid sputum." Lung auscultation showed crackles on the right and a chest radiograph revealed a patchy infiltrate in the right lung. Which of the following is the most appro-priate next step in management?

A. Obtain an expectorated sputum sample for culture.

B. Treat empirically with antibiotics.

C. Insert a nasogastric tube.

D. Treat with a proton pump inhibitor (PPI).

38.3 A 42-year-old man underwent open reduction and internal fixation of a com-minuted fracture of the right femur. He was doing well until the fifth postop-erative day, when he complained of pleuritic chest pain and developed fever of 101°F (38.3°C), heart rate of 118 beats/min, respiration of 30 breaths/min, blood pressure of 130/85 mm Hg, and oxygen saturation of 85% on room air. His left ankle became edematous, warm, and tender. Which of the following is a risk factor for his condition?

A. Having an IV in his arm for more than 3 days

B. Failure to adequately use his incentive spirometer

C. Urinary bladder catheterization

D. Prolonged immobility

38.4 A 50-year-old woman with diabetes was recuperating from left inguinal hernia repair. Her glycosylated hemoglobin (HbA_{1c}) prior to surgery was 10%. During postoperative follow-up a week after surgery, the surgical site was markedly erythematous, warm, and tender with pus. Which of the following is the next step in treatment?

    A. Apply topical antibiotic to the surgical site.

    B. Warm compresses alone will relieve the inflammation.

    C. Open the surgical site and drain the infected material.

    D. Send the patient home with prescription for oral antibiotics for 7 days.

ANSWERS

38.1 **B.** In the presence of severe hemodynamic changes and diffuse abdominal tenderness, intraperitoneal leak is the most common cause of fever in the first 36 hours after laparotomy.

38.2 **B.** This patient likely has aspiration pneumonia. She has risk factors including her age, functional status, recent general anesthesia, and advanced neurologic disease. She requires treatment with antibiotics which cover anaerobic bacteria. There is evidence that aspiration risk may *not* be reduced by placing a nasogastric tube before surgery but actually predisposes a person to aspiration pneumonia. Giving the patient a PPI does not treat and can increase risk of aspiration pneumonia. Expectorated sputum is unreliable for anaerobic cultures because of likely contamination by oral flora.

38.3 **D.** This patient has DVT and concomitant pulmonary embolism. Risk factors include prolonged immobility, vascular damage, and hypercoagulability.

38.4 **C.** Incision and drainage are the most important therapy for SSI. Antibiotics are used solely in cases of significant systemic involvement.

CLINICAL PEARLS

▶ Postoperative fevers in the first few days are common and usually resolve on their own.

▶ A thorough risk assessment, history, and physical are needed to determine if laboratory testing and antibiotics are warranted.

▶ The timing of the fever is useful in creating an effective differential diagnosis for postoperative fever.

▶ Removal of all unnecessary medication, catheters, lines, and tubes should be discontinued in the postoperative febrile patient.

REFERENCES

Beilman G, Dunn D. Surgical infections. In: Brunicardi FC, Anderson DK, Billiar TR, et al., eds. *Schwartz's Principles of Surgery*. 9th ed. New York, NY: McGraw-Hill Education; 2010.

Libman H, Wilson P. *Evaluation of Postoperative Fever, ACP Smart Medicine & AHFS DI Essentials*, editorial changes 2014-06-27. Philadelphia, PA: American College of Physicians; 2015.

Narayan M, Medinilla S. Fever in the postoperative patient. *Emerg Med Clin North Am*. 2013 Nov;31(4):1045-1058.

REFERENCES

You were busy seeing patients in your outpatient clinic when you heard a commotion coming from the waiting room. You went to check and found a very frantic mother and her 2-year-old son who is clutching his throat, coughing, drooling, and visibly struggling to breathe. The mother endorses that just a few minutes ago, the child was running around while eating grapes when she suddenly heard him gagging and wheezing. Her son has an appointment for well-child examination and he is apparently doing well. He has no significant history of respiratory illness. The toddler is still conscious but unable to talk, and his cough is becoming weaker. Breath sounds are decreased bilaterally, with wheezing and stridor heard on auscultation. You tried to ventilate the patient with the chin-lift maneuver but the chest fails to rise. You opened the mouth but you are unable to see any foreign object.

▶ What is the most likely diagnosis?
▶ What is the next step in the management of this patient?

ANSWERS TO CASE 39:
Acute Causes of Wheezing and Stridor in Children

Summary: A 2-year-old boy had acute onset of coughing, choking, drooling, and wheezing while eating grapes. He is unable to speak and his cough is weak. He was in a good state of health prior to the incident and has no history of respiratory illness. Physical examination reveals decreased breath sounds, wheezing, and stridor. There is no chest rise on ventilation attempt. No foreign object could be seen on his mouth.

- **Most likely diagnosis:** Foreign-body airway obstruction (FBAO)

- **Next step in the management for this patient:** Heimlich maneuver (subdiaphragmatic abdominal thrusts)

ANALYSIS

Objectives

1. Identify the illnesses, other than asthma, that cause acute wheezing in children.

2. Understand the steps in the diagnosis and management of a wheezing child.

Considerations

Acute onset of wheezing in an otherwise healthy child similar to the above case should raise the suspicion for **FBAO**. Witnessed swallowing followed by choking is not necessary for diagnosis, but as much information should be gathered surrounding the onset of symptoms. FBAO is common among children aged 6 months to 3 years, accounting for approximately 70% of cases. Small toys and objects, balloons, and food (eg, nuts, grapes, and candies) are high-risk objects for aspiration. Older children may be able to identify the object they swallowed and assume the posture of clutching their neck with their hand (**universal choking sign**). Symptoms such as weak cough, inability to speak or cry, high-pitched sounds, or no sounds during inhalation, cyanosis, choking, vomiting, drooling, wheezing, blood-streaked saliva, and respiratory distress are clues to the diagnosis of FBAO. Physical findings of unilateral wheezing, unequal or decreased breath sounds, and stridor are common. In children, the foreign body could lodge on either side of the airway. Eight out of 10 times, the foreign body lodges in one of the bronchi. If the foreign body lodges in the esophagus, acute wheezing is still possible when the obstruction compresses on the airways.

One should not attempt to remove the foreign object in a child who is actively coughing and able to vocalize. Blind finger sweep is not recommended because of the danger of further obstruction or injury. Although the patient mentioned above is still conscious, he seems to have ineffective coughing and is beginning to get tired. Ventilation should be attempted while opening the airway with the head-tilt maneuver, which could also relieve the obstruction. In the above case, an attempt to remove the foreign object was initiated when ventilation was unsuccessful.

If a child older than 1 year is no longer able to cough, vocalize or breathe a series of abdominal thrusts (Heimlich maneuver) should be the next step to try to expel the foreign body. In children less than 1 year, instead of abdominal thrust, a series of five back blows alternating with chest thrusts is performed. If the child continues to deteriorate even after 1 minute of resuscitative efforts and the above maneuvers fail to expel the foreign object, the emergency medical services (EMS) system should be activated while continuing cardiopulmonary resuscitation (CPR).

In the hospital setting, a bronchoscopic procedure is the treatment of choice. Chest x-ray is often normal, but in some cases shows a radiopaque foreign object or identifies localized hyperinflation and/or atelectasis. Most deaths from FBAO occur in children younger than 5 years; 65% are infants.

APPROACH TO:
Wheezing and Stridor

DEFINITIONS

HEIMLICH MANEUVER: Performed in children greater than 1 year and in adults by standing or sitting behind the person who is choking and placing the thumb side of one fist between the navel and the xiphoid process. The other hand grasps the fisted hand and a series of upward abdominal thrusts are delivered to create an "artificial cough" in a choking victim in an effort to dislodge the object blocking the airway.

STRIDOR: Wheezing coming from obstruction of the large airway that has a constant pitch and intensity throughout the entire inspiratory effort.

WHEEZING: A musical sound heard on pulmonary auscultation produced by the oscillating walls of airways that had been narrowed by mucus, inflammation, and so on.

CLINICAL APPROACH

Among the many causes of wheezing in children, asthma and viral infections are most common. Worldwide studies show that approximately 10% to 15% of infants wheeze in the first 12 months of life. The diagnosis of wheezing hinges on accurate history, physical examination, laboratory tests, and even response to treatments. It is also important to gather information regarding the age of onset, exposure to cigarette smoke, presence of allergic signs and symptoms, frequency of wheezing, association with vomiting or feeding, and other accompanying symptoms.

The etiology of **acute wheezing** in children could be infectious (eg, bronchiolitis) or mechanical obstruction (eg, FBAO). **Recurrent wheezing**, on the other hand, encompasses anomalies of the tracheobronchial tree (eg, bronchomalacia), cardiovascular disease (eg, vascular rings and slings), gastroesophageal reflux, and immunologic disorders (eg, bronchopulmonary dysplasia, cystic fibrosis). This case concentrates on acute onset of wheezing other than asthma in children (Case 56 provides a more detailed discussion of asthma).

Bronchiolitis

Bronchiolitis affects more than one-third of children less than 2 years and is the most common acute cause of wheezing, especially in infants who are 1 to 3 months old. Infants younger than 6 months are most severely affected, owing to smaller, more easily obstructed airways and a decreased ability to clear secretions. It is a viral infection causing nonspecific inflammation of the small airways and usually during the winter months. **Respiratory syncytial virus (RSV) accounts for 50% to 80% of cases**; the rest are caused by parainfluenza, adenovirus, influenza, *Mycoplasma pneumoniae*, *Chlamydia pneumoniae*, and metapneumovirus. These viruses and atypical bacteria elicit inflammatory and immune responses that produce mucus, edema, and cellular debris that block the small airways. Influenza vaccinations in infants and toddlers have reduced the incidence of bronchiolitis caused by the flu virus.

Initially, the child develops nasal congestion and rhinorrhea for 1 to 2 days, followed by low-grade fever, wheezing, cough, irritability, and varying degrees of dyspnea. As a result, the child may have poor oral intake and possibly dehydration.

Symptoms reach a peak in 2 to 5 days and gradually resolve in 1 to 2 weeks. Physical examination may reveal wheezing, fine crackles, prolonged expiratory phase, tachypnea, and increased work of breathing as evidenced by nasal flaring, intercostal retraction, and even apnea. Other physical findings may include otitis media, irritability, and hypothermia or hyperthermia.

The diagnosis of bronchiolitis is based on clinical presentation, the patient's age, seasonal occurrence, and findings from the physical examination. Tests are typically used to exclude other diagnoses, such as bacterial pneumonia, sepsis, or congestive heart failure, or to confirm a viral etiology and determine required infection control for patients admitted to the hospital.

Current literature does not support the routine use of laboratory tests as they do not alter clinical outcomes unless the child is less than 90 days with the need to rule out secondary bacterial infection. If the diagnosis is doubtful or the clinical presentation is concerning for other diagnoses, one may request a chest x-ray. Radiologic findings in individuals with bronchiolitis are variable and may include bronchial wall thickening, tiny nodules, linear opacities, and patchy atelectasis. Infiltrates and lobar consolidation are more consistent with pneumonia. RSV bronchiolitis is a self-limited disease and can be safely managed in an outpatient setting. However, disease manifestation can be variable, and risk factors for severe disease include preexisting cardiac or pulmonary disease, premature birth, very young age (<2-3 months), nosocomial RSV infection, and, in some studies, low socioeconomic status. Patients who are in severe respiratory distress, younger than 3 months or premature, those with comorbid conditions, lethargy, hypoxemia, or hypercarbia, and those with atelectasis or consolidation in chest radiograph need to be hospitalized. **The single best indicator of severity is low pulse oximetry.** Indicators of mild disease include good PO intake, age greater than 2 months, oxygen saturation greater than or equal to 94%, and normal age-based respiratory rate (<45 breaths/min for 0-2 months old, <43 breaths/min for 2-6 months old, and <40 breaths/min for 6-24 months old).

The Agency for Healthcare Research and Quality (AHRQ), in collaboration with the American Academy of Family Physicians (AAFP) and the American Academy of Pediatrics (AAP), recommends **supplemental oxygen if the SpO$_2$ is less than 90% and supportive care as the modes of treatment with clear evidence of effectiveness in RSV bronchiolitis.**

Supportive care should consist of supplemental humidified oxygen, fluids, and the suctioning of nasal and pharyngeal secretions. The most important therapy is humidified oxygen. Medications have a limited role in the management of bronchiolitis. Several drugs are commonly used, but little or inconclusive evidence supports the routine use of any drug in the management of bronchiolitis. Nebulized bronchodilators, cool mist, steroids, antibiotics, and ribavirin have insufficient evidence or have not been shown to help in previously healthy children. Administration of RSV immunoglobulin (RespiGam) and palivizumab (Synagis) just before the beginning of RSV season is proven effective preventive therapy for children younger than 2 years with increased risks from chronic lung disease, history of prematurity (<35-week gestation), or with congenital heart disease.

Croup

Croup is a very common cause of airway obstruction in children aged 6 months to 6 years, and is a leading cause of hospitalization for children younger than 4 years. It is **a viral infection that causes inflammation of the subglottic region** of the larynx that produces the characteristic barking cough, hoarseness, stridor, and different degrees of respiratory distress that are more severe at night. The croup syndrome encompasses laryngotracheitis, laryngotracheobronchitis, laryngotracheobronchopneumonitis, and spasmodic croup.

Croup usually occurs during fall and winter. The parainfluenza viruses (I, II, III) are responsible for as many as 80% of croup cases, with parainfluenza I accounting for most episodes and hospitalizations. Other pathogens include enterovirus, human bocavirus, influenza virus A and B, RSV, rhinovirus, and adenovirus in approximate order of frequency. In communities with low measles immunization rates, measles should be listed as a rare but possible cause. Influenza A has been implicated in children with severe respiratory compromise.

The prodrome is characterized by 12 to 72 hours of runny nose and low-grade fever followed by a barking cough and variable levels of respiratory distress, usually at night. Hypoxia only occurs in severe cases. These symptoms peak from 1 to 2 days, and in most cases, resolve in 1 week.

Diagnosis is made through clinical presentation. However, imaging studies confirm the diagnoses. Frontal neck x-rays show the "steeple sign," which is indicative of subglottic narrowing of the tracheal lumen. When the diagnosis is uncertain, computed tomography (CT) scan of the neck offers a more sensitive evaluation.

Treatment is geared toward the severity of the croup (the level of respiratory distress). The most reliable clinical features to test severity are resting stridor and chest wall retractions. Use of pulse oximetry can help assess severity.

Emergency management of croup should begin with assessment of airway obstruction; oxygen should be used liberally. Chest radiographs rarely are of use, but can be considered if other pulmonary conditions are strongly considered.

Lateral neck films can be considered if there is concern for epiglottitis or bacterial tracheitis. There is no proof that humidified air is of value and mist tents should be avoided. Hospitalization is appropriate if severe croup is clinically apparent. Severe croup is exemplified by cyanosis, decreased level of consciousness, progressive stridor, severe stridor, severe retractions, markedly decreased air movement, toxic appearance, severe dehydration, and social factors limiting adequacy of outpatient monitoring. Children who are hospitalized with croup should be monitored closely and frequent physical examination needs to be performed.

The current cornerstones of treatment are glucocorticoids and nebulized epinephrine. Steroids have proven beneficial in severe, moderate, and even mild croup. Dexamethasone 0.60 mg/kg by mouth or parenterally as a single dose is beneficial because of its long half-life and anti-inflammatory action, whereby laryngeal mucosal edema is decreased. They also decrease the need for salvage nebulized epinephrine. Nebulized racemic (mixture of d-isomers and l-isomers) or L-epinephrine is typically reserved for patients in moderate-to-severe distress. It works by adrenergic stimulation, which causes constriction of the precapillary arterioles, thereby leading to fluid resorption from the interstitium and improvement in the laryngeal mucosal edema. Its β_2-adrenergic activity leads to bronchial smooth muscle relaxation and bronchodilation. The following medications should be avoided: sedatives, opiates, expectorants, and antihistamines.

Epiglottitis

Epiglottitis is a bacterial infection of the supraglottic tissue and surrounding areas that causes rapidly progressive airway obstruction. It usually affects children younger than 5 years and is most commonly caused by bacteria, with *Streptococcus pyogenes* (β-hemolytic *Streptococcus* group A) and *Haemophilus influenzae* as the most frequent bacterial causes in children. With the introduction of the *H influenzae* type b (Hib) vaccine, there has been a 10-fold decrease in cases of childhood epiglottitis, with group A *Streptococcus* now the leading infectious etiology.

Within 24 hours, the patient with epiglottitis would appear "toxic" and develop fever, severe sore throat, muffled speech ("hot potato voice"), drooling, and dysphagia. The child usually is noticeably anxious and assumes the sniffi position, leaning forward on outstretched arms with chin thrust forward and neck hyperextended (tripod position) so as to increase the airway diameter.

With progression of airway obstruction, the patient may begin to have wheezing and stridor. **Epiglottitis is a medical emergency and visualization to confirm the presence of severely erythematous epiglottis is preferably done in the operating room with experienced surgeon or anesthesiologist.** Mortality rates as high as 10% can occur in children whose airways are not protected by endotracheal intubation. With endotracheal intubation, mortality is less than 1%.

Medical treatment begins by evaluating airway, breathing, and circulation. The patient should be kept in a calm environment to prevent sudden airway obstruction. Supplemental oxygen administration, a nonthreatening initial step, is easily accomplished with blow-by oxygen administered by a parent. Place the equipment needed for emergent airway management at the bedside. Keep the patient in view at all times. The clinician should avoid oral and throat examinations which can provoke anxiety and acute obstruction.

The radiographic finding that is characteristic of epiglottitis is the "thumb sign" or protrusion of the enlarged epiglottis from the anterior wall of the hypopharynx seen on a lateral neck x-ray. Blood tests should be considered after there is rapid access to ability to intubate, to reduce the risk of anxiety-provoking testing. A complete blood count (CBC) usually shows leukocytosis, neutrophilia, and bandemia.

If acute respiratory arrest occurs, ventilate the child with 100% supplemental oxygen, using a bag-valve-mask device, and arrange for intubation. When a child has a respiratory arrest and appropriate surgical personnel are unavailable, the attending physician may attempt intubation.

Alternative methods to gain immediate control of the airway, such as needle cricothyrotomy, are considered temporary until a more permanent procedure (eg, tracheostomy) can be performed. The best setting for an endotracheal intubation is in an operating room with the patient under general anesthesia.

Treatment consists of appropriate antibiotics (second- or third-generation cephalosporins or ampicillin/sulbactam) and airway management, usually in an intensive care unit (ICU) setting with a team ready to respond for intubation or tracheostomy.

Bacterial Tracheitis

Bacterial tracheitis is an uncommon life-threatening infection most often seen in 5- to 8-year olds. It often follows an upper respiratory infection that suddenly worsens with high fever, stridor, and cough. Patients appear toxic. Secretions are so thick that they threaten upper air way obstruction. Patients should be treated similarly to epiglottitis with patient ideally going to the operating room for sedation, intubation, and bronchoscopy for cultures and suctioning of thick secretions. X-rays can be done, but airway stabilization takes priority. If done, a steeple sign much like croup may be seen. *Staphylococcus aureus* is most commonly isolated. *S pyogenes*, *Moraxella catarrhalis*, *H influenzae*, and anaerobes are also seen. Ampicillin/sulbactam, third-generation cephalosporins with clindamycin cover most likely causative organisms. Vancomycin should be considered in communities with high rates of methicillin-resistance *S aureus*.

Abscesses

Deep abscesses of the neck are less common causes of acute wheezing, but they have the potential to be very serious. They are located in the peritonsillar, retropharyngeal, and pharyngomaxillary spaces.

Retropharyngeal abscess affects children of 2 to 4 years. The abscess is usually caused by extension of pharyngeal infection, penetrating trauma, iatrogenic instrumentation, or foreign body. Children with this condition are present with fever, drooling, dysphagia, odynophagia, stridor, and respiratory distress. Physical examination may indicate tender enlarged cervical lymphadenopathy, cervical spine range-of-motion limitation, possible stridor, and wheezing. Diagnosis is made by lateral neck films which show bulging in posterior pharynx (prevertebral soft tissue more abundant in children during expiration). Treatment utilizes antibiotics such as cephalosporins or antistaphylococcal penicillins. Incision and drainage is also an option.

Peritonsillar abscess is an infection of the superior pole of the tonsils and is more common in young teenagers. Fever, severe sore throat, muffled voice, drooling, trismus, and neck pain are typical symptoms. Enlarged tonsils with abscess, cervical adenopathy, and deviation of the uvula may be obvious on physical examination. CT scan of the neck is the most helpful diagnostic modality for identifying deep neck abscesses. The predominant pathogens are *S pyogenes*, *S aureus*, and anaerobes. The administration of ampicillin-sulbactam or clindamycin (if penicillin allergic) for 14 days is appropriate treatment. Drainage of the abscess is indicated either as first-line treatment or when antimicrobial agents fail to produce adequate result. Serious complications from deep abscesses result from airway obstruction, septicemia, aspiration, jugular vein thrombosis/thrombophlebitis, carotid artery rupture, and mediastinitis.

CASE CORRELATION

- See Cases 2 (Dyspnea), 24 (Pneumonia) and case 56 (Asthma).

COMPREHENSION QUESTIONS

39.1 A 7-month-old infant was brought by her mother to an outpatient clinic because of a 2-day history of fever, copious nasal secretions, and wheezing. The mother volunteered that the baby has been healthy and has not had these symptoms in the past. The infant's temperature is noted to be 100.7°F (38.1°C), her respiratory rate is 50 breaths/min, and her pulse oximetry is 95% on room air. Physical examination reveals no signs of dehydration, but wheezing is heard on bilateral lung fields on auscultation. The infant shows no improvement after three treatments with nebulized albuterol. Which of the following is the recommended treatment?

A. Continued nebulized albuterol every 4 hours.

B. Antihistamines and decongestants.

C. Antibiotics for 7 days.

D. Initiate Synagis.

E. Supportive care with hydration and humidified oxygen.

39.2 A 9-year-old girl is being seen in your office with fever and difficulty breathing. You are concerned about the diagnosis of epiglottitis. Which of the following is the most accurate statement regarding epiglottitis?

A. Child usually prefers to be in prone position.

B. Radiographic finding of "steeple sign."

C. Every effort should be made to visualize the epiglottis in the office to confirm the diagnosis.

D. Diagnosis is decreasing in incidence.

39.3 A 5-year-old child is brought into the office due to the mother's concern of difficulty breathing. On examination, the child appears toxic, has a high fever, cough productive of thick mucopurulent expectorant, and stridor with wheezing. Which of the following is the most likely condition and organism that requires antibiotic therapy?

A. Epiglottis-*H influenzae*

B. Tracheitis—*S aureus*

C. Epiglottis—*S pyogenes* (β-hemolytic *Streptococcus* group A)

D. Tracheitis—*S pyogenes* (β-hemolytic *Streptococcus* group A)

E. Retropharyngeal abscess—*S aureus*

39.4 A 12-year-old girl was brought to the emergency department because of severe sore throat, muffled voice, drooling, and fatigue. She had been sick for the past 3 days and is unable to eat because of painful swallowing. The parents deny any history of recurrent pharyngitis. The patient still managed to open her mouth and you were able to see an abscess at the upper pole of the right tonsil with deviation of the uvula toward the midline. Examination of the neck reveals enlarged and tender lymph nodes. Which of the following is the most appropriate management?

A. Analgesics for pain

B. Oral antibiotics

C. Nebulized racemic epinephrine

D. Incision and drainage of the abscess

E. Tonsillectomy and adenoidectomy

ANSWERS

39.1 **E.** Bronchiolitis is the most likely diagnosis in this case. There is no established treatment for bronchiolitis except for supportive management of the patient's symptoms. Because the infant did not respond to an albuterol trial, there is no justification for continuing its use. Antihistamines, decongestants, and antibiotics are not effective. Synagis is not helpful in the acute setting.

39.2 **D.** The incidence of epiglottitis has markedly reduced since the introduction of the Hib vaccine. Children with epiglottitis are more likely to be in the tripod position than prone. The "steeple sign" is seen in croup; the "thumb" sign is seen in epiglottitis. Visualization of the epiglottis should preferentially occur in an operating room, where immediate intubation or tracheostomy can occur.

39.3 **B.** Tracheitis matches the symptom description and is usually caused by *S aureus*. Group A streptococci are now the leading cause of epiglottis, but the symptom constellation is more likely due to tracheitis. Retropharyngeal abscess usually presents insidiously with neck pain with swelling, fever, dysphagia, and drooling.

39.4 **D.** This patient is suffering from peritonsillar abscess. Of the choices listed, incision and drainage is the most appropriate. Tonsillectomy is only indicated if there are confirmed cases of **recurrent** pharyngitis and peritonsillar abscess.

CLINICAL PEARLS

▶ Sufficient airflow is required for the airway to produce a wheezing sound. Disappearance of wheezing in a patient who initially presents with wheezing is an ominous sign that suggests complete blockage of the airway or imminent respiratory failure.

▶ Bronchiolitis is the most common lower respiratory disease of infants and the most common reason for hospitalization for infants younger than 1 year.

▶ Never perform a blind finger sweep of a foreign object aspirated by an infant or child.

▶ Epiglottitis and tracheitis are medical emergencies that require the ability to rapidly secure airways.

REFERENCES

Acevedo JL, Lander L, Choi S, Shah RK. Airway management in pediatric epiglottitis: a national perspective. *Otolaryngol Head Neck Surg.* 2009;140(4):548-551.

Dawson-Caswell M, Muncie HL. Respiratory syncytial virus infection in children. *Am Fam Physician.* 2011;83(2):141-146.

Gunn JD. Stidor and drooling. In: Tintinalli JE, Stapczynski S, Ma OJ, et al., eds. *Tintinalli's Emergency Medicine: A Comprehensive Study Guide.* 7th ed. New York, NY: McGraw-Hill Education; 2011. Available at: http://www.accessmedicine.com. Accessed May 11, 2015.

Zoorob R, Sidani M, Murray J. Croup: an overview. *Am Fam Physician.* 2011;83(9):1067-1073.

A 28-year-old white woman presents to your office with a chief complaint of constipation and abdominal pain. On further questioning, she reports she has had this problem since beginning college at the age of 18. Her symptoms have waxed and waned since this time, but never have worsened. She describes her abdominal pain as dull, crampy, and nonfocal but more prominent in the left lower quadrant, and improved with defecation. She denies radiation of pain, nausea, vomiting, fever, chills, weight loss, heartburn, or bloody or dark stool. She reports that over the last 3 months she is having cramps 7 to 10 times per month and having a bowel movement every 1 to 2 days that is hard and feels incomplete. She has tried over-the-counter remedies, including stool softeners and antacids, but only experienced minimal improvement in her symptoms. She only takes birth control pills and denies any use of herbal supplements or laxatives. Her family history is negative, including for colorectal cancer and inflammatory bowel disease, and she reports that her parents and siblings are healthy. She is currently engaged and reports significant stress in preparing for the wedding. On physical examination, you note her to be somewhat anxious, but otherwise in no apparent distress. Her vital signs and general physical examination are normal. Her abdomen has normal bowel sounds, no tenderness on superficial and deep palpation, and no rebound, rigidity, or guarding. Liver and spleen size are within normal limits and no masses are palpable. A pelvic examination is normal. The rectal examination shows normal sphincter tone, no masses, and brown stool that is occult blood negative.

▶ What is your most likely diagnosis?
▶ What is your next diagnostic step?
▶ What is the next step in therapy?

ANSWERS TO CASE 40:
Irritable Bowel Syndrome

Summary: A 28-year-old woman presents with a several-year history of crampy abdominal pain and constipation alternating with diarrhea. She denies any fever, weight loss, heartburn, or bloody stools. Her past medical history and family history are otherwise unremarkable. The physical examination, including abdominal and pelvic examination, are grossly within normal limits.

- **Most likely diagnosis:** Irritable bowel syndrome (IBS) (mixed subtype).

- **Most appropriate next diagnostic step:** In the absence of any alarm features, a complete blood count (CBC), C-reactive protein (CRP), celiac disease antibody testing for initial screening can be considered to confirm diagnosis by ruling out common conditions that mimic IBS.

- **Next step in therapy:** Trial of insoluble fiber supplementation, relaxation techniques, and exercise.

ANALYSIS

Objectives

1. Describe the epidemiology, clinical manifestations, and pathophysiology of IBS.

2. Learn the diagnostic approach to IBS and rationale for ordering diagnostic studies based on symptom subtype and/or presence of "alarm features."

3. Review current therapeutic strategies in the patient with IBS.

4. Recognize the role of psychosocial factors in IBS.

Considerations

This is a young woman with long-standing crampy abdominal pain and constipation. She denies any "alarm features" like weight loss, bloody stools, fever, and refractory diarrhea, and her family history is negative for colon cancer or inflammatory bowel disease. The chronicity and lack of worsening of her symptoms coupled with her young age points to a functional gastrointestinal (GI) disorder, such as IBS. The presence of fever, weight loss, or an abnormal physical examination would be other worrisome findings. Although not required, a reasonable workup in this case could include testing to rule out anemia, inflammatory disease, and celiac disease.

APPROACH TO:
Irritable Bowel Syndrome

DEFINITIONS

IRRITABLE BOWEL SYNDROME: This is a functional GI disorder characterized by chronic abdominal pain and altered bowel habits.

ROME III CRITERIA: Developed by an international working team to standardize patient selection for functional bowel disorder research, it is often used to determine diagnosis of IBS and other functional gastrointestinal disorders. The criteria are approximately 70% sensitive and 80% specific, with a positive predictive value of 40% and negative predictive value of 90%.

CLINICAL APPROACH

The prevalence of IBS is approximately 12% of the North American population and accounts for a large proportion of GI complaints seen both by primary care physicians and gastroenterologists. **IBS affects women up to two times more often than men** in North America. Patients typically present in the second or third decades of life, although virtually any age group can be affected. The pathophysiology of IBS remains unclear, but appears to be a combination of environmental and host factors. Environmental factors include early history of abuse or other psychosocial stressors, food intolerance, enteric infections, and antibiotic use. Host factors that affect symptoms include altered gut pain sensitivity, altered microbial flora, gastrointestinal permeability, gut immune hyperactivity, and dysregulation of the brain-gut axis through increased reactivity to stress. IBS also commonly coexists with other functional disorders such as fibromyalgia, lower back pain, and chronic headaches.

Patients with IBS may complain crampy abdominal pain with a predominant pattern of constipation, diarrhea, alternating constipation with diarrhea, or periods of normal bowel habits that alternate with either constipation and/or diarrhea. The location and the nature of the pain in IBS are subject to great variability. The pain often has variable intensity and is improved or relieved with defecation. The crampy pain usually does not wake a person up from sleep. Other gastrointestinal symptoms seen in IBS include the passage of mucus with stool, bowel urgency, bloating, and the sensation of incomplete stool evacuation. Up to 50% of people with IBS also suffer from upper GI symptoms such as dyspepsia, nausea, and gastroesophageal reflux.

Diagnosis

In an effort to objectively identify patients with IBS, the Rome criteria (Table 40–1) were developed and subsequently revised two times. Based on the presence of positive symptoms and the absence of structural or biochemical explanation of the symptoms, a patient may be diagnosed with IBS. Physicians are encouraged to avoid unnecessary and expensive studies and instead to use judicious cost-effective diagnostic testing.

Table 40–1 • ROME III DIAGNOSTIC CRITERIA FOR IRRITABLE BOWEL SYNDROME
Recurrent abdominal pain or discomfort at least 3 d/mo for the past 3 mo, associated with two or more of the following: • Improvement with defecation • Onset associated with a change in the frequency of stool • Onset associated with a change in form (appearance) of stool Criterion fulfilled for the previous 3 mo with symptom onset at least 6 mo prior to diagnosis

Data from the Rome Foundation. Available at: www.romecriteria.org/. Accessed May 12, 2015.

A thorough history should be obtained using open-ended, nonjudgmental questions. The physical examination should focus on ruling out organic pathologic processes that are inconsistent with IBS. Importance should be paid to all medications and dietary habits that may worsen or mimic the symptoms of IBS.

The differential diagnosis of IBS can be very broad. Patients should be asked for the presence of "alarm features," (Table 40–2) which include fever, anemia, involuntary weight loss greater than 10 lb, hematochezia, melena, refractory or bloody diarrhea, and a family history of ovarian cancer, colon cancer, celiac or inflammatory bowel disease. The **presence of alarm features usually points to an underlying organic etiology** and warrants a further workup.

In the patient with IBS (all subtypes) and the absence of alarm features, a complete blood count and age-appropriate colon cancer screening are appropriate initial tests. In IBS cases with diarrhea or mixed subtypes, testing for inflammation (CRP) and celiac disease testing (IgA tissue transglutaminase antibody or antiendomysial antibody) are recommended. Testing for bile malabsorption (fecal bile acids) can also be considered. Patients with severe constipation subtype may need physiologic testing. If there is a family history of ovarian cancer, a CA-125 can be obtained.

Treatment

IBS is a chronic, recurring condition with a wide range of symptoms. As with most chronic pain syndromes, the cornerstone of management is a therapeutic relationship between the physician and the patient. Setting goals for functional improvement, not cure also improve perceptions of success in a syndrome where

Table 40–2 • ALARM FEATURES WARRANTING FURTHER WORKUP
Unintentional or unexplained weight loss Unexplained fever Family history of colon or ovarian cancer Melena/blood in stool Age >60 with change in bowel habits to looser/increase frequency >6 wk Anemia Abdominal or rectal mass Markers of inflammatory bowel disease Markers of celiac disease

the patient's mental state actively influences symptoms. The treatment approach should be individualized, and will depend on the intensity of symptoms.

Based on the predominant symptom subtype, empiric therapy can be initiated to control a patient's symptoms.

Abdominal Pain

- Antispasmodics, such as dicyclomine and hyoscyamine, may be used on an as-needed basis, especially when pain is mild and infrequent.

- Low-dose tricyclic antidepressants (TCAs) should be considered when pain is more frequent and severe.

- Selective serotonin reuptake inhibitors (SSRIs) may be beneficial when depression or anxiety disorders are comorbid with IBS.

- Rifaximin, an antibiotic used for traveler's diarrhea, may be considered for patients without constipation symptoms.

- Probiotics and peppermint oil may be helpful for some.

Constipation-Predominant IBS

- Soluble fiber either via dietary fiber, synthetic fiber, or natural fiber, is recommended.

- Polyethylene glycol can improve symptoms of constipation, but has limited evidence for global functional improvement.

- Lubiprostone (Amitiza), which selectively activates intestinal chloride channels and increases fluid secretion is Food and Drug Administration (FDA) approved for IBS in women with constipation, but has a side effect of nausea in significant percentage of patients. Cost is often an issue with this medication.

- Linaclotide (Linzess) stimulated 3',5'-cyclic guanosine monophosphate (cGMP) production which increased intestinal motility and fluid secretion. Cost can be a factor in this medication also.

Diarrhea-Predominant IBS

- Loperamide may reduce the frequency of loose stools, as well as decrease bowel urgency.

- Alosetron (Lotronex) is FDA approved for severe diarrhea symptoms of at least 6 months but is currently restricted for use due to risk of ischemic colitis.

- Rifaximin (Xifaxan) is a gut-specific bacteriostatic agent FDA approved for traveler's diarrhea that can be used off label for nonconstipation IBS. Cost can be a barrier to using this medication.

Pharmacologic agents should be used as adjuncts in the overall treatment plan. A multifactorial approach, including modification of diet, exercise, psychological support, patient education and reassurance, and medication therapy is often required.

CASE CORRELATION

- See also Case 31 (Abdominal Pain and Vomiting in a Child).

COMPREHENSION QUESTIONS

40.1 A 65-year-old man reports a lifelong history of IBS with alternating bouts of constipation and diarrhea. He denies any so-called alarm symptoms, but does report that his symptoms have worsened over the last several months. He reports never having a colonoscopy before. Stool is negative for blood and leukocytes. Which of the following is the most important next step?

A. Esophagogastroduodenoscopy (EGD).

B. Begin trial of polyethylene glycol.

C. Explore possible underlying psychiatric symptoms.

D. Colonoscopy.

E. Increase fiber intake.

40.2 A 37-year-old woman reports a 10-year history of intermittent abdominal pain and constipation alternating with diarrhea. She has no weight loss, fever, or worrisome features on examination. Which of the following agents is clinically indicated as a first-line treatment for mild-to-moderate abdominal pain associated with IBS?

A. Amitriptyline

B. Lubiprostone

C. Dicyclomine

D. Fluoxetine

40.3 A 27-year-old graduate student in psychology is evaluated for intermittent abdominal pain. She is diagnosed with IBS. She asks whether there is a relationship between psychiatric disorders and IBS. Which of the following statements is most accurate?

A. IBS is usually caused by the underlying psychiatric disorder.

B. Psychiatric conditions may worsen coexisting IBS.

C. Successfully treating the psychiatric comorbidity causes remission of IBS.

D. No evidence supports a relationship between IBS and psychiatric disorders.

40.4 A 26-year-old college student has been increasingly stressed before final examinations. She has been using over-the-counter antacids more days out of the week than not for an upset stomach and feeling full immediately after eating. She typically has one bowel movement per week and there is no blood in the stool. She feels immediate relief after passage of stool and flatulence. For the patient with constipation-predominant IBS, which of the following is the best first-line therapy?

A. Hyoscyamine

B. Sertraline

C. Psyllium

D. Loperamide

40.5 A 25-year-old woman comes to your office worried that she might have IBS, which she heard about on the news. She reports abdominal pain and diarrhea for 3 months. She also reports observing blood in her stool several times. She is worried what impact her constantly having to use the bathroom is having on her job as a lawyer. Her physical examination is normal except for a hemoccult-positive test after a rectal examination. While looking over her records you notice that she has lost 20 lb since she last saw you 3 months ago. Which of the following is an appropriate next step?

A. Refer her for cognitive behavioral therapy.

B. Offer her symptomatic relief with loperamide.

C. Recommend that she take fiber for better bowel regulation.

D. Obtain colonoscopy.

ANSWERS

40.1 **D.** Age-appropriate cancer screening (colonoscopy) is indicated, even in the setting of an established diagnosis of IBS, because of the high pretest probability of detecting an underlying neoplasm.

40.2 **C.** Dicyclomine, an antispasmodic anticholinergic medication, can be used on an as-needed basis for mild-to-moderate abdominal pain associated with IBS. For more persistent and severe pain, low-dose TCAs, like amitriptyline, are beneficial. Lubiprostone is indicated in women with constipation-predominant IBS as a second-line agent.

40.3 **B.** Comorbid psychiatric disorders typically worsen IBS symptomatology, but have not been shown to cause IBS directly. Successfully treating an underlying psychiatric disorder may improve symptoms of IBS, but will not likely resolve all symptoms of IBS.

40.4 **C.** Fiber supplementation is considered first-line therapy in constipation-predominant IBS. It is effective and safe, and available without prescription.

40.5 **D.** This patient presents with alarm signs of blood in the stool and weight loss. Although psychiatric problems or irritable bowel syndrome are possible, more serious conditions should be evaluated and ruled out. A CBC, CRP, testing for celiac disease, and endoscopy or radiologic study assessing for inflammatory bowel disease would be prudent.

CLINICAL PEARLS

▶ The cornerstone of management of IBS is the therapeutic relationship between patient and the physician who can collaborate on an individualized plan of care that best manages the patient's symptoms. In the absence of alarm features, be prudent with laboratory testing.

▶ Alarm features may indicate an underlying organic pathology and require additional diagnostic workup that may include laboratory, radiologic, and/or endoscopic studies.

▶ Treatment should be symptom-specific and should include appropriate use of medication, dietary and lifestyle changes, and examination of any psychosocial factors that contribute to IBS symptoms.

REFERENCES

Chey WD, Kurlander MD, Eswaran S. Irritable bowel syndrome: a clinical review. *N Eng J Med.* 2015;313(9):949-958.

Owyang C. Irritable bowel syndrome. In: Kasper D, Fauci A, Hauser S, et al., eds. *Harrison's Principles of Internal Medicine.* 19th ed. New York, NY: McGraw-Hill Education; 2015. Accessed May 12, 2015.

Weinberg DS, Smalley W, Heidelbaugh JJ, Shahnez S. American Gastroenterological Association Institute guideline on the pharmacologic management of irritable bowel syndrome. *Gastroenterology.* 2014;147(5):1146-1148.

Wilkins T, Perpitone C, Alex B, Schade RR. Diagnosis and management of IBS in adults. *Am Fam Physician.* 2012;86(5):419-426.

A 20-year-old female college student is brought to the emergency room complaining of chest pain that started 45 minutes ago. She describes the chest pain as substernal, 10/10 in intensity, radiating to her jaw, and associated with headache, sweating, nausea, and palpitations. She was given oxygen, aspirin, and nitroglycerin by the emergency medical services (EMS) in route to the emergency department (ED) and received morphine on her arrival to the ED. The patient is accompanied by her roommate who mentioned that the patient came back from a concert about an hour ago and complained of feeling nauseated, anxious, and somewhat paranoid. The patient has no history of health problems and has not had similar episodes in the past. She is currently sexually active with one male partner and takes oral contraceptive pills (OCPs) for birth control. She reports drinking alcohol and smoking cigarettes occasionally. On questioning about use of illicit drugs, she hesitates, then says that she drank "a few beers," smoked "a few joints," and "took a capsule" at the concert. She swears that this is the first time she has used any illicit substances.

On examination, she is anxious and restless with heightened alertness. Her temperature is 101.0°F (38.3°C), pulse is 119 beats/min, respiratory rate is 24 breaths/min, blood pressure is 165/90 mm Hg, oxygen saturation of 97% on room air, height is 60 in, and her weight is 100 lb. Eye examination reveals dilated pupils bilaterally with sluggish light reflex along with occasional twitching of her right eye. Extraocular movements were found to be normal. Her heart examination reveals tachycardia with no murmurs. Respiratory examination reveals tachypnea with shallow breathing but lung fields are clear to auscultation. Neck is without carotid bruit or jugular venous distension. Distal extremity pulses are brisk and symmetrical. The remainder of her examination is unremarkable.

▶ What are the differential diagnoses for this case?
▶ What is your first diagnostic step?
▶ What is the next step in management of this patient?

ANSWERS TO CASE 41:
Substance Abuse

Summary: A 20-year-old female college student with no significant past medical history presents to the ED with symptoms of coronary ischemia and other symptoms that signify increased sympathetic activity after drinking alcohol and smoking and ingesting unknown substances.

- **Differential diagnosis:** Cocaine-induced myocardial ischemia, cocaine- and ecstasy-induced mental status changes (eg, anxiety, paranoia), panic attack, cardiac arrhythmia, and pulmonary embolism.

- **Next diagnostic step:** 12-lead electrocardiogram (ECG), markers of myocardial damage including serum troponin I, creatine kinase (CK), and MB isoenzyme (CK-MB) performed STAT, urine toxicology screen, blood alcohol level, comprehensive metabolic panel (electrolytes, glucose, kidney and liver function tests), complete blood count (CBC), prothrombin time (PT), partial thromboplastin time (PTT), international normalized ratio (INR), and a chest x-ray (CXR).

- **Next step in management:** The initial management of this patient will be the same as for any other patient presenting with acute chest pain, as she should be placed on telemetry and oxygen. Airway, breathing, and circulation should be ensured followed by administration of aspirin, sublingual nitroglycerin, and morphine. β-Blockers should be avoided initially, especially if cocaine intoxication is suspected, due to risk of unopposed α-constriction that can induce ischemia. Ruling out acute coronary syndrome with serial ECG and cardiac enzymes should occur every 8 hours over three intervals. She should be monitored closely for mental status changes, and withdrawal symptoms of potentially ingested illicit drugs.

ANALYSIS

Objectives

1. Know the etiology and epidemiology of substance abuse.

2. Know the most commonly used illicit and prescription drugs, their adverse and toxic effects, and the amount of time they remain in a patient's system.

3. Know the screening tools available, history taking, physical examination, and laboratory findings in patients with suspected illicit substance intoxication and substance abuse disorder.

4. Know the medications available to control acute toxicity and withdrawal symptoms, as well as treatment and relapse prevention.

5. Know the different behavioral therapies available for treatment of substance abuse.

Considerations

This is a healthy, young female who presents with acute chest pain unrelated to respiration and position but associated with nausea, fever, tachycardia, tachypnea, anxiety, heightened alertness, paranoia, and mydriasis. The events preceding her arrival include ingestion of alcohol and other likely illicit substances that might have caused her to have chest pain. After ruling out the cardiac causes of chest pain, it is very important to screen for signs and symptoms of acute illicit drug intoxication and drug abuse in this patient. Urine toxicology screening is performed to detect the most commonly abused illicit substances and if found positive, is an indication of recent substance use. When people consume two or more psychoactive drugs together, such as cocaine, ecstasy, and alcohol, the danger of experiencing adverse effects of each drug is compounded. In this patient, the history and physical examination suggest that she may have used combination of cocaine and alcohol which may have led to the formation of a third substance, Cocaethylene, which intensifies cocaine's euphoric effects. Cocaethylene is associated with a greater risk of coronary vasospasm than cocaine alone, resulting in myocardial ischemia and sudden death.

APPROACH TO:
Substance Abuse

DEFINITIONS

SUBSTANCE ABUSE: A maladaptive pattern of substance use leading to clinically significant impairment and ongoing use in spite of professional (eg, poor work or school performance), legal (eg, driving under the influence [DUI]), or interpersonal (eg, erratic behavior, fights, relationship losses) consequences.

SUBSTANCE DEPENDENCE: A maladaptive pattern of substance use leading to clinically significant impairment or distress, as manifested by the development of drug tolerance, withdrawal symptoms, inability to cut down on use and use despite the development of physical or psychological problems caused by the substance.

RELAPSE: Resumption of illicit drug use after an attempt or multiple attempts to quit.

DETOXIFICATION: A process that enables the body to rid itself of a drug.

CLINICAL APPROACH

Every year, the abuse of illicit drugs and alcohol rises. In 2012, drug overdose was the leading cause of injury death among people aged 25 to 64, causing more deaths than motor vehicle accidents. The drug overdose rate has more than doubled from 1999 to 2013. In 2013, 81.1% of the nearly 44,000 drug overdose deaths in the United States were unintentional, 12.4% were linked to suicide, and 6.4% were of undetermined intent. In 2011, drug abuse accounted for 2.5 million emergency department visits, with over 1.5 million of these cases attributable to prescription drugs. As of 2012, the percent of US persons of age 12 or older with illicit drug use in the past month (9.2%) or marijuana use in the past month (7.3%) was greater than previous years.

Primary care physicians are well positioned to identify patients at risk for drug abuse early in the course. Since addiction and dependence are equal opportunity afflictions, physicians should screen all new patients for substance abuse. Abrupt changes in behavior or functioning of the patient should also stimulate the physician to screen for substance abuse. As with many other chronic illnesses, early recognition and management of the substance abuse leads to better outcomes.

ASSESSMENT

Expectations From Substance Abuse and Reward Pathway

Several survey-based studies have shown that people abuse drugs to feel good, to get energy, to do better in school and work, and in some cases, due to curiosity. A feeling of euphoria is associated with all commonly abused drugs. The initial euphoric phase is followed by other effects, which differ with the type of the drug abused. With stimulants such as cocaine, ecstasy, and phencyclidine (PCP), the "high" is followed by overexcitement, and feelings of power and self-confidence. On the other hand, relaxation and satisfaction follow the euphoric phase in individuals abusing opiates. Thrill seeking, risk taking, and curious behavior, especially in the adolescent population, play a key role in initial experimentation and continued substance abuse.

The presence of a reward-reinforcement pathway is thought to be the cause of repeated self-administration of drugs to achieve the desired effects. The ventral tegmental area, nucleus accumbens, and frontal cortex of the brain form the stimulant, alcohol, sedative, and hypnotic reward pathway. The periaqueductal gray area, arcuate nucleus, amygdala, and locus coeruleus form the opioids reward system. These pathways are mediated by dopamine, γ-aminobutyric acid (GABA), and certain other peptides.

Etiology and Risk Factors

Vulnerability and affinity to addiction differ from person to person and is considered multifactorial in origin. Factors include gender, ethnicity, developmental stage, and socioeconomic environment. **Genetic susceptibility accounts for between 40% and 60% of a person's vulnerability to addiction.** Populations at increased risk of drug abuse include adolescents and persons with psychiatric disorders.

Epidemiology

According to the 2009 National Survey on Drug Use and Health, marijuana was the most commonly abused drug followed by psychotherapeutic medications. Marijuana is now legal in several states for medicinal or recreational purposes, which may increase the likelihood for abuse and dependence. Daily marijuana use has increased to 8.1 million Americans in 2013. The highest rate of use was among

18- to 25-year olds and males were more likely than females to be users of several different drugs. The highest rates of use were seen among American Indians or Alaska Natives followed by African Americans, Caucasians, Hispanics, and Asians. The rate of drug use was lower for college graduates than for those who did not graduate from high school. However, adults who had graduated from college were more likely to have tried illicit drugs in their lifetime than adults who had not completed high school. The rate of illicit drug use was higher for unemployed persons compared to those who were employed. The rate of current illicit drug use was approximately nine times higher among youths who smoked cigarettes than who did not. Among youths who were heavy drinkers, 69.9% also were current illicit drug users. **Table 41–1 includes the most commonly abused substance categories, street names, route of administration, intoxication effects, and potential health complications.**

History

Currently, **the United States Preventive Services Task Force (USPSTF) concludes that the current evidence is insufficient to assess the balance of benefits and harms of screening adolescents, adults, and pregnant women for illicit drug use.** This statement does not imply that clinicians should not screen patients for illicit drug use, but that there is a lack of evidence to determine the utility of screening. A few brief, standardized questionnaires have been shown to be valid and reliable in screening adolescent and adult patients for drug use/misuse.

Most clinicians perform alcohol and drug abuse screening as part of their routine social history. Electronic medical records often require this data to meet meaningful use criteria. If an individual is identified as having a substance abuse disorder, the history should be geared to determine what, how, and when the patient is using the drug. Information about co-occurring psychiatric or medical conditions and a personal or family history of substance abuse should be obtained. The clinician should ask open-ended questions and should remain nonjudgmental, respectful, and empathetic at all times. Information should also be elicited about health, family, social, career, financial, and legal impacts of the drug use.

Physical Examination

Some findings on the physical examination may aid in the diagnosis of illicit drug use. Eye examination is crucial, especially in an unconscious patient suspected to be under the influence of drugs. Dilated pupils may indicate stimulant or hallucinogen use or withdrawal from opioids. Constricted pupils are a hallmark of opioid use. Physical examination can also reveal damage to nasal mucosa or septum perforation due to insufflation, injection "track marks," or sequelae of cirrhosis due to viral hepatitis or alcohol abuse including spider angiomas, caput medusa, hepatomegaly, and/or ascites.

Laboratory Examination

Several laboratory tests are available for determining the presence of alcohol and other drugs in body fluids such as urine and blood. **Laboratory tests measure recent**

Table 41–1 • COMMONLY ABUSED ILLICIT AND PRESCRIPTION DRUGS

Category and Name	Commercial and Street Names	Route of Administration	Intoxication Effects and Potential Health Consequences
CANNABINOIDS			
Hashish	Boom, chronic, gangster, hash, hash oil, hemp	Swallowed, smoked	**Common features:** *euphoria, slowed thinking and reaction time, confusion, impaired balance and coordination and cough, frequent respiratory infections; impaired memory and learning; tachycardia, anxiety; panic attacks;* **tolerance, addiction**
Marijuana	Blunt, dope, ganja, grass, herb, joints, Mary Jane, pot, reefer, sinsemilla, skunk, weed	Swallowed, smoked	
DEPRESSANTS			
Barbiturates	*Amytal, Nembutal, Seconal, Phenobarbital* and barbs, red, phennies, tooies, yellows jackets	Injected, swallowed	**Common features:** *reduced anxiety; feeling of well-being; lowered inhibitions; slowed pulse and breathing; lowered blood pressure; poor concentration and fatigue; impaired coordination, memory, judgment;* **addiction;** *respiratory depression and arrest; death* **Also, for Barbiturates:** *sedation, drowsiness and depression, excitement, poor judgment, dizziness, life-threatening* **withdrawal** **Also, for Benzodiazepines:** *sedation, drowsiness and dizziness* **Also, for GHB:** *drowsiness, nausea and vomiting, headache, loss of consciousness, loss of reflexes, seizures, coma, death* **Also, for Methaqualone:** *euphoria and depression, poor reflexes*
Benzodiazepines	*Ativan, Halcion, Librium, Valium, Xanax* and candy, downers, sleeping pills, tranks	Swallowed, injected	
GHB	*γ-Hydroxybutyrate* and G, Georgia home boy, grievous bodily harm, liquid ecstasy	Swallowed	
Methaqualone	*Quaalude, Sopor, Parest* and ludes, mandrex, quad, quay	Injected, swallowed	
DISSOCIATIVE ANESTHETICS			
Ketamine	*Ketalar SV* and cat Valiums, K, Special K, vitamin K	Injected, snorted, smoked	**Common features:** *tachycardia, increased blood pressure, impaired motor function and memory loss; numbness; vomiting* **Also, for Ketamine:** *at high doses, delirium, depression, respiratory depression and arrest* **Also, for PCP and analogs:** *possible decrease in blood pressure and heart rate, panic, aggression and loss of appetite, depression, nystagmus*
PCP and analogs	*Phencyclidine* and angel dust, boat, hog, love boat, peace pill	Injected, swallowed, smoked	

OPIOIDS AND MORPHINE DERIVATIVES		
Codeine	*Codeine with Empirin or Fiorinal, Robitussin A–C, Tylenol with Codeine* and Captain Cody, doors & fours, loads, pancakes and syrup	Injected, swallowed	**Common features:** *pain relief, euphoria, drowsiness, miosis,* and nausea, constipation, confusion, sedation, respiratory depression and arrest, **tolerance, addiction,** unconsciousness, coma, death **Also, for Codeine:** less analgesia, sedation, and respiratory depression than morphine **Also, for Heroin:** staggering gait
Heroin	*Diacetyl-morphine* and brown sugar, dope, H, horse, junk, skag, skunk, smack, white horse	Injected, smoked, snorted	
Fentanyl and analogs	*Actiq, Duragesic, Sublimaze* and Apache, China girl, China white, dance fever, friend, goodfella, jackpot, murder 8, TNT, Tango and Cash	Injected, smoked, snorted	
Morphine	*Roxanol, Duramorph, MS-Contin* and M, Miss Emma, monkey, white stuff	Injected, swallowed, smoked	
Opium	*laudanum, paregoric:* big O, black stuff, block, gum, hop	Swallowed, smoked	
Oxycodone Hcl	Oxycontin and Oxy, OC, killer	Swallowed, injected	
Hydrocodone Acetaminophen	*Vicodin, Anexsia, Lorcet, Lortab, Norco* and Vike, Watson-387	Swallowed	
HALLUCINOGENS		
LSD	*Lysergic acid diethylamide* and acid, blotter, boomers, cubes, microdot, yellow sunshines	Swallowed, absorbed through mouth tissues	**Common features:** altered states of perception and feeling; nausea; persisting perception disorder (flashbacks) **Also, for LSD and Mescaline:** increased body temperature, heart rate, blood pressure; loss of appetite, sleeplessness, numbness, weakness, tremors; persistent mental disorders **Also, for Psilocybin:** nervousness, paranoia
Mescaline	Buttons, cactus, mesc, peyote	Swallowed, smoked	
Psilocybin	Magic mushroom, purple passion, shrooms	Swallowed	

(Continued)

Table 41–1 • COMMONLY ABUSED ILLICIT AND PRESCRIPTION DRUGS (CONTINUED)			
Category and Name	**Commercial and Street Names**	**Route of Administration**	**Intoxication Effects and Potential Health Consequences**
STIMULANTS			
Amphetamines	*Biphetamine, Dexedrine* and bennies, black beauties, crosses, hearts, LA turnaround, speed, truck drivers, uppers	Injected, swallowed, smoked, snorted	**Common features:** *increased heart rate, blood pressure, metabolism; feelings of exhilaration, energy, increased mental alertness and rapid or irregular heartbeat; reduced appetite, weight loss, heart failure, nervousness, insomnia* **Also, for Amphetamine:** *rapid breathing and tremor, loss of coordination; irritability, anxiousness, restlessness, delirium, panic, paranoia, impulsive behavior, aggressiveness,* **tolerance, addiction Also, for Cocaine:** *increased temperature and chest pain, respiratory failure, nausea, abdominal pain,* strokes, seizures, headaches, malnutrition, panic attacks, mydriasis **Also, for MDMA:** *mild hallucinogenic effects, increased tactile sensitivity, empathic feelings and impaired memory and learning, hyperthermia, cardiac toxicity, renal failure, liver toxicity* **Also, for Methamphetamine:** *aggression, violence, psychotic behavior* and memory loss, cardiac and neurological damage; impaired memory and learning, tolerance, addiction **Also, for Nicotine:** additional effects attributable to tobacco exposure; adverse pregnancy outcomes; chronic lung disease, cardiovascular disease, stroke, cancer, tolerance, addiction
Cocaine	*Cocaine hydrochloride* and blow, bump, C, candy, Charlie, coke, crack, flake, rock, snow, toot	Injected, smoked, snorted	
MDMA	*Methylenedioxy-methamphetamine* and Adam, clarity, ecstasy, Eve, lover's speed, peace, STP	Swallowed	
Methamphetamine	*Desoxyn* and chalk, crank, crystal, fire, glass, go fast, ice, meth, speed	Injected, swallowed, smoked, snorted	
Methylphenidate	*Ritalin* and JIF, MPH, R-ball, Skippy, the smart drug, vitamin R	Injected, swallowed, snorted	
Nicotine	cigarettes, cigars, smokeless tobacco, snuff, spit tobacco, bidis, chew	Smoked, snorted, taken in snuff and spit tobacco	

OTHER COMPOUNDS

Anabolic steroids	*Anadrol, Oxandrin, Durabolin, Depo-Testosterone, Equipoise, roids, juice*	Injected, swallowed, applied to skin	**Common features:** *No intoxication effects* and hypertension, blood clotting and cholesterol changes, liver cysts and cancer, kidney cancer, hostility and aggression, acne; in adolescents, premature stoppage of growth; in males, prostate cancer, reduced sperm production, shrunken testicles, breast enlargement; in females, menstrual irregularities, development of beard and other masculine characteristics, hirsutism, virilization
Dextromethorphan	*Found in some cough and cold medications; Robotripping, Robo, Triple C*	Swallowed	**Common features:** *Distorted visual perceptions to complete dissociative effects* and at higher doses see "dissociative anesthetics"
Inhalants	*Solvents (paint thinners, gasoline, glues), gases (butane, propane, aerosol propellants, nitrous oxide), nitrites (isoamyl, isobutyl, cyclohexyl), laughing gas, poppers, snappers*	Inhaled through nose or mouth	**Common features:** *stimulation, loss of inhibition; headache; nausea or vomiting; slurred speech, loss of motor coordination; wheezing* and unconsciousness, cramps, weight loss, muscle weakness, depression, memory impairment, damage to cardiovascular and nervous systems, sudden death

Data from Commonly Abused Drugs. (Revised October 2010). Retrieved from The National Institute on Drug Abuse (NIDA).

Table 41–2 • HOW LONG DO DRUGS STAY IN YOUR SYSTEM?	
Alcohol	3-10 h
Amphetamines	24-48 h
Barbiturates	up to 6 wk
Benzodiazepines	up to 6 wk with high-level use
Cocaine	2-4 d; up to 10-22 h with heavy use
Codeine	1-2 d
Heroin	1-2 d
Hydromorphone	1-2 d
Methadone	2-3 d
Morphine	1-2 d
Phencyclidine (PCP)	1-8 d
Propoxyphene	6-48 h
Tetrahydrocannabinol (THC)	6-11 wk with heavy use

National Institutes of Health. Medline Plus. Toxicology Screen.

substance use rather than chronic use or dependence. Table 41–2 highlights how long illicit substances can be detected via urine toxicology screening. There is no conclusive test to determine substance dependence. Useful laboratory tests in those suspected of substance abuse include breath or blood alcohol tests, urine toxicology, liver enzyme tests, electrolytes, renal function, CBC, PT/INR and PTT, and vitamin deficiency screening.

INTERVENTION

Treatment Approach

Substance abuse is a difficult-to-treat disorder and requires an understanding of natural history of recovery from addiction. Although, initial symptoms from withdrawal may not be very different from one class of drug to another, there are significant differences in complications and management of withdrawal from different substances. Therefore, it is crucial to identify the abused substance early in the treatment. The treatment is a long-term process regardless of the substance being abused that often requires many behavioral changes and multiple attempts to quit.

In the United States, treatment of drug addiction is provided in various settings with different medication and behavioral therapy options, which should be discussed with the patient at the initiation of the treatment. Considering the wishes and readiness of the patient to acquire treatment, the physician should recommend a comprehensive plan, preferably including both medication and behavioral therapy. General categories for drug treatment programs include detoxification and medically managed withdrawal, long-term residential treatment, short-term residential treatment followed by long-term outpatient treatment, or exclusively outpatient treatment. A one-time intervention in primary care settings with phone call follow-up demonstrated no significant benefit in decreasing substance abuse.

Medication and behavioral therapy, especially when combined, are important elements of an overall therapeutic process that often begins with detoxification. This includes management of the withdrawal symptoms, followed by treatment and relapse prevention. A key to preventing relapses is to minimize the withdrawal symptoms, which is often the first step of treatment in a patient who acknowledges his addiction. Tapering doses of long-acting agents for the abused drugs are often used to treat drug withdrawal. Antidepressants, anxiolytics, mood stabilizers, and antipsychotic medications may be critical for treatment success when patients have co-occurring psychiatric disorders.

Pharmacotherapy

Detoxification is an important first step in substance-abuse treatment with three goals: initiating abstinence, reducing withdrawal symptoms and severe complications, and retaining the patient in treatment. Ongoing treatment is needed thereafter to maintain abstinence. The aims are to restore normal cognitive and emotional function, to diminish cravings, and to prevent relapse. The medication also helps to make patients more receptive to the behavioral treatment and to avoid drug seeking and related criminal behavior. See Table 41–3 for substance withdrawal symptoms, medications used to treat withdrawal symptoms, long-term treatment, and relapse prevention.

Behavioral Therapies

Behavioral treatment is an important adjunct to addiction treatment. It helps to provide positive reinforcement to remain abstinent, to modify lifestyles related to drug abuse, and to help develop coping mechanisms to handle stressful situations. Common behavioral therapy models include cognitive behavioral therapy and the 12-step model, which is used by organizations such as Alcoholics Anonymous and Narcotics Anonymous.

Table 41–3 · ADDICTION: WITHDRAWAL SYMPTOMS AND PHARMACOLOGY FOR DRUG WITHDRAWAL AND RELAPSE PREVENTION

ADDICTIONS

Withdrawal Symptoms	Generic Name	(*Brand Name*) Treatment Characteristics
OPIOIDS		
Muscle cramps, arthralgia, anxiety, nausea, vomiting, malaise, drug seeking, mydriasis, piloerection, diaphoresis, rhinorrhea, lacrimation, diarrhea, insomnia, elevated blood pressure and pulse	Methadone	(*Dolophine, Methadose*) Long-acting synthetic opioid; given in dosage sufficient to prevent opioid withdrawal, block the effects of illicit opioid use, decrease opioid craving.
	Buprenorphine	(*Subtex, Suboxone*) Partial agonist at opioid receptors, lowers the risk of overdose, reduces or eliminates withdrawal symptoms, no euphoria and sedation caused by other opioids (including methadone).
	Naltrexone	(*Revie*) Long-acting synthetic opioid antagonist, used in outpatient settings, prevents an addicted individual from feeling the effects associated with opioid use which is the notion behind this treatment, diminished craving and addiction.
TOBACCO		
Headaches, irritability, craving, depression, anxiety, cognitive and attention deficits, sleep disturbances, and increased appetite	Nicotine replacement therapies	(*gums, patch, spray, lozenges*) Used in maintaining low levels of nicotine in the body and reduce the withdrawal symptoms.
	Bupropion	(*Welbutrin, Zyban*) Mild stimulant effects, blocks reuptake of norepinephrine and dopamine, marketed initially as an antidepressants, showed efficacy in reducing tobacco craving, promoting cessation without concomitant weight gain.
	Vareniciline	(*Chantix*) Partial agonist/antagonist at nicotinic receptors, minimal stimulation of nicotine receptor but not enough to stimulate dopamine release which is related to the rewarding effects of nicotine, reduces craving and ensures abstinence.

ALCOHOL

Symptoms	Medication	Description
<12 hours: insomnia, tremulousness, mild anxiety, gastrointestinal upset, headache, diaphoresis, palpitations, anorexia	Naltrexone	(Revie) Used to reduce relapse in heavy drinkers (defined as 4 or more drinks/day in women and 5 or more drinks/day in men), relapse reduction up to 36% in first 3 months, not very effective in maintaining abstinence.
12 to 24 hours: visual, auditory, or tactile hallucinations	Acamprosate	(Campral) Reduces withdrawal by acting on GABA and glutamate pathway, very effective in maintaining abstinence in dependent drinkers even in severe cases for several weeks to months.
24 to 48 hours: Generalized tonic-clonic seizures	Disulfiram	(Antabuse) Causes retention of acetaldehyde by interfering with the degradation of alcohol, flushing, nausea and vomiting experienced on alcohol intake, noncompliance is common.
48 to 72 hours: Delirium Tremens; hallucinations (predominately visual), disorientation, tachycardia, hypertension, low-grade fever, agitation, diaphoresis	Topiramate	(Topamax) Thought to have similar mode of action as acamprosate, not FDA approved for alcohol addictions treatment.
	Chlordiazepoxide, diazepam, lorazepam	(Librium, Valium, Ativan) Benzodiazepines (preferably long-acting); decreased severity of withdrawal symptoms; reduced risk of seizures and delirium tremens.
	Carbamazepine, valproate	(Tegretol, Depakote) Anticonvulsants; decreased severity of withdrawal symptoms.
	Atenolol, propranolol	(Tenormin, Inderal) Beta-blockers; used as adjunctive agents, improvement in vital signs; reduction in craving.
	Clonidine	(Catapres) Alpha-agonists; used as adjunctive agents, decreased severity of withdrawal symptoms.

STIMULANTS

Symptoms	Medication	Description
Paranoia, depression, somnolence, anxiety, irritability, difficulty to concentrate, psychomotor retardation, increased appetite	Methylphenidate, amantadine	(Ritalin, Symmetrel) Indirect dopamine agonists; treatment retention was improved in one study of each agent; data are very limited.
	Propranolol	(Inderal) Adrenergic antagonists; treatment retention was improved and cocaine use was reduced in patients with severe withdrawal symptoms.
	Desipramine, bupropion	(Norpramin, Welbutrin) Antidepressants; medications are well tolerated but do not appear to be effective during stimulant withdrawal.

COMPREHENSION QUESTIONS

41.1 An 18-year-old woman who is captain of her high school cheerleading squad presents to the clinic with her mother, who is concerned about her erratic behavior and emotional outbursts. She states that her daughter rarely sleeps on the weekends but sleeps heavily at the beginning of the week and is frequently late for school. She has no significant medical or psychiatric history. Her mother states that she has tried to discuss these issues, but her daughter gets angry and leaves home. She wants to have her daughter tested for drug use. You speak to the patient alone, and she endorses the symptoms her mother reports. Her vital signs are within normal limits and physical examination is unremarkable. She consents to a urine toxicology screen that is positive for methamphetamine, then she admits that she last used over a month ago and has only used twice in her life. What is the most appropriate next step in managing this patient?

A. Confront the patient in the presence of her mother that she has an addiction problem.

B. Refer the patient for an immediate psychiatric evaluation.

C. Prescribe oral propranolol to prevent withdrawal symptoms.

D. Offer behavioral therapy and drug rehabilitation to the patient alone.

E. Obtain an ECG, comprehensive panel, and CBC.

41.2 A 67-year-old man is brought to the ED by ambulance with altered mental status. His physical therapist accompanies him and states that he found the patient semiconscious on his bed. He mentioned that the patient had a femoral neck fracture secondary to fall 4 weeks ago. He went through inpatient rehab and was discharged last week. He has been receiving home physiotherapy three times a week. He has a history of hypertension, diabetes mellitus type 2, and depression. His current medications include lisinopril, metformin, glyburide, Prozac (fluoxetine), and MS-Contin (morphine sulfate). Examination revealed a semiconscious man with temperature of 98.4°F, blood pressure of 135/87 mm Hg, respiratory rate is 8 breaths/min, and pulse of 59 beats/min. Further examination revealed pin point pupils on eye examination and sinus bradycardia with no murmur, rubs, or gallops on heart examination. Lung examination revealed shallow breathing and decreased breath sounds on both sides. He was immediately placed on bag-mask ventilation. What is the most appropriate next step in managing this patient?

A. Obtain neurology consult.

B. Computed tomography (CT) scan of the brain without contrast.

C. Give IV naloxone.

D. STAT echocardiogram.

E. Transfer to intensive care unit (ICU).

41.3 A 30-year-old woman presents to the clinic complaining of feeling depressed and jittery. She has been feeling this way on and off for the last year, since her husband passed away in a car accident. She reports a recent increase in headaches, insomnia, loss of appetite, and increased irritability. When asked about substance abuse, she says she drinks wine at night to help her sleep. Further questioning leads her to disclose that she started drinking more after her husband's death and she currently drinks, on average, 1.5 bottles of wine each evening. She denies previous history of psychiatric disorder. The patient's physical examination is unremarkable with the exception of elevated blood pressure 140/90 mm Hg. You diagnose and counsel the patient about alcohol dependence. Which of the following statements regarding available treatments for alcohol dependence is most accurate?

A. Naltrexone and acamprosate are recommended as FDA-approved options for treatment of alcohol dependence in conjunction with behavior therapy.

B. Disulfiram is the first-line treatment to decrease relapse.

C. Admission to the hospital for inpatient detoxification is the next best step in management.

D. Fluoxetine (Prozac) and other selective serotonin reuptake inhibitors (SSRIs) are recommended for patients with comorbid depressive disorders.

ANSWERS

41.1 **D.** This patient should be presented with the results of the urine toxicology screen and options about substance abuse treatment while not in the presence of her parent. She appears reasonable and psychologically stable during the appointment, thus does not require an immediate psychiatric evaluation. An ECG and serologic evaluation will not likely add to the investigation of this patient, as she is asymptomatic upon presentation. Similarly, she does not appear acutely intoxicated, and propranolol has no role in the prevention of withdrawal symptoms for methamphetamine intoxication.

41.2 **C.** The treatment of choice for the acute opioid intoxication is the administration of an intravenous opioid antagonist (ie, naloxone). This patient has been taking oral morphine for pain control after his surgery and is now presenting with classic symptoms of acute opioid intoxication. A useful mnemonic to remember the sign and symptoms of opioid agents is MORPHINE-ABC (ie, Miosis, Out of it/sedation, Respiratory depression, Pneumonia/aspiration, Hypotension/hypothermia, Infrequency includes constipation, decreased bowel sounds, and urinary retention, Nausea, Emesis/euphoria, Analgesic, Bradycardia, Coma/altered mental status).

41.3 **A.** The pharmacologic treatment is used as an adjunct in treatment of alcohol dependence. Naltrexone, disulfiram, and acamprosate are FDA approved for this indication. Consistent, good-quality, patient-oriented evidence have found naltrexone or acamprosate to be the most effective treatment of alcohol dependence when used in conjunction with behavioral therapy. Limited-quality patient-oriented evidence is available for use of fluoxetine or other SSRIs for patients with comorbid depression disorder.

CLINICAL PEARLS

▶ No single treatment for illicit substance abuse is appropriate for all individuals.

▶ Individual and/or group counseling and other behavioral therapies are critical components of effective treatment for addiction.

▶ Medications are an important element of treatment for many patients, especially when combined with counseling and other behavioral therapies.

▶ Addicted or drug-abusing individuals with coexisting mental disorders should have both disorders treated in an integrated way.

▶ Medical detoxification is only the first stage of addiction treatment and by itself does little to change long-term drug use.

▶ Recovery from drug addiction can be a long-term process and frequently requires multiple episodes of treatment.

REFERENCES

Center for Substance Abuse Treatment. (n.d.). Incorporating alcohol pharmacotherapies into medical practice. *Treatment Improvement Protocol (TIP) Series 49*. HHS Publication No. (SMA) 09-4380. Rockville, MD: Substance Abuse and Mental Health Services Administration; 2009. (Retrieved from Agency for Healthcare Research and Quality).

Commonly Abused Drugs. (Revised October 2010). Retrieved from The National Institute on Drug Abuse (NIDA).

Diagnosis & Treatment of Drug Abuse in Family Practice. (2003). Retrieved from The National Institute on Drug Abuse (NIDA).

Drugs, Brains, and Behavior The Science of Addiction. (Revised August 2010). Retrieved from The National Institute on Drug Abuse (NIDA).

National Center for Biotechnology Information, US National Library of Medicine. (Bookshelf ID: NBK25909). *Appendix B Assessment and Screening Instruments*.

National Center for Biotechnology Information, US National Library of Medicine. (Bookshelf ID: NBK25606). *Specialized Substance Abuse Treatment Programs*.

National Center for Health Statistics. *Health, United States, 2013: With Special Feature on Prescription Drugs*. Hyattsville, MD. 2014.

Principles of Drug Addiction Treatment: A Research-Based Guide. 2nd ed. NIH Publication No. 09-4180. (Revised April 2009). Retrieved from The National Institute on Drug Abuse (NIDA).

Screening for Illicit Drug Use. (January 2008). Retrieved from US Preventive Services Task Force.

Substance abuse and mental health services administration. *Results from the 2009 National Survey on Drug Use and Health: Mental Health Findings.* Center for Behavioral Health Statistics and Quality, NSDUH Series H-39, HHS Publication No. SMA 10-4609. Rockville, MD: Substance Abuse and Mental Health Services Administration; 2010.

Thomas R, Kosten M. Management of drug and alcohol withdrawal. *N Engl J Med.* 2003; 348:1786–1795.

A 35-year-old woman presents to your office complaining of skipped or "irregular heartbeats" for the past few weeks. She paid little attention to her symptoms because she had been under job-related stress and she thought these symptoms would disappear. Instead, her occasional skipped beats increased in frequency to twice a day, lasting up to 2 minutes per episode. Her father, who suffered from heart disease, urged her to see a doctor. She denied chest pain, shortness of breath, or dizziness. She consumes about two cups of caffeinated coffee per day. She recently tried some over-the-counter (OTC) diet pills to lose weight, but stopped taking them when her symptoms became more frequent. On examination, she has a normal body mass index (BMI), her blood pressure is 130/85 mm Hg, heart rate is 92 beats/min, and temperature is 98.6°F (37°C). Head, ears, eyes, nose, and throat (HEENT) examination is normal. No conjunctival pallor or injection is noted. Neck examination is without thyromegaly, nodule, or mass and without jugular venous distension or bruit. Lung examination is bilaterally clear to auscultation. Cardiac examination reveals regular rate and rhythm with normal S_1 and S_2 and without midsystolic click or murmur. Abdominal examination is unremarkable. Examination of the extremities reveals palpable symmetric distal pulses in all four extremities. Neurologic examination reveals no resting tremor. Reflexes are normal.

► What is your most likely diagnosis?
► What is your next diagnostic step?
► What is the next step in therapy?

ANSWERS TO CASE 42:

Palpitations

Summary: A 35-year-old woman presents to your office with palpitations for 2 weeks that have increased in frequency. Her symptoms are not associated with chest pain, syncope, dyspnea, or dizziness. She has no pertinent past medical history. She has the potential triggers of caffeine consumption, diet pill use, and stress. Family history of heart disease is also noted. Her examination is normal.

- **Most likely diagnosis:** Cardiac dysrhythmia, benign.

- **Next diagnostic step:** Obtain 12-lead ECG.

- **Next step in therapy:** Restrict caffeine and alcohol; eliminate any amphetamine-based stimulants and/or diuretics; keep a diary of symptoms or possible triggers; follow-up with patient in 2 weeks. If symptoms persist, additional workup may be required.

ANALYSIS

Objectives

1. Define palpitations.

2. Identify benign rhythm disturbances and those associated with sudden cardiac death.

3. Identify the most common structural heart diseases associated with sudden cardiac death.

4. Develop a rational approach that takes into account cardiac and noncardiac causes for palpitations.

Considerations

This 35-year-old woman gives a history of frequent palpitations and otherwise appears healthy (normal physical examination) without a history of associated dizziness or syncope. Because she is also younger than the age of 50 (thus at low risk for coronary artery disease), she is most likely to have a nonthreatening cause for her symptoms and can be worked up on an outpatient basis.

This history is the most important part of the workup in this patient. We are given clues to noncardiac factors that may contribute to palpitations, including caffeine consumption, use of diet pills, job-related stress, and possibly stress surrounding her father's own health problems. However, stress should not be assumed to be the only cause of her symptoms. Anemia should be considered if there is a history of fatigue, light-headedness, gastrointestinal (GI) blood loss, or menorrhagia.

Family history can be very important because some dysrhythmias, such as familial prolonged QT syndrome, can run in families. A family history of premature cardiac death (or unexplained sudden death) should be sought, as hypertrophic cardiomyopathy is an autosomal dominant disorder and may not always demonstrate a heart murmur when the patient is examined.

If this woman were to have a midsystolic click associated with or without a late systolic murmur, the physician should consider the presence of **mitral valve prolapse** (MVP) syndrome. Usually asymptomatic, it is the **most common valvular heart defect** in the United States, occurring in 3% to 6% of the population. Because MVP is common, the presence of palpitations may or may not be comorbid with this condition. Nonetheless, patients may present with palpitations, fatigue, chest discomfort (not typical of angina), and dyspnea with this valvular finding. This symptom complex is defined as mitral valve prolapse syndrome. These patients may also present with panic attacks or manic-depressive syndromes. Two percent of patients with MVP will have complications resulting in progression to mitral regurgitation with subsequent left-sided two-chamber enlargement, atrial fibrillation (if the left atrium becomes enlarged), left ventricular dysfunction leading to heart failure, pulmonary hypertension, and infective endocarditis. For these reasons, a surface echocardiogram is recommended at baseline when suspicion for MVP is identified.

APPROACH TO:
Palpitations

DEFINITION

PALPITATIONS: A subjective sensation of unduly strong, slow, rapid, or irregular heartbeats that may be related to cardiac arrhythmias. The sensation may last seconds, minutes, hours, or days and is often intermittent. They are common, usually not dangerous, and may be the result of a change in the heart's electrical system.

CLINICAL APPROACH

Etiologies

Approximately 40% of patients complaining of palpitations have an underlying primary rhythm disturbance. An underlying mental health problem (anxiety or panic disorder) is the cause in 31% of symptomatic patients. Drugs (prescription, recreational, or over-the-counter) cause 6% of palpitations; intrinsic structural problems with the heart are the cause of 3%; 4% have noncardiac causes; and the remaining 16% have no identifiable cause.

The largest group has some type of primary rhythm disorder:

- Premature atrial contractions (PAC)—most common etiology of palpitations
- Premature ventricular contractions (PVC)
- Sinus tachycardia
- Sinus bradycardia
- Wolff-Parkinson-White (WPW) syndrome

- Sick sinus syndrome

- Supraventricular tachycardias (SVT)

- Ventricular tachycardia (VT)

These rhythm disturbances can be seen throughout childhood and adulthood.

Supraventricular tachycardia refers to any tachycardia that is not ventricular in origin. This definition includes physiologic sinus tachycardia which can be a normal reaction to stress and a variety of noncardiac conditions such as fever and hyperthyroidism. In the clinical setting however, it is used practically as a synonym for paroxysmal supraventricular tachycardia (PSVT). This term refers to those SVTs that have a sudden, almost immediate onset and regular rhythm. A person experiencing PSVT may feel their heart rate go from 60 to 200 beats/min instantaneously, often in response to a quick movement such as picking something up from the floor. Because physiologic sinus tachycardia has a gradual onset and atrial fibrillation (AF) and multifocal atrial tachycardia (MAT) are irregular rhythms, they are excluded from the PSVT category.

PSVTs are most commonly atrioventricular (AV) nodal reentrant tachycardias or part of WPW syndrome, which may be "concealed" (ie, not evident on the resting ECG). WPW syndrome is caused by an accessory track between the atria and ventricles that conducts electrical impulses in addition to the AV node. The classic ECG finding is a slurring on the upstroke of the QRS complex known as a delta wave. WPW can cause dangerous arrhythmias and lead to sudden cardiac death.

Brugada syndrome is an ion channel disorder that is most common in Asian males. Characteristic findings on an ECG include a right bundle branch block pattern and an elevation at the J point that is greater than 2 mm, with a slowly descending ST segment in conjunction with flat or negative T waves in the right precordial leads V_1, V_2, or V_3. It can cause dangerous arrhythmias that results in sudden death.

Sick sinus syndrome usually involves a dysfunction of the sinoatrial (SA) node that leads to bradycardia and can cause fatigue and syncope. Patients, however, can also have a tachycardia-bradycardia variety of sick sinus syndrome in which they also experience supraventricular tachycardia with its associated symptoms of palpitations and angina pectoris.

Patients with **long QT interval syndrome** are at increased risk for ventricular arrhythmias and sudden cardiac death (SCD). Long QT syndrome is caused by mutations in multiple genes and can have an **autosomal dominant pattern.** It is seen more commonly in females. Patients with this syndrome will present with either palpitations and/or syncope and have a family history of syncope or sudden death. Prolonged QT interval is defined as QT_C[1] 470 ms in men or greater than 480 ms in women. **Any patient with a QT interval greater than 500 ms is at increased risk for dangerous dysrhythmias.** Prolonged QT intervals may also be the result of the use of certain medications such as quinidine, procainamide, sotalol, amiodarone, and tricyclic antidepressants.

QT_C[1] is defined as measured QT interval corrected for heart rate:

$$QT_C = \frac{QT \text{ (in ms)}}{\sqrt{RR \text{ interval (in ms)}}}$$

Benign rhythm disturbances include premature atrial contractions, sinus tachycardia, and sinus bradycardia appropriate for activity/stress level, sinus pauses less than 3 seconds, and isolated unifocal PVCs. However, PVCs in the presence of known cardiac disease, metabolic disease, or the presence of worrisome symptoms (such as near syncope, syncope, or seizures) require aggressive workup because of the risk of ventricular tachycardia or fibrillation. PVCs occurring at rest and disappearing with exercise are usually benign, commonly seen in athletes, and require no investigation.

Psychiatric causes of palpitations are always considered in the differential diagnosis for palpitations and may be missed if not screened for in the initial history. Panic disorder is seen more often in women of childbearing age. Patients with panic attacks commonly present to emergency departments with complaints of chest pain, shortness of breath, and palpitations. They will report brief episodes of overwhelming panic or sense of impending doom associated with tachycardia, dyspnea, or dizziness. Still, these complaints may be identical to primary rhythm disturbances and deserve formal workup and cardiac risk stratification.

Cardiac or structural causes of palpitations include cardiomyopathy, atrial or ventricular septal defects, congenital heart disease, mitral valve prolapse, pericarditis, valvular heart disease (eg, aortic stenosis, aortic insufficiency), and congestive heart failure. The presence of restrictive, hypertrophic, or dilated cardiomyopathies may lead to sudden cardiac death.

Hypertrophic obstructive cardiomyopathy (HOCM) is the most common cause of sudden cardiac death in adolescents in the United States and is often not detected on routine physical examination. These patients may present with chest pain, syncope, and palpitations, but are commonly asymptomatic. Hypertrophic cardiomyopathy may be passed down as an autosomal dominant trait. A heart murmur, if present, will usually be systolic and will be accentuated by Valsalva maneuver. Echocardiography demonstrating a thickened intraventricular septum with ventricular obliteration remains the gold standard for diagnosis. There is no evidence to suggest routine echocardiography screening in athletes to detect HOCM, and such a practice has been shown not to be cost-effective.

Marfan syndrome should be suspected in patients who are tall and have scoliosis, pectus excavatum, long, thin digits (arachnodactyly), high-arched palate, and an arm span exceeding their height. Mitral valve prolapse may be seen in patients with Marfan syndrome. These patients often have aortic root dilations and are at risk for aortic arch aneurysm rupture. The diagnosis can be confirmed by echocardiography.

Noncardiac causes of palpitations may be suggested by the history and examination. Noncardiac etiologies include anemia, electrolyte disturbances, hyperthyroidism, hypothyroidism, hypoglycemia, hypovolemia, fever, pheochromocytoma, pulmonary disease, and vasovagal syncope. **Laboratory screening includes a complete blood count (CBC), comprehensive metabolic panel, and thyroid-stimulating hormone (TSH).** If a pheochromocytoma is suspected, a 24-hour urine collection for catecholamines and metanephrines is indicated.

Numerous medications and substances may contribute to palpitations including alcohol, caffeine (especially energy drinks), illicit drugs (cocaine), tobacco, decongestants (eg, pseudoephedrine, often found in OTC and herbal weight loss drugs), diuretics (causing electrolyte disturbances), digoxin, β-agonists (eg, albuterol), theophylline, and phenothiazine. Patients should be questioned about their use of OTC medications, herbs, and supplements, as they often will not provide this information unless specifically asked. It is always reasonable to ask the patient to bring the herbal preparations and supplements that they are taking to the clinic so that the physician can review the ingredients.

CLINICAL PRESENTATION

Evaluation of a patient presenting with palpitations should take into account numerous factors. The patient's age at symptom onset is important, as an **age older than 50 years should always lead to the consideration of coronary artery disease.** However, notwithstanding a patient's age, cardiac risk assessment should occur with every patient. Possible triggers should be pursued, such as medication use, exercise, and psychosocial stress. Physicians should pay particular attention to palpitations associated with syncope, as these are usually pathologic and hospitalization with cardiac monitoring and cardiology evaluation should be considered.

The clinical examination should focus on vital signs (blood pressure and heart rate), including orthostatic readings if suggested by history. The thyroid gland should be examined for abnormalities such as goiter, nodule, or bruit. The presence of resting tremor or brisk reflexes should also lead the physician to consider hyperthyroidism.

The cardiac examination should be thorough. The point of maximum impulse should be palpated, as displacement may suggest cardiomegaly. The rate and rhythm, along with any irregularities, should be noted, and an ECG should be obtained. For example, an irregularly irregular rhythm is suggestive of atrial fibrillation whereas an occasional extra beat may be PACs or PVCs. Extra sounds, such as the midsystolic click of mitral valve prolapse or any murmurs consistent with valvular pathology, should also be documented and an echocardiogram should be obtained.

A 12-lead electrocardiogram is appropriate in all patients with palpitations, even if they are symptom free during the physician encounter. The presence of left ventricular hypertrophy, atrial enlargement, atrioventricular block, old myocardial infarction, and delta waves (as seen in WPW syndrome) should trigger additional testing. Prolonged QT intervals increase the risk for dangerous rhythm disturbances and require a thorough review of medications that can cause this, as well as consultation with a cardiologist or cardiac electrophysiologist.

Other cardiac testing may be appropriate based on the history, examination, and results of the initial evaluation. **Ambulatory electrocardiographic rhythm monitoring** can be accomplished **for periods of 24 to 72 hours using a Holter monitor.** A cardiac **event monitor can be worn by a patient for up to 30 days** and might be useful when the palpitations do not occur daily. The monitor is worn continuously and activated by the patient when palpitations are felt.

An echocardiogram can be useful in identifying patients with suspected structural abnormalities of their heart chambers or heart valves, which could trigger heart rhythm disturbances. These findings could be missed on physical examination. A transesophageal echocardiogram should be performed to look for a thrombus prior to cardioversion. Exercise stress testing in age- and risk-appropriate patients may be important for identifying dysrhythmias triggered by exercise. This test may be of particular importance in patients with suspected coronary artery disease. Anyone with suspected structural problems should be evaluated by a surface echocardiogram prior to undergoing stress testing. Patients with suspected hypertrophic cardiomyopathy or severe aortic stenosis should avoid exercise stress testing, as they may develop heart rhythm disturbances which may be nonrecoverable. Finally, electrophysiology studies may be needed to recreate rhythm disturbances and identify hyperactive foci and accessory tracts such seen in WPW syndrome. These areas can subsequently be electrically ablated.

TREATMENT

The treatment of a given patient's symptoms is dependent on the etiology. If palpitations are medication related, the offending agent should be weaned or stopped. Anxiety may be treated by a combination of pharmacologic and nonpharmacologic interventions. If the problem is structural cardiac disease, referral to a cardiologist is usually indicated.

β-Blockers or calcium channel blockers are often used as first-line therapy for primary supraventricular rhythm disturbances. If symptoms are short-lived or episodic, short-acting negative chronotropics, such as short-acting β-blockers, can be used on an as-needed basis.

Symptomatic PSVT can often be self-treated by patients with recurrent episodes by several vagal stimulation techniques. Carotid sinus massage, Valsalva maneuver, and cold applications to the face (diver's reflex) can trigger vagus nerve stimulation, which may break an episode of SVT. When these are unsuccessful, IV adenosine is often administered. If the adenosine terminates the SVT, then the arrhythmia is most likely a reentry SVT. If it does not, then the rate may be slowed down with β-blockers or calcium channel blockers. At that point, consultation with a cardiologist should be sought.

Chronic atrial fibrillation should be treated with medication to keep the ventricular rate below 100 beats/min; these agents for rate control are often β-blockers or calcium channel blockers. A return to normal sinus rhythm may be attempted with electrical cardioversion or antiarrhythmic drugs, such as amiodarone, sotalol, or with class 1C drugs such as flecainide and propafenone. Class 1C drugs should not be used in the presence of structural cardiac disease or cardiac hypertrophy. A transesophageal echocardiogram (TEE) should be done prior to cardioversion in order to rule out the presence of a thrombus that might dislodge with the cardioversion. Rhythm control and rate control have similar rates of stroke and mortality. Rate control is often the preferred strategy for many patients. **Most patients with atrial fibrillation will also require anticoagulation**, as they are at an increased risk of embolic stroke from blood clots that form in the cardiac atrium, in accordance with the CHADS2-VASC risk calculation.

Ventricular arrhythmias can be extremely dangerous and usually require prompt treatment. Ventricular fibrillation is not compatible with life and needs to be treated immediately with electrical defibrillation. Patients with ventricular tachycardia, who are unstable, need to be electrically cardioverted. Amiodarone should be given to a patient with stable ventricular tachycardia and in patients who were converted back into a sinus rhythm through cardioversion. Lidocaine should be used in place of amiodarone in patients who are allergic to iodine. The most common cause of ventricular arrhythmias is ischemia.

An automatic implantable cardioverter-defibrillator (AICD) is indicated in patients with conditions that commonly result in ventricular fibrillation or tachycardia leading to sudden death. Some of these conditions are advanced dilated cardiomyopathy, long QT syndrome, hypertrophic cardiomyopathy, and Brugada syndrome.

CASE CORRELATION

- See also Case 20 (Chest Pain).

COMPREHENSION QUESTIONS

42.1 A 35-year-old man who has never had a physical examination comes to clinic. He recently moved to the area and needs to establish with a new physician. He has had no previous medical problems to date and no pertinent family history. He denies any changes in bowel or bladder habits and does not smoke or drink alcohol. When prompted he says that he has noticed a "fluttering" in his chest for past 3 months that spontaneously resolves. He has had increased stress at work and has been drinking six cups of caffeinated coffee a day to complete his workload. He has not had time to exercise and his diet consists of what he can find in the office cafeteria. He denies any history of anxiety. Which of the following is the most common underlying etiology of his palpitations?

A. Medication

B. Structural heart disease

C. Coronary artery disease

D. Primary rhythm disturbance

E. Idiopathic

42.2 A 42-year-old asymptomatic woman is noted to have an abnormal finding on ECG. Which of the following is an indication for referral to a cardiologist or cardiac electrophysiologist?

A. PVCs on a resting ECG that resolve with exercise

B. Delta waves on an ECG

C. Isolated unifocal PVCs found on ECG

D. Sinus arrhythmia

42.3 Which of the following patients should undergo an exercise stress test for evaluation of his palpitations?

A. A 60-year-old man with symptomatic PVCs but without syncope

B. A 35-year-old man with hypertrophic cardiomyopathy seen on an echocardiogram

C. A 32-year-old, tall, slender man with pectus excavatum and a midsystolic click on examination

D. A 68-year-old man with suspected aortic stenosis

42.4 A 16-year-old adolescent boy comes to your office for a sports physical. He is planning to try out for his high school football team but first needs medical clearance. He has no cardiovascular complaints and his history is unremarkable, except for a family history which includes an uncle dying suddenly while jogging at age 25. His physical examination is unremarkable except for a harsh systolic murmur loudest over his left lower sternal border which increases with the Valsalva maneuver. You obtain an ECG which shows left ventricular hypertrophy. Which of the following is the most appropriate next step in management?

A. An exercise stress test

B. An echocardiogram

C. A chest x-ray

D. A coronary catheterization

E. Reassurance that he is cleared to play football

42.5 You are called to the bedside of a patient who was complaining of chest pain. When you get there you find the patient confused and not answering questions. The nurse informs you that the patient was speaking coherently only several minutes ago. The patient's pulse is 180 beats/min, his systolic blood pressure is 60 mm Hg, and his diastolic blood pressure cannot be measured. Telemetry reveals supraventricular tachycardia. Which of the following is the most appropriate next step in the management of this patient?

A. Adenosine

B. Cardiology consultation

C. Emergent electrical cardioversion

D. Negative chronotropic agent

E. 12-lead ECG

ANSWERS

42.1 **D.** Primary rhythm disturbances are the most common cause of palpitations, making up approximately 40% of cases. Other common causes include psychiatric etiologies (eg, anxiety, panic disorder), medications, metabolic (eg, electrolytes, thyroid hormone imbalance), and structural heart disease. Many cases of palpitations remain undiagnosed in spite of appropriate evaluation.

42.2 **B.** The presence of delta waves indicates WPW syndrome and the presence of an accessory tract that can be ablated by an electrophysiologist.

42.3 **A.** A 60-year-old with PVCs, especially if they are of new onset, may be showing the initial presentation of coronary artery disease and should undergo stress testing. All of the other conditions listed are contraindications to stress testing.

42.4 **B.** This young man has signs suggestive of hypertrophic cardiomyopathy. The confirmatory test for it is an echocardiogram. Coronary catheterization and stress testing are tests for coronary artery disease and not recommended for this patient. A β-blocker or calcium channel blocker would worsen the patient's hemodynamic status. Adenosine is indicated for supraventricular tachycardia with a narrow QRS complex and not ventricular tachycardia.

42.5 **C.** This patient has ventricular tachycardia with clinical deterioration and hemodynamic instability. He needs immediate electrical cardioversion. If the patient was in a stable ventricular tachycardia, then medical cardioversion could be conducted using intravenous amiodarone.

CLINICAL PEARLS

▶ Patients with palpitations require an in-depth evaluation into potential cardiac etiologies, as psychosocial stress cannot be assumed as the sole etiology.

▶ Consider Marfan syndrome in a tall patient with long arms, long fingers, and wears glasses.

▶ A 24- to 72-hour Holter monitor is appropriate in a patient with frequent (eg, daily) palpitations; a 30-day event monitor is a better test in someone with infrequent episodes.

▶ Hypertrophic cardiomyopathy is the most common cause of sudden cardiac death in adolescents. An adolescent with a systolic heart murmur that increases in intensity with Valsalva maneuver should have his/her activity restricted until a diagnostic echocardiogram can be performed.

▶ Unexplained prolonged QT interval syndrome requires further evaluation.

REFERENCES

Batra AS, Hon AR. Consultation with the specialist: palpitations, syncope, and sudden death in children: who's at risk? *Pediatric Rev.* 2003; 24(8):269–275.

Bouknight DP, O'Rourke RA. Current management of mitral valve prolapse. *Am Fam Physician.* 2000; 61(11):3343–3350, 3353-3354.

Field JM, Hazinski MF, Sayre MR, et al. Part 1: executive summary: 2010 AHA guidelines for CPR and ECC. *Circulation.* 2010 Nov 2;122(18 suppl 3):S640–S656.

Lip GY, Halperin JL. Improving stroke risk stratification in atrial fibrillation. *Am J Med.* 2010; 123(6):484–488.

Marill KA, Ellinor PT. Case records of the Massachusetts General Hospital. Case 37-2005. A 35-year-old man with cardiac arrest while sleeping. *N Engl J Med.* 2005; 353(23):2492–2501.

Michaud GF, Stevenson WG. Supraventricular tachyarrhythmias. In: Kasper D, Fauci A, Hauser S, et al., eds. *Harrison's Principles of Internal Medicine.* 19th ed. New York, NY: McGraw-Hill Education; 2015. Available at: http://accessmedicine.mhmedical.com. Accessed May 25, 2015.

Miller JM, Zipes DP. Diagnosis of cardiac arrhythmias. In: Libby P, Bonow RO, Mann DL, et al., eds. *Braunwald's Heart Disease.* 8th ed. Philadelphia, PA: Saunders Elsevier; 2008:763–831.

Rowland T. Evaluating cardiac symptoms in the athlete: is it safe to play? *Clin J Sport Med.* 2005; 15(6):417–420.

Wexler RK, Pleister A, Raman S. Outpatient approach to palpitations. *Am Fam Physician.* 2011; 84(1):63–69.

Zipes D, Ackerman M, Mark Estes N, et al. Arrhythmias. *J Am Coll Cardiol.* 2005; 45:1354–1363.

The mother of a 16-year-old adolescent girl calls you when you are on call on a Saturday afternoon. The mother states that her daughter was either stung by a bee or bitten by a spider on her left arm several hours ago. The patient has no known history of previous allergic reactions to insect bites or stings. She is having no difficulty breathing or swallowing, nor has she been dizzy or light-headed. The mother's primary concern is that the area around the bite or sting is red and swollen. She says that the site of the injury was the midpoint of the forearm, and now it hurts, slightly itches, and there is redness and swelling extending in a circular pattern several centimeters in diameter. The red area is moderately warm to the touch, so her mother is concerned that it is infected. She gave her daughter some ibuprofen for the pain and would like you to phone in a prescription for an antibiotic as well as something to prevent the reaction from spreading.

► What is the most appropriate first step in treatment of this patient?
► What other treatments might be beneficial at this point?
► What immunization is appropriate for this patient?

ANSWERS TO CASE 43:
Sting and Bite Injuries

Summary: A 16-year-old adolescent girl has been stung by a wasp and is having a painful and itchy local reaction. Also included in the differential diagnosis for this case are nonvenomous insect bites (eg, mosquito) and spider bites. She has no history of previous allergic reactions. The patient's mother is calling and asking you to manage the situation over the phone by prescribing antibiotics.

- **Most appropriate antibiotic to use:** No antibiotic treatment is indicated, as this is a local reaction to a bee sting, with high likelihood for a histamine-mediated reaction, and a low likelihood of a bacterial infection.

- **Next step in therapy:** Local application of ice, oral administration of nonsteroidal anti-inflammatory drugs (NSAIDs) or acetaminophen for pain, and oral or topical antihistamines for itching.

- **Immunization that is appropriate:** Tetanus-diphtheria-pertussis (Tdap) booster, if not up-to-date.

ANALYSIS

Objectives

1. Know the insects that commonly cause bite and sting injuries.

2. Be able to differentiate local from systemic reactions to bites and stings.

3. Know the management of common insect bite and sting as well as animal bite injuries.

Considerations

This adolescent without a history of allergies has sustained a wasp sting, and no therapy is required other than symptomatic treatment. The insect order *Hymenoptera* includes wasps, yellow jackets, hornets, honeybees, bumblebees, and fire ants. These insects cause the majority of cases of sting- or bite-induced anaphylaxis and cause more mortality than all other types of insect bites and stings. Local reactions occur as a result of the toxic properties of the venom, whereas more severe reactions tend to be caused by allergic reaction to venom allergens.

Several types of bee stings result in the retention of the stinger in the victim, which can result in continued injection of the bee venom. Stingers should be promptly removed with caution, as grasping the base of the stinger may result in compression of a venom-containing sac, resulting in increased venom release. Thus, it is suggested that scraping or brushing the stinger off of the skin is preferable to grasping the stinger. However, **rapidly removing the stinger is preferable to taking the time to locate a scraping implement** if one (such as a credit card or driver's license) is not immediately at hand.

Spider bites may present in the same fashion as many insect and bee stings. Typically, the development of pruritus and histamine-mediated swelling within the first few hours of the bite are absent. Cellulitis is common, as is the development of an eschar at the site of the bite. Most spider bites, especially those associated with the brown recluse spider, are associated with methicillin-resistant *Staphylococcus aureus* (MRSA).

APPROACH TO:
Bites and Stings

DEFINITIONS

HYMENOPTERA: Order of insects which includes wasps, yellow jackets, hornets, honeybees, bumblebees, and fire ants, and make up the majority of insect stings.

LARGE LOCAL ALLERGIC REACTIONS: Erythema and warmth of the skin at the area of insect sting, mediated by immunoglobulin E (IgE) reactive to the *Hymenoptera* venom.

CLINICAL APPROACH
INSECT STINGS AND BITES

Local Reactions

Almost all *Hymenoptera* stings will result in a **local reaction**, which includes redness, swelling, pain, and itching at the site of the injury. These reactions **tend to occur almost immediately and last for hours to days.** The local tissue response is a consequence of a histamine-mediated reaction caused by the venom that is released by the sting. Local reactions can be treated with ice and antihistamines for itching. Tetanus prophylaxis should be provided for those who have not been vaccinated.

Delayed Reactions

Large local allergic reactions are mediated by IgE reactive to the *Hymenoptera* venom. These reactions are often confused with cellulitis, as large areas (≥ 10 cm in diameter) of redness and warmth develop over 24 to 48 hours. These reactions are not infectious and will not respond to antibiotics. These reactions are **best treated with oral steroids** initiated early after the sting, as these reactions may last up to 5 to 10 days. Tetanus prophylaxis should be reviewed and updated if necessary. A person with a history of a large local reaction to a bee sting is likely to have similar reactions to subsequent stings. However, the history of this type of reaction does not result in an increased risk of anaphylaxis to subsequent stings.

Anaphylaxis

Up to 4% of the population may have a systemic reaction to a *Hymenoptera* sting. Those who have had a previous systemic reaction have a 50% or greater risk of having a systemic reaction to future stings. These systemic reactions can vary from milder symptoms of nausea, generalized urticaria, or angioedema to severe and life-threatening hypotension, shock, airway edema, and death. Severe immediate-hypersensitivity reactions usually occur within minutes of the sting.

Treatment of anaphylaxis should include assessment and management of the ABCs (airway, breathing, and circulation), with intubation if necessary, IV access, and fluid resuscitation at 10 to 20 mg/kg (usually 500-1000 cc) as soon as possible. **Subcutaneous or intramuscular epinephrine should be administered as quickly as possible (0.3-0.5 mL of 1:1000 solution for adults; 0.01 mg/kg for children at 0.3 mg maximum dose)** and repeated in 5 to 10 minutes if needed. Antihistamines, steroids (if severe), and bronchodilators may be required as well. Anyone with an anaphylactic reaction should be observed in a hospital setting for 12 to 24 hours, as the symptoms can recur. Persons with known anaphylactic reactions should be prescribed epinephrine injector kits to carry with them for immediate access at all times. They should be instructed to avoid wearing perfumes, bright clothing, and avoid walking barefoot when in areas prevalent with bees. Desensitization therapy can also be offered to those with known anaphylaxis, as their risk of future severe reactions can be reduced by up to 50%.

Most spider bites do not cause significant injury or illness. When suspected, the area should be cleansed with warm soap and water, and a cool compress should be applied to the affected area. NSAIDs or acetaminophen are also recommended. When erythema, warmth, and pain develop around the site of injection, MRSA cellulitis should be considered, and the patient should be treated with either oral clindamycin or trimethoprim-sulfamethoxazole. If oral antibiotics do not adequately treat the cellulitis, abscess should be considered and if present, incision and drainage should be performed. In these cases, as well as for those resistant to oral antibiotics, intravenous vancomycin should be started.

ANIMAL BITES

Nearly 5 million animal bites occur in the United States each year. The most common animals involved are dogs and cats, while human bites are also common. Cat and rodent bites are notorious for being "injection"-type bites, while those from dogs and humans are commonly "crush"-type bites, based on the teeth involved in the bite.

The initial management of the patient who has been bitten should focus on the ABCs and on protection of the current injury (eg, splinting of fractures, protection of cervical spine, etc), as well as local wound care including control of bleeding and assessment of the injuries incurred. History should be gathered on the type of animal that caused the bite, the situation regarding the bite (whether provoked or unprovoked), and the vaccination status of the animal, particularly to document rabies vaccination status. Almost all cases of human rabies in the United States since 1960 have been caused by bats, skunks, dogs, foxes, and raccoons. Consultation with your local health department after animal bites is recommended.

Local cleaning of the wound(s) with soap and water, irrigation with sterile saline solution, and debridement of devitalized tissue should take place as soon as possible. For minor and superficial to shallow wounds, these treatments are often all that is required.

The risk of infection from an animal or human is dependent on numerous factors. Larger and deeper wounds are more likely to become infected than smaller, superficial wounds. Bite wounds on the hand tend to have an increased risk of infection due to thin skin and close proximity to small joint spaces. Host factors, such as the presence of chronic illnesses or immune suppression, also play a role in susceptibility to infection. Cat and human bites have a high risk of infection and should always be treated empirically with antibiotics, whereas only 20% of dog-bite wounds become infected.

Many different bacteria can be involved in bite wound infections. All cat bite wounds should be suspected to be contaminated with *Pasteurella multocida*. Both cats and dogs carry multiple species of staphylococci and streptococci, as well as anaerobic bacteria. Humans carry staphylococci, streptococci, *Haemophilus* species, *Eikenella* species, and anaerobic bacteria.

The treatment of bite wounds starts with local care—cleaning, irrigation, and debridement of crushed and infected tissue. The primary closure of bite wounds is controversial and should be limited to lacerations less than 12 hours old. Deep puncture and wounds with signs of infection should be well irrigated with sterile solution and not primarily closed. Tetanus vaccination should be updated in all patients as needed. Hepatitis B and HIV postexposure prophylaxis should be considered for patients who sustained a human bite from a high-risk person. Animal control authorities should be contacted for guidance regarding rabies vaccination.

All patients who sustained cat bites should be treated for 10 to 14 days with oral amoxicillin-clavulanate. Although clear evidence of efficacy is lacking for the treatment of dog and human bites, current recommendations are for antibiotic prophylaxis with amoxicillin-clavulanate for 5 to 7 days for patients with moderate-to-severe wounds. When cellulitis is present, longer courses of antibiotic therapy, usually 10 to 14 days, are required. Hospitalization, intravenous antibiotics, and surgical intervention may be required for more severe infections including osteomyelitis, septic joint infections, and in patients with complicating medical conditions including immunosuppression.

COMPREHENSION QUESTIONS

43.1 Which of the following therapeutic options is recommended in treating both bee stings and bite wounds?

A. Antibiotic prophylaxis with amoxicillin-clavulanate

B. Antihistamines for itching

C. Tetanus vaccination

D. Surgical wound debridement

43.2 A 22-year-old woman develops a progressively enlarging red, hot area on her leg following a sting from a yellow jacket. She states that the sting was sharp and of brief duration and she was able to fully remove the stinger with tweezers. She did not suffer any symptoms of systemic anaphylaxis. She has no previously known allergies. She sees you in the office a day after the sting and states that the area of the sting is still enlarging despite using over-the-counter corticosteroid cream and a first-generation antihistamine. Which of the following is the most appropriate next treatment for this patient?

A. Oral prednisone

B. Topical corticosteroid

C. Antibiotic directed against gram-positive cocci

D. Portable epinephrine kit for future stings

E. Reassurance

43.3 You see a 7-year-old boy a day after he was bitten by his pet dog. According to his mother, the dog bit the child after he surprised the dog and grabbed its tail. The dog has had all of its vaccinations, including rabies. The child has had no fever, has full movement of the injured limb, and has no sign of neurologic or vascular injury. The wound is on the child's forearm, is not deep, is not bleeding, but has developed 2 cm of erythema surrounding the site. Which of the following is the most appropriate treatment?

A. Hospitalization for IV antibiotic

B. Oral amoxicillin-clavulanate for 3 to 5 days

C. Oral amoxicillin-clavulanate for 7 to 14 days

D. Local care without any antibiotic

43.4 You see a 43-year-old man who was involved in a fist fight 2 days ago and sustained a deep laceration wound around his knuckles from where he struck the face of another man. He was intoxicated at the time and upon return home, he did not clean the wound and went straight to sleep. The injury site has now developed purulent drainage, pain, erythema, and the man has a low-grade fever. There is no rash and he has not noted any spreading of the erythema. An x-ray of the hand shows a hairline fracture of the fifth metacarpal head with swelling and bruising noted over the affected area. Which of the following is the most likely organism causing infection?

A. Methicillin-resistant *S aureus*

B. Streptococci

C. *Eikenella corrodens*

D. *Escherichia coli*

E. *Peptostreptococcus*

43.5 A mother brings in her 6-year-old child who was bitten on the hand while playing with a rabbit that was recently obtained from a neighbor. The child's wound is on the volar surface of the right second finger just distal to the proximal interphalangeal joint. Which of the following steps in the management of bite wounds is most effective in preventing wound infection?

A. Tetanus prophylaxis

B. Rabies prophylaxis

C. Saline irrigation and wound care

D. Prophylactic antibiotics

E. Irrigation and primary closure

ANSWERS

43.1 **C.** Tetanus vaccination is common to the management of both bee stings and bite wounds. Bee stings rarely become infected and do not require antibiotic therapy.

43.2 **A.** This patient is having a large, local reaction to her sting. This is an IgE-mediated reaction. It may respond to a course of oral steroids. There is at least a 50% chance that a similar reaction will occur if she was stung again, but she is unlikely to develop anaphylactic reactions in the future and does not need anaphylaxis prophylaxis. The patient should be informed that the localized reaction may take 5 to 10 days to completely resolve, and may resolve more quickly with treatment with oral steroids. Her history of a sting makes cellulitis less likely.

43.3 **C.** This child is developing cellulitis from the bite wound. Based on his presentation, he does not appear to require hospitalization. He can be treated with oral antibiotics for 1 to 2 weeks.

43.4 **C.** While each of these bacteria can be isolated in injuries from human bites, *Eikenella* species appear to be most common in closed fist injuries. For patients presenting after a "fist fight" with bite injuries, prophylaxis with amoxicillin-clavulanate is indicated due to inoculation with oral flora into the skin and subcutaneous tissues.

43.5 **C.** Rodents and lagomorphs (rabbits) are neither reservoirs of the rabies virus nor have been shown to transmit the rabies virus to humans. The most important step in preventing the infectious complications of bite wounds is proper wound care with inspection, irrigation, and debridement. Tetanus prophylaxis should be considered in all bite wounds. Antibiotic prophylaxis may also be indicated especially in high-risk bites (those located on the hand, late presentation, cat bites) and should be directed against staphylococci, streptococci, anaerobes, and *Pasteurella* species as appropriate.

CLINICAL PEARLS

► Anyone with a history of anaphylactic reactions should be given a prescription for an epinephrine injector kit and instructed in the importance of keeping it at hand. These prescriptions need to be updated often, as the medication expires in 6 to 12 months.

► Local cleaning of the wound(s) with soap and water, irrigation with saline, and debridement of devitalized tissue should take place as soon as possible.

► Human "bite" wounds are not always the result of a bite. A punch to the mouth can cause a serious inoculation and infection to the knuckles of the puncher.

► All cat and human bites should be empirically treated with amoxicillin-clavulanate due to high rates of infection, whereas approximately 20% of dog-bite wounds become infected.

► Cellulitis following spider bites should be treated with the suspicion of MRSA with oral clindamycin *or* trimethoprim-sulfamethoxazole.

REFERENCES

Brook I. Management of human and animal bite wounds: an overview. *Adv Skin Wound Care*. 2005; 18(4):197–203.

Chen E, Hornig S, Shepherd SM, Hollander JE. Primary closure of mammalian bites. *Acad Emerg Med*. 2000; 7:157–161.

Golden DBK. Stinging insect allergy. *Am Fam Physician*. 2003;67:2541–2546.

Manning SE, Rupprecht CE, Fishbein D, et al. Human rabies prevention—United States 2008: recommendation of the Advisory Committee on Immunization Practices; CDC. *MMWR Recomm Rep*. 2008;57:1–28.

Schneir AB. Bites and stings. In: Tintinalli JE, Stapczynski J, Ma O, et al. *Tintinalli's Emergency Medicine: A Comprehensive Study Guide*. 7th ed. New York, NY: McGraw-Hill Education; 2011. Available at: http://accessmedicine.mhmedical.com. Accessed May 25, 2015.

Schwab RA, Powers RD. Puncture wounds and bites. In: Tintinalli JE, Stapczynski J, Ma O, et al. eds. *Tintinalli's Emergency Medicine: A Comprehensive Study Guide*. 7th ed. New York, NY: McGraw-Hill Education; 2011. Available at: http://accessmedicine.mhmedical.com. Accessed May 25, 2015.

Suchard JR. "Spider bite" lesions are usually diagnosed as skin and soft-tissue infections. *J Emerg Med*. 2011; 41(5):473–481.

Turner TW. Do mammalian bites require antibiotic prophylaxis? *Ann Emerg Med*. 2004; 44:274–276.

A 60-year-old man is brought to the emergency room by ambulance because of slurred speech and left-sided weakness. His wife states the patient went to bed at approximately 11 PM the night before and was well. At 5 AM, the time they usually get up, she noticed that he had some difficulties talking and moving his left arm and leg. They arrived at the emergency department (ED) at 6 AM. He has history of long-standing hypertension (HTN), a heart attack 10 years ago, high cholesterol, and obesity. He is taking baby aspirin, an angiotensin-converting enzyme (ACE) inhibitor, and a statin on a daily basis. He consumed alcohol heavily in the past, but stopped drinking completely after the heart attack. He has smoked a half pack of cigarettes daily since his teenage years. His wife remembers that about 3 months ago he complained of mild bilateral leg pain during their morning walk and had to stop after 15 minutes. Also, she remembers that 1 month ago he had a "slight right eye blackout" for 5 minutes.

On presentation to the ED his blood pressure is 195/118 mm Hg, his pulse is 106 beats/min, his respiratory rate is 18 breaths/min, his temperature is 99.8°F (37.6°C), and his oxygen saturation is 97% on room air. Although his pupils are equally round and reactive and the ocular movements are intact, he is unable to turn his eyes voluntarily toward the left side. His neck is supple, there is no jugular venous distension, and there are no bruits. His lungs are clear, heart sounds regular without murmurs, and abdomen is nontender and unremarkable. His extremities are warm, but distal pulses in his feet are difficult to palpate. The neurologic examination reveals that he is awake, alert, and oriented, although he does not recognize that he is ill. He is right-handed, and shows loss of awareness and attention with respect to objects or stimuli on his left side. He has mild dysarthria, but his speech is fluent and he understands and follows commands appropriately. There is mild weakness on the left side of the face and left-sided homonymous hemianopsia, but there is no nystagmus or ptosis, and no tongue or uvula deviation. He is not able to move his left arm and leg, has hyperreflexia, and his left great toe is upgoing on Babinski test.

▶ What is the most likely diagnosis?
▶ What is your next diagnostic step?
▶ What is your next step in therapy?

ANSWERS TO CASE 44:
Cerebrovascular Accident/Transient Ischemic Attack

Summary: The patient is a 60-year-old, right-handed man with history of coronary artery disease, hypertension, and hypercholesterolemia, who presents to the emergency room with a 5-hour history of slurred speech and an inability to move his left arm and leg. He had an episode of amaurosis fugax (fleeting, painless, transient monocular vision loss) in his right eye 1 month prior to presentation of these symptoms. On physical examination, although he is alert and oriented, he has no awareness of his disability (anosognosia) and exhibits left-sided neglect, as well as significant hypertension, dysarthria, and left hemiparesis. He also has left-sided homonymous hemianopsia, conjugate rightward gaze deviation, left hemifacial weakness, and left hyperreflexia.

- **Most likely diagnosis:** Cerebrovascular accident (CVA).

- **First diagnostic step:** Obtain a STAT computed tomography (CT) scan of the brain without contrast.

- **Next step in therapy:** Determine advisability for acute treatment with thrombolytic agents.

ANALYSIS
Objectives

1. Recognize the significance of a correct diagnosis and evaluation of transient ischemic attacks (TIAs) and CVAs based on risk factors.

2. Recognize the conditions that can mimic a TIA or a stroke.

3. Understand that the clinical evaluation gives the most important clues about diagnosis of TIA or stroke.

4. Be familiar with the accepted approach for the early management of patients with ischemic stroke.

5. Be familiar with the current strategies for prevention of ischemic stroke and TIA.

Considerations

This 60-year-old patient has developed focal neurologic deficits, which is the common presentation of a patient with a stroke. Considering that he has a history of uncontrolled hypertension, hypercholesterolemia, and vascular manifestations of atherosclerosis such as coronary artery disease and peripheral vascular disease (lower extremity claudication), ischemic stroke is the most worrisome and probable diagnosis. Furthermore, he had a TIA (amaurosis fugax) 30 days prior to presentation, which places him at an even greater risk for an ischemic stroke. His neurologic deficits are compatible with an ischemic stroke in the territory of the right middle cerebral artery, which is his nondominant hemisphere, and the reason why he is not aphasic.

Of immediate importance, after securing ABCs (airway, breathing circulation), the clinician should confirm that the neurologic impairments are secondary to an ischemic stroke and not other conditions, specifically an intracranial hemorrhage. A brain CT without contrast should be obtained as soon as possible to exclude hemorrhage, tumor, abscess, and mass effect. Serum glucose, urine toxicology screen, coagulation studies, serum electrolytes, renal function tests, lipid profile, and a complete blood count (CBC) are also indicated. A 12-lead ECG should be obtained to exclude acute myocardial infarction or arrhythmia such as atrial fibrillation, and the patient should be placed on telemetry.

Since it has been more than 3 hours from the onset of symptoms, this patient is not a candidate for thrombolytic therapy. Although this patient's blood pressure is markedly elevated, in the setting of an acute ischemic CVA, blood pressure management should be cautious, as compensatory hypertension can be permitted to avoid increasing risk of ischemic injury from hypoperfusion.

This patient should be admitted to the hospital for further evaluation and management, preferably to a dedicated stroke unit if available. Aspirin should be given within 48 hours of the onset of stroke, and deep venous thrombosis (DVT) prophylaxis should be started with low-molecular-weight or unfractionated heparin. However, anticoagulation with heparin or warfarin for treatment of the infarction itself has a poor risk-benefit ratio and is not indicated. An evaluation of the patient's speech and swallowing function and an early physiotherapy consultation should be obtained. Further imaging with brain magnetic resonance imaging (MRI), magnetic resonance angiography (MRA), or CT angiography can help to clarify the etiology of the stroke and guide treatment. In this patient, carotid duplex ultrasonography is indicated because he had an episode of amaurosis fugax, caused by a blockage of the ophthalmic artery which branches from the internal carotid artery.

Management of this patient's chronic medical conditions, to reduce his risk of subsequent strokes, is critical. In this patient, these measures include tight control of his hypertension and hypercholesterolemia, along with immediate smoking cessation. Since this patient had a stroke while taking daily aspirin, an alternative antiplatelet agent should be considered to prevent another stroke.

APPROACH TO:
CVA/TIA

DEFINITIONS

TRANSIENT ISCHEMIC ATTACK: A transient episode of neurologic dysfunction caused by focal brain, spinal cord, or retinal ischemia, **without** acute infarction. There is no time cutoff that reliably distinguishes whether a symptomatic ischemic event will result in ischemic infarction.

TRANSIENT SYMPTOMS WITH INFARCTION (TSI): A transient episode of neurologic dysfunction associated with irreversible ischemic brain injury as evident by imaging changes even after resolution of symptoms.

ISCHEMIC STROKE: An infarction of the central nervous system with resultant neurologic deficit that persists beyond 24 hours or is interrupted by death within 24 hours.

HEMORRHAGIC STROKE: Central nervous system (CNS) damage secondary to intracerebral or subarachnoid hemorrhage. This is the etiology of 13% to 20% of strokes in the United States.

CLINICAL APPROACH

There are over a million people who suffer a stroke in the United States each year, and the incidence of TIA approaches 500,000 per year. Strokes remain the third leading cause of death in North America and are a major cause of disability. **TIA is defined as a transient episode of neurologic dysfunction caused by focal brain, spinal cord, or retinal ischemia, *without* acute infarction.** Most TIAs last for less than 1 hour. A stroke is presumed to have occurred if the symptoms persist for more than 24 hours. However, there is an unreliable correlation of symptom duration with actual infarction. **Patients with a TIA are at increased risk of a subsequent stroke.** The reported occurrence of a stroke after a TIA is as high as 5.3% within 2 days and 10.5% within 90 days. Patients with a TIA often require hospital admission, further evaluation, and the same long-term management as stroke patients. **An assessment called the $ABCD^2$ score (Age, Blood pressure, Clinical features, Duration of symptoms, and Diabetes)** can be used to identify patients at high risk of ischemic stroke in the first 7 days after TIA.

The $ABCD^2$ score is as follows:

Age ($\geq$60 years = 1 point)

Blood pressure elevation when first assessed after TIA (systolic $\geq$140 mm Hg or diastolic $\geq$90 mm Hg = 1 point)

Clinical features (unilateral weakness = 2 points; isolated speech disturbance = 1 point; other = 0 points)

Duration of neurologic symptoms ($\geq$60 minutes = 2 points; 10 to 59 minutes = 1 point; <10 minutes = 0 points)

Diabetes (present = 1 point)

Estimated 2-day stroke risk determined by the $ABCD^2$ score are as follows:

Score 0 to 3: Low stroke risk (1%)

Score 4 to 5: Moderate risk (4%)

Score 6 to 7: High risk (8%)

Hypertension is the single most important risk factor for stroke, and the incidence of stroke in the United States has decreased partly as a result of better efforts to control hypertension in the past few decades. Other risk factors include diabetes mellitus, older age, male sex, family history, dyslipidemia, tobacco abuse, alcohol abuse, cocaine abuse, and prothrombotic disorders. Many cardiovascular conditions also predispose people to stroke, usually through formation of an embolic clot. These conditions include atrial fibrillation, myocardial infarction, endocarditis, carotid stenosis, rheumatic heart disease, presence of a mechanical valve, advanced dilated cardiomyopathy, and a patent foramen ovale or atrial septal defect which can expose the systemic arterial system to a paradoxical embolus from a venous source. Sickle cell disease is also a risk factor for stroke and patients with this condition commonly experience their strokes as children.

Ischemic strokes are generally classified as being of thrombotic or embolic origin. Strokes that affect the small branches of the main arteries of the brain are termed lacunar infarcts or small-vessel strokes. These strokes often forewarn a larger, more debilitating stroke. The causes of the emboli are usually of cardiovascular origin and include the previously mentioned conditions as well as dissection of various vessels. While most emboli result from blood clots, emboli can also occur from vegetations from infective endocarditis, sterile vegetations from Libman-Sacks endocarditis (which occurs in systemic lupus erythematosus), and marantic endocarditis (which occurs with cancer).

DIAGNOSIS AND EVALUATION

Sudden onset of focal neurologic deficits is the usual presentation of stroke patients, although some patients can have a gradual worsening of symptoms. Unless there is a hemispheric infarction, basilar artery occlusion, or cerebellar stroke with edema, nearly all of the patients are alert. If the middle cerebral artery territory is affected, the patient will generally experience aphasia (when the dominant hemisphere is involved), contralateral hemiparesis, sensory loss, spatial neglect, and contralateral impaired conjugate gaze. When the territory of the anterior cerebral artery is affected, lower extremity deficits are more frequent than upper extremity deficits. These patients often have associated cognitive and personality changes. Vertebrobasilar stroke symptoms and signs include motor or sensory loss in all four extremities, crossed signs, disconjugate gaze, nystagmus, dysarthria, and dysphagia. If the cerebellum is affected by ischemic stroke, then ipsilateral limb and gait ataxia are commonly present.

What risk factors for stroke are not modifiable?

- Age
- Family history
- Gender
- Ethnicity
- Prior stroke, TIA, or heart attack

What risk factors for stroke are modifiable?

- Hypertension, including compliance with medications
- Cigarette smoking
- Diabetes mellitus

- Carotid or other artery disease

- Peripheral artery disease

- Atrial fibrillation

- Coronary heart disease

- Congestive heart failure

- Sickle cell disease

- Hyperlipidemia

- Poor diet

- Physical inactivity

- Obesity

Assessment of vital signs is important in the initial examination. Severe high blood pressure can be suggestive of hypertensive encephalopathy or intracranial hemorrhage. A fever may lead to consideration of an infectious cause. A rapid or irregularly irregular pulse may suggest atrial fibrillation as a potential cause of the stroke. A timely general physical examination and comprehensive neurologic examination should follow, as well as subsequent interval evaluations.

The differential diagnosis of acute neurologic signs and symptoms is broad. Along with CVAs, such symptoms can be caused by seizures, acute confusional states, delirium, syncope, metabolic and toxic encephalopathy (eg, hypoglycemia, poisoning), brain tumors, CNS infections, migraines, multiple sclerosis, and subdural hematoma. Migraines with neurologic symptoms can be especially difficult to differentiate from stroke since migraines do not have to be accompanied by a headache. However, the symptoms of stroke are usually of a much more rapid onset than those of a migraine. Stroke victims are also usually alert and aware of what is happening to them, unlike people suffering from delirium or various types of encephalopathies. When it is determined that a stroke is the cause of the presentation, **it is crucial to differentiate between ischemic and hemorrhagic stroke because of the implications on further treatment.**

The initial assessment should establish if the patient is eligible for thrombolytic treatment; establishing the time of symptom onset is the most important factor. The onset of symptoms is assumed to be the time that the patient was last known to be free of symptoms, such as when they went to bed.

Brain Imaging

A CT scan of the brain without contrast is the initial imaging test of choice in the evaluation of acute stroke. A CT scan of the brain may not show evidence of an ischemic stroke for up to 72 hours, but can immediately exclude most cases of intracranial hemorrhage, tumors, or abscesses. CT is also more readily available, cost-effective, and takes less time than MRI and can also be used to detect a hemorrhagic transformation of an infarct in a patient with an ischemic stroke whose symptoms deteriorate. If neurologic symptoms have resolved, MRI evaluation within 24 hours is the preferred imaging study due to its increased sensitivity for differentiating between a TIA and a TSI stroke.

Further imaging studies may be indicated to clarify the etiology of the stroke and to detect intracranial or extracranial arterial occlusions, which may affect treatment decisions. Evaluation of the cerebrovascular system can be accomplished with magnetic resonance angiography (MRA), CT angiography, catheter angiography, or transcranial Doppler ultrasonography.

Other Tests

A 12-lead ECG should be performed in all stroke patients to detect or rule out acute myocardial infarctions, which can either cause a stroke or result from a stroke. An ECG will also aid in the diagnosis of atrial fibrillation or other arrhythmia that may cause a stroke. Echocardiography may also be necessary to assess the structure of the heart. Transesophageal echocardiography is particularly useful in detecting cardiac sources of embolism, such as thrombus caused by myocardial infarction, endocarditis, rheumatic heart disease, valvular prostheses, and atrial septal defects. A carotid duplex ultrasonography evaluation is also recommended to evaluate for carotid plaques or stenosis.

Serum glucose, electrolytes, renal function tests, and urine toxicology screening are important to exclude hypoglycemia as well as metabolic and toxic encephalopathy. If the patient is on anticoagulant therapy, the prothrombin time, partial thromboplastin time, and platelet count should be measured and are required before considering thrombolytic therapy. A lipid panel, erythrocyte sedimentation rate, antinuclear antibodies (ANA), complete blood count, and serologic tests for syphilis are also often indicated. In young patients without an identifiable cause for a stroke, a workup for coagulation disorders or antiphospholipid syndrome may be indicated. A lumbar puncture is contraindicated if subarachnoid or intracranial hemorrhage is suspected.

TREATMENT

As in every critical patient, **the initial survey should assess the ABCs.** If hypoxia is detected, supplemental oxygen should be administered to maintain oxygen saturation above 92% and the cause of the hypoxia investigated (eg, partial airway obstruction, aspiration pneumonia, and atelectasis). An endotracheal tube should be placed if the airway is threatened. **A cardiac monitor should be placed to detect atrial fibrillation or any other arrhythmias.**

Unless a hypertensive encephalopathy, aortic dissection, acute renal failure, or pulmonary edema is present, the **treatment of arterial hypertension should be cautious.** Prior to intravenous thrombolytic treatment, blood pressure should be lowered if systolic blood pressure is greater than 185 mm Hg or 110 mm Hg. After thrombolytic treatment, systolic blood pressure should be kept less than 180 mm Hg and diastolic blood pressure less than 105 mm Hg. Pharmacologic treatments for hypertension in patients with acute ischemic stroke include intravenous labetalol, nicardipine, and sodium nitroprusside.

Fever and elevated serum glucose after a stroke are often associated with less favorable outcomes and should be controlled during the poststroke period. An infectious source for the fever should be investigated.

Except when thrombolytic therapy is given, **most patients with a nonhemorrhagic stroke should receive aspirin within the first 48 hours.** Urgent anticoagulation is not recommended.

Judiciously selected patients can benefit from intravenous administration of recombinant tissue-type plasminogen activator (rtPA) if they can be treated within 3 hours of the onset of ischemic stroke. The risk of hemorrhage associated with rtPA treatment is approximately 5% and there are numerous contraindications to the use of thrombolytic therapy, including recent surgery, trauma, gastrointestinal bleeding, myocardial infarction, use of certain anticoagulant medications, and uncontrolled hypertension. Depending on availability, some hospitals have the capability of direct intra-arterial thrombolysis in which the thrombolytic agent is delivered directly to the clot via canalization or even mechanical retrieval of thrombus. These modes of treatment may be considered in centers with experimental protocols or extensive experience.

Poststroke cerebral edema can be a serious complication and can lead to herniation of the brain stem resulting in death. Cerebral edema should be treated with mannitol or decompression neurosurgery, although there is insufficient evidence to show significant benefit for these treatments in improving outcomes.

Acute treatment in a dedicated stroke unit results in better outcomes and decreased mortality. Early poststroke treatment care includes mobilization once the patient is stable and evaluations of the patient's ability to speak and swallow. After a stroke, the patient is often immobile and needs intensive medical care in order to avoid malnutrition, skin breakdown, and infection. A patient's neurologic deficits commonly improve after a stroke and may continue to improve for up to 6 months to a year. Prior strokes also predispose patients to seizures, and some patients may initially present with a seizure as the first symptom of stroke. When thrombolytic therapy is not used, DVT prophylaxis should be provided. Family support and treatment of depression should also be initiated when appropriate.

PREVENTION OF STROKE IN PATIENTS WITH PREVIOUS ISCHEMIC STROKE OR TIA

A history of a previous TIA or CVA confers a high risk for future events. Aggressive risk factor control should be undertaken in these patients. All patients should be counseled to quit smoking and to reduce alcohol intake. Hypertensive patients should be treated per Joint National Committee on Prevention, Detection, Evaluation, and Treatment of High Blood Pressure, 8th report (JNC 8) guidelines (see Case 30). Elevated serum cholesterol should be treated with high-intensity lipid-lowering (statin) therapy. Tight diabetic control should aim for a hemoglobin A_{1c} level less than 8%. Antiplatelet agents such as aspirin (81-325 mg/d), the combination of aspirin and extended-release dipyridamole (Aggrenox), or clopidogrel (Plavix) should be started in patients with a history of noncardioembolic ischemic stroke or TIA.

Carotid endarterectomy (CEA) can reduce the risk of stroke in a patient with a history of previous TIA or CVA and symptomatic carotid artery stenosis of greater than 60% to 70%, and is typically not indicated when stenosis is less than 50%.

Noninvasive carotid balloon angioplasty and stenting is an alternative to CEA in select patients.

Anticoagulation with warfarin reduces the risk of stroke and stroke recurrence in patients with appropriate risk factors. It is indicated to reduce the risk of embolic strokes for patients with persistent or paroxysmal atrial fibrillation or advanced congestive heart failure. It is also indicated for patients with an ischemic stroke caused by a myocardial infarction and existence of a left ventricular thrombus, as well as for patients with rheumatic heart disease or a mechanical heart valve.

CASE CORRELATION

- See also Cases 32 (Dementia) and 34 (Migraine Headache).

COMPREHENSION QUESTIONS

44.1 A 72-year-old man is brought to the emergency department because of weakness and numbness of the right arm. The evaluating medical student asks the attending doctor about the diagnosis and management of transient ischemic attacks. Which of the following would be most commonly expected in a patient with a TIA?

A. Resolution of symptoms within 1 hour

B. Stroke within 90 days in less than 1% of patients

C. CT evidence of infarction

D. CT evidence of ischemia

E. MRI evidence of infarction

44.2 An 84-year-old African-American woman was found by her daughter-in-law walking down the street a few blocks from her house. The daughter-in-law noticed that she did not appear to know where she was and did not recognize her. Upon prompting, she seemed confused and would not speak. The patient experienced a CVA 1 year previously and had mild residual deficits on her left side. She takes medications for hypertension, hyperlipidemia, constipation, and gout. In the emergency room, the patient has a blood pressure of 195/106 mm Hg, pulse of 86 beats/min, respiratory rate of 18 breaths/min, and temperature of 97.9°F (36.6°C). She does not follow commands and is oriented only to person. She complains of headache, yet a CT of the brain does not show evidence of an acute hemorrhage. Which of the following is the most appropriate next step in management?

A. Lumbar puncture

B. Chest x-ray

C. IV labetalol

D. MRI of the brain

E. IV mannitol

44.3 An 82-year-old man with a suspected stroke is transferred to a major medical stroke center from an outside rural hospital. Four hours have elapsed since initial presentation. His blood pressure is 164/92 and he is awake, alert, oriented, and moving all four extremities. Which of the following should be considered in the management of this patient?

   A. Avoidance of acetaminophen

   B. Aggressive blood pressure management

   C. Thrombolysis

   D. Early mobilization and therapy

   E. A swallowing evaluation

44.4 A 65-year-old man was hospitalized due to sudden weakness of the right arm, which was diagnosed as an ischemic stroke. Carotid duplex ultrasonography revealed a 40% to 59% bilateral stenosis. Total cholesterol is 188 mg/dL and low-density lipoprotein (LDL) cholesterol is 98 mg/dL. Which of the following is the best strategy regarding prevention of future strokes in this patient?

   A. Warfarin

   B. Carotid endarterectomy

   C. Clopidogrel

   D. Long-acting nitrates

   E. Statin

44.5 A man is brought to the emergency room by ambulance. Coworkers at his office stated that he was acting normally until approximately 1 hour ago when he became confused and had trouble walking. One coworker thought that his right leg seemed especially weak. His vitals are temperature 97.4°F (36.3°C), pulse 118 beats/min, and blood pressure 90/65 mm Hg. The patient is arousable, but does not follow commands and is not oriented. He has a medical alert bracelet on his arm indicating that he is a diabetic and allergic to penicillin. A serum glucose level obtained at the bedside is 50 mg/dL. Which of the following should be your immediate first step in management?

   A. Immediately give the patient intravenous D50 or glucagon.

   B. Immediately obtain a CT scan to assess possibility for giving rtPA.

   C. Immediately perform a lumbar puncture to assess for subarachnoid hemorrhage.

   D. Immediately give the patient mannitol.

   E. Immediately start cardiopulmonary resuscitation (CPR) with chest compressions.

ANSWERS

44.1 **A.** TIA is a brief neurologic episode, typically less than 1 hour in duration that does not cause infarction. The occurrence of stroke after TIA is as high as 5.3% within 2 days and 10.5% within 90 days. Warfarin is indicated in specific circumstances, such as the presence of atrial fibrillation, but is not routinely used following a TIA.

44.2 **C.** IV labetalol should be started to achieve appropriate blood pressure control. Routine chest x-rays affect the clinical management in few patients with stroke, and are not recommended as routine initial workup. CT of the brain *without* contrast can exclude most cases of intracranial hemorrhage, tumors, or abscesses, and is the initial test of choice in the workup of suspected stroke but it can miss up to 15% of subarachnoid hemorrhages. When a subarachnoid hemorrhage is suspected but not seen on CT, a lumbar puncture is indicated for diagnosis.

44.3 **D.** Early mobilization of stroke patients should be started when they are considered medically stable. In the setting of an acute stroke, management of high blood pressure should be cautious. Thrombolytic therapy can be beneficial in selected patients, but carries significant risks and has numerous contraindications. Fever should be treated and a workup performed to determine its etiology, as it carries an increased risk of morbidity and mortality. At this point, 4 hours after symptoms, when the patient is speaking without difficulty, a swallowing evaluation is not immediately warranted.

44.4 **C.** Patients with stroke but no detected sources of embolism benefit from antiplatelet agents not anticoagulants. Aspirin, clopidogrel, or a combination of aspirin and dipyridamole are acceptable regimens. For patients with recent TIA or ischemic stroke and ipsilateral severe (>70%) carotid artery stenosis, carotid endarterectomy is recommended. When the degree of stenosis is less than 50%, there is no indication for CEA. Patients with a history of symptomatic cerebrovascular disease should be treated with high-intensity statin therapy.

44.5 **A.** The patient has severe hypoglycemia and needs to be treated immediately with intravenous glucose or glucagon. If the patient does not recover with glucose or glucagon infusion, then other tests, such as a CT scan, may be warranted. Be aware that hypoglycemia can mimic many of the symptoms of a stroke, including focal weakness. Mannitol is used in cases of cerebral edema and not for raising blood sugar. The patient is tachycardic, likely from hypoglycemia, and does not require CPR.

CLINICAL PEARLS

▶ Hypertension is the single most important modifiable risk factor for stroke.

▶ Although most strokes are cerebral infarctions, it is crucial to differentiate between ischemic and hemorrhagic stroke because of the implications on further treatment.

▶ Judiciously selected patients can benefit from intravenous administration of rtPA.

▶ CT of the brain without contrast is the initial imaging test of choice in most suspected strokes.

▶ Unless a hypertensive encephalopathy, aortic dissection, acute renal failure, or pulmonary edema is present, the treatment of arterial hypertension should be cautious.

REFERENCES

Adams H, Adams R, Del Zoppo G, Goldstein LB. Guidelines for the early management of patients with ischemic stroke: 2007 guidelines update. A scientific statement from the Stroke Council of the American Heart Association/American Stroke Association. *Stroke*. 2007; 38:1655–1711.

Aiyagari V, Gorelick PB. Management of blood pressure for acute and recurrent stroke. *Stroke*. 2009; 40:2251–2256.

Donnan G, Fisher M, Macleod M, Davis S. Stroke. *Lancet*. 2008; 371(9624):1612–1623.

James PA, Oparil S, Carter BL, et al. 2014 evidence-based guideline for the management of high blood pressure in adults: report from the panel members appointed to the Eighth Joint National Committee (JNC 8). *JAMA*. 2014; 311(5):507–520.

Johnston SC, Rothwell PM, Nguyen-Huynh MN, et al. Validation and refinement of scores to predict very early stroke risk after transient ischaemic attack. *Lancet*. 2007; 369(9558):283.

NASCET Steering Committee. North American Symptomatic Carotid Endarterectomy Trial. *Stroke*. 1991; 22(6):711–720.

Simmons BB, Cirignano B, Gadegbeku AB. Transient ischemic attack: part I. Diagnosis and evaluation. *Am Fam Physician*. 2012; 86(6):521–526.

Simmons BB, Gadegbeku AB, Cirignano B. Transient ischemic attack: part II. Risk factor modification and treatment. *Am Fam Physician*. 2012; 86(6):527–532.

Smith WS, Johnston S, Hemphill J, III. Cerebrovascular diseases. In: Kasper D, Fauci A, Hauser S, et al., eds. *Harrison's Principles of Internal Medicine*. 19th ed. New York, NY: McGraw-Hill Education; 2015. Available at: http://accessmedicine.mhmedical.com. Accessed May 25, 2015.

van der Work HB, van Gijn J. Acute ischemic stroke. *New Engl J Med*. 2007; 357(6):572–579.

A 39-year-old homeless man presents to the emergency department (ED) with a nonproductive cough and subjective fever. He says that his illness has been worsening over the past 2 weeks, originally starting with dyspnea on exertion and now he is short of breath at rest. On questioning, he tells you that he lives in a homeless shelter when he can, but he frequently sleeps on the streets. He has used IV drugs (primarily heroin) "on and off" and has been sexually promiscuous with both men and women without barrier protection for many years. He denies any significant medical history, and only gets medical care when he comes to the ED for an illness or injury. On review of systems, he complains of chronic fatigue, weight loss, and diarrhea. On examination, he is a thin, disheveled man appearing much older than his stated age. His temperature is 100.4°F (38.0°C), his blood pressure is 100/50 mm Hg, his pulse is 105 beats/min, and his respiratory rate is 24 breaths/min. His initial oxygen saturation is 89% on room air, which comes up to 94% on 4 L of oxygen by nasal cannula. Significant findings on examination include dry mucous membranes, a tachycardic but regular cardiac rhythm, a soft and non-tender abdomen, and generally wasted-appearing extremities. His pulmonary examination is significant for tachypnea and fine crackles bilaterally, but there are no visible signs of cyanosis on extremities. His chest x-ray reveals diffuse, bilateral, interstitial infiltrates that look like "ground glass."

▶ What is the most likely cause of this patient's current pulmonary complaints?
▶ What underlying illnesses does this patient most likely has?
▶ What diagnostic testing and treatment should be started?

ANSWERS TO CASE 45:
HIV, AIDS, and Other Sexually Transmitted Infections

Summary: A 39-year-old, homeless, IV drug abuser is seen with fever, cough, dyspnea, and fatigue. He is found to be tachypneic, febrile, and hypoxemic. His chest x-ray reveals bilateral interstitial infiltrates.

- **Most likely cause of current illness:** *Pneumocystis jiroveci* (formerly known as *Pneumocystis carinii*) pneumonia.

- **Most probable underlying illness:** AIDS.

- **Recommended current testing and treatment:** Complete blood count (CBC), serum electrolytes, arterial blood gas; HIV enzyme-linked immunosorbent assay with confirmatory Western blot; CD4/CD8 cell count; HIV RNA assay; sputum culture for *P jiroveci and acid-fast bacilli*; urine culture for *Chlamydia* and *Neisseria gonorrheae*; serum rapid plasma reagin (RPR); start treatment with oral trimethoprim-sulfamethoxazole (TMP-SMX); and consider starting highly active antiretroviral therapy (HAART) with appropriate case management including intensive drug abuse treatment, counseling, and social work.

ANALYSIS
Objectives

1. Know the common risks and modes of transmission of human immunodeficiency virus (HIV)/acquired immunodeficiency syndrome AIDS.

2. Be aware of common presentations of persons infected with HIV.

3. List the most common sexually transmitted infections (STIs).

4. Describe common treatment regimens for STIs.

Considerations

The case described is that of a 39-year-old man who is homeless, an intravenous drug abuser, bisexual, and sexually promiscuous. He has had chronic fatigue and weight loss, and now presents with fever, tachypnea, and hypoxemia. It is likely that he is infected with the HIV virus, and has an opportunistic infection, *P jiroveci* pneumonia. HIV infects the helper and cytotoxic T cells of the immune system, which are defined by the presence of the cell-signaling proteins CD4 and CD8 respectively, and causes a decline in both their number and their function in supporting the immune system. This decline in functional helper and cytotoxic T cells disables the cell-mediated arm of the immune system and leaves the body vulnerable to infection from multiple opportunistic organisms. This advanced stage of the HIV infection, in which such opportunistic infections occur, is known as AIDS.

P jiroveci (formerly known as *P carinii*) pneumonia is an AIDS-defining illness in persons infected with HIV. *P jiroveci* is a fungus that may colonize many people, but typically causes disease only in those with profound immune deficiencies, such as AIDS infections or cancers treated with chemotherapy. *P jiroveci* pneumonia usually presents with nonproductive cough, fever, and dyspnea that worsens over a few days to a few weeks. Patients usually are found to be febrile, tachypneic, and hypoxic, and their lung examination may be unremarkable (other than tachypnea). The presence of a bilateral interstitial infiltrates on chest x-ray, often described as having a "ground-glass" appearance, is classic for *P jiroveci* pneumonia. The identification of the organism in sputum, either spontaneously produced or induced, is diagnostic, but treatment is usually started prior to definitive diagnosis in those with a classic clinical picture and high suspicion.

As *P jiroveci* pneumonia occurs after the CD4 and CD8 counts have markedly reduced, patients often will have signs and symptoms of other AIDS-related complications as well. In patients with AIDS, it is common to see additional comorbid conditions including oral or esophageal candidiasis, chronic infectious diarrhea, Kaposi sarcoma, wasting syndrome, and weight loss. Although it presents in the setting of advanced disease, *P jiroveci* pneumonia remains a common presenting illness in patients who did not know that they were infected with HIV, and is a frequent initial opportunistic infection in those with known HIV disease. The incidence of *P jiroveci* pneumonia is decreasing in the United States with more widespread awareness of HIV disease, broader usage of antiretroviral therapy, and prophylactic use of TMP-SMX in patients with CD4 counts of less than 200 cells/μL.

APPROACH TO:
HIV, AIDS, and Other Sexually Transmitted Infections

DEFINITIONS

ACQUIRED IMMUNODEFICIENCY SYNDROME: The advanced stage of the HIV infection, in which opportunistic infections occur with specific criteria for its designation.

HUMAN IMMUNODEFICIENCY VIRUS: A retrovirus that infects the helper T cells of the immune system, which are defined by the presence of the cell-signaling protein CD4, and causes a decline in both their number and their effectiveness.

CLINICAL APPROACH

HIV/AIDS

Epidemiology

As of 2013, over 35 million people in the world are living with HIV infection and/ or AIDS. Over 1.5 million people died of AIDS-related illnesses worldwide in 2013, with a disproportionate share of the deaths occurring in sub-Saharan Africa. HIV disease is caused by the human retroviruses, HIV-1 and HIV-2. HIV-1 is more common worldwide, whereas HIV-2 has been reported in western Africa, Europe, South America, and Canada.

As of 2011, 1.2 million people in the United States were estimated to be infected with HIV, with **approximately 25% of persons unaware of their infection.** The highest prevalence of HIV occurs in men who have sex with other men and in IV drug users, although the occurrence in heterosexual sexual contact is increasing. African Americans are disproportionately affected with infection, both in total numbers of cases and in development of new infections.

Transmission

HIV is transmitted from person to person through contact with infected blood and body fluids. Sexual contact is the most common mechanism of transmission and, while anal intercourse has the highest rate of transmission, HIV can be acquired through vaginal and oral intercourse as well. Heterosexual transmission of HIV now accounts for 27% of new infection and 86% of cases in infected women. The risk of HIV transmission is also increased by the presence of genital or anal lesions caused by other sexually transmitted diseases, such as gonorrhea, syphilis, and genital herpes. The risk of transmission can be reduced by the proper and consistent use of latex condoms (either male or female condoms). Because HIV can pass through lambskin condoms, these are not recommended. Male circumcision has also been shown to decrease the rate of HIV transmission. Due to the large amount of undiagnosed HIV infections, the Centers for Disease Control and Prevention (CDC) expanded screening recommendations, which are summarized in Table 45–1.

Sharing needles by IV drug users is the third most common source of transmission of HIV behind male-to-male and heterosexual transmission. Vertical transmission from an infected woman to her baby has been found to occur during pregnancy, during the process of delivery of a baby, and rarely from breast-feeding.

Table 45–1 • CDC HIV SCREENING RECOMMENDATIONS
For patients in all health-care settings
• HIV screening is recommended for patients in all health-care settings after the patient is notified that testing will be performed unless the patient declines (opt-out screening). • Persons at high risk for HIV infection should be screened for HIV at least annually. • Separate written consent for HIV testing should not be required; general consent for medical care should be considered sufficient to encompass consent for HIV testing. • Prevention counseling should not be required with HIV diagnostic testing or as part of HIV screening programs in health-care settings.
For pregnant women
• HIV screening should be included in the routine panel of prenatal screening tests for all pregnant women. • HIV screening is recommended after the patient is notified that testing will be performed unless the patient declines (opt-out screening). • Separate written consent for HIV testing should not be required; general consent for medical care should be considered sufficient to encompass consent for HIV testing. • Repeat screening in the third trimester is recommended in certain jurisdictions with elevated rates of HIV infection among pregnant women.

Reproduced from Branson BM, Handsfield HH, Lampe MA, et al. Revised recommendations for HIV testing of adults, adolescents and pregnant women in health-care settings. MMWR Recomm Rep. 2006;55(RR-14):1-17.

Blood and blood-product transfusions have been linked to infection, although the routine screening of donor blood for HIV now makes this an extremely rare event.

Health-care workers have been infected with HIV through accidental punctures with needles or by infected blood entering through open skin wounds or mucous membranes. The risk of transmission to health-care workers is low and is related to the viral load of the patient, the amount of blood to which the worker is exposed, and the depth of the inoculum. Postexposure risk of developing HIV infection can be reduced by immediate and careful cleaning of the exposure/puncture site along with postexposure prophylactic (PEP) treatment with antiretroviral therapy started within 72 hours after exposure. Regimens for PEP include two to three antiretroviral medications taken for 28 days.

Clinical Course of HIV Infection

Following initial exposure to HIV, some patients will complain of nonspecific symptoms, such as low-grade fever, fatigue, sore throat, or myalgias. This illness typically occurs 6 to 8 weeks following the infection and is commonly self-limited. The primary infection is also known as acute seroconversion syndrome, as the symptoms are thought to be related to the development of antibodies to the virus.

Following the resolution of the primary infection symptoms (if any occur), there is a period of clinical latency. During this time, most infected persons are asymptomatic, although some may develop lymphadenopathy. This period can last from 6 months to up to 10 years following the transmission of the virus. However, while the patient is asymptomatic during this period, a relentless decline in helper and suppressor T-cell number and immune function usually occurs in the untreated patient, with the result that many patients initially present with profound immunodeficiency and opportunistic infections.

Clinical Categorization of HIV/AIDS Infections

The CDC defines four clinical stages for adults aged greater than or equal to 13.

Stage 1: No AIDS-defining illness and either CD4 cell count greater than or equal to 500 cells/μL or percentage of total lymphocytes greater than 29

Stage 2: No AIDS-defining illness and either CD4 cell count of 200 to 499 cells/μL or percentage between 14 and 28

Stage 3: (AIDS) CD4 cell count less than or equal to 200 cells/μL or percentage less than 14 and documentation of AIDS-defining condition (Tables 45–2 and 45–3)

Stage 4: Unknown laboratory parameters with an AIDS-defining condition

For classification purposes, a patient's **HIV is defined by the highest clinical stage in which the patient has ever qualified.**

Diagnostic Evaluation

The standard screening test for HIV infection is the detection of HIV antibodies using the enzyme-linked immunosorbent assay (ELISA). **Samples that are repeatedly positive on ELISA testing must be confirmed by Western blot testing,** an

Table 45-2 • SOME EXAMPLES OF HIV-RELATED CONDITIONS THAT ARE NOT AIDS DEFINING

Bacillary angiomatosis
Oropharyngeal candidiasis
Persistent, recurrent, or difficult-to-treat vaginal candidiasis
Cervical dysplasia or carcinoma in situ
Oral hairy leukoplakia
Idiopathic thrombocytopenic purpura
Listeriosis
Pelvic inflammatory disease (especially if complicated by tubo-ovarian abscess)
Peripheral neuropathy
Herpes zoster, two or more episodes involving more than one dermatome

Data from Centers for Disease Control and Prevention. 1993 Revised classification system for HIV infection and expanded surveillance case definition for AIDS among adolescents and adults. MMWR Recomm Rep. 1992;41(RR-17):1-19.

electrophoresis assay that detects antibodies to HIV antigens of specific molecular weights.

When HIV is diagnosed, a complete history and physical examination should be performed. Emphasis should be placed on identifying possible mechanisms of exposure, comorbid conditions, presence of STIs, determining the presence of AIDS-defining conditions, reducing risky behaviors, and assisting with coping

Table 45-3 • EXAMPLES OF AIDS-DEFINING CONDITIONS

Candidiasis of bronchi, trachea, or lungs
Coccidioidomycosis (disseminated or extrapulmonary)
Cytomegalovirus disease
Disseminated or extrapulmonary histoplasmosis
Burkitt lymphoma
M avium complex (disseminated or extrapulmonary)
Pneumonia, recurrent
Toxoplasmosis of brain
Esophageal candidiasis
Extrapulmonary *Cryptococcus*
HIV-related encephalopathy
Intestinal isosporiasis (>1-mo duration)
Immunoblastic lymphoma
Mycobacterium tuberculosis (any site)
Progressive multifocal leukoencephalopathy
Wasting syndrome caused by HIV
Invasive cervical cancer
Intestinal cryptosporidiosis (>1-mo duration)
Herpes simplex: chronic ulcer, bronchitis, pneumonitis, or esophagitis
Kaposi sarcoma
Primary brain lymphoma
P jiroveci pneumonia
Recurrent *Salmonella* septicemia

Data from Centers for Disease Control and Prevention. Guidelines for the prevention and treatment of opportunistic infections among HIV-exposed and HIV-infected children: recommendations from the National Institutes of Health, the HIV Medicine Association of the Infectious Diseases Society of America, the Pediatric Infectious Diseases Society, and the American Academy of Pediatrics, 2009. MMWR Recomm Rep. 2009;58(RR-11):1-166.

strategies. **HIV infection is reportable to local health authorities, but partner notification laws vary by state,** so it is important to know both local and state regulations.

Before instituting therapy, laboratory testing should include HIV genotype testing to identify strains that may be resistant to therapy. A quantitative assay of HIV RNA levels (viral load) can help to assess disease activity. CD4 and CD8 lymphocyte counts and viral load should be measured at baseline and every 3 to 6 months thereafter to monitor for disease staging, progression, and the risk of complications and opportunistic infections. A CBC, comprehensive metabolic panel, and urinalysis should be performed at baseline and periodically thereafter to monitor for complications of HIV and of the medications that are used in treatment. Serology for toxoplasmosis and cytomegalovirus should also be obtained to identify organisms at risk for reactivation following immunosuppression.

Screening for other sexually transmitted diseases (syphilis, hepatitis B and C, N gonorrhea, *Chlamydia trachomatis*, herpes simplex) **should be performed** initially and repeated, if needed, because of any ongoing risks identified. Hepatitis A and B vaccination should be offered to those who lack immunity. A purified protein derivative (PPD) test should be done, and if initially negative, repeated annually. However, a PPD may be falsely negative if the patient is very immunosuppressed or very ill. If positive, a chest x-ray and Quantiferon Gold test should be performed for confirmation of potential active tuberculosis disease. Women should have regular Papanicolaou (Pap) smears and human papillomavirus (HPV) testing to evaluate for cervical dysplasia or cancer.

Late Disease

HIV and its comorbid opportunistic infections can affect every organ system in the body. Some infections, such as tuberculosis and pneumococcal pneumonia, also affect healthy people but are greatly increased in incidence and severity in the presence of HIV disease. Many mildly pathologic organisms, such as *Candida* species, cause unusual, severe infections in parts of the body, such as the esophagus and lungs, which they would rarely if ever affect without coinfection with HIV. Moreover, some AIDS-defining conditions, such as Kaposi sarcoma, can occur in persons with normal T-cell counts while other infections, such as cytomegalovirus retinitis and cryptococcal meningitis, are only seen in the presence of extreme immunodeficiency and very low T-cell counts. Many cancers are common in HIV-positive people, some of which, such as cervical carcinoma, are found in the non–HIV-infected population while others, such as primary central nervous system (CNS) lymphoma, are extremely rare outside of persons infected with HIV. Moreover, HIV infection damages the body directly and leads to such conditions as HIV-related dementia and HIV-associated nephropathy. Without antiretroviral therapy, AIDS is a universally fatal disease.

Treatment

Because of the complexity of treatment regimens and frequently changing treatment guidelines, **patients with HIV/AIDS should be referred, in almost all cases, to a physician with expertise in treating these conditions, including an infectious disease specialist.** In general, HAART, the combination of several antiretroviral drugs aimed at controlling the viral load of HIV and preventing HIV from multiplying, is used in patients who have AIDS (by laboratory or clinical criteria), who have symptoms of disease, or who are pregnant (to reduce the risk of vertical transmission). Updated guidelines on HIV/AIDS treatment and monitoring can be obtained by going to **http://www.aidsinfo.nih.gov.**

Prophylactic treatments to reduce the risk of infection are also important in immunosuppressed patients. HIV patients should receive annual attenuated influenza vaccination and should be offered pneumococcal vaccination (preferably before the CD4 count falls to less than 200 cells/μL). **Live virus vaccines are contraindicated in both HIV patients, if CD4 counts are less than 200, and their close (household) contacts.** Prophylaxis against *P jiroveci* pneumonia should be instituted using TMP-SMX when the CD4 count falls to less than 200 cells/μL or if there is a history of oropharyngeal candidiasis. *Mycobacterium avium*–intracellulare complex prophylaxis, using azithromycin or clarithromycin, is recommended if the CD4 count falls to less than 50 cells/μL.

OTHER SEXUALLY TRANSMITTED INFECTIONS

Chlamydia

Infection with *C trachomatis* is the most frequently reported sexually transmitted infection in the United States. *Chlamydia* can be passed from person to person by vaginal, anal, or oral intercourse. Infections are frequently asymptomatic, making screening necessary to identification. The United States Preventive Services Task Force (USPSTF) recommends screening for *Chlamydia* in all sexually active women age 24 or younger and in older women who are at increased risk for infection. Risk factors for infection include having multiple sexual partners, young age, history of other STI, and non-Hispanic Black race. The risk of transmission can be reduced by the proper use of latex condoms with every sexual encounter. Untreated *Chlamydia* infections in women can lead to ascending infections (ie, pelvic inflammatory disease [PID]), with an increased risk of ectopic pregnancy or infertility. *Chlamydia* can also cause cervicitis in women and epididymitis in men. It can cause urethritis and pharyngitis in men and women.

Testing for *Chlamydia* can be performed by collecting samples directly from the cervix, pharynx, or urethra, or by *C trachomatis* nucleic acid amplification testing of properly collected urine samples. Patients diagnosed with *Chlamydia* and their sexual partner(s) should be treated to reduce the risk of complications and to prevent further spread of the disease. Common treatment regimens for uncomplicated infection include azithromycin 1 g single dose PO or doxycycline 100 mg PO twice a day for a week. Doxycycline should not be used in a pregnant woman.

Gonorrhea

Gonorrhea is the common name for infection caused by *N gonorrhoeae*. This may also pass from person to person by vaginal, oral, or anal intercourse. Gonorrhea frequently leads to symptoms and signs of urethral infection in men, including dysuria and penile discharge. In women, the infection may be asymptomatic until complications, such as PID, occur. Because of this, the USPSTF recommends routinely screening sexually active women age 24 and less and older women at risk for gonorrhea. Testing for gonorrhea is performed similarly to, and usually in tandem with, testing for *Chlamydia* by sampling the cervix, urethra, anus, or pharynx or collecting urine for *N gonorrhoeae* nucleic acid amplification. Because of frequent coinfection, persons with gonorrhea should also routinely be treated for *Chlamydia*. The recommended treatment for gonorrhea is ceftriaxone 250 mg IM × 1 dose (along with treatment for *Chlamydia* as described earlier).

Syphilis

Syphilis is the manifestation of infection by the spirochete *Treponema pallidum*. Syphilis infections may be symptomatic or asymptomatic (latent). Symptomatic syphilis is often divided into three stages based on the symptom and length of time from exposure.

- Primary: Characterized by a painless ulcer, or chancre, at the site of infection (usually on the genitalia)

- Secondary: Characterized by skin rash, neurologic symptoms, or ophthalmologic abnormalities

- Tertiary: Characterized by cardiac or granulomatous lesions (gummas)

Commonly, syphilis is diagnosed on serologic testing of an asymptomatic person and this is called latent syphilis. If latent syphilis can be diagnosed within a year of infection, it is known as "early latent;" all other latent syphilis is either "late latent" or "latent syphilis of unknown duration."

Syphilis can be diagnosed either by direct identification of the *Treponema spirochete* or by serologic testing. Spirochetes can be identified by dark-field microscopy of tissue or exudate from a chancre. Serologic testing can be either a nontreponemal test, such as the RPR or Venereal Disease Research Laboratory (VDRL) test or a treponemal test, such as the fluorescent treponemal antibody absorbed (FTA-ABS) test. In general, initial screening is done with the RPR or VDRL test and confirmation testing done with the FTA-ABS. Screening for syphilis is recommended for all pregnant women in order to lower the risk of congenital syphilis. Screening should be performed for anyone with another STI or otherwise at high risk for infection.

Penicillin G is the recommended treatment for syphilis in all stages. The dosage, preparation used, and length of treatment will vary based on the stage of the disease. For penicillin-allergic patients, doxycycline, tetracycline, or ceftriaxone may be used as alternatives.

Herpes

Genital herpes is a viral infection caused by herpes simplex virus (HSV) type 1 or type 2. Most cases of recurrent genital herpes are caused by HSV-2. Clinically, HSV causes painful vesicles or ulcers. However, most persons infected with HSV-2 have not been clinically diagnosed because of the presence of mild or unrecognized infection. These persons may shed virus and therefore may transmit the infection to others while being asymptomatic.

HSV infections may be diagnosed by culture or polymerase chain reaction (PCR) testing of samples from clinically evident lesions. Serologic antibody testing to both HSV-1 and HSV-2 is also available, although both false positive and false negative and cross-reactivity may occur. Testing positive for HSV-1 alone can also be difficult to interpret, as this is a common nonsexually transmitted infection of childhood.

Antiviral therapy is available for HSV infections. Treatment can be used both for the acute management of symptomatic outbreaks and for suppression to reduce the frequency of outbreak or the risk of viral transmission to an uninfected partner. Pregnant women with a history of HSV should be placed on suppressive therapy late in pregnancy to reduce the risk of symptomatic outbreak or viral shedding at the time of delivery, so as to reduce the risk of neonatal herpes in the newborn. Women with clinically evident genital herpes at the time of delivery should be offered cesarean delivery.

Trichomoniasis

Trichomoniasis, or "trich," is a very common, curable sexually transmitted infection caused by the protozoan *Trichomonas vaginalis*. This infection is asymptomatic in approximately 70% of those infected. Symptomatic women may have vaginal itching, burning, or discharge. On examination, the physician may see a "frothy" discharge and the characteristic erythematous "strawberry" cervix. Symptomatic men may have urethral itching, burning, or discharge.

The diagnosis of trichomoniasis can be made by the direct visualization of the motile, flagellated trichomonads and many white blood cells on a wet mount of vaginal or penile discharge. Trich can be treated with a single, 2-g dose of oral metronidazole for the identified patient and sexual partner(s). Tinidazole is an alternative treatment.

HPV

HPV infection is the most common sexually transmitted infection. It can be passed during anal, vaginal, or oral intercourse or by skin to skin contact during sexual activity. There are many strains of HPV and the manifestation of the infection, if any, is related to the specific viral strain, the site of infection and host factors. **Most infections with HPV are asymptomatic and cleared by the body's immune system.** HPV infections can lead to genital warts, cervical cancer in women, penile cancer in men, and anal or oropharyngeal cancers in both.

Because of the ubiquity of the virus and the health risks related to exposure, vaccination against HPV is recommended routinely for both adolescent girls and boys. HPV vaccination has been shown to reduce the incidence of genital warts and of cervical cancer.

> ## CASE CORRELATION
> - See also Case 22 (Vaginitis).

COMPREHENSION QUESTIONS

45.1 A 42-year-old woman who is known to be HIV positive is found to have a CD4 count of 125 cells/mm³ and is taking HAART. She has not experienced any AIDS-defining illness. She continues to use IV heroin and abuse alcohol on a daily basis. She does not regularly take her antiretroviral medication and is often lost to follow-up. Which of the following treatments is most appropriate at this time?

    A. Initiate fluconazole for candidiasis prophylaxis.

    B. Initiate antiviral treatment for herpes zoster prophylaxis.

    C. Initiate TMP-SMX for *P jiroveci* pneumonia prophylaxis.

    D. Initiate clarithromycin for *M avium*–intracellulare complex prophylaxis.

45.2 A 25-year-old previously healthy man presents to the emergency room after experiencing a generalized tonic-clonic seizure that lasted 30 seconds. He has been experiencing headaches over the past 6 months but no other associated symptoms. His mother states that she witnessed him to have two previous seizures. The patient has a history of being sexually promiscuous and using IV illicit drugs. The result of his last HIV test is unknown. On neurologic examination, he is noted to have increased tone on the right and decreased right arm swing when walking. The remainder of his neurologic examination is unremarkable. A computed tomography (CT) scan of the head with contrast reveals that he has a ring-enhancing lesion measuring 15-mm over the left motor strip region and a 12-mm ring-enhancing lesion in the left basal ganglia. Which of the following would be an AIDS-defining condition in this patient?

    A. Glioblastoma multiforme

    B. Subarachnoid hemorrhage

    C. Herpes zoster encephalitis

    D. Listeriosis with brain abscess

    E. Primary brain lymphoma

45.3 A 22-year-old woman tests positive for gonorrhea from routine screening during a well-woman examination. She was asymptomatic at the time of the testing. She has no known drug allergies. Which of the following treatments would be recommended for her?

    A. Penicillin G 1.2 million units IM × 1

    B. Ceftriaxone 250 mg IM × 1

    C. Ciprofloxacin 250 mg PO × 1 dose

    D. Ceftriaxone 250 mg IM × 1 and azithromycin 1 g PO × 1

45.4 A 45-year-old man has STI screening done at a screening fair at a local free clinic. He has never been tested for STIs before and is completely asymptomatic. He tests negative for HIV, gonorrhea, and *Chlamydia* but is notified that he has a positive RPR. What is the next appropriate step for him?

A. Treatment with penicillin G

B. FTA-ABS testing

C. Notification of his STI to the local health department

D. Repeat his STI panel as this is likely a false-positive test

ANSWERS

45.1 **C.** With this level of cell count, the patient should continue antiretroviral therapy and start *P jiroveci* pneumonia prophylaxis. The level is not yet low enough to recommend *M avium*–intracellulare complex prophylaxis.

45.2 **D.** Primary brain lymphoma is an AIDS-defining condition. Glioblastoma multiforme and subarachnoid hemorrhage may present with these symptoms, but are not AIDS-defining conditions. Listeriosis and herpes zoster encephalitis can be associated with HIV, but are not AIDS-defining conditions.

45.3 **D.** Patients who test positive for gonorrhea should be treated for both gonorrhea and *Chlamydia*. Ceftriaxone 250 mg IM is the appropriate treatment for gonorrhea and azithromycin is the appropriate treatment for *Chlamydia*. Her sexual partner(s) should also be offered treatment.

45.4 **B.** He has tested positive on his initial screening test for syphilis with a nontreponemal test. A confirmatory test with a treponemal test should be performed prior to making the diagnosis or implementing treatment. If he is confirmed as positive, he should then be treated with penicillin and notification should be made to the health department.

CLINICAL PEARLS

▶ Because of the complexity of the drug regimens and the ever-changing guidelines, persons with HIV should be comanaged with an infectious disease specialist or other physician with expertise in treating HIV.

▶ The risk of transmission of HIV to health-care workers by accidental needle sticks from HIV-infected patients is very low. It is important to report these injuries promptly, as early prophylactic treatment can significantly lower the risk of developing HIV disease.

▶ Someone who tests positive for gonorrhea should be treated for both gonorrhea and *Chlamydia*, because of the high risk of coinfection.

REFERENCES

AIDS Education and Training Centers. *Peer Education Trainer's Manual.* 2015 ed. Available at: http://www.aidsetc.org/resource/peer-education-trainers-manual. Accessed March 14, 2015.

Armstrong C. CDC updates guidelines on diagnosis and treatment of sexually transmitted diseases. *Am Fam Physician.* 2011; 84(1):123–125.

Centers for Disease Control and Prevention. Available at: http://www.cdc.gov/hiv/library/reports/surveillance. Accessed March 14, 2015.

Centers for Disease Control and Prevention. Sexually transmitted diseases. Available at: http://www.cdc.gov/std/. Accessed May 9, 2015.

Chu C, Selwyn PA. Diagnosis and initial management of acute HIV infection. *Am Fam Physician.* 2010; 81(10):1239–1244.

Cohen MS, Shaw GM, McMichael AJ, Haynes BF. Acute HIV-1 infection. *N Engl J Med.* 2011;364:1943–1954.

Fauci AS, Lane H. Human immunodeficiency virus disease: AIDS and related disorders. In: Kasper D, Fauci A, Hauser S, et al., eds. *Harrison's Principles of Internal Medicine.* 19th ed. New York, NY: McGraw-Hill Education; 2015. Available at: http://accessmedicine.mhmedical.com. Accessed May 25, 2015.

Khalsa AM. Preventive counseling, screening, and therapy for the patient with newly diagnosed HIV infection. *Am Fam Physician.* 2006; 73(2):271–280.

Mattei PL, Beachkofsky TM, Gilson RT, Wisco OJ. Syphilis: a reemerging infection. *Am Fam Physician.* 2012; 86(5):433–440.

Roett MA, Mayor MT, Uduhiri KA. Diagnosis and management of genital ulcers. *Am Fam Physician.* 2012; 85(3):254–262.

World Health Organization. Global health observatory Data. Available at: http://www.who.int/gho/hiv/en/. Accessed March 14, 2015.

World Health Organization. Guidelines on post-exposure prophylaxis for HIV and the use of co-trimoxazole prophylaxis for HIV-related infections among adults, adolescents, and children. Available at: http://www.who.int/hiv/pub/guidelines/arv2013/arvs2013supplement_dec2014/en/. Accessed March 14, 2015.

A 33-year-old African-American man presents to the office for an acute visit with nausea and diarrhea present for the past week. Along with these symptoms, he has had a low-grade fever, some right upper quadrant (RUQ) abdominal pain, and has noticed that the whites of his eyes appear yellow. He has no significant medical history and takes no medications regularly. He denies alcohol, tobacco, or IV drug use at any time in his life. He works as a pastor in a local church that went on a mission to build a medical clinic in a rural area of Central America about 5 weeks ago. He had a mild case of traveler's diarrhea while there, recovered within a week, and has otherwise felt well. On examination, he is a well-developed man who appears to be moderately ill. His temperature is 99.8°F (37.6°C), his blood pressure is 110/80 mm Hg, his pulse is 90 beats/min, and his respiratory rate is 14 breaths/min. He has a prominent yellow color to his sclera and under his tongue. His mucous membranes are moist. Lung and cardiac examinations are unremarkable. His abdomen examination reveals normal bowel sounds yet moderate tenderness in the RUQ. His liver edge is palpable just below the costal margin and his spleen is not palpable. There are no abdominal masses palpated, and no rebound tenderness or guarding. On rectal examination, he has clay-colored soft stool that is fecal occult blood test negative.

▶ What is the most likely diagnosis?
▶ When and how did he most probably contract this illness?
▶ How can you confirm the diagnosis?
▶ What is the treatment at this point?

ANSWERS TO CASE 46:
Jaundice

Summary: A 33-year-old man with no significant medical history develops diarrhea, abdominal pain, and jaundice about a month after traveling to Central America. He is noted to have scleral icterus and tender hepatomegaly.

- **Most likely diagnosis:** Acute infection with hepatitis A.

- **Most probable timing and source of infection:** Ingestion of contaminated food or water while on his mission to Central America 5 weeks earlier.

- **Test to confirm the diagnosis:** Anti–hepatitis A immunoglobulin (Ig) M.

- **Treatment of acute hepatitis A:** Supportive care and symptomatic treatment for the patient; report infection to local health department; consider giving hepatitis A vaccine or Ig prophylaxis to close household or sexual contacts. Hepatitis A immunization will not be required for the patient.

ANALYSIS

Objectives

- Develop a differential diagnosis for adults with jaundice, with and without pain.

- Know the symptoms, management, complications, and modes of transmission of hepatitis A, B, and C.

- Be able to interpret the results of hepatitis viral serology tests.

Considerations

This presentation of nonbloody diarrhea along with nonspecific, crampy abdominal pain is most often caused by viral gastroenteritis, and is self-limited. However, this patient has several signs and symptoms that serve as clues to point to other potential diagnoses. Of particular importance, the complaint of yellow eyes should prompt an evaluation for causes of jaundice.

Bilirubin is a breakdown product of red blood cells. During the breakdown of hemoglobin, bilirubin is formed and bound to albumin, which carries it to the liver. In the liver, a portion of the bilirubin is made water soluble by conjugation to a glucuronide. This "conjugated bilirubin" is excreted in the bile and then largely excreted in the stool. Unconjugated bilirubin in the liver remains mostly bound to albumin and to a lesser degree high-density lipoproteins.

Most cases of **jaundice can be characterized as having prehepatic, hepatic, or posthepatic causes.** Prehepatic jaundice most often results from hemolysis of red blood cells, which overwhelms the liver's ability to conjugate and clear the bilirubin through its normal pathways. This results in a state of hyperbilirubinemia that is primarily unconjugated.

Hepatic causes of jaundice can lead to either unconjugated or conjugated hyperbilirubinemia. Viruses including hepatitis and alcohol reduce the liver's ability to transport bilirubin *after* it has been conjugated, resulting in a conjugated hyperbilirubinemia.

Posthepatic jaundice is usually caused by obstruction to the flow of bile through the bile ducts. This can be caused by bile duct stones, strictures, or tumors that narrow or block the ducts. Posthepatic jaundice is, therefore, a conjugated hyperbilirubinemia.

APPROACH TO:
Jaundice

DEFINITIONS

CAPUT MEDUSAE: Dilated superficial paraumbilical veins that usually result from shunting associated with severe portal hypertension and liver failure.

SPIDER ANGIOMA/TELANGIECTASIAS: Dilated, small, superficial veins with the distribution of the superior vena cava that appear as red, blue, or purple web-like formations, most often seen on the face, neck, upper trunk and abdomen, and lower extremities. The persistent dilation of blood vessels is due to increased serum estrogen levels, which remain elevated due to the inability of the impaired liver to conjugate estrone.

CLINICAL APPROACH

History and Examination

The most important information in the diagnostic evaluation of the patient with jaundice is derived from the history and should include questions focused on identifying the most common etiologies. Specific information should include when the jaundice commenced and whether it is of acute or gradual onset. The presence of gastrointestinal symptoms including abdominal pain, nausea, vomiting, diarrhea, or changes in stool or urine color is significant. Skin pruritis is common in patients with jaundice and this symptom may precede the onset of jaundice.

Associated constitutional symptoms, including unintentional weight loss or the development of lymphadenopathy should prompt the clinician to consider an underlying malignancy. Fever, shaking chills, and right upper quadrant abdominal pain can be signs of acute cholangitis, cholecystitis, or choledocholithiasis. Anorexia, fatigue, myalgias, and flu-like symptoms commonly indicate viral hepatitis. Bruising or bleeding disorders may suggest severe hepatic dysfunction that is interfering with the production of clotting factors. Increasing abdominal girth may be caused by ascites and peripheral edema by obstruction of venous return from the lower extremities and hypoalbuminemia.

A complete review of the past medical history is mandatory. **Any medications, whether prescription, nonprescription, or herbal supplements, should be reviewed.**

Acetaminophen and aspirin are widely used over-the-counter agents that in toxic amounts can cause hepatocellular damage. Numerous herbal agents (eg, Jamaican bush tea, Kava Kava, and Ma Huang) have also been associated with liver damage.

The **social history is of critical importance in a patient with jaundice.** The abuse of alcohol is the most common cause of cirrhosis in the United States. Intravenous drug use, transfusions of blood or blood products, and unsafe sexual practices can lead to infection with hepatitis B or C. Viral hepatitis has also been linked to tattooing when unsterilized or shared equipment is used. Travel history, especially the location and timing of any international travel, and recent exposure to persons with jaundice or contaminated foods (eg, raw oysters, contaminated produce) can lead to the consideration of hepatitis A.

A comprehensive physical examination is also paramount in the workup of the patient with jaundice. Along with a general physical examination, certain areas should be emphasized. Jaundice typically remains undetected on examination until the serum bilirubin level is at least greater than twice the normal upper limit, approaching 4 mg/dL. The yellow pigmentation may initially be detected as a yellowing of the sclera, especially in persons with darker skin types. Yellow discoloration can also commonly be seen in oral mucosal membranes such as under the tongue and hard palate.

Examination of the skin should document the jaundice and also look for clues to its cause. The stigmata of alcohol abuse (eg, caput medusae, spider angioma) or IV drug use (eg, needle track marks, ruptured veins, cellulitis) should be noted. Large hematomas, by themselves, could be a cause of jaundice as the blood reabsorbs. Evidence of easy bruising or bleeding should also be documented and quantified.

Abdominal examination must include the evaluation of the general contour of the abdomen, the presence of ascites or hepatosplenomegaly, and any rebound guarding or localized tenderness. A grossly enlarged liver with nodular contour may suggest malignancy, cirrhosis, or hepatitis. Hepatomegaly may occur due to underlying liver disease or hepatic congestion due to right-sided heart failure. Right upper quadrant tenderness can be associated with acute hepatitis but also with acute gallstone disease. Splenomegaly may suggest portal hypertension from cirrhosis, malignancy, or splenic sequestration of damaged red blood cells.

Laboratory Testing

The most important initial laboratory evaluation of jaundice is the serum bilirubin level, which is usually reported as a total bilirubin level. Direct and indirect concentrations can also be readily obtained. The degree of jaundice generally correlates with the level of serum bilirubin concentration. **The reported direct bilirubin is a measurement of the conjugated bilirubin level.** Unconjugated bilirubin can be determined by subtracting the direct bilirubin from the total bilirubin.

The relative relationship of conjugated and unconjugated bilirubin in a jaundiced person can be indirectly evaluated by performing a urinalysis. **Conjugated bilirubin is excreted in the urine, whereas unconjugated bilirubin is bound to albumin and exempted from glomerular filtration.** A high bilirubin level in the urinalysis in a jaundiced patient suggests a conjugated hyperbilirubinemia; absence of bilirubin on the urinalysis suggests an unconjugated hyperbilirubinemia. An overproduction or impaired conjugation or uptake of bilirubin generally results in unconjugated hyperbilirubinemia. Conversely, a decreased excretion or biliary obstruction typically leads to conjugated hyperbilirubinemia.

UNCONJUGATED HYPERBILIRUBINEMIA

Unconjugated hyperbilirubinemia, usually identified as an incidental finding when liver enzymes are tested for some other reason, in a patient without jaundice or known underlying hepatic dysfunction, is often caused by **Gilbert syndrome.** Gilbert syndrome is a congenital reduction of conjugation of bilirubin in the liver due to an autosomal recessive gene involved in glucuronidation. It occurs in approximately 5% of the population and is of no health significance. Patients generally present with normal physical examination and routine laboratory tests, except for icterus and mild unconjugated (2-4 mg/dL) hyperbilirubinemia. It is also more commonly diagnosed in males due to higher daily bilirubin production. Occasionally, the bilirubin level will increase during times of stress, illness, fasting, and then recover to its baseline, slightly elevated level (usually <3 mg/mL), after the illness resolves. In a patient with mildly elevated unconjugated bilirubinemia, otherwise normal liver enzymes, thyroid-stimulating hormone (TSH), and complete blood count (CBC), and who is otherwise well, no further workup is indicated.

Hemolysis can cause an unconjugated hyperbilirubinemia in proportion to the amount of hemolysis that occurs. It is most often diagnosed by the identification of anemia along with the presence of red cell fragments on peripheral smear, and elevated serum lactate dehydrogenase and haptoglobin. The serum bilirubin level typically remains below 5 mg/dL in hemolytic conditions such as spherocytosis, thalassemias, sickle cell disease, glucose-6-phosphate dehydrogenase deficiency, malaria, thrombotic thrombocytopenic purpura (TTP), and hemolytic uremic syndrome (HUS). The treatment is to treat the underlying cause of the hemolysis.

CONJUGATED HYPERBILIRUBINEMIA

Hepatitis A is an acute viral infection of the liver primarily transmitted via fecal-oral contamination and accounts for 30% of acute viral hepatitis in the United States. Contaminated food and water are the primary sources of infection, although risks also include drug use (both injection and noninjection), male-male sexual contact, household and sexual contact with another infected individual, and working in a daycare setting. Hepatitis A virus (HAV) is also more widespread among those who live in low socioeconomic areas likely due to inadequate sanitation and hygiene practices. Hepatitis A infection is widespread in Africa, Asia, Greenland, Middle East, Mexico, and Central and South America. Travelers to these areas are at risk for infection and should be immunized prior to travel with two separate immunizations 6 months apart.

Hepatitis A causes a self-limited illness characterized by jaundice, fever, fatigue, malaise, nausea, vomiting, anorexia, right upper quadrant abdominal discomfort, and clay-colored stools. Common physical findings include jaundice and hepatomegaly. HAV infection can lead to fulminant hepatic failure in those who have chronic hepatitis B or C infection. The average incubation period is 25 to 50 days and transmission is possible 2 weeks prior to the development of symptoms and for 1 week after jaundice appears. While the symptoms can resemble a mild flu-like illness, or even be asymptomatic in younger patients, there is an approximately 0.1% to 1% fatality rate which increases in those over age 40. The icteric phase commonly lasts for 6 to 8 weeks. Most persons will recover from the associated fatigue within 3 months, although some people have an illness that will last up to 6 months. While there is no specific treatment for hepatitis A, supportive care and symptomatic treatments are indicated. Patients who develop fulminant hepatitis should be hospitalized in a facility with liver transplant capability.

Hepatitis A is diagnosed based on the presence of a conjugated hyperbilirubinemia, elevated serum transaminases, and positive antibody titers. An acute infection causes an elevation of anti-HVA IgM. In the absence of HAV symptoms, an elevated IgM anti-HAV may indicate a false-positive result, asymptomatic infection, or prolonged presence of the immunoglobulin after the initial infection. An elevated anti-HAV IgG but negative IgM indicates a history of a previous hepatitis A infection but not an acute illness. Additional laboratory findings may include nonspecific elevations of acute-phase reactants including serum alkaline phosphatase, platelets, and erythrocyte sedimentation rate (ESR).

Effective measures in preventing HAV transmission include adequate hand washing, avoidance of contaminated foods and water, and proper food handling and preparation. Hepatitis A vaccination is recommended for children aged 12 to 18 in identified high-risk counties, travelers to endemic areas, persons with chronic liver disease or chronic clotting-factor disorders, men who have sex with men, IV drug users, HIV-infected individuals, and workers with a high risk of exposure including food handlers, in addition to anyone who desires immunity to hepatitis A. Household or sexual contacts of persons infected with hepatitis A and previously unvaccinated can be offered postexposure prophylaxis with hepatitis A vaccination or Ig. Ig is preferred in patients for whom vaccine is contraindicated, adults greater than 40 years, immunocompromised individuals, and those who have been diagnosed with chronic liver disease.

Hepatitis B has infected over 2 billion people worldwide and there are currently 350 million chronic carriers, of whom a million will die from hepatitis B virus (HBV)–associated liver disease each year. Areas of the world with intermediate-to-high rates of infections are Eastern Europe, Asia, sub-Saharan Africa, Middle East, and the Pacific islands. Hepatitis B is a viral infection transmitted via contact with contaminated blood or body fluids. Sexual contact (eg, men having sex with men, multiple partners, and sexual contact with an infected person) and needle sharing are common mechanisms of infection in the United States. Hepatitis B may also be vertically transmitted from mother to baby. The incubation period from exposure to clinical symptoms is 6 to 24 weeks. Only 50% of infections with hepatitis B are symptomatic. Up to 5% of the world's population is affected with chronic HBV infection and approximately 1% of infections result in hepatic failure and death. Along with the acute-phase symptoms, which are similar to hepatitis A, hepatitis B can cause a chronic infection. The risk of developing **chronic hepatitis B is inversely related to the age at infection**—90% of infected infants, 20% to 50% of children younger than age 5, and less than 5% infected adults—develop chronic hepatitis B, which can lead to cirrhosis and hepatocellular carcinoma. **Hepatitis B causes up to 80% of cases of hepatocellular carcinoma worldwide.**

Serologic evaluation is necessary to determine the presence and type of hepatitis B infection. Hepatitis B surface antigen (HBsAg) is present in both acute and chronic infections and viral load is associated with risk of transmission to others. HBsAg typically becomes detectable in 1 to 10 weeks following HBV exposure and disappears in 4 to 6 months in those who subsequently recover and clear the virus spontaneously. Persistent detection of HBsAg after 6 months postexposure generally indicates chronic HBV infection. Hepatitis e antigen (HBeAg) is accepted as a marker for HBV replication and degree of infectivity. Patients with the HBeAg are 100 times more infectious than those lacking this antigen. **Antibody to the surface antigen (anti-HBs) in the absence of HBsAg is seen in resolved infections and is the serologic marker produced after hepatitis B vaccination.** An IgM antibody to the hepatitis B core antigen (anti-HBcAg IgM) is diagnostic of an acute HBV infection. Anti-HBcAg IgM is the only serologic marker detectable during the window period of seroconversion. A measurable level of HBsAg with a negative anti-HBcAg IgM is diagnostic of chronic hepatitis B. Figures 46–1 and 46–2 show the serologic studies associated with acute hepatitis B infection and chronic hepatitis B infection, respectively.

Acute hepatitis B infection is treated supportively. Persons with chronic hepatitis B may be candidates for antiviral therapy and should be referred to a hepatologist, both to evaluate the appropriateness of therapy and to monitor for the development of hepatocellular carcinoma, cirrhosis, and other potential complications of antiviral therapy.

Hepatitis B vaccination is universally recommended for children. Vaccination is also recommended for adults at high risk of disease, including health-care and public safety workers, household contacts of patients with HBV, IV drug users, persons with chronic liver disease, individuals requiring periodic blood or blood

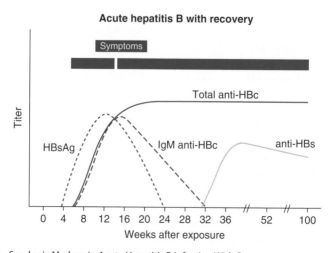

Figure 46–1. Serologic Markers in Acute Hepatitis B Infection With Recovery.

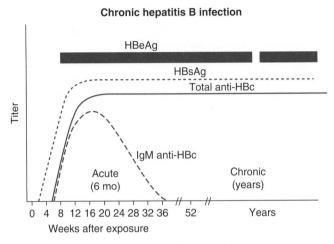

Figure 46–2. Serologic Markers in Chronic Hepatitis B Infection.

product transfusions, and patients receiving dialysis. Postexposure prophylaxis with hepatitis B Ig and/or vaccination is recommended for all unvaccinated persons who are exposed to infected bodily fluids or secretions.

Hepatitis C (HCV) is the most common cause of chronic liver disease in the United States, with more than 3 million infected persons. Infection is most prevalent in persons born between 1945 and 1965, the majority of whom were likely infected during the 1970s and 1980s. Approximately 2% to 3% (130-170 million) of the world population has been infected with the HCV. Transmission occurs via exposure to infected blood or body fluids via sexual contact and use of illicit drugs, sharing of needles and other drug paraphernalia, tattooing, accidental exposure of health-care workers, or by vertical transmission. Blood or blood-product transfusion and organ transplantation from infected donors were common sources of exposure prior to 1992.

HCV can be detected in the blood within 1 to 3 weeks of exposure, followed by an acute hepatitis C infection between 2 and 12 weeks of postexposure, with liver cell injury detectable in 4 to 12 weeks. Most infections are asymptomatic, yet hepatitis C can also cause an acute illness with jaundice, abdominal pain, malaise, and anorexia. **Of those infected with hepatitis C, 60% to 80% will develop a chronic infection**, with measurable levels of hepatitis C virus RNA (HCV RNA) for more than 6 months.

Chronic hepatitis C can lead to cirrhosis, hepatic decompensation, and hepatocellular carcinoma. Up to 30% of those with chronic HCV infection will develop cirrhosis during a 20- to 30-year time frame, making hepatitis C the current leading cause for liver transplantation in the United States. Patients with HCV infection should avoid alcohol consumption, acetaminophen, and nonsteroidal anti-inflammatory drugs (NSAIDs), and should receive hepatitis A and B vaccinations to prevent rapid disease progression and risk of coinfection. The progression of chronic HCV infection can be assessed by the amount of inflammation and cirrhosis seen on liver biopsy, which is commonly performed to evaluate extent of fibrosis and to determine candidacy for antiviral treatment with ribavirin and/or interferon. Treatment and cure results are highly variable depending on virus genotype, patient risk factors, and chronic health conditions. Treatment goals are to reduce long-term complications of chronic infection by inducing a sustained remission of HCV. There is currently no vaccination available for hepatitis C.

Hepatitis D is a rare cause of viral hepatitis in the United States that uses the viral envelope of hepatitis B to infect its host and thus requires coinfection of hepatitis B and D. It is commonly encountered in patients infected with HIV. Approximately 5% of HBV carriers may be coinfected with hepatitis D worldwide. It is endemic in the Mediterranean, Middle East, the Pacific islands, and South America. The clinical manifestations of HBV and hepatitis D virus (HDV) coinfection typically resemble that of an HBV infection. In coinfection, 10% or less will become chronically infected. Interferon is the only approved drug for treating chronic hepatitis D. Hepatitis B vaccine is the mainstay in HDV prevention. There is currently no vaccination available for hepatitis D.

Hepatitis E is transmitted via the fecal-oral route and while it is rare in the United States, it has a high prevalence in Asia, Africa, Middle East, and Central America. The incubation period is 4 to 5 weeks. The clinical signs and symptoms of hepatitis E virus (HEV) infection are generally more severe compared to those seen in HAV with a greater likelihood of prolonged cholestasis. It has a very high mortality rate, mostly in the third trimester for pregnant women. Malnourished individuals or those with underlying liver disease are also more likely to develop fulminant hepatitis. Diagnosis of acute HEV infection can be confirmed by detection of HEV in serum or stool or IgM anti-HEV. Treatment is supportive. Ig prophylaxis is available in countries where HEV is endemic, but its efficacy remains unproven. There is currently no vaccination available for hepatitis E.

Alcohol abuse can cause an acute severe hepatitis, chronic fatty liver disease, hepatitis, cirrhosis, and fibrosis. Alcohol leads to a conjugated hyperbilirubinemia by impairing bile acid secretion and uptake. Common physical findings include ascites, jaundice, cutaneous telangiectasias, palmer erythema, testicular atrophy, gynecomastia, and malnutrition. **Transaminase levels from alcohol abuse typically show an aspartate aminotransferase (AST) out of proportion to the alanine aminotransferase (ALT), commonly with a ratio of 2 or greater;** γ-glutamyl transferase (GGT) levels are often abnormal in alcohol hepatitis; viral hepatitis usually causes greater elevations of the ALT (see Case 41 for a more thorough discussion of alcohol abuse).

Physical obstructions of bile drainage can also cause conjugated hyperbilirubinemia. Common etiologies of obstruction include gallstones that become impacted in the bile ducts, postoperative biliary strictures, or extrinsic compression of the bile ducts by tumors, such as pancreatic cancer. Pancreatic cancer is the most common cause of painless jaundice in a patient with biliary obstruction. Imaging of the bile system with ultrasound, computed tomography (CT) scan, or magnetic resonance imaging (MRI) or magnetic resonance cholangiopancreatography (MRCP) is usually diagnostic. Endoscopic retrograde cholangiopancreatography (ERCP) can be diagnostic and, in some cases, therapeutic.

Nonalcoholic fatty liver disease (NAFLD) results from deposition of fat within the hepatocytes, commonly from obesity, diabetes mellitus, hyperlipidemia, and hypertriglyceridemia. Rapid weight loss and protein-calorie malnutrition may also lead to NAFLD. One of the leading causes of liver disease, up to 25% of persons with NAFLD may have underlying cirrhosis. While most cases are asymptomatic and detectable only via elevated serum transaminases, symptoms may mimic those of acute viral hepatitis. There are currently no acceptable treatments for NAFLD, yet appropriate nutrition, weight management, and avoidance of alcohol are recommended.

COMPREHENSION QUESTIONS

46.1 A 32-year-old man with asthma and hypertension comes in for evaluation of an elevated bilirubin level that was detected on blood work required for a preemployment physical. The bilirubin level was 2.5 mg/dL (normal up to 1.0 mg/dL) with an elevated unconjugated component. He feels well and generally drinks one beer per night. He is monogamous with his wife and has no history of IV drug abuse and has one tattoo. His sclerae are anicteric and there are no signs of jaundice. His liver enzymes, electrolytes, TSH, and CBC are normal. Which of the following is the next step in the evaluation of this patient?

A. Reassurance

B. Counsel on alcohol abstinence

C. Abdominal ultrasound

D. Hepatitis serologies

E. Referral to a hepatologist

46.2 A 45-year-old woman was diagnosed 6 months ago with acute hepatitis B infection. She is unaware of how she contracted the virus. She takes no medications and since the diagnosis, she has started taking a multivitamin and has started exercising. She now has the following serologies: HBsAg negative; anti-HBsAg positive; HBeAg negative; anti-HBcAg positive. Which of the following is the correct diagnosis?

A. Chronic active infection with low infectivity

B. Chronic active infection with high infectivity

C. Resolved acute infection

D. Resolved acute infection but contagious to sexual contacts

E. Resolved infection but at risk for reinfection in the future

46.3   A 60-year-old retired Navy captain comes to the doctor after a 15-lb unintentional weight gain over the past 4 months. His medical history is significant for osteoarthritis and his only complaint is fatigue. He has smoked a pack of cigarettes daily since his early 20s and consumes two to three alcoholic beverages several times per week. On examination, he is slightly jaundiced, with no hepatomegaly or RUQ tenderness to palpation. He has mild shifting dullness in his abdomen, and significant lower extremity edema. His skin is noted to have several faded tattoos. Which of the following antibodies would most likely be present in this patient?

A.   Anti-HAV IgG

B.   Anti-HBc IgM

C.   Anti-HBs IgG

D.   Anti-HBe IgM

E.   Anti-HCV IgG

46.4   A 21-year-old college student plans to take a trip to Thailand with his friends in a couple of months. He confesses that he has experimented with illicit drugs including smoking marijuana as well as intranasal and intravenous cocaine and heroin. He is excited about the upcoming trip and wants to find out which immunizations he will need prior to his departure. Which of the following vaccinations and serologic tests will you recommend?

A.   Hepatitis A vaccination, hepatitis A and B serologies

B.   Hepatitis A and B vaccination, hepatitis A and B serologies

C.   Hepatitis B vaccination, hepatitis B and C serologies

D.   Hepatitis A and B vaccination, hepatitis B and C serologies

ANSWERS

46.1   **A.** This is a classic case of Gilbert disease, a benign mild elevation of unconjugated bilirubin. In the face of otherwise normal history, examination, and liver enzymes, no further workup is indicated. People with Gilbert syndrome can have icteric sclera and jaundice that worsens with stress or illness.

46.2   **C.** These serologies are consistent with resolved hepatitis B infection and ongoing immunity; the HBsAg antibodies indicate immunity. This patient has both negative surface and e antigens, so is not at risk to spread the disease to others.

46.3   **E.** The patient has chronic hepatitis C that has progressed to cirrhosis causing the edema, weight gain, and ascites. Hepatitis A does not proceed to cirrhosis. Anti-HBs is present in people immunized to hepatitis B. Anti-HBe IgM reflects viral infectivity of hepatitis B. Anti-HBc IgM reflects exposure to hepatitis B 4 to 36 weeks after exposure.

46.4 **D.** Both hepatitis A and B vaccination are recommended with travel to Asia. This patient has a high likelihood of hepatitis B and C infection given his history of intranasal and intravenous drug use. Vaccination recommendations can change and it is best to review travel recommendations at www.cdc.gov/travel. An appointment with a primary care physician or travel clinic should be made 4 to 6 weeks prior to taking any international trips to determine the appropriate vaccinations needed and general health information. However, if a patient has not been immunized against hepatitis A, two separate vaccines 6 months apart are required to confer immunity.

CLINICAL PEARLS

▶ The acute onset of painless jaundice in a patient older than age 50 should prompt an examination for pancreatic cancer (malignancy in the head of the pancreas causing compression of the bile ducts).

▶ All pregnant women should be screened for the presence of HBsAg. If positive, treating the newborns with hepatitis B immunoglobulin (HBIg) and vaccination can reduce the risk of vertical transmission.

▶ One of the greatest risks for the development of cirrhosis in those with chronic hepatitis C is alcohol use. Anyone with chronic hepatitis C should be counseled to avoid all alcohol intake.

▶ All persons born between 1945 and 1965 should be screened for hepatitis C.

▶ Nonalcoholic fatty liver disease is a leading cause of cirrhosis in patients with obesity, diabetes mellitus, and hyperlipidemia.

REFERENCES

Centers for Disease Control and Prevention. Diagnosis and management of food-borne illnesses. *MMWR Morb Mortal Wkly Rep.* 2004; 53(RR-04):1–33.

Centers for Disease Control and Prevention. Traveler's health. Available at: http://www.CDC.gov/travel. Accessed March 26, 2015.

Dienstag JL. Acute viral hepatitis. In: Kasper D, Fauci A, Hauser S, et al., eds. *Harrison's Principles of Internal Medicine.* 19th ed. New York, NY: McGraw-Hill Education; 2015. Available at: http://accessmedicine.mhmedical.com. Accessed May 25, 2015.

Roche SP, Kobos R. Jaundice in the adult patient. *Am Fam Physician.* 2004; 69:299–304.

United States Preventive Services Task Force. Hepatitis C: screening. June 2013. Available at: http://www.uspreventiveservicestaskforce.org/Page/Topic/recommendation-summary/hepatitis-c-screening. Accessed March 26,2015.

Ward RP, Kugelmas M, Libsch KD. Management of hepatitis C: evaluating suitability for drug therapy. *Am Fam Physician.* 2004; 69(6):1429–1436.

Wilkins T, Malcolm JK, Raina D, Schade R. Hepatits C: diagnosis and treatment. *Am Fam Physician.* 2010; 81(11):1351–1357.

Wilkins T, Tadkod A, Hepburn I, Schade RR. Nonalcoholic fatty liver disease: diagnosis and management. *Am Fam Physician.* 2013;88(1):35–42.

Workowski KA, Levine WC. Sexually transmitted diseases treatment guidelines, 2002. *MMWR Morb Mortal Wkly Rep.* 2002; 51(RR-06):1–80.

World Health Organization. Hepatitis. Available at: http://www.who/int/csr/disease/hepatitis/whocdscslryo20022/en/index3.html. Accessed March 26, 2015.

A 52-year-old man presents to the office with approximately 2 weeks of upper abdominal pain. His symptoms are difficult for him to describe, but include some "discomfort" in the epigastric region that comes and goes. He has had some "heartburn" and nausea, but no vomiting or diarrhea. He has noticed that his stools appear darker than they used to be, has not had bloody stools or rectal bleeding, and has recently noticed early satiety. He tried taking an over-the-counter antacid (calcium carbonate), which only minimally helped to relieve his symptoms. He takes an over-the-counter nonsteroidal anti-inflammatory drug (NSAID) "once or twice" a day because of arthritis in his knees. He does not smoke cigarettes or drink alcohol. On examination, he is pale appearing, but in no acute discomfort. He is afebrile, his blood pressure is 120/80 mm Hg, his pulse is 95 beats/min, and his respiratory rate is 14 breaths/min. Head, ears, eyes, nose, and throat (HEENT) examination is notable only for pale conjunctiva. Cardiac and pulmonary examinations are unremarkable. His abdomen has normal bowel sounds and moderate tenderness in the epigastrium with slight guarding but no rebound. Rectal examination reveals normal sphincter tone, no masses, and dark black stool that tests positive on fecal immunochemical (FIT) testing.

▶ What is the most likely diagnosis?
▶ What evaluation and treatment are indicated at this point?
▶ What can be suggested to reduce the risk of recurrence of this problem?

ANSWERS TO CASE 47:
Dyspepsia and Peptic Ulcer Disease

Summary: A 52-year-old man presents with vague upper abdominal discomfort, nausea, and early satiety. He is a daily NSAID user. He appears pale on examination, suggesting that he may be anemic. He has mild abdominal tenderness and melanotic stool on examination that should raise suspicion for an upper gastrointestinal (GI) bleed.

- **Most likely diagnosis:** Bleeding peptic ulcer.

- **Evaluation and treatment at this point:** Given that this patient has a high likelihood of having an upper GI bleed, hemodynamic stability should be ensured immediately. Two large-bore IVs should be placed, IV fluids started, and the patient should be transported to the emergency department. Initial testing should include a STAT complete blood count (CBC), blood type and screen, consultation for an esophagogastroduodenoscopy (EGD; upper GI endoscopy), discontinuation of his NSAID, and testing for *Helicobacter pylori*. He should be treated with a proton pump inhibitor (PPI) and antibiotics for *H pylori*, if tests confirm its presence. He may require a blood transfusion if found to be significantly anemic.

- **Reduce risk of recurrence by:** Discontinuation and avoidance of NSAIDs or aspirin or if unable to completely discontinue, use of a PPI along with the NSAID; eradication of *H pylori*.

ANALYSIS

Objectives

1. Learn the common presenting signs and symptoms of peptic ulcer disease (PUD), functional dyspepsia, and gastroesophageal reflux disease (GERD).

2. Learn the risk factors for the development of PUD.

3. Learn how to diagnose and treat PUD and GERD, as well as to know the risks of pharmacotherapy.

4. Understand the role of *H pylori* in PUD, including methods for testing for and treatment of PUD.

5. Know the "alarm symptoms" and "extraesophageal symptoms" for GERD and PUD.

Considerations

The Rome III Committee defines *dyspepsia* as one or more of the following symptoms: postprandial fullness, early satiety, and epigastric pain or burning. Approximately 15% to 25% of dyspepsia is caused by peptic ulcer disease, while 70% is attributable to functional (nonulcer) dyspepsia, or dyspepsia without an identifiable organic cause. Reflux esophagitis accounts for 5% to 15% of cases of dyspepsia,

Table 47–1 • "ALARM" SYMPTOMS FOR WHICH EARLY UPPER GI ENDOS-COPY IS RECOMMENDED
Unintentional weight loss
Progressive dysphagia
Recurrent/persistent vomiting
Odynophagia
Unexplained anemia
Gastrointestinal bleeding/hematemesis
Family history of cancer, specifically upper GI cancer
History of gastric surgery
Jaundice

while gastric or esophageal cancer are found in fewer than 2% of cases. Peptic ulcer disease is a condition of the gastrointestinal tract characterized by mucosal damage (eg, from NSAIDs or aspirin), then chronic exposure of the damaged mucosa to pepsin and gastric acid secretion. It usually occurs in the stomach and proximal duodenum. Less commonly, it occurs in the lower esophagus, the distal duodenum, or the jejunum, as in unopposed hypersecretory states including Zollinger-Ellison syndrome, with hiatal hernias (Cameron ulcers), or in ectopic gastric mucosa (eg, Meckel diverticulum). Symptoms of functional dyspepsia are essentially the same as those of PUD, with no evidence of structural disease to explain the symptoms, thus it is a diagnosis of exclusion.

Gastroesophageal reflux disease, the most common gastrointestinal condition, is a chronic digestive condition in which stomach contents and acid leak backwards from the stomach into the esophagus. A presumptive diagnosis can be accurately made in the setting of classic symptoms of heartburn and regurgitation.

Diagnostic endoscopy should be considered for patients with new-onset dyspepsia older than age 50 or who have symptoms that may be associated with upper GI malignancy (Table 47–1). The cutoff age may be more appropriate at 40 or 45 for Asian or African-American patients. For persons younger than age 50 and without alarm symptoms, testing for H $pylori$ via immunoglobulin G (IgG) serology, rather than the 13-C urea breath test or stool antigen as initial testing, is recommended due to low cost and ease of collection. For those who test positive, treating the H $pylori$ infection via combination antibiotic and acid-suppression therapy is indicated. For persons who test negative, empiric therapy with a PPI for 4 to 8 weeks is a cost-effective intervention. Endoscopy or reconsideration of the diagnosis should be considered for those who continue to be symptomatic following these interventions.

APPROACH TO:

Dyspepsia and Peptic Ulcer Disease

DEFINITIONS

H$_2$ ANTAGONIST: Class of medications that are competitive antagonists of histamine binding to gastric parietal cell H$_2$ receptors, which prevent activation of the pathway that mediates release of acid into the gastric lumen.

PROTON PUMP INHIBITOR: Class of medications that suppress gastric acid production by irreversibly inhibiting the H^+/K^+ ATPase proton pump in gastric parietal cells.

CLINICAL APPROACH

PUD is a term generally used to describe both duodenal and gastric ulcers. **Duodenal ulcers are more prevalent overall, whereas gastric ulcers are more common in NSAID users.** Risk factors for the development of PUD include *H pylori* infection, the use of NSAIDs and aspirin, cigarette smoking, alcohol consumption and personal or family history of PUD. Black and Hispanic populations have a higher likelihood of developing PUD as well. The lifetime risk of developing PUD in the United States is approximately 10%. Table 47–2 summarizes other causes of PUD.

History and Examination

Dyspepsia symptoms are common and there is significant overlap between the symptoms of PUD, GERD, and functional dyspepsia. Patients with symptoms primarily of heartburn or acid regurgitation are more likely to have GERD. **Classic symptoms associated with PUD include epigastric abdominal pain that is improved with the ingestion of food, or pain that develops a few hours after eating.** Nocturnal symptoms are also common with PUD, when the circadian stimulation of acid secretion is maximal prior to awakening. The symptoms of PUD are often gradual in onset and may present for weeks or months. Patients often self-medicate with over-the-counter acid-suppression medications which usually provide some relief, prior to presenting to the physician.

Table 47–2 • CAUSES OF PEPTIC ULCERS		
Causes	Etiology	Comments
Common causes	*Helicobacter pylori* infection NSAIDs	Gram-negative, motile spiral rod found in 48% of patients with peptic ulcer disease 5% to 20% of patients who use NSAIDs over long periods develop peptic ulcer disease NSAID-induced ulcers and complications are more common in the elderly, those with concomitant *H pylori* infection, or those on steroids or anticoagulants
Other/rare causes	Other medications Acid-hypersecretory states/gastrinomas (eg, Zollinger-Ellison syndrome) Malignancy Stress	Steroids, bisphosphonates, potassium chloride, chemotherapeutic agents (eg, intravenous fluorouracil) Multiple gastroduodenal, jejunal, or esophageal ulcers that are difficult to heal Gastric cancer, lymphomas, lung cancers After acute illness, multiorgan failure, ventilator support, extensive burns (Curling ulcer), or head injury (Cushing ulcer)

Data from Kurata JH, Nogawa AN. Meta-analysis of risk factors for peptic ulcer. Nonsteroidal anti-inflammatory drugs, Helicobacter pylori, and smoking. J Clin Gastroenterol. 1997;24:2-17.

The examination of the patient with dyspepsia should both attempt to confirm the suspicion of PUD and to rule out other diagnoses that may present with abdominal pain. Most patients with dyspepsia and GERD will have unremarkable abdominal examinations, while PUD may only have the examination finding of mild-to-moderate epigastric tenderness. The presence of GI bleeding may be documented by fecal occult blood testing; however, the bleeding from PUD may be episodic and a single negative fecal occult blood test does not completely rule out an upper gastrointestinal bleed. Signs of anemia (eg, pale conjunctiva and skin, tachycardia, orthostatic hypotension) should be evaluated and treated according to severity and underlying risk factors. If a patient with known coronary artery disease becomes symptomatic and has a hemoglobin level less than 7 g/dL, then blood transfusion should be considered.

Helicobacter pylori

H pylori is a corkscrew-shaped gram-negative bacillus that is the causative agent of most non–NSAID-related ulcers, and is associated with the development of gastric cancer. **The presence of the organism is associated with a five to seven times increased risk of the development of PUD.** *H pylori* infection is commonly acquired during childhood and is more common in developing countries. **Serologic testing for anti–*H pylori* antibodies (eg, IgG, IgM)** is inexpensive, noninvasive, readily available, and is the first test that should be performed in a previously uninvestigated patient. It is a highly sensitive and specific test, yet **cannot distinguish an active infection from a treated infection.** Once the test is positive, it will almost always stay positive and should not be repeated. **Stool antigen testing**, has an excellent positive predictive value and is most often used 8 to 14 weeks posttreatment to test for eradication in cases suspected refractory to treatment. For this test to be most accurate, patients must not have been treated with PPIs for at least 2 weeks prior to stool collection. Active *H pylori* infection can be confirmed by 13-C **urea breath testing**. This test is performed by having the patient ingest a carbon-labeled urea compound, which is then metabolized by urease from the *H pylori* organism. The labeled CO_2 released by this process is measured in exhaled breath. This test is highly sensitive and specific, is the most expensive option, and should be reserved for patients who have been treated and with inconclusive stool antigen testing.

The **gold standard** for diagnosis of *H pylori* is **endoscopy with gastric mucosal biopsy.** The bacterium can either be visualized microscopically using a variety of staining methods, cultured, or detected by rapid testing of the specimen. Endoscopy also allows for direct visualization of ulcers and evaluation for the presence of malignancy or other pathology in the esophagus, stomach, or duodenum. Endoscopy is invasive, expensive, requires conscious sedation, and should be considered when a patient has high suspicion for esophageal or gastric complications of PUD or GERD, rather than purely for diagnosis of *H pylori*.

Complications of PUD

Approximately 25% of patients with PUD have a serious complication such as hemorrhage, perforation, or gastric outlet obstruction. Silent ulcers and complications are more common in older patients and in patients taking chronic NSAIDs and aspirin.

Clinically relevant upper gastrointestinal bleeding occurs in 15% to 20% of patients with PUD, is the most common indication for surgical intervention, and is the most common cause of death. The risk of rebleeding in PUD is the greatest within 48 hours of initial bleed and the risk of death increases proportionally with advanced age, medical comorbidities, and hemodynamic status.

Complications of GERD

Up to 40% of patients with chronic GERD will experience heartburn and regurgitation on a monthly basis. Most patients with GERD will have nonerosive reflux disease (NERD), while others will progress to erosive esophagitis. Caucasian men aged 45 or greater who have chronic GERD, smoke cigarettes, and drink alcohol are at the greatest risk of development of Barrett esophagus, which is a precursor for esophageal adenocarcinoma. Patients with Barrett esophagus should be placed on lifelong PPI therapy and should undergo surveillance upper endoscopy to monitor for the development of esophageal adenocarcinoma.

Management of Suspected PUD

A CBC should be obtained to determine a baseline hemoglobin value and should be repeated every 6 to 8 hours to monitor for anemia and gastrointestinal blood loss, even in the setting of negative fecal occult blood. Liver transaminases and serum amylase and lipase levels should be obtained when biliary or pancreatic disease is suspected. An electrocardiography (ECG) should be performed upon initial evaluation to rule out cardiac ischemia, since upper abdominal pain can be an atypical sign of acute coronary syndrome. A chest x-ray should be obtained to rule out abdominal visceral perforation, characterized by free air under the diaphragm. Abdominal ultrasonography is indicated when cholecystitis is suspected. A pregnancy test should be obtained on all reproductive-age women, and endocervical cultures obtained when suspicion of pelvic inflammatory disease is high. Patients with significant anemia, hemodynamic instability (eg, hypotension, tachycardia, orthostasis), or a suspected acute abdomen should be immediately hospitalized. Urgent surgical evaluation should be obtained if an acute abdomen is present.

Dyspepsia in patients younger than age 50 with no alarm symptoms can be managed with a noninvasive *H pylori* "test-and-treat" protocol with serologic testing followed by acid suppression using a PPI if symptoms remain. A negative test rules out *H pylori* infection in dyspeptic patients. If positive, appropriate treatment to eradicate the infection, along with a PPI to suppress acid production, should be prescribed (Table 47–3 lists *H pylori* treatment regimens).

Management of GERD

Patients who experience classic GERD symptoms often begin self-directed acid-suppressive therapy with either an H_2 antagonist or a PPI. Over-the-counter formulations of these medications have a 2-week limit on therapy, then physician consultation is advised. The "test and treat" strategy for GERD posits starting with the lowest possible dose of an H_2 antagonist once daily to control symptoms, then increasing frequency and potency to a PPI if symptoms are not adequately controlled (step-up therapy). If a patient is on chronic PPI therapy, they should be "stepped down" to an H_2 antagonist if possible.

Table 47–3 • *HELICOBACTER PYLORI* TREATMENT REGIMENS

Drug	Dose
Triple Therapy (7-14 days)	
Bismuth subsalicylate *plus*	2 tabs QID
Metronidazole *plus*	250 mg QID
Tetracycline	500 mg QID
Ranitidine bismuth citrate *plus*	400 mg BID
Tetracycline *plus*	500 mg BID
Clarithromycin or metronidazole	500 mg BID
Omeprazole (or lansoprazole) *plus*	20 mg BID (30 mg BID)
Clarithromycin *plus*	250 or 500 mg BID
Amoxicillin or	1 g BID
Metronidazole (in penicillin-allergic patients)	500 mg BID
Quadruple Therapy (10-14 days)	
Omeprazole (or lansoprazole)	20 mg (30 mg) daily
Bismuth subsalicylate plus	525 mg QID
Metronidazole plus	250 mg QID
Tetracycline	500 mg QID

Data from Del Valle J. Peptic ulcer disease and related disorders. In: Fauci AS, Braunwald E, Kasper DL, et al., eds. Harrison's Principles of Internal Medicine. *17th ed. New York, NY: McGraw-Hill; 2008:1863.*

When a patient requires acid-suppressive therapy for 8 weeks to control symptoms and cannot undergo step-down therapy or stop medication, then they should undergo upper endoscopy to rule out potential complications. Patients with heartburn or regurgitation should be advised to avoid smoking, alcohol, spicy foods, citrus foods, fatty foods, large meals, fatty meals, chocolate, peppermint, and should avoid eating or drinking 3 to 4 hours prior to recumbency. Elevation of the head of the bed 6 to 8 inches and avoiding tight clothing around the waist may also help to improve symptoms.

Generally PPIs have greater efficacy in suppressing acid production and hastening ulcer healing than H$_2$ blockers. Those with no evidence of active infection can be treated with acid suppression alone for 4 to 8 weeks. If symptoms resolve, no further testing is indicated. Along with treatment, offending agents, such as NSAIDs and tobacco, should be discontinued. Most patients with *H pylori* infection who have been treated successfully will require chronic acid suppressive therapy to combat symptoms of dyspepsia. Chronic acid suppressive therapy with PPIs has been associated with increased risk of community-acquired pneumonia; *Clostridium difficile*–associated diarrhea; demineralization of bone; and decreased absorption of calcium, magnesium, and iron.

Patients older than age 50 or those with alarm symptoms for either PUD or GERD should be referred for upper GI endoscopy to exclude complications of esophageal stricture, erosive disease, or malignancy. Endoscopy is preferred over radiographic procedures such as barium esophagram due to direct visualization and the ability to perform biopsy. Endoscopy also can be therapeutic, as a stricture could be readily dilated, and a visible source of bleeding can be identified and cauterized. **Any patient 50 years or older who has hematemesis, hematochezia, or melena should undergo a colonoscopy regardless of the upper endoscopic findings,** to evaluate for a lower gastrointestinal cause of bleeding including diverticulosis, vascular malformation, or malignancy.

Surgical treatment for PUD is rarely indicated, yet may be warranted in cases of severe hemorrhage that cannot be controlled via endoscopy, or in cases of perforation or obstruction.

CASE CORRELATION

- See Case 23 (Lower GI Bleeding) and Case 40 (Irritable Bowel Syndrome).

COMPREHENSION QUESTIONS

47.1 A 30-year-old woman with no significant medical history presents asking for advice. She recently attended a health fair where she tested positive for *H pylori* on a blood test. She denies any recent abdominal discomfort, nausea, vomiting, diarrhea, or melena. Occasionally, she uses over-the-counter acid-suppressive therapy after eating spicy foods or drinking alcohol when she develops dyspepsia and heartburn, and her symptoms resolve within a week. Which of the following is the most appropriate advice to give this patient regarding *H pylori*?

A. Based on this test result, it is not possible to tell if she has an active infection.

B. She should undergo stool antigen testing to prove infection.

C. She should undergo upper endoscopy to prove infection.

D. She should be prescribed a PPI for 8 weeks.

E. She should be prescribed triple therapy to treat infection.

47.2 A 62-year-old man presents to clinic with increasing shortness of breath and fatigue over the last several days. Cardiac examination reveals regular rate and rhythm and lungs are clear to auscultation bilaterally. No jaundice, jugular venous distention (JVD), or peripheral edema is noted. Mucous membranes are pink with no evidence of cyanosis and capillary refill is brisk. CBC reveals a microcytic anemia and a gastric ulcer is diagnosed on upper GI endoscopy. Gastric mucosa biopsy confirms an *H pylori* infection. His last colonoscopy was 10 years ago and was unremarkable. Which of the following is the next most appropriate step in the workup of this patient?

A. Barium esophagram

B. Abdominal ultrasound

C. Colonoscopy

D. Urea breath test

E. Stool antigen test

47.3 A 41-year-old man presents for evaluation of upper GI discomfort present over the last 2 months. He says that he has a "full" sensation in the epigastric region. He recently began smoking again due to increased stress at work. He denies blood in his stool, denies vomiting, and has had no dysphagia. He has lost 10 lb in the last few weeks unintentionally, which he attributes to not eating. His mother has hemorrhoids, and no family member has ever had colon cancer. He has never had a colonoscopy. Which of the following is the most appropriate next step in workup of this patient?

A. *H pylori* "test-and-treat"

B. PPI therapy for 8 weeks

C. Fecal occult blood test

D. Upper endoscopy

E. Colonoscopy

47.4 A 19-year-old woman arrives at the emergency room with a 15-hour history of nausea, vomiting, and severe epigastric abdominal pain that awoke her from sleep. She admits to heavy alcohol consumption the prior evening that is common for her on the weekends. She takes no medications and does not take NSAIDs regularly. Her blood pressure is 100/60 mm Hg, pulse rate is 130 beats/min, respiratory rate is 14 breaths/min, and her temperature is 39°C (102.2°F). An acute abdominal series upon admission displayed a substantial amount of free air under the right hemidiaphragm. Which of the following is the most likely diagnosis?

A. Perforated peptic ulcer

B. Alcohol-related gastritis

C. Appendicitis

D. Gastroenteritis

E. Kidney stones

47.5 A 36-year-old man presents to your office for follow-up after having been recently admitted to the hospital for hypoxia due to an acute asthma attack. A chest x-ray performed on admission was unremarkable. Upon admission, he was given intravenous corticosteroids and started on a PPI for stress ulcer prophylaxis. He was discharged home on a tapering course of oral corticosteroids and advised to continue the PPI until steroid therapy was completed. Which of the following complications from PPI therapy is most likely to occur in this patient?

A. Community-acquired pneumonia

B. Osteoporosis

C. Hypermagnesemia

D. Elevated ferritin

E. *C difficile*-associate diarrhea

ANSWERS

47.1 **A.** *H* pylori serologic testing cannot distinguish active infections from old infections nor can they diagnose the presence of ulcers. Treating a positive serum test in an asymptomatic person is not indicated. Stool antigen testing, upper endoscopy, daily PPI therapy, or triple therapy is not indicated.

47.2 **C.** The presence of blood in the stool or anemia in a patient older than age 50, even when an ulcer is found, is an indication for colonoscopy, as this may also represent a presentation of a concomitant colon cancer. The urea breath test may be beneficial after completion of treatment to confirm eradication of the infection.

47.3 **D.** This patient presents with the alarm symptom of weight loss. He should be referred for early endoscopy.

47.4 **A.** The acute abdomen and free air under the diaphragm indicates a perforated viscus. This patient has perforated ulcer with hemodynamic instability. Additional workup includes a chemistry panel, CBC, and urgent laparotomy.

47.5 **E.** Given that this patient was recently admitted to the hospital and started on PPI therapy, his greatest immediate risk is of the development of *C difficile*–associate diarrhea. While community-acquired pneumonia can be seen concomitantly with asthma exacerbations, and is associated with PPI use, the patient had a negative chest x-ray on admission. If he developed pneumonia subsequently, it would be classified as a health-care–associated pneumonia. PPIs can cause hypomagnesemia, hypocalcemia, hypophosphatemia, and decreased iron absorption. While chronic steroids and PPIs can lead to osteoporosis, the time course is likely too short in this case to develop these complications.

CLINICAL PEARLS

▶ Persons who require long-term NSAID therapy and/or aspirin should be monitored for signs and symptoms of dyspepsia and peptic ulcer disease.

▶ Persons with chronic symptoms of dyspepsia who have not been taking NSAIDs or aspirin, or those from Mexico, Central America, Africa, or other endemic areas should be tested for *H pylori* infection via IgG serologic testing and treated if positive.

▶ Commonly held beliefs, such as ulcers being caused by stress or spicy foods, are incorrect. The vast majority of ulcers are caused by *H pylori* and NSAIDs.

▶ Patients who experience heartburn and regurgitation should be treated with acid-suppressive therapy in a step-up fashion, with attempts at step-down therapy when symptoms are controlled.

▶ Acid-suppression therapy carries long-term risks of community-acquired pneumonia; *C difficile*–associated diarrhea; demineralization of bone; decreased absorption of calcium, magnesium, and iron; and interaction with the metabolism of clopidogrel.

REFERENCES

Chey WD, Wong BCY. The Practice Parameters Committee of the American College of Gastroenterology. Management of *Helicobacter pylori* infection. *Am J Gastroenterol.* 2007; 102:1808–1825.

Del Valle J. Peptic ulcer disease and related disorders. In: Kasper D, Fauci A, Hauser S, et al., eds. *Harrison's Principles of Internal Medicine.* 19th ed. New York, NY: McGraw-Hill Education; 2015. Available at: http://accessmedicine.mhmedical.com. Accessed May 25, 2015.

Fashner J, Gitu AC. Diagnosis and treatment of peptic ulcer disease and *H. pylori* infection. *Am Fam Physician.* 2015; 91(4):236–242.

Heidelbaugh JJ, Gill AS, Harrison RV, Nostrant TT. Atypical presentations of gastroesophageal reflux disease. *Am Fam Physician.* 2008; 78(4):483–488.

Heidelbaugh JJ, Kim AH, Chang R, Walker PC. Overutilization of proton pump inhibitors: what the clinician needs to know. *Ther Adv Gastroenterol.* 2012; 5(4):219–232.

Katz PO, Gerson LB, Vela MF. Guidelines for the diagnosis and management of gastroesophageal reflux disease. *Am J Gastroenterol.* 2013; 108(3):308–328.

Lanza FL, Chan FKL, Quigley EMM. The Practice Parameters Committee of the American College of Gastroenterology. Prevention of NSAID-related ulcer complications. *Am J Gastroenterol.* 2009; 104:728–738.

Loyd RA, McClellan DA. Update on the evaluation and management of functional dyspepsia. *Am Fam Physician.* 2011; 83(5):547–552.

Talley NJ, Vakil N. Guidelines for the management of dyspepsia. *Am J Gastroenterol.* 2005; 100:2324–2337.

An 18-month-old girl is brought to the office by her mother for an acute visit because of a rash. She had a subjective high fever for the past 3 days, along with some mild respiratory symptoms of cough and rhinorrhea. She was given acetaminophen for the fever, but no other medications. The fever has gone down in the past day, but today she developed an erythematous rash that developed suddenly starting on the trunk and spread to the extremities. The child has no significant medical history and no known sick contacts, although she attends day care 3 days a week. On examination, she is mildly fussy but is easily consolable in her mother's lap. On examination, her rash in the areas mentioned above consists of small macules and papules that blanch on palpation. The remainder of her examination is unremarkable.

▶ What is the most likely diagnosis?
▶ What is the most likely cause of this illness?
▶ What is the appropriate treatment?

ANSWERS TO CASE 48:
Fever and Rash

Summary: An 18-month-old girl is brought in for evaluation of a rapidly spreading rash that started after 3 days of fever. She has diffuse, blanching, erythematous macules and papules but otherwise appears well.

- **Most likely diagnosis:** Roseola

- **Most likely cause of the illness:** Human herpes virus 6 (HHV-6)

- **Treatment:** Supportive care only, as the rash is likely to completely resolve in 24 to 48 hours

ANALYSIS

Objectives

1. Be able to identify common rashes associated with viral infections in children.

2. Know the appropriate management of febrile illness associated with rashes in children.

Considerations

This toddler has a history of fever, and rash that is diffuse, erythematous macules and papules. The rash is most likely due to roseola, caused by HHV-6. HHV-6 is a ubiquitous virus that infects most children between 6 months and 3 years, although most infections are asymptomatic. The virus has an incubation period of 1 to 2 weeks and causes a prodromal illness associated with mild respiratory symptoms and a sudden high fever (39°C-40°C), which in rare cases can cause febrile seizures. After a few days of inoculation, the fever typically resolves and the erythematous rash appears.

APPROACH TO:
Fever and Rash

DEFINITIONS

ENANTHEM: An eruption on a mucous membrane as a symptom of a disease

EXANTHEM: An eruption on the skin as a symptom of a disease

CLINICAL APPROACH

Febrile illness and rashes are extremely common presentations in family medicine and pediatric offices. In most cases, these presentations represent mild, self-limited illnesses that require no specific therapy. However, some cases will represent serious infections that require urgent intervention. Rashes associated with fever may be caused by viruses, bacteria, spirochetes, drug reaction, or autoimmune diseases.

The patient history should attempt to identify any exposures that may cause these syndromes, focusing on duration of the illness, other associated constitutional symptoms, sick contacts, history of recent travel, use of medications, or exposure to animals and insects (eg, ticks). A review of immunization status is critical, as many diseases preventable by vaccines can cause fever and rash. **Immunization does not always guarantee complete lifelong immunity**, but should confer a less severe presentation of the disease.

A thorough physical examination with a complete skin examination should be performed. Examination findings can both lead to a specific diagnosis and identify complications of the causative agent. For example, the presence of exudative pharyngitis along with fever and rash may suggest scarlet fever caused by a group A *Streptococcus* infection, while wheezes or rhonchi on lung examination in a patient with crops of vesicles at different stages may lead to a diagnosis of varicella (chicken pox) complicated by pneumonitis.

The ability to accurately describe skin lesions is necessary for classification and in forming a differential diagnosis. Understanding the definitions of macules, papules, pustules, and vesicles allows for increased accuracy in diagnosis and ability to cogently discuss challenging cases with colleagues. See Case 13 for definitions of many of the terms used to describe common skin lesions.

COMMON VIRAL INFECTIONS

Roseola

Human herpes virus 6 is a ubiquitous virus that infects most children before the age of 3, although most infections are asymptomatic. The virus has an incubation period of 1 to 2 weeks and causes a prodromal illness associated with mild respiratory symptoms and a high fever that can range from 101°F to 106°F (37.9°C to 41.1°C). This prodromal illness typically does not last for longer than 5 days. **Following defervescence, a characteristic erythematous maculopapular rash appears suddenly** on the trunk and spreads rapidly to the extremities, with sparing of the face. The rash commonly disappears in 1 to 2 days. The diagnosis is primarily clinical, based on the history and examination. Due to the short-lived nature of the disease, no treatment is usually required other than reassurance.

Varicella

The varicella zoster virus is a highly contagious virus that causes two clinical syndromes, chicken pox and shingles (zoster). **Chicken pox** is the more common childhood infection, but can also occur in adolescents and adults, can cause severe disease and complications in adult cases, and is seen more commonly in winter or early spring months. A typical case of chicken pox in children begins with the development of a rash in clusters followed by malaise, fever (38°C-42°C), and anorexia. The initial exanthem is often **papules or vesicles on an erythematous base**, described as "dewdrops on a rose petal." The vesicles then progress to shallow, crusted erosions and ulcerations. Patients may also develop enanthems, with lesions on the oral, nasal, or gastrointestinal mucosa. In rare cases, serious complications may develop, which include encephalitis, meningitis, and pneumonitis.

Superinfection of the vesicles with bacteria, most commonly group A *Streptococcus* and *Staphylococcus aureus*, is a particularly common and potentially dangerous complication. The contagious period continues 4 to 5 days after the appearance of the rash or until all lesions have crusted over. It takes an average of 10 to 21 days after contact with an infected person for someone to develop chicken pox. The diagnosis of varicella is usually clinical, but may be confirmed with Tzanck smear or identification of the virus by DNA polymerase chain reaction (PCR). Antiviral therapy using acyclovir, valacyclovir, or famciclovir may shorten the course of the illness in patients older than 2 years if started within 24 hours of onset of the exanthem. Varicella vaccination is now universally recommended at 12 to 15 months with a booster dose at 4 years. While the vaccine has significantly reduced the incidence of childhood chicken pox, breakthrough infections can occur in vaccinated individuals. However, these infections are usually much less severe, with fewer vesicles and little to no fever. The varicella vaccine is a live, attenuated virus and should not be given to immunocompromised or pregnant patients.

Shingles, or herpes zoster, is a reactivation of the varicella virus, which remains dormant in the dorsal root ganglia following the initial infection. The reactivated virus causes a vesicular eruption, usually along a single dermatome that does not cross the midline. The reaction can occur at any age, but is more common in the elderly or immunosuppressed. The rash can be extremely painful and can result in chronic postherpetic neuralgia that can last long after resolution of the rash. Antiviral therapy started within 72 hours of onset of the rash may reduce the incidence of the postherpetic neuralgia. A herpes zoster vaccine is now recommended for people over 60 and has been shown to decrease the likelihood of development of zoster.

Erythema Infectiosum

Parvovirus B19 causes a characteristic syndrome known as erythema infectiosum or **fifth disease.** This virus tends to infect children younger than 10 years and occurs most commonly in the winter or spring months and is primarily spread by infected respiratory droplets. The child usually presents with a prodrome of mild fever and upper respiratory symptoms prior to outbreak of the rash that typically lasts between 4 to 14 days. The rash usually starts as confluent erythematous macules on the face, which usually spares the nose and periorbital regions. This gives the classic **"slapped cheek" appearance** that is commonly diagnostic of the infection. The facial rash usually lasts for 2 to 4 days and is followed by a lacy, pruritic exanthem on the trunk and extremities that usually lasts for 1 to 2 weeks, but can have a relapsing course for several months. Parvovirus B19 in adults and older adolescents tends to cause a more severe illness, with rheumatic complaints including arthralgias. In patients with sickle cell disease, parvovirus B19 infection can lead to an aplastic crisis with anemia and leukopenia. The virus can also be transmitted from mother to fetus during pregnancy, resulting in fetal hydrops and pregnancy loss.

COMMON BACTERIAL INFECTIONS

Group A β-Hemolytic Streptococcus

Group A β-hemolytic *Streptococcus* (GABS) is associated with numerous diseases, particularly in children. It is the causative agent of streptococcal pharyngitis and its complications, which include rheumatic fever and postinfectious glomerulonephritis. It can also cause impetigo, erysipelas, and cellulitis. Invasion and multiplication within the fascia can lead to necrotizing fasciitis.

The rash of **scarlet fever** usually starts approximately 2 days after the onset of sore throat and fever. The rash consists of punctate, raised, erythematous eruptions that can become confluent (Pastia lines) and feel like sandpaper. The rash tends to start on the upper trunk and spreads to the rest of the trunk and the extremities. The exanthem can also be associated with an enanthem, causing the appearance of a "strawberry tongue." The rash fades and desquamation typically occurs 4 to 5 days after the first appearance of the rash.

GABS infections can be confirmed by rapid antigen testing or culture via a pharyngeal swab. Serologic tests commonly demonstrate marked leukocytosis with neutrophilia with normal or increased eosinophilia, and elevated erythrocyte sedimentation rate (ESR), C-reactive protein (CRP), and antistreptolysin O titer. The first-line treatment for GABS infections is penicillin, with cephalosporins or macrolides as alternatives in the penicillin-allergic patient. Patients are commonly no longer contagious within 48 hours after starting antibiotics and should be counseled that they can return to school or work if afebrile and on antibiotics for at least 24 hours. Exposed individuals should be monitored for fever and other symptoms for at least a week and should receive treatment if they have a positive throat culture. Household and close contacts with similar symptoms should be empirically treated.

Neisseria meningitidis

Neisseria meningitidis (meningococcus) can cause an acute, life-threatening infection, often associated with a rash, and is spread through respiratory secretions. Meningococcemia causes a severe illness with high fevers, hypotension, and altered mental status. Most people with meningococcemia progress to develop frank bacterial meningitis, with associated signs of meningeal irritation. The **rash of meningococcemia often starts as an erythematous maculopapular eruption that does not blanch with compression which progresses to form petechiae.** The petechiae may coalesce into purpura in a condition known as purpura fulminans that can result in gangrene and amputation of limbs when associated with disseminated intravascular coagulation. Other complications include adrenal hemorrhage, deafness, and cerebral and renal infarctions.

Persons with suspected meningococcemia should be immediately hospitalized and quarantined, usually in the intensive care unit. The ABCs (airway, breathing, and circulation) should be urgently evaluated, blood and cerebrospinal fluid cultures collected, and empiric antibiotic therapy instituted until an organism is isolated via culture and drug sensitivities are obtained. **Treatment should not be delayed by performing a lumbar puncture, as early and appropriate antibiotic treatment markedly improves the outcome of meningococcal infections.** A common empiric regimen for presumed meningitis in infants less than 30 days old is ampicillin plus gentamicin, while for adults, vancomycin plus ceftriaxone should be used. Antibiotic coverage can be later tailored based on culture results. The first choice for culture-proven meningococcal meningitis is penicillin G. A meningococcal vaccine is now recommended for routine childhood immunization and also should be offered to patients at risk for the disease (eg, asplenia, those living in dormitories or military barracks). Close contacts of someone with meningococcal infection should be offered prophylaxis with ciprofloxacin or rifampin.

TICK-BORNE DISEASES

Rocky Mountain Spotted Fever

Rocky Mountain spotted fever (RMSF) is an acute, life-threatening infection caused by the organism *Rickettsia rickettsii*, which is transmitted via various species of tick. The infection occurs more often in the summer months, when people are more likely to be outdoors. Despite its name, RMSF is most common in the southeastern United States, but does occur throughout the United States, Canada, Mexico, Central America, and parts of South America. The early phase of the illness causes nonspecific signs and symptoms such as fever, headache, myalgias, arthralgias, and fatigue. Some patients, especially children, may complain of abdominal pain. **The classic exanthem is a macular, papular, or petechial eruption that starts on the wrists and ankles and spreads both centrally and to the palms and soles.** The rash usually develops between the third and fifth day of the illness. Serologic evaluation often reveals a low white blood cell count, low platelet count, hyponatremia, and elevated liver transaminases. The diagnosis is confirmed with serology, but this is not helpful in the acute setting. Due to its severity, a high suspicion for RMSF should be maintained and likely cases of the illness treated empirically with doxycycline. Early treatment is important as there is an associated risk of fatal outcome after day 5 of the illness and therapy should be continued for at least 3 days after the patient becomes afebrile.

Lyme Disease

Lyme disease is endemic in many areas of the United States, including New England and the mid-Atlantic region. The causative spirochete, *Borrelia burgdorferi*, is transmitted via the bite of deer ticks of the *Ixodes* species. Because the ticks are very small, infected persons are often unaware of a history of a tick bite. The characteristic rash, **erythema migrans**, develops 3 to 30 days following infection. The exanthem is typically an expanding erythematous macule with central clearing, often described as appearing like a "bull's eye." Early dissemination of the disease can present as multiple secondary erythema migrans, diffuse arthralgias and myalgias, Bell palsy, aseptic meningitis, carditis, and rarely as complete heart block. Late disease is most characteristically marked by polyarthritis. Diagnosis is confirmed via serologic antibody testing. The treatment of choice for Lyme disease is doxycycline, amoxicillin, or cefuroxime. Patients treated with appropriate antibiotic therapy in the early stages of Lyme disease commonly recover completely and without lasting sequelae. Approximately 10% to 20% of patients who presented late in the disease, despite appropriate antibiotic therapy, may have persistent or recurrent symptoms known as posttreatment Lyme disease syndrome.

Table 48–1 provides a summary of some of the most common causes of the presentation of rash and fever in children.

Table 48–1 • INFECTIOUS CAUSES OF FEVER AND RASH

Disease	Causative Organism	Rash	Other Symptoms
Roseola	HHV-6	Erythematous, maculopapular rash, starting on the trunk and sparing the face	Prodromal high fever
Chicken pox	Varicella-zoster virus	Papules or vesicles on an erythematous base "dew drops on a rose petal"	Fever and malaise
Shingles	Varicella-zoster virus	Vesicular rash in a dermatomal pattern	Postherpetic neuralgia
Erythema infectiosum	Parvovirus B19	Erythematous macular rash on cheeks "slapped cheek," followed by a lacy, reticulated rash over trunk and extremities	Prodromal fever and upper respiratory infection (URI) symptoms, arthritis in adults
Measles	Measles virus	Erythematous maculopapular rash starting at the forehead and moving down the body	Koplik spots, fever, and malaise
Rubella	Rubella virus	Erythematous macular rash starting at the face and neck and moving to the trunk and extremities	Prodromal fever, sore throat, and malaise; congenital rubella syndrome
Small pox	Variola virus	Macules, papules, or pustules at the same stage of development	Fever, myalgias, and malaise
Hand-foot-and-mouth disease	Coxsackie virus	Vesicular enanthem on tongue, on lips, and in mouth; maculovesicular rash on hands, feet, buttocks, and groin	Fever
Scarlet fever	Group A *Streptococcus*	Erythematous papular rash starting on neck and moving to trunk and extremities, "strawberry tongue" enanthem	Pharyngitis and fever
Rheumatic fever	Group A *Streptococcus*	Erythema marginatum—erythematous, serpiginous macules with pale centers	Carditis, polyarthritis, subcutaneous nodules, and Sydenham chorea
Meningococcemia	*Neisseria meningitidis*	Erythematous maculopapular rash progressing to form petechiae	Meningitis, fever, myalgias, hypothermia, and hypotension
Toxic shock syndrome	*Staphylococcus aureus*	Diffuse erythematous macular rash with peeling palms and soles	Fever, vomiting, diarrhea, and hypotension

(*Continued*)

Table 48–1 • INFECTIOUS CAUSES OF FEVER AND RASH (CONTINUED)			
Disease	Causative Organism	Rash	Other Symptoms
Typhoid fever	*Salmonella enterica*	Maculopapular rash on lower chest and abdomen "rose spots"	Fever, myalgias, diarrhea, abdominal pain, and hepatosplenomegaly
Rocky Mountain spotted fever	*Rickettsia rickettsii*	Maculopapular rash starting on the wrists and ankles and involving the palms and soles	Fever, headache, myalgias, and malaise
Lyme disease	*Borrelia Burgdorferi*	Erythema migrans— erythematous macule with central clearing "bull's eye"	Malaise, Bell palsy, meningitis, arthritis, carditis, and heart block
Ehrlichiosis	*Anaplasma phagocytophilum, Ehrlichia chaffeensis*	Erythematous maculopapular rash	Fever, headache, myalgias, nausea, and vomiting

COMPREHENSION QUESTIONS

48.1 A 4-year-old boy is brought to your office by his mother for evaluation of a rash on his face that his mother first noticed the day prior to presentation. His mother comments that it looks like somebody "slapped him." The mother reports that he has had a cold for the last couple of days. The child's physical examination is unremarkable except for an erythematous macular rash over both cheeks. The mother admits that the child is behind on his immunization schedule. Which of the following is the most likely cause?

A. Varicella-zoster virus

B. Parvovirus B19

C. Human herpes virus 6

D. Rubella virus

E. Child abuse and you should contact social services immediately

48.2 A 6-year-old girl is brought to your office by her mother because of a rash first noticed 1 week ago. Her mother reports that several children in her child's school have chicken pox but that her child has received all of her immunizations including two doses of the varicella vaccine. You observe the child actively playing with the toys in your waiting room before both the mother and child are brought back to the examination room. The child has a temperature of 100.4°F (38.0°C), a pulse of 90 beats/min, a blood pressure of 100/70 mm Hg, and a respiration rate of 20 breaths/min. The physical examination is unremarkable except for approximately 20 vesicles on erythematous bases sparsely scattered on the child's trunk and limbs. Which of the following is the most appropriate treatment?

A. Supportive care

B. Antiviral therapy

C. Antibiotic therapy

D. Immune globulin

48.3 You are on duty when an 18-year-old man is brought to the emergency room (ER) from his college dorm by his roommate. He is confused and cannot give a history. He has a temperature of 104.0°F (40.0°C), pulse of 110 beats/min, blood pressure of 90/60 mm Hg, and a respiration rate of 24 breaths/min. His head cannot be moved because of severe nuchal rigidity. Multiple petechiae are observed on his buttocks and legs. What is the most appropriate advice to give to this patient's roommate?

A. Reassurance that he does not require prophylaxis.

B. Take acyclovir for prophylaxis.

C. Take penicillin for prophylaxis.

D. Take rifampin for prophylaxis.

E. Take cefuroxime for prophylaxis.

48.4 A 7-year-old boy is brought to a hospital in Charlotte, North Carolina with a fever of 104.0°F (40.0°C). A maculopapular rash is seen on his wrists and ankles but the palms and soles are spared. His laboratory results show leukopenia, hyponatremia, and elevated liver transaminases. His parents say that he was on a camping trip 1 week ago but they vigorously used insect repellants and filtered all of their water. His father came in contact with poison oak, but the boy denies any pruritus. Which of the following is the best treatment for this patient's rash?

A. Penicillin

B. Acyclovir

C. Ceftriaxone

D. Vancomycin

E. Doxycycline

ANSWERS

48.1 **B.** This question describes erythema infectiosum, or fifth disease, which is caused by parvovirus B19. It often has a prodrome of fever and upper respiratory systems mistaken by the mother in this question as a "cold." This child also has the classic "slapped cheek" rash of erythema infectiosum and, while the child does need to be caught up on his immunizations, the child has the classic symptoms of fifth disease and not of the diseases for which children are immunized.

48.2 **A.** The child has chicken pox caused by the varicella-zoster virus. While the child did receive two doses of the varicella vaccine and the vaccine is effective, sporadic breakthrough cases do occur. However, the cases are usually much less severe and have fewer complications than in unimmunized patients. Supportive care is advised, as this illness in this stage will be self-limited; after a week, antivirals likely have no benefit. Antibiotics and immune globulin have no role in the treatment of this patient.

48.3 **D.** The patient has meningitis and meningococcemia caused by *N meningitidis*. The patient is severely affected and is in septic shock. All people in close contact with the patient should receive ciprofloxacin or rifampin prophylaxis.

48.4 **E.** The patient has Rocky Mountain spotted fever and should be treated with doxycycline. The disease is commonly found in North Carolina and is carried by ticks that the boy could have picked up during the camping trip. RMSF has a characteristic rash that starts on the wrists and ankles and can eventually involve the palms and soles. Typically, the rash of RMSF spreads centripetally from the wrists and ankles to involve the trunk and extremities.

CLINICAL PEARLS

▶ Shingles that approaches the eye (herpes zoster ophthalmicus), because of a reactivation involving the trigeminal nerve, should be evaluated by an ophthalmologist. A clue that the eye may become involved is seeing characteristic lesions approaching the tip of the nose.

▶ Many vaccine-preventable illnesses, including measles, rubella, and varicella, have characteristic rashes associated with them. Always get a vaccination history on children presenting with fever and rash. Also, consider the possibility that immigrants from other countries may not be vaccinated if they present with similar symptoms.

REFERENCES

Chen LF, Sexton DJ. What's new in Rocky Mountain spotted fever. *Infect Dis Clin North Am.* 2008; 22(3):415–432.

Cohen JI. Herpes zoster. *N Engl J Med.* 2013; 369:255–263.

Dandache P, Nadelman RB. Erythema migrans. *Infect Dis Clin North Am.* 2008; 22(2):235–260.

Ely JW, Stone MS. The generalized rash: part I. Differential diagnosis. *Am Fam Physician.* 2010; 81(6):726–734.

Ely JW, Stone MS. The generalized rash: part II. Diagnostic approach. *Am Fam Physician.* 2010; 81(6):735–739.

Folster-Holst R, Kreth HW. Viral exanthems in childhood—infectious (direct) exanthems. Part 1: classic exanthems. *J Dtsch Dermatol Ges.* 2009; 7(4):309–316.

Folster-Holst R, Kreth HW. Viral exanthems in childhood—infectious (direct) exanthems. Part 2: other viral exanthems. *Dtsch Dermatol Ges.* 2009; 7(5):414–419.

Mann K, Jackson MA. Meningitis. *Pediatr Rev.* 2008; 29(12):417–429.

McKinnon HD, Howard T. Evaluating the febrile patient with a rash. *Am Fam Physician.* 2000; 62: 804–816.

Shapiro ED. Lyme disease. *N Engl J Med.* 2014; 370:1724–1731.

Survey JT, Reamy BV, Hodge J. Clinical presentation of parvovirus B19 infection. *Am Fam Physician.* 2007; 75(3):373–376.

Zerr DM, Meier AS, Selke SS, et al. A population-based study of primary human herpesvirus 6 infection. *N Engl J Med.* 2005; 352(8):768–776.

A 32-year-old woman presents for evaluation of a lump that she noticed in her right breast on self-examination. She says that while she does not perform breast self-examination often, she thinks that this lump is new. She denies nipple discharge or breast pain, although the lump is mildly tender on palpation. She has never noticed any breast masses previously and has never had a mammogram. She has no personal or family history of breast disease. She takes oral contraceptive pills (OCPs) regularly, but no other medications. She does not smoke cigarettes or drink alcohol. She has never been pregnant. On examination, she is a well-appearing, somewhat anxious, and thin woman. Her vital signs are within normal limits. On breast examination, in the lower outer quadrant of the right breast, there is a 2-cm, firm, well-circumscribed, freely mobile mass without overlying erythema that is mildly tender to palpation. There is no skin dimpling, retraction, or nipple discharge. While no other discrete breast masses are palpable, the bilateral breast tissue is noted to be firm and glandular throughout. There is no evidence of axillary, supraclavicular, or cervical lymphadenopathy. The remainder of her physical examination is unremarkable.

▶ What is the most likely diagnosis of this breast lesion?
▶ What is the first step in evaluation?
▶ What is the recommended follow-up for this patient?

ANSWERS TO CASE 49:

Breast Diseases

Summary: A 32-year-old woman presents for evaluation of a lump in her right breast that she found on breast self-examination (BSE). The lump is estimated to be 2 cm in size, firm, and freely mobile. There is no lymphadenopathy noted on physical examination.

- **Most likely diagnosis:** Breast cyst.

- **First step in evaluation:** Needle aspiration of cyst.

- **Follow-up:** If aspiration of the cyst results in complete resolution of the mass, and if the fluid is clear/yellow, then follow-up clinical examination in 1 to 2 months is recommended to ensure no recurrence; if aspiration does not make the mass disappear, if the fluid is bloody, or if the lesion recurs, then further evaluation with ultrasound and biopsy of the lesion is indicated.

ANALYSIS

Objectives

1. Learn how to workup a breast mass.

2. Know the risk factors for breast cancer.

3. Know how to manage benign breast diseases.

Considerations

A palpable breast mass is a potentially frightening finding for a woman. In 2013, an estimated 232,340 new cases of invasive breast cancer and 64,640 in situ breast cancer were diagnosed, with 39,620 expected deaths. Breast cancer incidence rates are highest in non-Hispanic white women, followed by African-American women, and are lowest among Asian/Pacific Islander women. Nearly one in eight women will be diagnosed with breast cancer in their lifetime.

The evaluation of the breast mass should definitively answer the question of whether or not the lesion is benign or malignant. Statistically, most palpable breast masses are benign cysts or fibroadenomas, not cancers. Unfortunately, a definitive determination of whether or not a lesion is benign or malignant cannot be made solely by history or physical examination.

Certain factors have been identified as increasing a woman's risk of breast cancer:

- A family history of breast cancer in a first-degree relative (eg, parent, sibling), especially if the cancer occurred in a premenopausal woman and was bilateral, is associated with an increased risk that could indicate deleterious *BRCA1/BRCA2* genes.

- Early age at menarche (<12 years), late age of menopause (>55 years), and nulliparity or first live birth after the age of 30 years.

- The use of hormones, either estrogen alone or combined with progesterone, are considered to confer higher risks, although recent studies question whether oral contraceptives pose any significant risk.

- Lifestyle considerations, including obesity, physical inactivity, and alcohol use (>3 drinks per day).

- History of previous breast disease, especially biopsies showing atypical hyperplasia, carcinoma in situ, or prior breast cancer.

In the case presented, there are several clues that suggest the likelihood of a benign process. While breast cancer can occur at any age, approximately 70% of breast cancers occur in women older than age 50. The possibility of malignancy in a woman in her thirties cannot ever be excluded, but the likelihood of cancer is lower compared to a woman in her fifties. The characteristics of the lesion are most consistent with a benign, likely cystic, lesion. It is described as well-circumscribed, firm, mobile, tender, and with no overlying skin changes. Lesions that are hard, fixed in place, nontender, have indistinct borders, or have overlying skin dimpling/retraction are highly suggestive of malignancy. It is important to note that no individual characteristic on examination is diagnostic of a benign or malignant lesion, and an appropriate evaluation is imperative.

APPROACH TO:
Diseases of the Breast

DEFINITIONS

ACROMEGALY: A condition that results from the excessive production of growth hormone by a pituitary adenoma. Among the numerous physical effects of the excessive growth hormone, menstrual irregularities and breast discharge may result.

GALACTORRHEA: The spontaneous release of milk from the breast, not associated with childbirth or nursing.

FIBROADENOMA: A benign noncancerous lesion of the breast composed of fibrous and glandular tissue.

DUCT ECTASIA: Inflammation of a mammary duct below the nipple, which can lead to duct obstruction, a tender mass, and duct discharge.

INTRADUCTAL PAPILLOMA: A benign tumor growth into a mammary duct, often with a resultant palpable small mass and duct discharge.

CLINICAL APPROACH

Palpable Breast Mass

Following a complete history, with an emphasis on factors that may confer an increased risk of breast cancer, a careful examination of both breasts should be performed. The complete clinical breast examination (CBE) should include a visual inspection for skin changes, dimpling, retraction, and asymmetry in both the seated and supine positions, and should note the presence and quality of any nipple discharge (eg, color, presence of blood, etc). Starting in their 20s, women should be instructed on the benefits and limits of the BSE. Women should be aware of how their breasts normally appear and feel and should be encouraged to report any changes to their physician. In women with breast implants, it is reasonable for them to do BSEs, and it is helpful to have the surgeon help to identify the borders of the implants. For women who choose to perform the BSE, the optimal time to conduct the assessment is when the breasts are not tender or swollen. The BSE has been shown to increase the likelihood of discovering a palpable lesion, raising anxiety, increasing the number of biopsies, and has not been shown to decrease mortality.

Examination by palpation should be performed in a systematic manner to include all quadrants of the breast, as well as the superficial, intermediate, and deep breast tissue. Specific characteristics of any palpable lumps, including size, location, tenderness, mobility, firmness, and distinction of the mass from the surrounding tissue should be noted, both to assist in developing a diagnosis and to allow for serial examinations to determine if the mass is changing. The breast examination should also include palpation of the axilla and supraclavicular regions to identify the presence of any palpable or enlarged lymph nodes. The characteristics of the mass and the age of the woman will provide initial clues toward likely diagnosis (Table 49–1).

The identification of a new solid breast mass particularly in women older than 35 years should prompt **triple assessment, including a clinical breast examination, imaging (mammography and/or ultrasound), and pathologic assessment via core biopsy or surgical excision.**

For women younger than 35 years, suspected lesions characteristic of fibroadenoma or fibrocystic changes can be assessed by ultrasonography, and rarely mammography followed by fine-needle aspiration (FNA) with histologic evaluation. **Ultrasonography** can be used as an adjunct to mammography in an effort to determine if the lesion is solid or cystic. It can also be used in women with large and/or dense breasts or in women with persistent breast pain without evidence

Table 49–1 • TYPICAL CHARACTERISTICS OF BREAST LUMPS ON PHYSICAL EXAMINATION		
Characteristic	More Likely Benign	Suspicious for Malignancy
Consistency	Soft	Firm/hard
Surface	Smooth, regular	Irregular
Mobility	Mobile	Fixed or tethered
Symptoms	Tender	Painless
Age	<30 y	>50 y

Data from Lippman ME. Breast cancer. In: Fauci AS, Braunwald E, Kasper DL, et al., eds. Harrison's Principles of Internal Medicine. 17th ed. New York, NY: McGraw-Hill; 2008:564.

of mass via mammography. For pregnant females with a new breast complaint, targeted ultrasonography is the first-line choice for imaging.

Fine-needle aspiration can be both diagnostic and therapeutic and is performed if the mass is cystic and symptomatic. An FNA that identifies fluid that is clear, yellow, or green-tinged and that results in complete resolution of the mass is diagnostic of a benign cyst. In this setting, the fluid can be discarded and no further workup is necessary. Cystic lesions that resolve after FNA do not require further evaluation unless they recur. If CBE, FNA, or imaging suggest benign disease, then the CBE should be repeated within 4 to 6 weeks to evaluate for potential recurrence of the lesion.

If the breast mass does not completely resolve, if the fluid withdrawn is bloody, if no fluid is aspirated, if the lesion has a complex nature (containing cystic and solid components), or if the lesion recurs on follow-up CBE, then further evaluation is indicated via stereotactic core-needle or excisional biopsy. FNA can be performed on solid lesions; however, it should be used for lesions most likely to be cystic, which may require ultrasonography for characterization. It is the least invasive and most simple procedure, but also has the highest risk of false-negative or nondiagnostic results.

Core-needle biopsy and **mammotome** biopsy use larger cutting needles to obtain larger tissue samples. These are usually performed using ultrasound or mammographic guidance by a radiologist or surgeon. These procedures have a greater likelihood of providing a diagnostic sample yet are more invasive and costlier than FNA. Although **surgical excision** is the most invasive and expensive diagnostic method, it is indicated when stereotactic biopsies detect **atypical ductal hyperplasia** and can be therapeutic by offering complete removal of the lesion.

Breast Pain

Breast pain (mastalgia) is the most frequent breast-related complaint for which women present for evaluation. The etiology of chronic mastalgia is unknown and likely multifactorial. Similar to the presentation of a breast lump, the patient's primary fear, whether spoken or unspoken, is whether or not the pain is a manifestation of breast cancer. Thus, the evaluation of the woman with mastalgia should include a history to evaluate for an increased breast cancer risk, a careful breast examination, and a screening mammography in women for whom it is routinely indicated. Any abnormalities detected in the primary evaluation should be evaluated as outlined above. **Breast pain is not a common presentation of breast cancer,** particularly when the pain is bilateral.

Most cases of breast pain are categorized as cyclic mastalgia, noncyclic mastalgia, or extramammary pain. **Cyclic mastalgia** is usually diffuse, bilateral, often radiates to the axilla and upper arm, and is related to the woman's menstrual cycle. Pain generally occurs during late luteal phase and resolves with onset of menses. In some cases, it can be unilateral. **Noncyclic mastalgia** may be either continuous or intermittent, and is not associated with the menstrual cycle. It is more commonly unilateral and more prevalent in postmenopausal women. **Extra-mammary pain** is defined as breast pain secondary to other etiologies including chest wall pain, yet often the underlying cause may be difficult to determine.

Common Causes of Mastalgia

The etiology of most cases of chronic mastalgia is unknown. Common causes include the following:

- Pregnancy
- Mastitis
- Thrombophlebitis
- Cyst
- Benign tumors
- Cancer
- Musculoskeletal cause
- Stretching of Cooper ligaments
- Pressure from brassiere
- Fat necrosis from trauma
- Hidradenitis suppurativa
- Medications such as OCPs, antidepressants, antipsychotics, and antihypertensives

Laboratory testing is usually unnecessary in the evaluation of mastalgia, although a pregnancy test should be performed in reproductive-age women. Hormonal contraceptives or hormone replacement therapy may be causes of breast pain and consideration should be given to discontinuation or reduction of estrogen dosages. An appropriately fitted supportive bra and lifestyle changes including tobacco cessation and stress reduction techniques, are often successful in alleviating symptoms. While nonsteroidal anti-inflammatory drugs (NSAIDs) are often beneficial in providing pain relief, evening primrose oil, caffeine reduction, and various vitamin supplements have not been shown to provide significant relief. Other low-risk treatments with possible efficacy include soy protein, a low-fat and high-carbohydrate diet, and chasteberry extract. For women with unrelenting pain in spite of the above modifications, **danazol**, an antigonadotropin, is Food and Drug Administration (FDA) approved for the treatment of breast pain, but is relatively expensive and has numerous side effects (eg, hair loss, acne, weight gain, and irregular menses). Other options include **tamoxifen, toremifene,** and **bromocriptine**, which are hormonal therapies with significant risks that have some evidence for efficacy in refractory cases.

Nipple Discharge and Galactorrhea

Nipple discharge is usually caused by a benign process. Up to 25% of women will have this symptom during their life. Nipple discharge that occurs only with nipple stimulation, that is clear, yellow, or green, and that appears from multiple ducts is usually physiologic and does not require extensive investigation. This discharge often resolves when efforts are made to reduce nipple stimulation, including ceasing efforts to check to see if the discharge will still occur.

Nipple discharge that is spontaneous, persistent, bloody, from a single duct, associated with a mass, and occurs in women over 40 years is more likely to represent a pathologic process and requires prompt evaluation. In this setting, the most common causes of discharge include intraductal papillomas, duct ectasia, cancers, and infections. If the discharge is not obviously bloody, then testing for occult blood via a guaiac-based assay should be performed.

Following the initial history and physical examination, mammography should be performed in all women with a spontaneous or bloody nipple discharge and in any woman in whom routine breast cancer screening is indicated. For most women, this should commence at age 40. All palpable breast masses should be evaluated appropriately and promptly. The **treatment of most cases of unilateral, spontaneous, or bloody nipple discharge is surgical excision of the terminal duct** involved, allowing for both resolution and diagnosis.

Galactorrhea is a discharge of milk or a milk-like secretion from the breast in the absence of parturition or beyond 6 months postpartum in a non–breast-feeding woman. The secretion may be milky or serous (yellow) appearing, intermittent or persistent, scant or abundant, free-flowing or expressible, and unilateral or bilateral. If the clinician is uncertain whether the discharge represents benign galactorrhea, then the discharge should undergo histologic and microscopic analysis, which will commonly contain fat globules and few cells. The condition is more common in women who are 20 to 35 years and in previously pregnant women. Galactorrhea is associated with stress, physical irritation, numerous medications, hypothyroidism, chronic renal failure, hypothalamic-pituitary disorders, hormone-secreting neoplasms (most commonly pituitary adenomas), or may be idiopathic, but **is not associated with breast cancer.**

Numerous pharmacologic agents can cause galactorrhea via blockade of dopamine and histamine receptors, depletion of dopamine stores, inhibition of dopamine release, and stimulation of lactotrophic hormones. Common medications and classes of medications associated with galactorrhea include serotonin reuptake inhibitors (SSRIs), tricyclic antidepressants (TCAs), angiotensin-converting enzyme (ACE) inhibitors, atenolol, verapamil, antipsychotics, H_2 (histamine) receptor antagonists, and opiates. Estrogen in oral contraceptives can cause galactorrhea by suppressing the hypothalamic secretion of prolactin inhibitory factor and by direct stimulation of the pituitary lactotrophs.

Offending medications should be discontinued when possible. Prolactin and thyroid-stimulating hormone (TSH) levels should be obtained to evaluate for endocrine abnormalities. Evaluation of serum electrolytes and renal function can assess the woman with galactorrhea for renal failure, Cushing disease, and acromegaly. Imaging of the pituitary to evaluate for a pituitary adenoma with magnetic resonance imaging (MRI) is indicated if the prolactin level is significantly elevated.

Treatment of galactorrhea is geared at addressing the underlying condition. For example, women with hypothyroidism should be treated with levothyroxine. Treatment should also be aimed toward the severity of the prolactin level and pending fertility status. Dopamine agonists are the treatment of choice in most patients with hyperprolactinemia. Bromocriptine is the preferred agent for treatment of hyperprolactin-induced anovulatory infertility. Surgical resection rarely is required for prolactinomas and other pituitary adenomas unless the woman experiences significant hypothalamic-pituitary-gonadal axis disruption or visual deficits commensurate with compression of the optic chiasm (homonymous hemianopsia).

COMPREHENSION QUESTIONS

49.1 A 34-year-old woman presents with a history of intermittent clear-yellow breast nipple discharge for 2 months. She had been taking antipsychotic medication for a history of schizophrenia, but has not taken the medication in 3 months. Laboratory studies reveal normal TSH, free T3, and free T4 levels, and her thyroid gland is not palpable. A urine pregnancy test is negative. Which of the following is the most appropriate advice to give to this woman?

A. It is likely that the nipple discharge will become bloody.

B. Due to her clinical presentation, the likelihood of breast cancer is greater than 50%.

C. This condition is common in patients who take antipsychotic medications.

D. Unless her free T3 level becomes elevated, there is no reason for concern.

49.2 A 52-year-old woman presents to her family physician with a palpable breast lump. An attempt at FNA does not result in aspiration of fluid. Her mammogram is normal. Her mother was diagnosed with breast cancer at age 45. She does not smoke but socially drinks alcohol. She currently takes low-dose estrogen contraception pills and takes 1200 mg of calcium daily. She began her menstrual periods at age 10 and she had her first child at age 24. Which of the following is the appropriate next step in evaluation of this patient?

A. Repeat clinical examination in 4 to 6 weeks.

B. Repeat mammogram routinely in 1 year.

C. Referral for biopsy.

D. Discontinuation of her hormone replacement therapy.

49.3 A 29-year-old woman presents with the complaint of nipple discharge from the left breast. On further questioning, she states that the discharge is milky in color. She is a G2P2 with her last delivery 3½ years ago. She breast-fed both children for 9 months. She takes no medications and has regular menstrual periods. On examination, a small amount of nonbloody milky discharge can be expressed from several ducts from the left nipple, while no discharge is expressed from the right breast. Which of the following is the best initial diagnostic step for this patient?

A. Pregnancy test.

B. Refer to a breast specialist for evaluation for unilateral nipple discharge.

C. TSH, free T4, and prolactin levels.

D. Follicle-stimulating hormone (FSH), luteinising hormone (LH), and gonadotropin-releasing hormone (GnRH) levels.

E. Send the discharge for histologic and pathologic evaluation.

49.4 A 33-year-old woman presents with the complaint of a palpable, firm, mobile, 2.5-cm mass in the 12 o'clock position on her right breast. She states that it has been present for almost 6 months, enlarges with her menstrual cycle, and becomes most painful with the onset of her menses. She smokes approximately 8 to 10 cigarettes daily, drinks three to four cups of caffeinated coffee daily, and rarely drinks alcohol. She has no family history of breast cancer. Which of the following is the most appropriate initial evaluation of this mass?

A. Surgical excision

B. Mammogram

C. Ultrasound

D. FNA

ANSWERS

49.1 **C.** Nipple discharges that are spontaneous, unilateral, persistent, bloody, and associated with a mass are more likely to represent pathologic processes and need to be evaluated for malignancy. While most cases are benign (eg, papilloma, duct ectasia), evaluation and surgical intervention are usually required. In this case, the galactorrhea represents a side effect of antipsychotic medication, will not become bloody, likely has no relation to thyroid hormone levels (especially in an euthyroid patient), and does not increase her risk of breast cancer.

49.2 **C.** A biopsy is the next most appropriate step in this setting. A negative mammogram is not diagnostic of a benign process and does not rule out the possibility of having breast cancer. A tissue diagnosis is needed in this setting especially with a known first-degree relative with breast cancer and early age of menarche to evaluate for potential malignancy.

49.3 **A.** The evaluation and management of most cases of galactorrhea can be handled by the primary care physician. A pregnancy test should be the first evaluation. If pituitary adenoma is diagnosed, then the patient can be referred for specialty care. Milky discharge from multiple ducts in the nonlactating breast may occur in certain syndromes—it is usually due to an increased secretion of pituitary prolactin. Hypothyroidism can also cause hyperprolactinemia. Psychiatric agents such as chlorpromazine- and estrogen-containing agents such as the oral contraceptive pills may also cause milky discharge.

49.4 **C.** Ultrasound is the most appropriate first step in evaluation of this lesion, which is likely a fibroadenoma. This modality can characterize whether or not the lesion is cystic or solid. If it is cystic, then FNA is the next step. If solid, then mammography is the next step.

CLINICAL PEARLS

▶ Approximately 1% of breast cancer occurs in men. A new palpable mass in a man's breast should prompt a diagnostic evaluation.

▶ Remember that the question in the mind of just about every woman presenting with a breast-related complaint is, "Do I have breast cancer?" The job of the physician is to both manage the presenting complaint and to provide the appropriate diagnostic workup and reassurance.

▶ BSEs should be discussed with all female patients of childbearing age, focusing on benefits versus limitations, and risk of unnecessary procedures.

▶ All breast masses require some form of evaluation and should never simply be dismissed.

REFERENCES

American Cancer Society. Breast cancer facts and figures. Available at: http://www.cancer.org/research/cancerfactsstatistics/breast-cancer-facts-figures/. Accessed April 5, 2015.

Bleyer A, Welch HG. Effect of three decades of screening mammography on breast-cancer incidence. *N Engl J Med.* 2012;367:1998–2005.

Branch-Elliman W, Golen TH, Gold HS, et al. Risk factors for Staphylococcus aureus postpartum breast abscess. *Clin Infect Dis.* 2012; 54(1):71–77.

Davidson N. Breast cancer and benign breast disorders. *Goldman's Cecil Medicine.* 24th ed. Philadelphia, PA: Elsevier/Saunders; 2012.

Dickson G. Gynecomastia. *Am Fam Physician.* 2012; 85(7):716–722.

Klein S. Evaluation of palpable breast masses. *Am Fam Physician.* 2005; 71:1731–1738.

Leung A, Pacaud D. Diagnosis and management of galactorrhea. *Am Fam Physician.* 2004; 70(3): 543–550.

Lippman ME. Breast cancer. In: Kasper D, Fauci A, Hauser S, et al., eds. *Harrison's Principles of Internal Medicine.* 19th ed. New York, NY: McGraw-Hill; 2015. Available at: http://accessmedicine.mhmedical.com. Accessed May 25, 2015.

Nelson M, Cole T, Valerio AF, et al. *Diagnosis of Breast Disease.* 13th ed. *Institute for Clinical Systems Improvement.* 2010.

Salzman B, Fleegle S, Tully AS. Common breast problems. *Am Fam Physician.* 2012;86(4):343–349.

Santen RJ, Mansel R. Benign breast disorders. *N Engl J Med.* 2005;353(3):275–285.

U.S. Preventive Services Task Force. Screening for breast cancer: U.S. Preventive Services Task Force recommendation statement. *Ann Intern Med.* 2099; 151(1):716–726.

A 28-year-old nulliparous woman presents for evaluation of irregular menstrual cycles for the past year. They occur on average only once every 2 or 3 months and she has gone as long as 4 months without a cycle. Currently, she states her last cycle occurred 11 weeks ago. Her cycles have been "mostly" regular, usually occurring every 30 days. Her menarche occurred at age 13, and she has never been on hormonal contraception. She does not smoke, does not drink alcohol, and does not exercise. She is sexually active in a monogamous relationship with a male partner who uses condoms for contraception. On review of systems, she reports a 30-lb weight gain in the past 18 months, but denies other constitutional symptoms. On examination, she is noted to be obese, with a body mass index (BMI) of 36, and her other vital signs are within normal limits. She has fine hair growth on her face and a velvety thickening of the skin on her neck. Her general physical examination is unremarkable. A pelvic examination reveals normal external genitalia, no vaginal or cervical discharge, no cervical motion tenderness, and no uterine or adnexal masses.

▶ What is the most likely diagnosis?
▶ What is the initial step in evaluation of this condition?
▶ What therapy can best regulate her menstrual cycle?

ANSWERS TO CASE 50:

Menstrual Cycle Irregularity

Summary: A 28-year-old woman presents for evaluation of irregular menstrual cycles over the past year. She is obese, has gained 30 lb, and is found to be hirsute. She has acanthosis nigricans, a skin condition characterized by dark, velvety discoloration in body creases whereby the skin becomes thickened. Her pelvic examination is unremarkable.

- **Most likely diagnosis:** Anovulatory menstrual cycles secondary to polycystic ovary syndrome (PCOS)

- **Initial laboratory test:** Pregnancy test

- **Treatment to regulate cycle:** Oral contraceptive pills

ANALYSIS

Objectives

1. Learn the common causes of irregular menstrual cycles.

2. Develop an understanding of a rational workup of menstrual cycle abnormalities.

3. Learn the management of common menstrual cycle disorders.

Considerations

Menstrual cycles are considered normal if they occur at regular intervals of 21 to 35 days in length. During their reproductive years, most women will at some point experience early, late, or missed menstrual cycles, and it will be considered to be normal. When this occurs on a rare occasion and pregnancy is ruled out, watchful waiting is usually indicated, with resumption of normal menstrual cycles almost always occurring.

The differential diagnosis of persistent menstrual cycle irregularities is broad. Pregnancy must be ruled out in a woman with a significant menstrual pattern change. After pregnancy is excluded, numerous neuroendocrine and genitourinary conditions must be considered.

In a normal (highly simplified) menstrual cycle, the hypothalamus secretes gonadotropin-releasing hormone (GnRH), which stimulates the anterior pituitary to secrete follicle-stimulating hormone (FSH) and luteinizing hormone (LH). As the FSH level rises, it causes an ovarian follicle to mature and release estrogen which induces endometrial proliferation. A mid-cycle LH surge causes ovulation, and the follicle is transformed into the corpus luteum that secretes progesterone, which compacts and matures the endometrium. If pregnancy does not occur, the production of progesterone abruptly decreases, resulting in sloughing of the endometrium and a menstrual bleed.

In our case of an obese, hirsute woman with ongoing weight gain and irregular menses, PCOS should be the initial consideration after pregnancy has been excluded. PCOS is defined as a syndrome of insulin resistance and androgen excess and has substantial metabolic impact. It is associated with infertility, hirsutism, acne, obesity, and the metabolic syndrome. PCOS is diagnosed via the Rotterdam criteria, requiring two of the following three manifestations:

- Hyperandrogenism, evidenced by hirsutism or elevated serum androgen levels (eg, testosterone, androstenedione, or dehydroepiandrostenedione [DHEA])

- Oligomenorrhea with cycle length greater than or equal to 35 days

- Multifollicular ovaries on pelvic ultrasound, defined as 12 or more small follicles in an ovary

Anovulation is the menstrual cycle irregularity associated with PCOS. Without ovulation, there is a failure of luteal production of progesterone, resulting in an absence of normal menstruation. Women with PCOS can have induced menstrual bleeding by providing periodic supplemental progesterone or by using combination oral contraceptive pills (estrogen and progesterone). Weight loss is very important in women with PCOS to increase fertility, as a loss of even 2% to 5% of body weight can greatly increase rates of pregnancy. Insulin resistance in PCOS is treated with metformin and thiazolidinediones. Infertility secondary to PCOS is treated with clomiphene citrate, aromatase inhibitors, and gonadotropins.

APPROACH TO:
Menstrual Cycle Irregularity

DEFINITIONS

AMENORRHEA: Absence of menstrual bleeding for 6 or more months when a woman is not pregnant

MENOMETRORRHAGIA: Heavy menstrual flow or prolonged duration of flow occurring at irregular intervals

MENORRHAGIA: Excessive menstrual flow, or prolonged duration of flow (>7 days), occurring at regular intervals

METRORRHAGIA: Bleeding occurring at irregular intervals

CLINICAL APPROACH

A thorough history is the initial component of the evaluation of menstrual irregularities. The history of presenting complaint should examine both the specific abnormality that is occurring and when it was first noted. Encouraging the woman with menstrual irregularities to use a menstrual calendar can be very valuable in this setting. Associated symptoms including weight gain or loss, galactorrhea, and heat or cold intolerance, should be documented. A complete past medical history should be obtained, including a complete reproductive health history detailing age at menarche, history of any previous menstrual cycle abnormalities, medications (especially anticoagulants, phenytoin, antipsychotics, tricyclic antidepressants [TCAs], and corticosteroids), contraception, infections, surgeries, and sexual practices along with pregnancies and their outcomes is required. A social history focusing on psychosocial stressors, substance use, exercise, eating habits, and sexual activity should be documented.

The general physical examination should attempt to identify medical conditions that can cause menstrual abnormalities. Extremes of body mass index—both obese and underweight conditions—can directly affect menstruation. Hirsutism and/or acne should prompt the clinician to consider a workup for androgen excess. The thyroid gland should be examined for size, consistency, and the presence of nodules. Skin and hair changes may also occur with thyroid and other endocrine conditions. Breasts should be examined for galactorrhea. Unexplained bruising or easy bleeding may occur with concomitant coagulopathies.

The pelvic examination is a critical component in the evaluation of the woman with menstrual irregularities. Initial efforts should be made to determine whether the blood is coming from the uterus or another anatomic site, as urethral, rectal, vaginal wall, or cervical bleeding can easily be mistaken for menstrual abnormality. Signs of pelvic infection should be noted and cultures collected, as cervicitis may predispose to cervical bleeding. A Papanicolaou (Pap) smear should be performed according to current cervical cancer screening guidelines. A bimanual examination should note the size and consistency of the uterus and the presence of any uterine or adnexal masses or tenderness. In women who have never been sexually active, the pelvic examination should be conducted carefully. Unless the bleeding is severe, in which case examination under anesthesia may be warranted, the examination may be deferred until after a trial of medical therapy. A pelvic ultrasound may also be considered to evaluate for potential anatomic abnormalities including uterine fibroids or masses, adnexal masses, or tumors.

Abnormal Bleeding Associated With Regular Menstrual Cycles

Menorrhagia with regular intervals between bleeding is suggestive that regular ovulation is occurring. This implies that the endocrine pathways are functioning normally and that the problem may be anatomic within the genital or hematologic system. **Leiomyomata** (uterine fibroids), especially those that are submucosal in the uterus, are a common cause of heavy uterine bleeding. They create an increased endometrial surface area with a resultant increase in menstrual bleeding. **Endometrial polyps** may cause menorrhagia by a similar mechanism. **Coagulopathy that is inherited (most commonly von Willebrand disease) or due to medications (eg, warfarin) is also a common cause of abnormal menstrual bleeding.** Liver disease, thrombocytopenia, and hematologic disorders predisposing to bleeding may also contribute.

Reduced volume of menstrual bleeding associated with regular ovulation is a less common occurrence. **Asherman syndrome** occurs with scarring within the uterine cavity caused by trauma from uterine curettage. It can result in the reduction in the size of the uterus as the walls become scarred and adherent to each other. This may result in minimal or even absent menstruation in the setting of normal hormonal function. A scarred and obstructed cervical os can cause a similar clinical picture.

Abnormal Bleeding Associated With Irregular Menstrual Cycles

Bleeding that is unpredictable in terms of timing and flow is known as dysfunctional uterine bleeding (DUB) and generally implies an abnormality within the hypothalamic-pituitary-ovarian axis. This pattern commonly occurs shortly after menarche and as a woman approaches menopause. At other times, it signals anovulation. In this setting, the endometrium is continuously stimulated by estrogen and sloughs off irregularly. Chronic anovulation should be evaluated with serum prolactin and LH levels.

Continuous estrogen stimulation can also lead to endometrial hyperplasia and endometrial carcinoma. **Risk factors for endometrial carcinoma include a history of anovulatory menstrual cycles, obesity, nulliparity, age older than 35, the use of tamoxifen, or of unopposed exogenous estrogen.**

The **evaluation of a woman with DUB is dependent on age and risk factors.** In the period after menarche, watchful waiting is usually indicated, with correction of the problem usually occurring within 1 to 2 years. In women younger than 35 years who are not at increased risk of endometrial cancer, treatment including hormonal cycling may be offered without workup beyond the history and physical examination.

Further evaluation is indicated for women with risk factors for endometrial cancer, women younger than age 35 with continued symptoms despite treatment, and postmenopausal women with uterine bleeding. The standard workup includes a pelvic ultrasound and an endometrial biopsy. **Transvaginal pelvic ultrasound** provides information on uterine size and the presence of masses, and can assess the thickness of the endometrium, which correlates with the risk of hyperplasia. An **endometrial biopsy** can be performed quickly and easily in the office setting, using a thin, disposable, sampling device. The combination of sonographic measurement of endometrial thickness and endometrial biopsy is highly sensitive and specific for the diagnosis of endometrial cancer. **Hysteroscopy** (endoscopic evaluation of the uterine cavity) can directly visualize endometrial masses, polyps, or other abnormalities, and allows for directed biopsy. It is often performed with **dilation and curettage** (D&C), which sharply removes almost the entire endometrial lining for diagnostic and therapeutic purposes.

When the workup does not reveal malignancy, **anovulatory bleeding is usually responsive to treatment with either combined estrogen and progestin oral contraceptives (OCPs) or progestin alone.** A progestin can be given for 7 to 10 days with a subsequent withdrawal bleed expected to occur within a week following the completion of the course. Both of these regimens have been shown to reduce the risk of developing endometrial hyperplasia and carcinoma. When medical treatments fail, or when symptoms are severe, surgical options may be required. Hysterectomy provides definitive treatment and is necessary in the case of a malignancy. Endometrial ablative procedures are also available and widely used.

CASE CORRELATION

- See also Case 11 (Health Maintenance in Adult Female) and Case 29 (Health Maintenance, Adolescent).

COMPREHENSION QUESTIONS

50.1 A 42-year-old obese G2P2 woman presents for evaluation of irregular menstrual bleeding for a year. She has had painless vaginal bleeding in various amounts at various times of the month. She has a history of smoking a half a pack of cigarettes per day for 10 years. She has two children, is on no medications, and has no significant medical history. She took an oral contraceptive agent for 5 years during her teen years. Her examination reveals her uterus to be slightly enlarged, but without masses or tenderness. The remainder of her examination is unremarkable. A pregnancy test is negative. Which of the following is the most significant risk factor for her having endometrial cancer?

A. Smoking

B. Parity

C. Body habitus

D. History of oral contraceptive use

50.2 A 35-year-old woman has had irregular menstrual cycles since high school. She frequently misses cycles and has never been pregnant. When she has cycles, they are very light and last for only a few days. She has had mild-to-moderate comedonal and pustular acne since late adolescence and in recent years has developed some hair growing under her chin. She denies taking any medications or history of other gynecologic or medical problems. Which of the following is the most appropriate evaluation for the initial workup of her problem?

A. Serum TSH

B. Serum karyotype

C. Serum estradiol

D. Urine cortisol

E. Serum FSH

50.3 A 28-year-old woman complains of irregular spotting between cycles for the past 2 months. She has been previously healthy and has never been pregnant. She has been sexually active for the past 6 months with the same male partner. On examination, her only positive findings are a mildly enlarged and moderately tender uterus. Her pregnancy test is negative. Which of the following is the most probable diagnosis?

A. Uterine leiomyoma

B. Cervical carcinoma

C. Endometritis

D. Endometrial cancer

E. Urinary tract infection

ANSWERS

50.1 **C.** This patient's obesity is the most significant risk factor for endometrial cancer, due to chronically elevated unopposed estrogen levels stored in adipose tissue. Parity is protective for endometrial cancer. Risk factors for endometrial cancer include anovulatory menstrual cycles, obesity, nulliparity, age greater than 35, and use of tamoxifen or unopposed exogenous estrogen. Interestingly, smoking is a negative risk factor for endometrial cancer.

50.2 **A.** Estrogen does not have a role in the initial workup for anovulation; serum karyotype is useful for premature ovarian failure but not for anovulation. Urine cortisol may help in the diagnosis of Cushing disease, but not generally indicated unless the patient has other stigmata of corticosteroid excess such as abdominal striae, easy brusability, and buffalo hump. TSH is indicated in DUB workup. Both total serum testosterone levels and prolactin are useful. Thus, in general, a pregnancy test, TSH, and prolactin level are the initial tests for the evaluation of menstrual irregularities.

50.3 **C.** Endometritis is a common cause of vaginal spotting. It is generally a polymicrobial infection caused by an ascending infection of normal vaginal flora. Commonly isolated organisms include gonorrhea, *Chlamydia trachomatis, Ureaplasma urealyticum, Peptostreptococcus, Gardnerella vaginalis,* and the group B *Streptococcus* species. The patient's history makes cervical cancer less likely. Leiomyoma or polyps are possible, but less likely with her history of recent spotting and sexual activity. Endometrial cancer would also be unlikely in a patient with previously regular menses. While a urinary tract infection may cause hematuria in cases of severe cystitis, it would not cause uterine enlargement or tenderness. The diagnosis of endometritis can be confirmed with an endometrial biopsy showing inflammatory cells, in particular plasma cells.

CLINICAL PEARLS

▶ The first test performed on a woman with menstrual cycle irregularities should be a pregnancy test.

▶ A history of anovulatory cycles does not confer absolute protection against pregnancy. Ovulation may occur intermittently and irregularly. If the woman does not want to become pregnant, she should be counseled on contraceptive options.

▶ Women with PCOS should be treated and monitored appropriately, due to an elevated risk of concomitant factors with cardiometabolic syndrome.

REFERENCES

Ely JW, Kennedy CM, Clark EC, Bowdler NC. Abnormal uterine bleeding: a management algorithm. *J Am Board Fam Med*. 2006;19:590–602.

Hall JE. Disorders of the female reproductive system. In: Kasper D, Fauci A, Hauser S, et al., eds. *Harrison's Principles of Internal Medicine*. 19th ed. New York, NY: McGraw-Hill Education; 2015. Available at: http://accessmedicine.mhmedical.com. Accessed May 25, 2015.

Hickey M, Higham JM, Fraser I. Progestogens with or without estrogen for irregular uterine bleeding associated with anovulation. *Cochrane Database Sys Rev*. Sept 12, 2012;9:CD001895.

Norman RJ, Dewailly, D, Legro RS, Hickey TE. Polycystic ovary syndrome. *Lancet*. 2007; 370:685–697.

Osayande AS, Mehulic S. Diagnosis and initial management of dysmenorrhea. *Am Fam Physician*. 2014;89(5):341–346.

Radosh L. Drug treatments for polycystic ovary syndrome. *Am Fam Physician*. 2009; 79(8):671–676.

Sweet MG, Schmidt-Dalton TA, Weiss PM. Evaluation and management of abnormal uterine bleeding in premenopausal women. *Am Fam Physician*. 2012; 85(1):35–43.

Teede H, Deeks A, Moran L. Polycystic ovary syndrome: a complex condition with psychological, reproductive, and metabolic manifestations that impacts on health across the lifespan. *BMC Med*. 2010; 8:41.

Wong CL, Farquhar C, Roberts H, Proctor M. Oral contraceptive pill as treatment for primary dysmenorrhea. *Cochrane Database Syst Rev*. Apr 15 2009;CD002120.

A 30-year-old obese woman presents to your office with a chief complaint of recurrent yeast infections and increased thirst. She also has noticed increased urinary frequency, but believes this is related to her yeast infection. Over the last several years, she has gained more than 40 lb despite having tried numerous diets, most recently a low-carbohydrate, high-fat diet. The patient's only other pertinent history is that she was told to "watch her diet" during pregnancy because of excessive weight gain. Her baby had to be delivered at 38 weeks via cesarean section because he weighed more than 10 lb (>4500 g). Her family history is unknown, as she was adopted. On physical examination, her blood pressure is 145/92 mm Hg, her pulse is 72 beats/min, and her respiratory rate is 16 breaths/min. Her height is 65 in and her weight is 223 lb (body mass index [BMI] = 37.1). Her physical examination reveals darkened skin that appears to be thickened on the back of her neck and moist, reddened skin beneath her breasts. Her pelvic examination reveals a thick, white, vaginal discharge. A wet preparation from the vaginal discharge reveals branching hyphae consistent with *Candida* species. A urinalysis is negative for leukocyte esterase, nitrites, protein, and glucose.

▶ What is the most likely primary diagnosis for this patient?
▶ What physical findings are suggestive of the diagnosis and have implications for management?
▶ What diagnostic studies should be ordered at this time?

ANSWERS TO CASE 51:
Diabetes Mellitus

Summary: A 30-year-old obese woman presents with a recurrent yeast infection, polydipsia, and polyuria. She has gained over 40 lb despite efforts to lose weight, and was told to "watch her diet" during a recent pregnancy. On examination, she has a BMI of 37.1, acanthosis nigricans, *Candida* vaginitis, and a negative urinalysis.

- **Most likely diagnosis:** Type 2 diabetes mellitus.

- **Significant physical findings:** Obesity, acanthosis nigricans, blood pressure that is elevated for a diabetic (JNC 8 blood pressure goal in the diabetic patient is <140/90 mm Hg), *Candida* vaginitis, and likely *Candida* skin infection under her breasts.

- **Diagnostic studies:** Fasting serum glucose measurement or glycosylated hemoglobin level (HbA_{1C}); follow-up testing should include a comprehensive metabolic panel including electrolytes, blood urea nitrogen (BUN), and creatinine; fasting lipid panel; urine microalbumin/creatinine ratio.

ANALYSIS

Objectives

1. Know the diagnostic criteria for diabetes mellitus, including classic signs and symptoms, physical findings, and diagnostic studies.

2. Know the pathophysiologic and epidemiologic differences between types 1 and 2 diabetes mellitus.

3. Learn the treatment options for diabetic patients.

4. Be aware of the acute emergencies that can occur in diabetic patients and how to manage them.

Considerations

Diabetes mellitus is one of the most common medical problems encountered in medical practice, and was the seventh leading cause of death in the United States in 2011. In 2012, there were an estimated 29.1 million diabetics in the United States and the number is increasing both in the United States and worldwide. It was estimated that of the 29.1 million people, 21 million were diagnosed, and 8.1 million were undiagnosed. Diabetes affects all ethnic groups, but there is a disproportionate burden of disease in African Americans, Native Americans, and Hispanics. The global epidemic of obesity has led to a dramatic increase in the number of type 2 diabetics presenting with disease in their teens and twenties. While some diabetics exhibit the classic symptoms of polyuria, polydipsia, polyphagia, and weight loss, many patients are diagnosed when asymptomatic.

The complications of diabetes are myriad. Diabetics are 6 to 10 times more likely than nondiabetics to be hospitalized for cardiovascular disease and 15 times more likely to be hospitalized for peripheral vascular disease. It is the leading cause of blindness in working-age adults in the United States, most of which is preventable. It is also the leading cause of end-stage renal disease requiring dialysis and of nontraumatic amputations. The American Diabetes Association (ADA) estimates the annual cost of diabetes in the United States, including direct medical costs and lost productivity, at $245 billion per year.

Other common complications of diabetes include neuropathic, gastrointestinal, and immunologic disease. Peripheral neuropathy, leading to reduced sensation or pain, can lead to the development of injuries, ulcerations, infections, or amputations of the extremities. Gastroparesis can be a chronic problem that causes nausea and vomiting and impairs the patient's ability to maintain an adequate nutritional status. Poorly controlled diabetics suffer relative immunosuppression that makes them more prone to opportunistic infections, including bacterial and fungal skin and genitourinary infections.

Impaired glucose tolerance or elevated serum glucose levels may be present for years prior to a formal diagnosis of type 2 diabetes mellitus. In the case presented, the history of excessive weight gain during pregnancy with fetal macrosomia and advice to "watch her diet" should prompt the clinician to suspect a history of gestational diabetes. Women who have gestational diabetes are at a threefold increased risk of developing diabetes later in life.

The symptoms of polydipsia and polyuria should lead the clinician to an increased suspicion for the possibility of diabetes. High serum glucose levels function as an osmotic diuretic, resulting in frequent urination. Patients with diabetes also may present with polyphagia, as their insulin deficiency prevents food intake from being properly metabolized, resulting in a state of hunger for which they will frequently eat but not feel satiated.

DIAGNOSIS

The American College of Endocrinology diagnostic criteria for diabetes are any of the following:

1. A fasting plasma glucose greater than or equal to 126 mg/dL (no caloric intake for at least 8 hours)

2. A plasma glucose greater than or equal to 200 mg/dL 2 hours after a 75-g glucose load (ie, glucose tolerance test)

3. Random plasma glucose greater than or equal to 200 mg/dL plus symptoms (eg, polydipsia, polyuria)

4. Glycosylated hemoglobin (HbA_{1c}) greater than or equal to 6.5%

HbA_{1c} is used to estimate the average glucose levels over the past 3 months in those who are diagnosed with diabetes for appropriate monitoring and goal setting. A HbA_{1c} less than 6% is considered as a normal value, while values between 6% and 6.5% are considered "pre-diabetes." In patients with hemoglobinopathies (eg, sickle cell anemia), recent blood loss, or a recent drastic change in diet (eg, no or extremely low-carbohydrate diet), serum fructosamine levels should be obtained, and indicate average glucose levels over a 2- to 3-week period.

Measurement of C-peptide and insulin levels can be used to distinguish type 2 from type 1 diabetes when the history, physical examination, and other tests, such as serum ketones and osmolality, are not enough. Other tests recommended by the ADA are fasting lipid profiles (at the time of diagnosis and, at least, annually thereafter), serum creatinine, urinalysis, urine microalbumin: creatinine ratios (at time of diagnosis in type 2 diabetics and annually thereafter; in type 1 diabetics who have had disease for 5 years and annually thereafter), annual dilated eye examinations, regular foot examinations, electrocardiography (ECG) (in adults), and, in type 1 diabetics, thyroid disease screening with a thyroid-stimulating hormone (TSH).

The absence of glucose on urinalysis does not exclude a diagnosis of diabetes and should not delay a blood glucose measurement. **Glucosuria occurs when the blood glucose level is greater than the renal "threshold" level, often estimated at a serum level of 180 mg/dL, the level that approximates a glycosylated hemoglobin level of 8.0%.** Overt signs of insulin resistance (eg, acanthosis nigricans, elevated blood pressure, obesity) also make the diagnosis of type 2 diabetes more likely.

The general approach to managing diabetes mellitus is aimed at secondary prevention of macrovascular (eg, accelerated coronary artery disease, accelerated cerebral and peripheral vascular disease) and microvascular (eg, retinopathy, nephropathy, and neuropathy) complications.

APPROACH TO:
Diabetes Mellitus

DEFINITIONS

AACE/ACE: American Association of Clinical Endocrinologists and American College of Endocrinology—Organization who devised the current clinical practice guidelines for a comprehensive care plan for diabetes mellitus.

TYPE 1 DIABETES: Often referred to as juvenile diabetes, the exact pathophysiologic mechanism is unknown, yet thought to be likely an autoimmune disorder. Current theories support the notion that either an infection or an environment or genetic trigger causes the body to mistakenly attack pancreatic β-cells that make insulin.

CLINICAL APPROACH

Diabetes mellitus is a general term for several different variations of disease along a spectrum that result in high blood glucose levels that, if uncontrolled over a period of time, eventually lead to microvascular and macrovascular complications. The major classifications of diabetes mellitus are types 1 and 2 diabetes and gestational diabetes.

Type 1 Diabetes

Type 1 diabetes (insulin-dependent diabetes mellitus [IDDM]) is a chronic disease of carbohydrate, fat, and protein metabolism due to a lack of insulin, resulting from autoimmune destruction of insulin-producing pancreatic β cells. Due to the lack of insulin, which is required for glucose and carbohydrate metabolism, type 1 diabetics are prone to metabolize fats, with the resultant production of ketones. This process leads to **diabetic ketoacidosis (DKA)**, a syndrome characterized by hyperglycemia, high levels of serum acetone, and β-hyroxybutyrate, and an anion gap metabolic acidosis. DKA often occurs during times of physical stress, such as an infection or myocardial infarction, or when the patient does not properly take his or her insulin. DKA is a medical emergency requiring hospitalization, vigorous intravenous hydration with normal saline, correction of the acidosis and electrolyte disturbances, aggressive insulin management, and evaluation for the underlying cause of the condition.

Type 2 Diabetes

Type 2 diabetes (previously called adult-onset diabetes mellitus [AODM], but still commonly called non–insulin-dependent diabetes mellitus [NIDDM]) patients, in contrast to type 1 diabetics in whom there is a lack of insulin, exhibit **insulin resistance in peripheral tissues often related to visceral adiposity and obesity,** and may have hyperinsulinemia. Type 2 diabetics often manifest signs of insulin resistance for many years prior to the diagnosis of overt diabetes. This type of diabetes accounts for at least 90% of the diagnosed cases, and virtually all cases of undiagnosed diabetes in the United States.

Type 2 diabetes has a stronger familial predisposition than type 1 diabetes, as type 2 diabetics often have a family history of the disease. The genetic factors are multifactorial and have not been accurately identified. It is strongly associated with obesity and its complications including cardiometabolic syndrome, hyperinsulinemia, hypertension, dyslipidemia, hyperglycemia, and central obesity.

Uncontrolled type 2 diabetics can achieve extremely high blood sugars without developing ketosis and acidosis. This type of diabetes is more prone to hyperosmolar states due to the high blood sugar levels. **Hyperosmolar hyperglycemic nonketotic syndrome (HHNS)** occurs when blood glucose levels become substantially elevated, often approaching 1000 mg/dL. This may be the presenting symptom of some cases of type 2 diabetes, or may result from either a concurrent illness or failure to take medications. Serum osmolarity is elevated (>320 mOsm/kg) and the patient has a large fluid deficit (up to 9 L). In severe cases, coma or death can occur due to electrolyte abnormalities, dehydration, and the toxic effects of metabolic acidosis. HHNS must be managed with hospitalization, aggressive rehydration with normal saline and correction of electrolyte abnormalities, treatment of underlying illnesses, and the judicious use of insulin.

Gestational Diabetes

Gestational diabetes mellitus (GDM) occurs in approximately 7% of all pregnancies, resulting in over 200,000 cases annually in the United States, with a prevalence of 1% to 14%. During pregnancy, elevated levels of human placental lactogen, estrogen, and progesterone produced by the placenta act as insulin antagonists leading to increased insulin resistance and carbohydrate intolerance. Maternal and fetal complications related to GDM are numerous. Maternal complications include hyperglycemia, diabetic ketoacidosis (DKA), increased urinary tract infection (UTI) risk, increased pregnancy-induced hypertension/preeclampsia, and retinopathy.

Fetal effects include congenital malformations, macrosomia, respiratory distress syndrome, hypoglycemia, hyperbilirubinemia, hypocalcemia, polycythemia, and hydramnios. Women with GDM are more prone to develop non–pregnancy-related type 2 diabetes and should be screened with a glucose tolerance test postpartum and should undergo annual diabetic screening.

Risk factors for GDM include age greater than 25 years, member of a high-incidence ethnic group (eg, Native American, African American, Hispanic American, South or East Asian, Pacific Islander), BMI of 25 or greater, history of glucose intolerance, previous history of GDM, and history of diabetes mellitus in a first-degree family member.

The American College of Obstetricians and Gynecologists recommends screening all women for gestational diabetes between 24 and 28 weeks' gestation with an oral 50-g 1-hour glucose tolerance test (GTT). If the 1-hour glucose challenge is greater than 135 to 140 mg/dL, then an oral 100-g 3-hour GTT should be performed. The 3-hour GTT requires serum glucose levels be obtained at fasting, 1-, 2-, and 3-hour intervals. The diagnosis of GDM is made based on two or more abnormal results, defined as glucose levels of 95, 180, 155, and 140 mg/dL, respectively. GDM is treated with strict dietary management via patient education and nutritional counseling and when necessary, oral diabetic agents with or without insulin. Increased surveillance for fetal demise in pregnant women with GDM is mandatory, particularly when fasting glucose levels exceed 105 mg/dL or when pregnancy becomes postterm.

MANAGEMENT

The overall goals for the diabetic patient are to achieve a "controlled" status:

1. Strict glycemic control with a goal of hemoglobin A_{1c} of less than or equal to 7.0%

2. Low-density lipoprotein cholesterol (LDL-C) level less than or equal to 100 mg/dL

3. Blood pressure less than or equal to 140/90 mm Hg (*JNC 8 guidelines*)

4. Lifestyle modifications including a diet consisting of low carbohydrates and low saturated fats and physical activity counseling (at least 150 min/wk of moderate-intensity aerobic physical activity [50%-70% maximum heart rate] and resistance training [3 times/wk])

The **treatment for type 1 diabetes centers on insulin administration.** In most cases, combination therapy using short-acting insulin prior to meals and long-acting basal insulin confers the greatest outcomes in minimizing complications. Insulin pump therapy, which provides a continuous subcutaneous infusion of short-acting insulin, is also an alternative for patients with labile glucose control. Insulin management requires careful and frequent self-monitoring of glucose, often with adjustment of insulin dosage based on the glucose levels, amount of physical activity, and caloric/carbohydrate intake (Table 51–1).

Patients with type 2 diabetes mellitus and those at risk of developing diabetes should be educated on the importance of appropriate calorie-restricted and

Table 51-1 · INSULIN PREPARATIONS			
Type of Insulin	Onset of Action	Peak of Action	Duration of Action
Rapid acting (lispro or aspart insulin)	15 min	30-90 min	3-5 h
Short acting (regular insulin)	30-60 min	60-120 min	5-8 h
Intermediate acting (neutral protamine hagedorn [NPH] insulin)	13 h	7-15 h	18-24 h
Long acting (glargine insulin; insulin detemir)	1 h	None	24 h

Data from the National Institutes of Health. Available at: http://diabetes.niddk.nih.gov/dm/pubs/medicines_ez/insert_C.htm. Accessed May, 2009.

low-carbohydrate diet and exercise as key components of their management. In some cases, this strategy may be all that is required to achieve appropriate glycemic control. An initial goal that is achievable by many patients is a 10% weight loss. When lifestyle changes alone do not result in adequate glycemic control, oral agents should be considered as first-line treatment in patients with a glycosylated hemoglobin level less than 9.0%. For severely obese patients, gastric bypass surgery may be considered when standard treatments fail to improve glycemic control.

Medications for the prevention of diabetes mellitus are currently not recommended but can be considered when lifestyle modifications prove unsuccessful. Several mediations are available for treating type 2 diabetes (Table 51–2). Metformin is the drug of choice to begin with unless contraindications are present.

Biguanides (eg, metformin) act on the liver to **decrease glucose output during gluconeogenesis.** Secondary actions include improved insulin sensitivity in the liver and muscle and a hypothesized decrease in intestinal absorption of glucose. Metformin can lower the HbA_{1c} by 1.5% to 2%. The UKPDS showed a significant reduction in cardiovascular events, diabetes-related deaths, and all causes of mortality in patients taking metformin. Other advantages to metformin include no potential risk of hypoglycemia, reduced serum insulin levels, potential modest weight loss, and a reduction in triglycerides and LDL cholesterol. The efficacy, safety, and improved outcomes make it a popular first-line agent in type 2 diabetes.

The most common side effects of metformin are gastrointestinal, including nausea and diarrhea. These side effects may be reduced by starting at low doses and taking the medication with meals. The most dangerous side effect attributable to metformin is the development of lactic acidosis. This risk is potentially fatal and is increased by renal insufficiency and chronic kidney disease, thus metformin use is contraindicated in those with a serum creatinine greater than or equal to 1.5 mg/dL in men and greater than or equal to 1.4 mg/dL in women, hepatic insufficiency, or congestive heart failure. Metformin should be withheld 48 hours prior to any imaging that requires iodinated contrast. Metformin is classified as category B in pregnancy and thought to be safe in nursing mothers. It is the oral agent of choice in type 2 diabetes in children older than age 10.

Sulfonylureas were the first oral agents available for the treatment of type 2 diabetes. Their principal action is to function as **insulin secretagogues** that stimulate

Table 51–2 • ORAL HYPOGLYCEMICS

Descriptions for both lifestyle modifications and metformin	Intervention	% Decrease in HbA$_{1c}$	Advantages	Disadvantages
Tier 1: well-validated core **Step 1:** initial therapy	lifestyle: to decrease weight and increase activity	1.0-2.0	Broad benefits	Insufficient for most within first year
	Metformin	1.0-2.0	Weight neutral	GI side effects, contraindicated with renal insufficiency
Step 2: additional therapy	insulin	1.5-3.5	No dose limit, rapidly effective, improved lipid profile	One to four injections daily, monitoring, weight gain, hypoglycemia, analogues are expensive
	Sulfonylurea	1.0-2.0	Rapidly effective	Weight gain, hypoglycemia (especially with glibenclamide or chlorpropamide)
Tier 2: less well validated	TZDs	0.5-1.4	Improved lipid profile (pioglitazone), potential decrease in MI (pioglitazone)	Fluid retention, CHF, weight gain, bone fractures, expensive, potential increase in MI (rosiglitazone)
	GLP-1 agonist	0.5-1.0	Weight loss	Two injections daily, frequent GI side effects, long-term safety not established, expensive
Other therapy	Glucosidase inhibitor	0.5-0.8	Weight neutral	Frequent GI side effects, TID dosing, expensive
	Glinide	0.5-1.5	Rapidly effective	Weight gain, TID dosing, hypoglycemia, expensive
	Pramlintide	0.5-1.0	Weight loss	Three injections daily, frequent GI side effects, long-term safety not established, expensive
	DPP-4 inhibitor	0.5-0.8	Weight neutral	Long-term safety not established, expensive

Abbreviations: CHF, chronic heart failure; DPP, dipeptidyl peptidase; GI, gastrointestinal; GLP, glucagon-like peptide; MI, myocardial infarction; TID, three times daily; TZD, thiazolidinedione.
Data from Nathan DM, Buse JB, Davidon MD, et al. Medical management of hyperglycemia in type 2 diabetes: a consensus algorithm of initiation and adjustment of therapy. Diabetic Care. 2008;31(12):1-11.

pancreatic β-cells to secrete insulin. Advantages include a potential 2% reduction in HbA_{1c}, once- or twice-a-day dosing, and relatively low cost. Disadvantages include poor response in 20% of patients, a tendency of users to gain weight, and a tendency for the medications to lose effectiveness over time. As insulin secretagogues, sulfonylureas carry a risk of causing hypoglycemia.

Sulfonylureas and insulin are considered to be the best validated second-line add-on therapy. The following medications are less well validated. Further studies are necessary to determine how these agents may play a role in the overall long-term management of type 2 diabetics.

The principal action of **thiazolidinediones (TZDs), or glitazones** (eg, rosiglitazone), is to **improve insulin sensitivity in muscle and adipose tissue.** Secondary actions include decreased hepatic gluconeogenesis and increased peripheral glucose utilization. Among their advantages is a modest decrease in serum triglyceride and increase in high-density lipoprotein (HDL) cholesterol levels. Since they are metabolized in the liver, they can be used in patients with renal impairment. They also do not, when used by themselves, cause hypoglycemia. Disadvantages include edema and weight gain, which is of significant concern in patients with congestive heart failure, liver disease and cirrhosis, chronic kidney disease, and chronic lower extremity edema. Since their release, several members of this class of medication have been withdrawn from the market due to increased risk of cardiovascular events. Thus, there is controversy over whether or not the benefits of this class of medications outweigh potential risks.

Meglitinides (eg, nateglinide) are **short-acting secretagogues** that increase insulin secretion from the pancreas and work in a similar fashion to sulfonylureas. These medications are taken no more than 1 hour prior to meals due to the rapid onset and short duration of action. They are useful in patients whose blood glucose values vary at mealtime but who have controlled fasting glucose levels. They reduce HbA_{1c} levels from 0.5% to 2%. The disadvantages include a risk of hypoglycemia, especially if the medication is taken but no meal is then eaten, and expense. They should not be used in patients with hepatic dysfunction.

α-**Glucosidase inhibitors** (eg, acarbose) **delay carbohydrate absorption** by inhibiting α-glucosidase in the small intestine, which decreases postprandial hyperglycemia. They reduce HbA_{1c} levels by 0.7% to 1.0%. This class of medication may offer benefits to patients with erratic eating habits, as hypoglycemia will not occur if meals are skipped. The principal side effects are gastrointestinal, including flatulence. These medications are contraindicated in cases of ketoacidosis and in patients with hepatic dysfunction.

Pramlintide is an amylinomimetic agent that has physiologic actions equivalent to those of human amylin, a glucoregulatory hormone synthesized by pancreatic β-cells and released with insulin in response to a meal. It inhibits inappropriately high glucagon secretion during episodes of hyperglycemia (eg, after a meal) in patients with type 1 or 2 diabetes mellitus and does not impair normal glucagon response to hypoglycemia. It is administered subcutaneously and does not require dose adjustments for renal or hepatic impairment, but requires titration to balance hypoglycemia and preprandial glycemic control. It reduces HbA_{1c} levels by 0.5% to 1.0%. Known side effects include hypoglycemia, nausea, and diarrhea, often dosing.

GLP-1 agonists, or glucagon-like peptide-1 incretin mimetics (eg, exenatide), are synthetic peptides that stimulate insulin release. This class can be used as adjunctive therapy for type 2 diabetics with inadequate glycemic control while also taking either metformin, a sulfonylurea, and/or a thiazolidinedione/glitazone. They reduce HbA_{1c} levels by 0.5% to 1.0%. A distinct benefit of this class is early satiety, which can improve dietary management. This class should be avoided in patients with diabetic gastroparesis. Side effects include hypoglycemia when added to a sulfonylurea (but not when added to metformin), nausea, vomiting, diarrhea, and acute pancreatitis.

DPP-4 inhibitors, or dipeptidyl peptidase-4 inhibitors (eg, sitagliptin), work via an enzyme that inactivates incretin hormones GLP-1 and glucose-dependent insulinotropic polypeptide (GIP). GIP and GLP-1 stimulate insulin synthesis and release from pancreatic β-cells in a glucose-dependent manner. GLP-1 also decreases glucagon secretion from pancreatic α-cells in a glucose-dependent manner, leading to reduced hepatic glucose production. This class can be used as monotherapy and as an adjunct to diet and exercise for management of type 2 diabetes mellitus in patients whom hyperglycemia cannot be controlled by diet and exercise alone. They can also be used in combination with metformin, a sulfonylurea, or a thiazolidinedione as second-line therapy for management of type 2 diabetes mellitus in patients who do not achieve adequate glycemic control with diet, exercise, and metformin, sulfonylurea, or thiazolidinedione monotherapy. The DPP-4 inhibitors have been shown to reduce HbA_{1c} levels by 0.5% to 0.8%. The principal side effects include upper respiratory tract symptoms and severe hypersensitivity (eg, requires titration to balance hypoglycemia and preprandial glycemic control anaphylaxis and/or angioedema).

The goal of diabetic management is to safely and consistently lower the average serum glucose levels to reduce the risk of macrovascular and microvascular complications. The goal of treatment is to achieve a HbA_{1c} of less than 7%, although some authorities advocate 6.5% as a goal. Other treatments are equally important to achieve tight glucose control in the effort to reduce adverse events, including heart attacks and strokes. The JNC 8 concluded that a blood pressure goal of less than 140/90 mm Hg reduces cardiovascular events. Diabetes is considered a coronary heart disease risk equivalent for decisions regarding lipid management. The LDL cholesterol goal is less than 100 mg/dL. All diabetics should be advised to be immunized with the pneumococcal vaccine and to get an annual influenza vaccination. They should be screened annually for diabetic neuropathy with a monofilament examination of the feet, should have annual microalbumin screening for diabetic nephropathy, and an annual dilated ophthalmologic evaluation to screen for diabetic retinopathy.

MANAGEMENT OF HYPOGLYCEMIA

Hypoglycemic symptoms are related to the central and sympathetic nervous systems. Decreased levels of glucose lead to deficient cerebral glucose availability that can manifest as confusion, difficulty with concentration, irritability, hallucinations, focal impairments (eg, hemiplegia), and eventually coma and death. Stimulation of the sympathoadrenal nervous system leads to sweating, palpitations, tremulousness, anxiety, and hunger. Causes of hypoglycemia include fasting, exogenous insulin, elevated C-peptide levels, autoimmunity, sulfonylurea abuse, and hormonal deficiency (eg, hypoadrenalism, hypopituitary, glucagon deficiency).

When hypoglycemia is suspected and the patient is conscious and cooperative, juice, soda, candy, or some other sugar-containing product can rapidly alleviate the symptoms on a temporary basis. If the person is not able to take something by mouth, rapid administration of intramuscular glucagon can be effective. In the hospital setting, or when intravenous access is available, a rapid injection of 50% dextrose (D_{50}) quickly restores normal serum and brain glucose levels. Following any of these therapies, the patient should be closely monitored, as the hypoglycemia may recur (especially if the patient uses a long-acting insulin or oral hypoglycemic agent), unless additional glucose and/or carbohydrates are administered.

COMPREHENSION QUESTIONS

51.1 A 16-year-old adolescent girl has had an increased craving for sweets. She often consumes two to three ice cream sundaes and four large sodas a day, but has still managed to maintain her weight. Friends often notice her using the bathroom more frequently to urinate but she denies any episodes of purging and states that she just has to urinate after drinking so much cola. On physical examination, she is 5 ft 8 in and 110 lb and her thyroid is not palpable. Which of the following test results is diagnostic of diabetes mellitus?

A. A single glucose reading of 124 mg/dL

B. A 2-hour oral glucose tolerance test greater than 200 mg/dL with a 100-g glucose load

C. A random glucose greater than 200 mg/dL with symptoms such as polydipsia or polyuria

D. A HbA_{1c} of 6.3%

51.2 A 7-year-old boy is brought to the office with symptoms of polydipsia, polyphagia, polyuria, and weight loss of 8 lb. For the past 24 hours, he has had abdominal pain and vomiting. A urinalysis performed in the office shows the presence of glucose and ketones. A finger-stick blood glucose is 530 mg/dL. Which of the following is the most appropriate initial management in this patient?

A. Discharge home with oral metformin and a prompt referral to a dietician.

B. Hospitalization with administration of intravenous normal saline and 5% dextrose, and regular insulin.

C. Discharge home with a prescription for insulin, advice to hydrate aggressively, and office follow-up in 24 hours.

D. Hospitalization with determination of electrolytes and potential anion gap acidosis, and administration of intravenous normal saline and regular insulin.

E. Hospitalization with immediate endocrinology consults for insulin dosing.

51.3 An 83-year-old man was diagnosed with type 2 diabetes mellitus 3 months ago. He has modified his diet and tries to walk at least half a mile every evening. He drinks a glass of wine with lunch and dinner daily. For the past week, he has felt dizzy upon standing and has fallen on two occasions, but has never lost consciousness. After the last episode of falling, he presented to the local emergency room (ER) where his blood pressure was 155/76 mm Hg, heart rate was 74 beats/min, and respiratory rate was 16 breaths/min. A finger stick showed a random glucose level of 64 mg/dL. Which of the following classes of medications has the lowest incidence of causing hypoglycemia when used as single-agent therapy?

A. Biguanide

B. Insulin

C. Sulfonylurea

D. Meglitinide

51.4 A 39-year-old G1P0 woman who is a new patient presents to the office at 10 weeks' gestation. She is known to have type 2 diabetes mellitus and currently takes metformin. Her last HbA_{1c} was 10.4% 1 month ago. Her urinalysis is negative for ketones and leukocytes, and reveals only trace protein. She has no other medical problems and does not drink or smoke. On physical examination, she is 5 ft 4 in and weighs 202 lb with a BMI of 34.7. She inquires about the risk of diabetes to her fetus. Compared to gestational diabetes mellitus, this patient is at an increased risk for developing which of the following?

A. Fetal malformations

B. Fetal macrosomia

C. Polyhydramnios

D. Shoulder dystocia

E. Diabetic gastroparesis

51.5 A 56-year-old man with cardiometabolic syndrome presents to discuss his diabetic management regimen. His last HbA_{1c} was 8.8% and he currently takes metformin twice daily. He adamantly does not want to take insulin. He has seen a lot of commercials for new diabetic agents and wants to try one that will help to curb his appetite. Which of the following agents will likely cause early satiety?

A. Acarbose

B. Rosiglitazone

C. Nateglinide

D. Pramlintide

E. Exenatide

ANSWERS

51.1 **C.** Diabetes mellitus can be defined by measurement of an 8-hour fasting glucose more than 125 mg/dL; a random glucose of 200 mg/dL or more with classic symptoms or a 2-hour GTT of 200 mg/dL or more after a 75-g glucose load. Recently, the ADA recommended that an HbA_{1c} of greater than or equal to 6.5% can be used for diagnosing diabetes.

51.2 **D.** This is a classic presentation of diabetic ketoacidosis, a common initial presentation of type 1 diabetes mellitus, and is a medical emergency. This child requires immediate hospitalization, determination of electrolytes and potential anion gap metabolic acidosis, intravenous normal saline, and insulin. Intravenous dextrose should not be administered until the fluid deficit is corrected with normal saline, and the anion gap has been reversed. Metformin will not clinically improve this patient. An endocrinologist is not required for dosing of insulin.

51.3 **A.** Biguanides (metformin) are effective medications for the treatment of type 2 diabetes; they do not cause hypoglycemia when given as monotherapy. Insulin and insulin secretagogues carry a risk of hypoglycemia as a complication of therapy.

51.4 **A.** Gestational diabetes is more likely to lead to fetal macrosomia and polyhydramnios. Both gestational and pregestational diabetes are associated with shoulder dystocia. Pregestational diabetes is associated with greater fetal malformations due to the higher serum glucose levels during organogenesis (5- to 10-week gestational age), whereas gestational diabetes tends to be associated with hyperglycemia after 20-week gestation, when the fetal organs have already formed. Preterm labor occurs at same frequency in diabetics as nondiabetics.

51.5 **E.** Exenatide has been shown to cause early satiety and should be avoided in patients with diabetic gastroparesis. The other medications may cause nausea, diarrhea, or other gastrointestinal side effects, but do not cause early satiety.

CLINICAL PEARLS

▶ Diabetes is one of the most common diseases encountered in clinical practice, and is often diagnosed in asymptomatic patients. The criteria for diagnosis have been lowered to decrease macrovascular and microvascular complications, including death.

▶ Type 2 diabetes accounts for more than 90% of all cases of diabetes in the United States. The increasing prevalence of obesity greatly contributes to more patients who will develop diabetes over the course of their lives.

▶ Biguanides are the mainstay of oral diabetic agents in patients with type 2 diabetes due to tolerability, low cost, efficacy, and demonstrated reduction in morbidity and mortality.

▶ Newer oral diabetic agents can play an important role in adjunctive therapy when modest reductions in HbA_{1C} are the goal.

▶ Long-acting insulin should be considered in patients with type 2 diabetes who have insulin resistance and cardiometabolic syndrome.

REFERENCES

American College of Obstetricians and Gynecologists. ACOG guidelines at a glance: gestational diabetes mellitus. *Obstet Gynecol.* 2013;122:406-416.

American Diabetes Association (ADA). Diagnosis and classification of diabetes mellitus. *Diabetes Care.* 2014;37(suppl 1):S81-S90.

American Diabetes Association (ADA). Executive summary: standards of medical care in diabetes—2014. *Diabetes Care.* 2014;37(suppl 1):S5-S13.

Evert AB, Boucher JL, Cypress M, et al. Nutrition therapy recommendations for the management of adults with diabetes. *Diabetes Care.* 2014;37(suppl 1):S120-S143.

Handelsman Y, Bloomgarden ZT, Grunberger G, et al. American Association of Clinical Endocrinologists and American College of Endocrinology—Clinical Practice Guidelines for Developing a Diabetes Mellitus Comprehensive Care Plan—2015. *Endocr Pract.* 2015;21(suppl 1):1-87.

James PA, Oparil S, Carter BL, et al. Evidence-based guideline for the management of high blood pressure in adults. Report from the panel members appointed to the Eighth Joint National Committee (JNC 8). *JAMA.* 2014;311(5):507-520.

Patel P, Macerollo A. Diabetes mellitus: diagnosis and screening. *Am Fam Physician.* 2010;81(7): 863-870.

Petznik A. Insulin management of type 2 diabetes mellitus. *Am Fam Physician.* 2011;84(2):183-190.

Powers AC. Diabetes mellitus: diagnosis, classification, and pathophysiology. In: Kasper D, Fauci A, Hauser S, et al., eds. *Harrison's Principles of Internal Medicine.* 19th ed. New York, NY: McGraw-Hill Education; 2015. Available at: http://accessmedicine.mhmedical.com. Accessed May 25, 2015.

Powers AC. Diabetes mellitus: management and therapies. In: Kasper D, Fauci A, Hauser S, et al., eds. *Harrison's Principles of Internal Medicine.* 19th ed. New York, NY: McGraw-Hill Education; 2015. Available at: http://accessmedicine.mhmedical.com. Accessed May 25, 2015.

Zoungas S, Chalmers J, Neal B, et al. Follow-up of blood-pressure lowering and glucose control in type 2 diabetes. *N Engl J Med.* 2014;371:1392-1406.

A 74-year-old African-American woman presents with the complaint that she has been developing nontraumatic bruises all over her extremities for the last several days. She has also noticed that her stools seem to be a lot darker, almost like "coffee grounds." She recently relocated to your area to live with her daughter. While this is her initial visit to your office, she has had refills available for all of her current medications and previously been at her baseline state of health. Her past medical history is significant for hypertension, postmenopausal state, an irregular heartbeat that she doesn't remember the exact name for, arthritis, and "a touch of diabetes." Her prescribed medications include hydrochlorothiazide and warfarin. Her over-the-counter medications include aspirin which she started taking since moving to your city, a multivitamin, acetaminophen for her arthritis, and ibuprofen for when her knees really bother her. She also admits to regularly drinking herbal teas.

▶ What is the differential diagnosis for this patient's presentation?
▶ What diagnostic studies are indicated?
▶ Why are the elderly at an increased risk for the development of adverse drug reactions?

ANSWERS TO CASE 52:
Adverse Drug Reactions and Interactions

Summary: A 74-year-old woman presents with easy bruising and dark stools for several days. She is new to your practice, and takes an antihypertensive medication and an anti-coagulant. She is also taking numerous over-the-counter medications.

- **Differential diagnosis:** Includes an adverse drug interaction involving warfarin and aspirin, nonsteroidal anti-inflammatory drugs (NSAIDs), and acetaminophen. Other (much less likely) possibilities include bleeding from a gastrointestinal malignancy, liver disease, or hematologic abnormality (eg, acute leukemia or severe thrombocytopenia).

- **Necessary diagnostic studies:** This patient should have a guaiac-based test for occult blood in the stool conducted in the office, a STAT complete blood count (CBC), a prothrombin time (PT) with international normalized ratio (INR), a comprehensive metabolic panel, and an electrocardiography (ECG). It would be appropriate to consider this patient for observation status in the hospital while her studies are pending if she is orthostatic, or if other signs suggest blood or volume loss that could predispose her to syncope.

- **Reasons for increased risk of drug reactions in the elderly:** Polypharmacy, decline in renal and hepatic function, and pharmacodynamic considerations including change in body composition and volume of distribution that develop with normal aging.

ANALYSIS

Objectives

1. Understand the scope and risk of the problem of drug interactions and adverse effects.

2. Learn strategies to reduce the risks of adverse drug interactions.

3. Know why the elderly are particularly vulnerable to potential adverse drug reactions.

Considerations

The extensive use of multiple medications, or polypharmacy—including prescribed, over-the-counter, herbal, and homeopathic products—makes adverse drug reactions and interactions a significant public health concern. Approximately 40% of people age 60 and older take at least five medications daily, and will experience an average of one adverse drug event each year and two-thirds of these patients will require medical attention because of it. Approximately **6.5% of hospital patients experience a documented adverse event secondary to medications.** Physiologic changes and the use of multiple medications simultaneously for multiple medical conditions place aging individuals and the elderly at increased risk of adverse events and drug-drug interactions. **An estimated 3% to 11% of hospital admissions in the elderly are related to adverse drug reactions.**

The patient presented above has numerous risks for the development of adverse events related to her various medications. In addition to her age, the use of warfarin is another risk, as its use should be closely monitored via serial PT/INR measurements. Warfarin also has numerous drug-drug interactions, including an increased risk of bleeding and bruising with the concomitant use of aspirin, NSAIDs, and/or acetaminophen.

Due to her age, the presence of bruising (suggesting an increased PT/INR), and the possibility of melena or hematochezia, this patient should have a fecal occult blood test (FOBT) performed and she should be screened for anemia with a CBC with platelet count. A negative FOBT test does not rule out lower gastrointestinal malignancy, thus if suspicion is high, she should undergo additional testing including colonoscopy. Due to her age and comorbid conditions, she should have a comprehensive metabolic panel to evaluate her glucose, electrolytes, and renal and liver functions, and an ECG to evaluate for signs of ischemia. With the possibility of significant abnormalities on these tests that may require urgent management, it would be reasonable to place her in observation status in the hospital for monitoring and treatment.

If she is found to have a prolonged PT/INR, several therapeutic options are available, depending on the clinical situation and the magnitude of the abnormality. For over-anti-coagulated patients with mildly elevated INR values (eg, 3-4) without evidence of bleeding, temporary discontinuation of warfarin or dose reduction is sufficient. For more elevated INR values in the setting of acute bleeding or spontaneous bruising, oral vitamin K along with stopping the warfarin will correct most abnormalities within a few days. When the INR value is very high (eg, >10), or if there is evidence of acute bleeding and hemodynamic compromise, then intravenous vitamin K and replacement of coagulation factors with a transfusion of fresh-frozen plasma (FFP) will rapidly reverse the coagulopathy.

APPROACH TO:
Adverse Drug Reactions and Interactions

DEFINITION

BEERS LIST: The Beers criteria for potentially inappropriate medication use in older adults (commonly referred to as the *Beers list*) is a guideline for healthcare providers to improve the safety in medication prescribing for older adults, to minimize unnecessary medications, and to minimize polypharmacy and drug interactions.

CYTOCHROME P450 (CYP): An enzyme system found mostly in the liver (but also in the small intestine, lungs, and kidneys) that is composed of more than 50 isoenzymes, and which is responsible for the metabolism of numerous medications. The **CYP isoenzymes can be induced**, resulting in increased drug metabolism and reduced therapeutic benefit of a medication, **or blocked**, resulting in decreased drug metabolism and potential for drug toxicity.

STOPP and START TOOLS: The Screening Tool of Older People's Prescriptions (STOPP) and Screening Tool to Alert to Right Treatment (START) are lists of potentially inappropriate and interactive medications with therapeutic alternatives.

CLINICAL APPROACH

Etiologies of Adverse Drug Effects

Adverse drug effects (ADEs) are defined as any effects experienced beyond the intended therapeutic scope of the drug that have a negative impact on the patient. Adverse drug effects can range from minor symptoms such as nausea or diarrhea, to severe or life threatening including cardiac arrhythmias precipitated by antiarrhythmic or stimulant medications. Other side effects of medications have been found to be beneficial. For example, peripheral α-adrenergic blockers, initially used as antihypertensives, have been found to minimize lower urinary tract obstructive symptoms from benign prostatic hyperplasia and is the most efficacious therapy for this condition. Another example is minoxidil, also an antihypertensive agent, which was found by some users to result in hair growth, so it is now marketed as a treatment for hair loss.

Drug interactions account for 5% to 10% of adverse reactions. Drug interactions may be caused by pharmacokinetic effects, resulting in a change in either the drug's concentration or the drug's effect. Some of these interactions may be predictable, as a consequence of chemical effects secondary to enzymatic effects, protein binding, renal or hepatic interactions, and pharmacodynamic interactions. For example, warfarin may interact with several other medications and dietary factors to increase the active form of this drug to toxic levels, resulting in over-anticoagulation with resultant bruising and hemorrhage.

Drugs also may have additive or synergistic effects caused by using two or more agents designed to produce a desired effect (eg, lowering blood pressure), yet they produce an effect greater than anticipated. An example of this is using a β-adrenergic blocking agent with certain calcium channel blockers (eg, diltiazem, verapamil). Both medications can decrease heart rate, but by different mechanisms of action. Combining the two agents may result in profound bradycardia and hypotension.

Other **interactions may be more directly related to the chemical properties** of the medications or the solutions in which they are delivered. For example, mixing glargine insulin with other insulin types in the same syringe may result in precipitation of the insulin product, rendering them ineffective. Similarly, some intravenous medications must be administered individually to avoid precipitation and potentiation, while others can be combined.

To avoid misuse of medications in the elderly, and to identify high-risk medications, an expert consensus panel developed a widely used list of medications that should be avoided, called the **Beers criteria.** Many of these medications are sedating or have anticholinergic effects that increase the risk of falls. Others have narrow therapeutic indexes, increasing the risk of developing toxic serum levels. **The STOPP/START criteria** have been used to detect adverse drug effects that are either causal or contributory to acute hospitalization in older people at a rate 2.8 times more frequently than compared to Beers criteria. It is imperative that clinicians are aware of equally effective therapeutic alternatives. If a patient is already on these medications, lowering the dose to the minimum effective dose is another way of minimizing risk. To date, there is no effective evidence that use of the Beers criteria, or the START/STOPP criteria reduce morbidity, mortality, or health-care costs.

Drug Metabolism

Medications with a high first-pass hepatic clearance may be particularly susceptible to adverse events caused by alterations in hepatic metabolism. Diseases that change the effective circulatory volume, including congestive heart failure, may also alter the rate of drug or metabolite elimination due to the effects on hepatic and renal blood flow.

The **CYP cytochrome system** plays a significant role in many real or potential adverse drug events. Although more than 50 CYP isoenzymes have been identified, six of these isoenzymes metabolize 90% of drugs. Alcohol has effects on the 2E1 isoenzyme, which can produce a hepatotoxic metabolite of acetaminophen. Because of this, the chronic use of alcohol and acetaminophen can induce liver damage, and an acetaminophen overdose, which is already potentially toxic to the liver, has worse outcomes when the patient has been drinking alcohol.

Grapefruit has a substantial impact on the cytochrome P450 3A4 system. Medications that have been found to interact with grapefruit include statins, anti-arrhythmic agents, immunosuppressants, and calcium channel blockers. Expert opinion posits that patients should refrain from grapefruit for 72 hours prior to taking medications that may interact with it, or to avoid it altogether if a patient takes one of these drug classes chronically.

Drugs that have a significant first-pass effect may have an effect on metabolism in the liver or absorption in the intestine. For example, increased levels of the 3A isoenzyme may result in alterations in the level, and therefore therapeutic effect, of cyclosporine.

Many drugs are bound to serum albumin. When multiple agents are competing for the same albumin-binding sites, there is a potential to have greater amounts of unbound medication, resulting in higher circulating free drug levels. This causes particular concern for drugs that have a smaller volume of distribution, rapid onset of action, or narrow therapeutic index.

Renal considerations are related to interaction of drugs at renal sites and decreased renal function. Renal interactions are often a result of alterations in the elimination of water-soluble drugs because of competition for the renal tubular system. These effects may be either positive or negative. An example of a beneficial effect is the concomitant administration of probenecid with penicillin. Probenecid decreases renal excretion of penicillin, resulting in an increased level and therapeutic effect of the antibiotic.

Other renal considerations include decreased kidney function secondary to either disease processes, such as hypertension or diabetes mellitus, chronic kidney disease, or from the natural decline in renal function that occurs with aging.

Many medications have recommendations for alteration in dosing amount and/or interval based on the patient's creatinine clearance. Creatinine is a byproduct of muscle metabolism and older patients may have falsely elevated calculated creatinine clearance rates because they have decreased muscle mass. Creatinine clearance is calculated using the following equation:

$$\text{Creatinine clearance} = \frac{[(140 - \text{age}) \times (\text{ideal body weight in kg})] \times (0.85 \text{ for women})}{72 \times \text{serum creatinine (mg/dL)}}$$

Interventions to Reduce the Risk of Adverse Drug Events

There are many possible interventions to reduce the risk of adverse drug events or interactions, especially in the older population, including the following:

- Always use the Beers criteria or STOPP/START criteria when considering medications in the elderly.

- Only prescribe medications that are clearly indicated, yet do not avoid a necessary medication.

- When a patient presents with a new complaint, consider the potential for ADEs in the differential.

- Obtain a history of adverse drug events related to previous and current medications on all patients.

- Maintain a current list of all medications that a patient is taking, including prescribed, over-the-counter, herbal, and homeopathic. Perform medication reconciliation at every visit.

- **Instruct your patients to bring in all of their medications regularly to make sure your medication list is accurate.**

- Routinely perform drug interaction surveys on patients taking multiple medications. Consider working with pharmacists and using computerized tools available to perform these surveys. Consider rational reductions and discontinuation of medication in elderly patients after consultation with the patient, family, and pharmacists.

- Have knowledge of renal, hepatic, and circulatory issues that affect your patients.

- Consider issues related to individual patients, such as unique genetic or ethnic factors.

- Document and report suspected all ADEs.

COMPREHENSION QUESTIONS

52.1 A 62-year-old man with hypertension, hypercholesterolemia, and benign prostatic hypertrophy (BPH) presents to his physician with increasing muscle aches in his thighs and shoulders and complains of dark, tea-colored urine. These symptoms started about 10 days ago. He has been drinking plenty of fluids as part of a new diet, specifically grapefruit juice. On routine laboratory evaluation, his serum transaminases are elevated to nearly three times the normal limit, serum creatinine is 1.4 mg/dL (baseline 1.2 mg/dL), and urinalysis reveals 1+ proteinuria. His only medications are lisinopril, simvastatin, and a baby aspirin. Which of the following is the most likely diagnosis in this patient?

A. Drug-induced hepatitis from long-term simvastatin

B. Postrenal azotemia and proteinuria due to BPH

C. Acute kidney injury secondary to aspirin and lisinopril

D. Hepatic enzyme inhibition leading to elevated circulating drug levels

52.2 A 73-year-old man has diabetes mellitus, coronary heart disease, stage 3 chronic kidney disease, and chronic obstructive pulmonary disease (COPD). He has newly diagnosed atrial fibrillation and meets criteria for anticoagulation with warfarin. His current medications include metformin, glipizide, losartan, metoprolol, and ipratropium. Which of the following is the most important consideration in avoiding adverse drug reactions in the elderly?

A. Increased glomerular filtration rate

B. Polypharmacy

C. Increased cardiac stroke volume

D. Increased hepatic blood flow

E. Age and functional status

52.3 A 36-year-old woman presents to your office after appearing very distressed after having a positive pregnancy test. She says that she has taken her oral contraceptive pills (OCPs) consistently at the same time every day for the past year. She has no significant past medical history except for mild depression. The only medication she takes is a prescribed OCP, but admits that she also take vitamins and herbal supplements. Which of the following additional information would be most helpful in discovering why her OCP may have failed?

A. Which OCP she is taking

B. Which herbal supplements she is taking

C. Her number of sexual partners

D. If she has ever been pregnant before

E. What time of day she takes her OCP

ANSWERS

52.1 **D.** Grapefruit juice inhibits the cytochrome P450 3A4 system that metabolizes simvastatin. This patient has rhabdomyolysis from increased circulating levels of simvastatin. Simvastatin may increase transaminases, but associated cases of hepatitis and liver failure are very rare. The combination of aspirin and lisinopril has not been shown to cause acute kidney injury; a creatinine level of 0.2 mg/dL above baseline levels does not confer acute kidney injury. Moderate proteinuria and a mild elevation in serum creatinine do not constitute postrenal azotemia and proteinuria due to BPH in this patient.

52.2 **B.** A multitude of factors result in the elderly being particularly vulnerable to adverse drug events. Included among these are polypharmacy, decreased renal and hepatic function, decreased cardiac output, and pharmacokinetic and pharmacodynamic considerations.

52.3 **B.** Asking which herbal supplements a patient takes is imperative. St. John's wort, a common herbal antidepressant, can induce CYP3A4 and CYP3A5 causing increased metabolism of estradiol and lowering efficacy of OCPs.

CLINICAL PEARLS

▶ Along with the biochemical changes that occur with aging, several physical conditions may also affect medication compliance. Arthritic patients may have difficulty opening prescription caps (especially childproof caps). Reduced vision may interfere with the ability to properly use a medication. Memory difficulties may cause trouble adhering to regimens involving multiple medications. All of these factors, and many others, need to be considered when prescribing medications to the elderly.

▶ In elderly patients with new symptoms, consider adverse drug events highly in your differential.

▶ Many practices have pharmacists as a component of the patient-centered medical home (PCMH) model of health care. Pharmacists can be invaluable members of the patient care team in reviewing medications, herbal supplements, vitamins, and potential interactions.

REFERENCES

American Geriatrics Society 2012 Beers Criteria Update Expert Panel. American Geriatrics Society updated Beers Criteria for potentially inappropriate medication use in older adults. *J Am Geriatr Soc.* 2012;60(4):616-631.

Blanco-Reina E, Ariza-Zafra G, Ocana-Riola R, Leon-Ortiz M. 2012 American Geriatrics Society Beers criteria: enhanced applicability for detecting potentially inappropriate medications in European older adults. A comparison with the Screening Tool of Older Person's Potentially Inappropriate Prescriptions. *J Am Geriatr Soc.* 2014;62(7):1217-1223.

Gallagher P, Ryan C, Byrne S, Kennedy J, O'Mahony D. STOPP (Screening Tool of Older Person's Prescriptions) and START (Screening Tool to Alert doctors to Right Treatment). Consensus validation. *Int J Clin Pharmacol Ther.* 2008;46(2):72.

Hamilton H, Gallagher P, Ryan C, et al. Potentially inappropriate medications defined by STOPP criteria and the risk of adverse drug events in older hospitalized patients. *Arch Intern Med.* 2011;171(11):1013-1019.

Hill-Taylor B, Sketris I, Hayden J, et al. Application of the STOPP/START criteria: a systematic review of the prevalence of potentially inappropriate prescribing in older adults, and evidence of clinical, humanistic and economic impact. *J Clin Pharm Ther.* 2013;38(5):360-372.

Lynch T, Price M. The effect of cytochrome P450 metabolism on drug response, interactions, and adverse effects. *Am Fam Physician.* 2007;76:391-396.

Oates JA. The science of drug therapy. In: Brunton LL, ed. *Goodman and Gillman's the Pharmacological Basis of Therapeutics.* 11th ed. New York, NY: McGraw-Hill Education; 2006:117-136.

O'Mahoney D, O'Sullivan D, Byrne S, et al. STOPP/START criteria for potentially inappropriate prescribing in older people: version 2. *Age Ageing.* 2015;44(2):213-218.

Pretorius RW, Gataric G, Swedlund SK, Miller JR. Reducing the risk of adverse drug events in older adults. *Am Fam Physician.* 2013;87(5):331-336.

Steinman MA, Hanlon JT. Managing medications in clinically complex elders: "There's got to be a happy medium." *JAMA.* 2010;304(14):1592.

Stump AL, Mayo T, Blum A. Management of grapefruit-drug interactions. *Am Fam Physician.* 2006;74(4):605-608.

WEBSITE RESOURCES

The **BEERS criteria** can be found at: www.americangeriatrics.org/files/documents/beers/2012AGSBeersCriteriaCitations.pdf

The **STOPP criteria** can be found at: www.biomedcentral.com/content/supplementary/1471-2318-9-5-S1.doc

The **START tool** can be found at: www.ageing.oxfordjournals.org/content/36/6/632.full.pdf

A previously healthy 48-year-old accountant presents to his primary care office with severe low back pain that began the previous day after he helped his daughter move into her college dorm. He denies any trauma or previous back injury. He describes the pain as generally "achy," and sometimes characterized as being "sharp" when he moves suddenly. The pain is located in his lower back and radiates down the back of both legs to the middle of his posterior thighs. He has been continent of both bowel and bladder and denies any weakness in his legs. He denies fever, chills, weight loss, or malaise. He finds it very difficult to stand for prolonged periods of time because he can't find a comfort position. He states that this is the worst back pain he has ever experienced, and it has not been relieved with acetaminophen or ibuprofen. His past medical history is significant for hypertension; his only medications are metoprolol and a baby aspirin daily. He does not smoke or use illicit drugs, and only drinks alcohol on occasion. On physical examination, he is well-developed, overweight, and in moderate discomfort. On neuromuscular examination, he has moderate tenderness bilaterally in his lumbar paraspinous muscles, and his lumbar flexion and extension are limited by pain. Strength and sensation are within normal limits and equal and symmetrical bilaterally, as are his deep tendon knee and ankle reflexes. Straight leg raise testing is negative bilaterally and gait is within normal limits.

▶ What is the most likely diagnosis?
▶ What is the most appropriate workup?
▶ What is the best treatment plan?

ANSWERS TO CASE 53:

Acute Low Back Pain

Summary: A previously healthy 48-year-old man presents with acute onset of low back pain after strenuous activity. His neurologic examination is unremarkable and he denies any systemic complaints.

- **Most likely diagnosis:** Acute low back pain, lumbosacral strain.

- **Workup:** No formal workup is required unless symptoms persist after conservative treatment for at least 1 month.

- **Treatment:** Rest, nonsteroidal anti-inflammatory drugs (NSAIDs), and muscle relaxants.

ANALYSIS

Objectives

1. Develop a differential diagnosis for acute low back pain and explore it with the history and physical.

2. Learn the "red flag" symptoms of low back pain and how to investigate them.

3. Learn the effective treatments for musculoskeletal back pain.

Considerations

Acute low back pain is one of the most common reasons for a visit to the doctor in the United States. While approximately 85% of patients who present with isolated low back pain will never be given a specific anatomic reason for the pain, over 90% of patients will fully recover within 2 weeks of symptom onset.

Since the differential diagnosis of low back pain is broad, the role of the clinician is to determine if the pain is caused by a systemic disease, if it is associated with neurologic compromise, and to consider psychosocial factors that may lead to chronic back pain and complicate the recovery or efficacy of treatment.

This patient's history includes pertinent positive findings of being overweight and a recent history of repetitive lifting and twisting that are associated with lumbosacral strain. His signs, symptoms, and physical examination are all consistent with a localized musculoskeletal condition. His age and lack of systemic symptoms are pertinent negative findings. He is not depressed and denies a history of substance abuse. This clinical scenario is best managed by symptomatic therapies for 4 to 6 weeks, without imaging, with close follow-up in 1 month if symptoms do not resolve. Education in proper lifting techniques and exercise therapy to improve core and back strength and flexibility may help to prevent future strain and injury.

APPROACH TO:
Low Back Pain

DEFINITIONS

HERNIATED DISC: Rupture of the fibrocartilage between the vertebrae leading to leakage of the nucleus pulposus that may impinge on the nerve roots causing pain.

SCIATICA: A sharp or burning pain that radiates along the path of the sciatic nerve (L4-S2) usually caused by a herniated disk of the lumbar region of the spine, which typically radiates to the buttocks and to the posterior thigh.

CLINICAL APPROACH

Acute low back pain should be evaluated in a systematic manner to avoid missing important "red flag" symptoms (Table 53–1) and unnecessary imaging, treatments, or referrals. The first step is to generate a differential diagnosis (Table 53–2) and to understand the common signs and symptoms of its components.

History, Physical, and Evaluation

The history in the patient presenting with acute low back pain must triage minor back conditions from those requiring urgent evaluation via a methodologic and consistently sound approach. Patients presenting with **cauda equina syndrome** have increasing neurologic deficits and leg weakness, bowel and/or urinary incontinence, anesthesia or paresthesia in a saddle distribution, and bilateral sciatica. Physical findings include pain elicited by straight leg raise test, reduction in anal sphincter tone, and decreased bilateral ankle reflexes. These patients require immediate evaluation with lumbosacral magnetic resonance imaging (MRI), corticosteroids to

Table 53–1 • RED FLAG SYMPTOMS IN LOW BACK PAIN
Unrelenting night pain
Unrelenting pain at rest
Neuromotor deficit
Unexplained fever
Greater than 6 weeks duration
Age >70
Loss of bowel or bladder control
Progressive focal neurologic deficits
Suspicion of ankylosing spondylitis
Trauma
History or suspicion of cancer
Osteoporosis
Chronic corticosteroid use
Immunosuppression
Alcohol abuse
Intravenous drug use

Table 53–2 • DIFFERENTIAL DIAGNOSIS OF LOW BACK PAIN

Condition (prevalence)

Mechanical low back pain (~97%)
- Lumbar strain, sprain (70%)
- Degenerative facets or disks (10%)
- Herniated disk (4%)
- Compression fracture (4%)
- Spinal stenosis (3%)
- Spondylolisthesis (2%)
- Spondylolysis (<1%)

Nonmechanical spinal conditions (1%)
- Cancer (primary or metastatic) (0.7%)
- Inflammatory arthritis (0.3%)
- Infection (0.01%)

Visceral disease (2%)
- Pelvic organs: prostatitis, PID, endometriosis
- Renal disease: nephrolithiasis, pyelonephritis, perinephric abscess
- Aortic aneurysm
- Gastrointestinal disease: pancreatitis, cholecystitis, peptic ulcer

Abbreviation: PID, pelvic inflammatory disease.
Data from Kinkade S. Evaluation and treatment of acute low back pain. Am Fam Physician. 2008;75:1181-1188, 1190-1192; Deyo RA, Weinstein JN. Low back pain. N Engl J Med. 2001;344(5):363-370.

decrease pain and inflammation, and commonly immediate surgical decompression of the entrapped cauda equina to prevent further neurologic deterioration.

Fevers, point tenderness directly over the vertebrae, recent infections, and a history of intravenous drug use can point toward an **infectious** process like osteomyelitis, septic discitis, paraspinous abscess, or epidural abscess. These infections should be promptly considered and evaluated by complete blood count (CBC), erythrocyte sedimentation rate (ESR), cultures from blood and abscess contents, cerebral spinal fluid (CSF), and MRI and require long courses of intravenous antibiotics and sometimes surgical drainage. An underlying **cancer** is much more likely if the patient has a history of cancer with a likelihood of metastasis to bone (eg, prostate, hematologic, breast, lung), unexplained weight loss, worsening pain at night, failure to improve after 1 month of conservative therapy, or an age greater than 50. To further evaluate patients with these risk factors, a CBC, ESR, and plain radiographs of the lumbar sacral spine should be obtained initially. Abnormalities in these tests should be further evaluated by MRI and/or a bone scan.

The history should also help to differentiate less urgent but important causes of low back pain. Sciatica is the classic sign of a **herniated disc.** It is typically characterized by a sharp or burning back pain that radiates down the back and side of the leg and distal to the knee. It improves on lying down and increases with Valsalva maneuver, sneezing, or coughing. Additional symptoms of radiculopathy may include anesthesia, dysesthesia, hyperesthesia, and paresthesia that are confined to a specific lumbosacral dermatome. Sciatica can be examined by performing both a straight leg raise test (91% sensitive, 26% specific) and a contralateral leg raise test (29% sensitive, 88% specific), along with sensory, strength, and reflex testing of the lower extremities (L4—knee strength and reflex; L5—great toe and foot dorsiflexion; and S1—plantar flexion and ankle reflexes). Greater than 90% of lumbar disc compression of nerve roots occurs at L4-L5 and L5-S1. MRI is not recommended for patients with sciatica unless the symptoms last for more than 1 month or if the patient is not a candidate for an epidural corticosteroid injection or surgical intervention.

Conservative treatment for sciatica involves anti-inflammatories including NSAIDs or acetaminophen, muscle relaxants including cyclobenzaprine, possibly short-course oral corticosteroids, and activity modifications. Given the lack of proven efficacy and potential adverse drug reactions, opioid use is generally reserved for patients who have severe pain and who have exhausted nonnarcotic treatment options. Physical therapy may be appropriate for individuals with persistent moderate symptoms of 3 weeks or more, since the majority of the patients are likely to experience spontaneous improvement in the first 2 weeks. Surgical options may be considered in those who suffer from disabling radicular pain of 6 weeks or more or with progressive neuropathic deficits.

Spinal stenosis is a congenital or acquired condition of spinal canal narrowing with or without concomitant facet hypertrophy that exerts pressure on the spinal cord and nerve roots. **Degenerative arthritis and spondylolisthesis are the most common acquired causes of lumbar spinal stenosis.** Congenital causes include dwarfism, spina bifida, and myelomeningocele. It presents as lower back and leg pain, leg weakness, and pseudoclaudication that occurs after walking various distances, while the vascularity of the legs remains uncompromised. The majority of patients with spinal stenosis are symptomatic only when engaged in activities. Pain is often relieved by sitting, performing lumbar flexion (bending over), squatting, or a laying down. It is more common in patients over 60 and its rules of evaluation are the same as for a herniated disc. Spinal stenosis is initially treated with NSAIDs and muscle relaxants, physical therapy, and epidural corticosteroid injections. Surgical therapy is reserved for patients who have failed conservative treatment or those with progressive neurologic deficits.

Vertebral compression fractures are more common in older people and those with osteoporosis or chronic corticosteroid use. These commonly occur after low-impact trauma or with no trauma history at all. Patients typically present with acute onset of back pain after certain sudden movements such as lifting, bending, or coughing. The pain often follows the distribution of the contiguous nerve and radiates bilaterally into the anterior abdomen or pelvis, also known as the "girdle of pain." The fractures are generally well localized to the thoracolumbar segment (T12-L2) of the spine. Vertebral compression fractures are best initially evaluated by plain film radiographs of the thoracolumbar spine. They can be treated medically with pain control, physical therapy, and with calcitonin and bisphosphonates, as well as treatment of the underlying osteoporosis. Spinal bracing and surgical management with balloon kyphoplasty can be considered and may have better outcomes than medical management in those with severe pain.

Psychosocial factors and emotional distress should also be evaluated in the patient with low back pain. Depression, fear avoidance (fear that activity will cause permanent damage), job dissatisfaction, current involvement in litigation, reliance on passive treatments, or somatization are predictors of slow recovery and increase the risk for developing chronic low back pain. Acknowledgement and management that includes treatment of such factors as applicable may be effective adjuvant therapy.

The vast majority of patients seeking medical evaluation with back pain will be diagnosed with **lumbosacral strain.** The exact anatomic cause of the pain is often unknown, but it is often hypothesized that there may be an incomplete tear in the annulus fibrosus that may leak fluids creating local inflammation, or it may bulge posteriorly and irritate certain lumbar roots. Irritation of the surrounding muscles, tendons, ligaments, or the joint capsule may be concomitantly involved in this painful process.

Treatment of Acute Mechanical Back Pain

The treatment of acute mechanical back pain (<4 weeks) centers on the use of NSAIDs, acetaminophen, muscle relaxants, heat, and early mobility. No significant benefit has been observed with the use of opioids, systemic corticosteroids, or bed rest. Bed rest for any length of time has not been shown to improve pain and may lengthen the duration of pain and prolong recovery. For those with moderate-to-severe pain, combination therapy of a muscle relaxant and an NSAID may be more effective than monotherapy. Due to their sedative effects, muscle relaxants are typically recommended for nighttime dosing. In general, patients should be encouraged to resume normal daily activities as tolerated with reasonable restrictions on bending and lifting until the pain resolves. Specific exercises have not been proven to be beneficial in speeding recovery. Massage therapy and spinal manipulation may be of some benefit for acute pain; physical therapy has some benefit for short-term pain relief, but most studies do not show long-term benefit. Although acupuncture and yoga may be reasonable options for chronic back pain, their effectiveness in acute back pain remains unproven. Spinal traction has not been shown to be helpful for chronic back pain with or without sciatica. For prevention, exercise has been proven to help prevent first episodes of back pain and recurrences in certain subgroups of workers. Lumbar support braces have not been shown to prevent low back pain.

CASE CORRELATION

- See also Case 3 (Joint Pain).

COMPREHENSION QUESTIONS

53.1 A 45-year-old man with no significant past medical history presents with severe back pain after lifting heavy boxes at work 2 days ago. Other than his back pain, his review of symptoms is negative. The pain radiates from his lower back down his right posterior thigh to his great toe when you perform both a straight leg raise and the contralateral leg raise tests. His strength, sensation, and reflexes are intact and symmetrical. Which of the following imaging studies should be done first in the evaluation of this patient?

A. Plain radiographs

B. MRI

C. Computed tomography (CT) scan

D. No imaging indicated

E. Bone scan

53.2 A 58-year-old white woman presents complaining of low back pain for exactly 1 month after a fall. She has no history of fever, unexplained weight loss, diabetes, or cancer. Her past medical history is significant for mild persistent asthma and nicotine dependence. She had a hysterectomy for uterine fibroids at age 40. Which of the following characteristics should prompt further evaluation of her pain?

A. History of corticosteroid use

B. Caucasian ethnicity

C. Time course of back pain

D. History of cocaine use

E. Premenopausal age

53.3 A 67-year-old man with coronary artery disease, dyslipidemia, and eczema comes to you complaining of lower back pain and left leg pain. The pain is worse when he stands for long periods of time, but improves when he bends forward to push his shopping cart around the grocery store. He indicates that his feet "burn" and "ache" after walking different distances every day. His lower extremity neuromuscular examination is unremarkable. Which of the following is the most appropriate treatment for this patient?

A. Emergent spinal cord decompression

B. Epidural corticosteroid injection

C. Kyphoplasty

D. Bed rest for 4 days

E. Tramadol

ANSWERS

53.1 **D.** The patient has signs and symptoms of a herniated disc. There is no evidence that imaging within the first month has any morbidity benefit.

53.2 **A.** The patient's history is suspicious for a vertebral compression fracture that could be secondary to osteoporosis. Osteoporosis commonly develops in postmenopausal women, and can occur in patients who have received corticosteroid therapy. The time course of her pain is 4 weeks; 6 weeks and greater is a "red flag" symptom for further evaluation with radiographic imaging. While osteoporosis is more common in Caucasian women, it is not considered a "red flag." Postmenopausal women are at greater risk for osteoporosis rather than premenopausal women. Smoking and alcohol dependence are risk factors for osteoporosis; there is no evidence that cocaine use contributes to the development of osteoporosis.

53.3 **B.** The patient's history is classic for spinal stenosis. Often patients find relief by sitting or stooping. NSAIDs, physical therapy, and epidural corticosteroid injections are used to relieve pain. Surgical decompression is used in cauda equina syndrome, and kyphoplasty is useful in vertebral fractures. Bed rest is not used in the conservative treatment of back pain for any cause and has been shown to increase the duration of pain.

CLINICAL PEARLS

▶ "Red flag" symptoms in low back pain should prompt an immediate diagnostic workup.

▶ Cauda equina syndrome is a surgical emergency that should be evaluated immediately by MRI.

▶ A herniated disc can be treated conservatively for 4 weeks before radiographic imaging has any proven benefit.

▶ Lumbosacral strain is common, generally resolves within a few weeks, and is treated with NSAIDs and muscle relaxants. Bed rest likely provides no significant benefit and may prolong pain and slow recovery.

REFERENCES

Balague F, Mannion AF, Pellise F, Cedraschi C. Non-specific low back pain. *Lancet*. 2012;379(9814): 482-491.

Casazza BA. Diagnosis and treatment of acute low back pain. *Am Fam Physician*. 2012;85(4):343-350.

Chou R, Huffman LH. Diagnosis and treatment of low back pain: a joint clinical practice guideline from the American College of Physicians and the American Pain Society. *Ann Intern Med*. 2007;147: 478-491.

Delitto A, George SZ, Van Dillen LR, et al. Low back pain: clinical practice guidelines linked to the International Classification of Functioning, Disability, and Health from the Orthopaedic Section of the American Physical Therapy Association. *J Orthop Sports Phys Ther*. 2012;42(4):A1-A57.

Kamper SJ, Apeldoorn AT, Chiarotto A, et al. Multidisciplinary biopsychosocial rehabilitation for chronic low back pain: Cochrane systematic review and meta-analysis. *BMJ*. 2015;350h444.

Klineberg E, Mazanec D, Orr D, Demicco R, Bell G, McLain R. Masquerade: medical causes of back pain. *Cleve Clin J Med*. 2007;74(12):905.

Last AR, Hulbert K. Chronic low back pain: evaluation and management. *Am Fam Physician*. 2009;79(12):1067-1074.

Lemeunier N, Leboeuf-Yde C, Gagey O. The natural course of low back pain: a systematic critical literature review. *Chiropr Man Therap*. 2012;20(1):33.

An 18-month-old male child is brought to your office by his mother for a routine well-child examination. This is his first visit to your office, as he has been seen for regular well-child examinations at another clinic since his birth. The child is the product of a spontaneous vaginal delivery at term without complications. His personal and family medical histories are unremarkable and his immunizations are up-to-date. He has one older sister of age 6, who is in the first grade, with normal growth and development. The child lives at home with both biological parents and his sister. There are no pets in the home and no one smokes. Overall, he eats a well-balanced diet, although mom reports he is sometimes a picky eater.

The child's mother notes that she is concerned about his development because he still does not speak single words and only babbles, and her other child was using many words by this age. On further history, you discover that he often disregards the calling of his name, but does startle to loud noises. The child's mother has read about autism on the internet and is concerned that her son may have this diagnosis. She also states that because of her concern, if he needs any immunizations today, she does not want them to be given for fear that this might worsen her son's condition.

On physical examination, the patient is in the 50th percentile for height, and 75th percentile for weight and head circumference. His entire physical examination is unremarkable. On developmental screening, you observe that he walks and runs well, and mom reports that he can walk up steps and kick a ball forward. During the examination, he only babbles and utters no discrete words. When given a toy car, he puts it in his mouth, but never demonstrates rolling the car along the floor. When you call the child's name, tap him on the shoulder, say "Look!" and point to a toy in the corner, you are unable to get his attention.

► By what age should an infant use single words?
► What is your next step in the evaluation of this patient?
► Should immunizations be delayed in this patient?

ANSWERS TO CASE 54:
Developmental Disorders

Summary: An 18-month-old child is brought in for a routine well-child examination and found to have a delay in language and social skill development.

- **Age by which a child should use single words:** Most children will say "mama/dada" indiscriminately by 9 months and use two words other than "mama/dada" by 12 months. No single identifiable words by 16 months are a red flag for the presence of an autism spectrum disorder (ASD).

- **Next step in evaluation of this patient:** Your screening of this patient notes developmental delays concerning for an ASD. You should complete your screening of this patient with a level 1 standardized autism-specific screening tool, such as the Screening Tool for Autism in Toddlers and Young Children (STAT). Due to the concerns noted on examination, you should refer the patient for a comprehensive ASD evaluation, early intervention/early childhood education services, and an audiology evaluation.

- **Timing of immunizations:** Despite current controversy, there is no evidence that immunizations are implicated as a cause of autism, thus the parents should be counseled that the routine immunizations are recommended. Many concerns have been raised that the measles-mumps-rubella (MMR) vaccine may precipitate autism, based on reports of parents who first detected autism in their children following MMR vaccination and a study of 12 autistic patients in which their physicians reported similar suspicions, which has since been retracted for falsification of methods. Subsequent studies have failed to show any evidence of a link between MMR vaccination and the development of autism. To date, there is no evidence to support that the use of thimerosal (a mercury-containing preservative) in vaccines causes autism.

ANALYSIS

Objectives

1. Learn the diagnostic criteria for autism spectrum disorders and the differential diagnosis of pervasive developmental disorder.

2. Know the key clinical signs of ASDs.

3. Be able to formulate a strategy for the assessment and management of ASDs.

Considerations

This 18-month-old child presents with significant language delay and social skills delay. These two findings are highly suspicious for ASD, therefore he should promptly undergo a comprehensive autism assessment. There is no description of stereotyped movement or findings, yet these are not necessary for the diagnosis of ASD. However, this child should also undergo a formalized audiology evaluation. Since he startles to loud noises, a significant hearing deficit is not likely.

APPROACH TO:
Pervasive Developmental Disorders

DEFINITIONS

JOINT ATTENTION: An infant demonstrates enjoyment in sharing with another individual an object/event by looking back and forth between the individual and the object/event.

SOCIAL RELATEDNESS: Internal drive to connect with others and share similar feelings.

CLINICAL APPROACH

ASDs include three of the pervasive developmental disorders identified in the DSM-IV and include autistic disorder (AD), Asperger syndrome (AS), and pervasive developmental disorder not otherwise specified (PDD-NOS).

In March 2014, the Centers for Disease Control and Prevention (CDC) released data on **the prevalence of ASD** in the United States, estimating **1 in 68 children—1 in 42 boys and 1 in 189 girls.** Family studies also estimate a recurrence risk of as much as 5% to 6% when there is an older sibling with an ASD.

As evidenced by prevalence statistics, most physicians will care for several children with an ASD during the course of their career. Furthermore, as a result of increased media attention intended to raise awareness about these disorders and the early signs, more and more parents will begin to raise concerns to their child's physician. Primary care physicians must be able to recognize the key clinical features of these disorders, to formulate a systematic plan to assess them, and to know how to assist families with the ongoing treatment and care of a child with an ASD.

ASDs are phenotypically heterogenous neurodevelopmental disorders that are the result of a combination of environmental and genetic factors. Evidence supports multiple gene involvement with environmental factors influencing the wide variation in phenotypic expression. Environmental factors implicated include exposures to teratogens in utero and maternal illnesses during pregnancy, but no studies have verified a causal role.

Common features shared by all ASDs include severe deficits in social skills and limited, repetitive, and stereotyped behavior patterns. However, only AS and PDD-NOS are characterized by significant language delays.

Although there is no pathognomonic feature, ASDs are universally characterized by deficits in social relatedness, and the early social deficits, such as delayed or absent joint attention appear to be reliable red flag symptoms. However, these characteristics frequently go unnoticed by parents and it is commonly a delay in speech that prompts them to raise a concern with their child's physician.

In order to diagnose ASD, a child must demonstrate abnormal behavior before age 3 and must have delays in the areas of social interaction, language used for social communication, and symbolic or imaginative play. Deficits include the following:

1. **Impaired social interaction:**

   a. Deficient use of nonverbal behaviors such as facial expressions, eye contact, and gestures

   b. Lack of peer relationships appropriate to developmental age

   c Does not spontaneously seek social relatedness through shared emotions, interests, or achievements with others

2. **Impaired communication:**

   a. Delay in/lack of spoken language development.

   b. If the child does have adequate speech, there is an impaired ability to sustain or begin a conversation with others.

   c. Repetitious, scripted, or stereotyped use of language.

   d. Lack of or severely delayed pretend play skills.

3. **Restricted, repetitive, and stereotyped patterns of behavior, interests, and activities:**

   a. Repetitive, nonfunctional, atypical behaviors such as hand flapping, finger movements, rocking, and twirling

   b. Restricted patterns of interest that is atypical in either intensity or focus

   c. Inflexible adherence to nonfunctional rituals

   d. Preoccupations with parts of objects

Children with AS may go unnoticed until they are school age and begin to demonstrate difficulties with peer and teacher interactions. Children with AS have only mild or limited speech delay, but if observed closely their language has often developed atypically. These children show deficits in the use of social language, such as choosing a topic of conversation, tempo, facial expression, or body language. Speech is also often pedantic and limited to only a few topics that hold an all-consuming interest to the child.

Neurogenetic comorbid conditions and mental retardation have also been found to be associated with ASDs, although the most recent data indicate the percentages to be much less than previously thought, estimated at 10% and 50%, respectively. Neurogenetic syndromes that may play a causative role in ASDs or otherwise may be associated, as well as other PDDs, must be considered in a clinician's differential diagnosis (Table 54–1).

Management

The key to successful management of ASDs is early diagnosis leading to early intervention. **Surveillance for ASDs should occur at every preventive visit throughout**

Table 54-1 • NEURODEVELOPMENTAL CONDITIONS ASSOCIATED WITH ASDs		
Condition	Etiology	Characteristics
Rett syndrome	X-linked dominant disorder (fatal to male fetus)	Microcephaly, seizures, and hand-wringing stereotypies
Childhood disintegrative disorder	Unknown	Normal development until 2-4 y, then severe deterioration of motor and social functioning
Fragile X syndrome	Most common genetic cause of AD and retardation in males	Mental retardation (MR), macrocephaly, large pinnae, large testicles, hypotonia, and hyperextensible joints
Neurocutaneous disorders Tuberous sclerosis Neurofibromatosis	*Autosomal dominant, half of cases are new mutations* Autosomal dominant, but most cases are new mutations	*Café-au-lait spots, axillary freckling, neurofibromas, ocular Lisch nodules* Hypopigmented macules, fibroangiomata, kidney lesions, CNS hamartomas, seizures, MR, ADHD
Phenylketonuria	Inborn error of metabolism	Routinely tested for by newborn screening; MR/AD preventable with dietary modification
Fetal alcohol syndrome	Exposure to alcohol in utero	Characteristic facies; associated with AD and other developmental disorders
Angelman syndrome	Loss of maternally expressed ubiquitin-protein ligase gene	Global developmental disorder, hypotonia in early childhood, wide-based ataxic gait, seizures, and progressive spasticity
Childhood schizophrenia	Unknown	Thought disorder, delusions, and hallucinations

childhood utilizing standard developmental screening tools. The Ages and Stages Questionnaires are common standardized tools that assess developmental milestones from 2 months through 6 years. This includes eliciting a family history of ASDs, parental and other caregiver concerns, developmental history, and making accurate observations of the child. All children should also be screened with the Modified Checklist for Autism in Toddlers (M-CHAT) at the 18- and 24-month visits. If concerns for an ASD are raised during well-child visits, then a screening tool specifically designed for ASDs should be used. Prior to 18 months, screening tools that target social and communication skills may be helpful for detecting early signs of ASDs.

Red flag symptoms indicating the need for immediate evaluation include the following:

- No babbling or pointing by 12 months

- No single words by 16 months

- No two-word phrases by 24 months

- Loss of language or social skills at any age

When a child demonstrates two or more risk factors or a positive screening result occurs, the clinician should take immediate action. The following steps should be accomplished simultaneously:

- Refer the child for a comprehensive ASD evaluation.

- Refer the child to early intervention/early childhood education services.

- Obtain an audiologic evaluation.

Children with ASDs who begin treatment at a younger age have significantly better outcomes, making early identification and intervention critical. The goals of treatment are to improve language and social skills, decrease maladaptive behaviors, support parents and families, and foster independence.

CASE CORRELATION

- See also Case 5 (Well-Child Care).

COMPREHENSION QUESTIONS

54.1 A mother brings her 5-year-old son to your office because his teacher is concerned that he has attention-deficit hyperactivity disorder (ADHD). The teacher has noticed that the child frequently makes long-winded speeches about boats in class and is often rocking back and forth in his seat. On further history taking, the child's mother states that he is very independent with few friends, and has always been interested in boats, preferring them over all other toys. You observe that his speech is monotone and restricted in volume and rate and he never makes eye contact with you or his mother. Which of the following statements is most accurate regarding this child?

A. An Asperger-specific screening tool appropriate for the child's age is the next important step.

B. The most important issue for today's visit is to screen the child for abuse and neglect.

C. This child should be started on oral amphetamine salts, which will lead to improved behavior.

D. This parent should be reassured, as this child's behavior and development is most likely a normal variant.

E. It is probable that one of his vaccinations is responsible for this child's clinical findings.

54.2 Which of the following statements is most accurate?

A. A previously healthy, normally developing 3-year-old child begins to lose bladder control and will no longer speak in sentences, but you should not be too concerned because this began after the birth of her younger sibling and she just wants more attention from her parents.

B. No use of single words by 12 months in a child is reason for immediate referral to speech therapy.

C. Children with ASDs will rarely grow up to be independent adults.

D. You counsel the parents of a 6-year-old boy with autism that their second child is at increased risk for having an ASD.

54.3 Which of the following observations during a clinical examination is concerning for the presence of an ASD?

A. You walk into the examination room and find a 36-month-old child pretending to have tea with her imaginary friend.

B. A 12-month-old child walks over to the sink, and points toward the faucet, but only utters "Uh," and does not say water.

C. A 2-year-old child is holding tightly to a tattered old blanket, which his mother says he will not leave the house without.

D. You tap an 18-month-old child on the shoulder and say, "Look!" and point to a toy in the corner of the room, but the child ignores you and continues to spin the wheels on his toy car.

ANSWERS

54.1 **A.** While at first glance the concerns of this child's teacher and mother may sound typical for ADHD, your clinical suspicion should be that the child has Asperger syndrome, based on a history of monotone, restricted speech limited to only one topic of interest, lack of eye contact, lack of peer relationships appropriate to developmental age, and the repetitive, nonfunctional, atypical behavior of rocking and twirling. Appropriate steps at this time include a complete history and physical examination accompanied by an Asperger-specific screening tool and immediate referral to a developmental pediatrician for a complete evaluation. You should reassure the child's mother that immunizations are not implicated in the cause of developmental disorders and administer any vaccines needed. You should not delay your diagnostic workup for a developmental disorder for any reason. Although immunizations are important, for this child's situation, evaluation of the developmental problems is of higher priority.

54.2 **D.** Family studies estimate a recurrence risk of as much as 5% to 6% when there is an older sibling with an ASD. Red flag symptoms indicating the need for an immediate evaluation for an ASD include loss of language or social skills at any age and no use of single words by 16 months. Although most children with an ASD will retain their diagnosis and exhibit residual signs of their disorder into adulthood, children with ASDs who begin treatment at a younger age have significantly better outcomes, and one of the goals of treatment is to foster independence.

54.3 **D.** The child in answer choice (D) demonstrates a deficit in joint attention, one of the most distinguishing characteristics of very young children with ASDs. It is the lack of pretend play skills, rather than their presence choice (A), that is concerning for an ASD. As demonstrated in answer choice (B) at about 12 to 14 months, a typically developing child will begin to request a desired object that is out of reach by pointing, and, depending on the child's speech skills, may utter simple sounds or actual words. Similar to answer choice (C), most children will form attachments during their early development with a stuffed animal, special pillow, or blanket. However, children with ASDs may prefer hard items such as ballpoint pens, keys, or flashlights.

CLINICAL PEARLS

▶ Screening tools for autism spectrum disorders, pervasive developmental disorders (NOS), and developmental delay are simple and easy to use in the office setting.

▶ Common features shared by all the ASDs include severe deficits in social skills and limited, repetitive, and stereotyped behavior patterns. However, only AD and PDD-NOS are characterized by significant language delays.

▶ Red flag symptoms indicating the need for immediate evaluation for an ASD include no babbling or pointing by 12 months, no single words by 16 months, no two-word phrases by 24 months, and loss of language or social skills at any age.

▶ When a child demonstrates two or more risk factors or a positive screening result occurs, take immediate action.

REFERENCES

Ages and Stages Questionnaires. Available at: http://www.agesandstages.com. Accessed April 12, 2015.

Carbone PS, Farley M, Davis T. Primary care for children with autism. *Am Fam Physician.* 2010;81(4): 453-460.

Centers for Disease Control and Prevention. Prevalence of autism spectrum disorder among children aged 8 years—autism and developmental disabilities monitoring network, 11 sites, United States, 2010. *MMWR Surveill Summ.* 2014;63(2):1-21. Available at: http://www.cdc.gov.mmwr/pdf/ss/ss6302.pdf. Accessed April 12, 2015.

Harrington JW, Allen K. The clinician's guide to autism. *Pediatr Rev.* 2014;35(2):62-78.

Hurley AM, Tadrous M, Miller ES. Thimerosal-containing vaccines and autism: a review of recent epidemiological studies. *J Pediatr Pharmacol Ther.* 2010;15(3):173-181.

Johnson CP, Myers SM; American Academy of Pediatrics, Council on Children with Disabilities. Identification and evaluation of children with autism spectrum disorders. *Pediatrics.* 2007;120:1183-1215.

Johnson CP, Myers SM; American Academy of Pediatrics, Council on Children with Disabilities. Management of children with autism spectrum disorders. *Pediatrics.* 2007;120:1162-1182.

Modified Checklist for Autism in Toddlers (M-CHAT). Available at: http://www.m-chat.org/mchat.php. Accessed April 12, 2015.

Screening Tool for Autism in Toddlers and Young Children (STAT). Available at: http://www.vkc.mc.vanderbilt.edu/vkc/triad/training/stat/. Accessed April 12, 2015.

Shah PE, Dalton R, Boris NW. Pervasive developmental disorders and childhood psychosis. In: Kliegman RM, Behrman RE, Jenson HB, Stanton BF, eds. *Nelson Textbook of Pediatrics.* 18th ed. Philadelphia, PA: Saunders Elsevier; 2007:133-138.

Smeeth L, Cook C, Fombonne E, et al. MMR vaccination and pervasive developmental disorders: a case-control study. *Lancet.* 2004;364:963-969.

A 46-year-old woman presents to your office complaining of a right hand tremor that has been steadily worsening over the past 2 years. She works as a literary agent and states that this tremor is increasingly impairing her ability to work, since this is affecting her dominant hand. She tells you in a slightly quivering voice, "I am often required to take my clients out to lunch, and I get embarrassed when I cannot eat and drink normally. Sometimes, I cannot even drink from a cup without shaking." She finds that a glass of wine with her meal sometimes helps minimize the tremor. On examination, her blood pressure is 125/85 mm Hg, her pulse is 84 beats/min, and her respiratory rate is 16 breaths/min. Neurologic examination reveals a mild head tremor, but no resting tremor of the hands. When she holds a pen by its tip at arm's length however, a coarse bilateral tremor becomes readily visible, which is more pronounced on the right side. The rest of her examination is unremarkable.

► What is the most likely diagnosis?
► What further evaluation needs to be performed?
► What pharmacologic interventions may be beneficial?

ANSWERS TO CASE 55:
Movement Disorders

Summary: A 46-year-old woman presents with a classic essential tremor. It manifests during action and remits when the limb is relaxed, unlike the tremor of Parkinson disease. She is very disturbed by the tremor as it is leading to a great deal of social embarrassment, often interfering with her work. She has found that alcohol helps to reduce the symptoms.

- **Most likely diagnosis:** Essential tremor.

- **Further evaluation necessary:** Ensure that medications, thyroid disease, alcohol, or other neurologic diseases are not causing the tremor.

- **Beneficial pharmacotherapy:** Propranolol, primidone, and gabapentin.

ANALYSIS

Objectives

1. Become familiar with the presenting signs and symptoms of the most common movement disorders.

2. Become familiar with the management of common movement disorders.

3. Be able to gauge the severity of disease and understand potential side effects of therapies.

Considerations

Essential tremor is the most common of all movement disorders, affecting 1.3% to 5% of persons over the age of 60. A complete history is crucial in making an appropriate diagnosis of essential tremor. It usually appears after the age of 50 and often interferes with common tasks and activities of daily living. Close to one-half of all patients with an essential tremor have a family history of tremor, although this is not a strict criterion for diagnosis. Tremor is often attenuated with the use of alcohol. It is important to ask about the consumption of caffeine, cigarette smoking, stimulant use (eg, pseudoephedrine) and to inquire about prescription medications (eg, fluoxetine, lithium, theophylline, valproic acid, haloperidol, metoclopramide) that are known to cause or enhance physiologic tremor.

When essential tremor is suspected, the patient should be observed while performing goal-directed tasks such as finger-to-nose testing or reaching for and drinking from a glass. Evaluating handwriting samples can help to identify the time of tremor onset and progression of disease. Tremor commonly affects the hands in 95%, the head in 34%, and the lower extremities in 20% of patients. In evaluating patients who present with tremor, thyroid and liver function tests are indicated. Additional testing includes serum ceruloplasmin and copper levels when patients are less than age 40 for evaluation of Wilson disease, a disorder of copper metabolism.

Pharmacotherapy constitutes the main approach to treatment of essential tremor. First-line therapies include the β-blocker propranolol and the anticonvulsant primidone, which are equally efficacious in reducing tremor symptoms. Topiramate and gabapentin are other anticonvulsants that can be used as second-line agents. The patient's report of symptoms and functional ability, rather than the severity of tremor detected on physical examination, should serve as guides for adjustment of therapy. It is also important to monitor patients for side effects of these medications. Propranolol is associated with fatigue, headaches, bradycardia, impotence, and depression. Primidone can cause an acute reaction consisting of nausea, vomiting, confusion, or ataxia in many patients. As with therapy for Parkinson disease, both deep brain stimulation and ablation of the ventral intermediate nucleus of the thalamus (Vim nucleus) are effective in patients with tremor that is refractory to medical treatment.

APPROACH TO:
Movement Disorders

DEFINITIONS

CHOREA: Unpredictable, involuntary, irregular, brief movements that are jerky, writhing, or flowing.

HYPERKINESIAS: Movement disorders characterized by extra or exaggerated movements.

HYPOKINESIAS: Movement disorders characterized by overall slowness of movement (bradykinesia), lack of movement (akinesia), or difficulty in initiating movement.

CLINICAL APPROACH

A movement disorder can be defined as any condition that disrupts normal voluntary movement of the body or that consists of one or more abnormal movements. They can be classified as hypokinesias or hyperkinesias (Table 55–1). Although less frequently encountered by family physicians than other chronic diseases, they

Table 55–1 • CLASSIFICATION OF MOVEMENT DISORDERS	
Hypokinetic Disorders	**Hyperkinetic Disorders**
Parkinson disease Secondary or acquired parkinsonism (can be caused by neuroleptics, hydrocephalus, head trauma) Progressive supranuclear palsy (PSP) Multiple system atrophy (Shy-Drager syndrome, olivopontocerebellar atrophy, striatonigral degeneration)	Tremor (essential tremor, dystonic tremor, drug-induced tremor, physiologic tremor) Tic disorders (Tourette syndrome) Chorea (Huntington disease) Myoclonus Dystonia Ataxia

are fairly common, especially in the aging population. Parkinson disease, for example, affects 1% of those over 60 and 2% of those over 85 years.

Movement disorders present a special challenge to family physicians for many reasons. Signs and symptoms can often be subtle and may not be detected on routine physical examinations. The normal process of aging is associated with changes in movement that may be mistaken for a more serious problem. **Laboratory and radiologic testing are often of limited value in the diagnosis of movement disorders.**

Management of tremor is equally challenging. Movement disorders have a great impact on other medical conditions as well as on the psychological well-being of patients and their families. Educating both the patient and family about the disease process and available treatment options can provide better understanding and management of the disorder. Although pharmacotherapy and surgeries are often administered by specialists, family physicians play an integral role in helping patients to cope with the broad impact of their disease.

Parkinson Disease

Parkinson disease is the most common neurodegenerative disease, and can cause significant disability and decreased quality of life. Symptoms appear as neurons and dopamine are lost from the substantia nigra (part of the basal ganglia) and intracytoplasmic inclusions (Lewy bodies) proliferate. Dopamine depletion in the substantia nigra ultimately leads to increased inhibition of the thalamus and decreased excitation of the motor cortex, which gives rise to parkinsonian symptoms such as bradykinesia. The **cardinal physical signs of the disease are distal resting tremor, micrographia, cogwheel rigidity, bradykinesia, postural instability, shuffling gait, and asymmetric onset.** Expressive language is typically not affected, but clarity and volume of speech may be compromised.

Pharmacotherapy is the mainstay of treatment for Parkinson disease, and has been shown to reduce both morbidity and mortality. The goals of treatment are to slow down progression and symptomatic therapy. For symptomatic early disease, first-line treatments are levodopa for motor impairment, dopamine agonists such as pramipexole and ropinirole to lower risk of motor complications, and monoamine oxidase type B (MAO-B) inhibitors. Amantidine may be used early on in the disease course but has limited evidence in improving outcomes. Anticholinergics (eg, benztropine, trihexyphenidyl) can also be utilized in young patients with severe tremor, but their use is often limited by side effects.

Tremor is best treated with dopamine agonists, levodopa, and anticholinergics. For motor fluctuations and dyskinesia, dopamine agonists and/or MAO-B inhibitors (eg, selegiline, rasagiline), or catechol-O-methyltransferase (COMT) inhibitors (eg, entacapone, tolcapone) can be added. Deep brain stimulation of the subthalamic nucleus has been shown to ameliorate symptoms in patients with advanced disease. Physical therapy and exercise may have modest benefits in slowing a patient's functional disability in Parkinson disease.

Common comorbid problems associated with Parkinson disease include depression, dementia, fatigue, excessive daytime sleepiness, and psychosis. Hallucinations affect up to 40% of patients with Parkinson disease. Psychosis is usually drug-induced and can be managed initially by reducing the dose of antiparkinsonian medications. In patients with debilitating psychotic symptoms and hallucinations, antiparkinsonian drugs may be discontinued in the reverse order of their effectiveness. Anticholinergics should be stopped first, followed by amantadine, then COMT inhibitors, and dopamine agonists. Discontinuing levodopa is typically not an option for most patients with Parkinson disease; however, dose reduction may be considered as a last resort to minimize symptoms. Consultation with a subspecialist for optimal medical management is often required. Since the functional impairment of Parkinson disease is progressive, discussion of advance directives is appropriate with all patients. Education and support are important ways patients can cope with their illness.

Tourette Syndrome

Tourette syndrome (TS) is the most common tic disorder, usually developing during childhood or early adolescence. Inheritance through an autosomal dominant pattern is thought to play a major role in its etiology. The diagnosis requires the presence of vocal tics such as grunting and multiple motor tics occurring several times a day for at least 1 year, onset generally between 2 and 15 years but no later than age 21, and having tics that cannot be explained by other medical conditions or medication side effects. Additionally, a family history of tics or similar symptoms also supports the diagnosis of TS. There are a number of different types of tics ranging from simple noises to echolalia (repetition of words), coprolalia (excessive use of obscene words), and palilalia (repetition of phrases or words with increasing rapidity). Tics may be temporarily suppressed during mental concentration but generally worsen during periods of stress, excitement, boredom, or fatigue. The majority of affected children also suffer from coexisting attention-deficit hyperactivity disorder (ADHD), obsessive-compulsive disorder (OCD), learning disorder, conduct disorder/oppositional defiant disorder, or migraine headaches.

Education and counseling of patient and family is most important, and may be the only treatment necessary. Explanation of tics, obsessions, and compulsions, and appreciation that these are not voluntary to patients, family, teachers, and coworkers is often very helpful. Patients frequently will suppress tics most of day and need to "release" tics upon return from school or work.

Pharmacotherapy should be considered if there is continued functional impairment despite education and behavioral therapy. Treatment of comorbid ADHD and OCD can reduce Tourette symptoms. Clonidine is considered the first-line treatment due to its long-term safety and its ability to improve symptoms of comorbid ADHD and OCD. Another α-receptor blocker, guanfacine, appears safe and effective for tics in patients with ADHD, but can cause significant hypotension and must be dosed cautiously.

Neuroleptics including pimozide and haloperidol are more effective for tics than clonidine but have greater risk of long-term side effects. Botulinum toxin injection into the affected muscles may be effective for the treatment of refractory phonic tics. Deep brain stimulation surgery is a final option available for refractory symptoms and requires subspecialty evaluation.

Huntington Disease

The most common cause of chorea among adults occurs is Huntington disease. Huntington disease is inherited in an autosomal dominant pattern, and affects men and women in equal numbers. It is caused by a trinucleotide (CAG) expansion in the Huntington gene located on chromosome 4. Onset may be at any age, although symptoms first appear between 35 and 50 years with progressive neuronal loss and dysfunction over the following 10 to 20 years. The two types of movement abnormalities pathognomonic for Huntington disease are chorea and abnormal voluntary movements. The presence of chorea is required at the time of diagnosis of Huntington disease. Initially, chorea involves mostly the face, trunk, and limbs. With time, the chorea becomes more widespread and affects the diaphragm, larynx, and pharynx. Abnormal voluntary movements include uncoordinated fine motor movements, gait disturbances, abnormal eye movements, dysarthria, dysphagia, and rigidity. Difficulties with voluntary movements get worse with time. Weight loss and cachexia are common among Huntington disease patients caused by the hyperkinetic movements and altered cellular metabolism leading to increased energy expenditure. Cognitive problems include difficulties with memory, visuo-spatial abilities, and poor judgment. A global dementia may be present in patients with advanced disease. The most common psychiatric problem is depression, which affects up to one-half of patients. Patients with Huntington disease are at significantly higher risk for suicide.

There is currently no treatment available to slow the progression of Huntington disease. Treatment should target the prevalent signs and symptoms, and be adjusted according to disease severity. Physiotherapy for gait and balance issues, a high calorie diet for increased metabolic requirement, and speech and swallowing therapy for managing dysphagia and aspiration are few of the supportive measures available for Huntington disease patients. Tetrabenazine, a dopamine depleting agent, can be helpful for chorea but has limited outcomes data. Side effects of tetrabenazine include depression, sedation, akathisia, and parkinsonian symptoms. Chorea that is unresponsive to tetrabenazine can be treated with neuroleptics. Benzodiazepines and antidepressants may be indicated for insomnia, anxiety, and depression. The primary counseling responsibility of the family physician is to understand the role of genetic testing and to offer it to affected and asymptomatic individuals in a responsible manner. Optimal care usually requires input from a multidisciplinary team which includes neurologists and therapists.

CASE CORRELATION

- See also Case 32 (Dementia).

COMPREHENSION QUESTIONS

55.1 An 18-year-old male patient is noted to have motor tics and involuntary, obscene vocalizations. Which of the following medications is indicated in the treatment of this disorder?

A. Trihexyphenidyl

B. Phenytoin

C. Carbamazepine

D. Haloperidol

E. Levodopa

55.2 A 21-year-old woman develops auditory hallucinations and persecutory delusions over the course of 3 days. She was hospitalized and started on haloperidol 2 mg three times daily. Within a week of treatment, she developed stooped posture and a shuffling gait. Her head was slightly tremulous and her movements became slowed. Her medication was changed to thioridazine, and trihexyphenidyl was added. Over the next 2 weeks, she became much more animated and reported no recurrence of her hallucinations. Which of the following is the most likely diagnosis?

A. Hyperparathyroidism

B. Adverse effect of neuroleptic

C. Encephalitis

D. Hypermagnesemia

E. Tourette syndrome

55.3 Which of the following represents the decrement in speech commonly exhibited by the patient with parkinsonism?

A. Progressively inaudible speech

B. Neologisms

C. Expressive aphasia

D. Receptive aphasia

E. Word salad

55.4 A 67-year-old woman with known Parkinson disease is brought to the clinic by her health-care provider. She is confined to a wheelchair and completely dependent on others. You notice large grossly abnormal movements in both the arms and legs. The patient has to be strapped to the wheelchair to avoid falling out and can't keep her shoes on due to the jerking movements. Bed rails have had to be installed on her bed to prevent her from falling out at night. She is not able to tell the correct month or the year. She has not had a change in her medication in 6 months. Which of the following medication adjustments would benefit her most?

A. Add haloperidol.

B. Decrease levodopa/carbidopa.

C. Increase levodopa/carbidopa.

D. Add donepezil.

E. Add entacapone.

ANSWERS

55.1 **D.** The clinical scenario described is associated with Tourette syndrome. A variety of drugs may help suppress the tics that are characteristic of this syndrome. These include haloperidol, pimozide, trifluoperazine, and fluphenazine. Antiepileptics such as carbamazepine and phenytoin are not useful. Levodopa is the drug of choice in treating advanced Parkinson disease. Trihexyphenidyl and benztropine are useful in suppressing the parkinsonism that may develop with haloperidol administration, but are not useful in the management of Tourette syndrome.

55.2 **B.** Butyrophenones, the most commonly prescribed of which is haloperidol, routinely produce some signs of parkinsonism if they are used at high doses for more than a few days. This psychotic young woman proved to be less sensitive to the parkinsonian side effects of thioridazine than she was to haloperidol. Adding the anticholinergic drug trihexyphenidyl may have also helped to reduce the patient's symptoms.

55.3 **A.** Language is not disturbed in Parkinson disease, as it is with aphasias. The clarity and volume of speech is what suffers. Handwriting is similarly disturbed, as the patient has increasingly smaller and less legible penmanship as he or she continues to write. This is referred to as micrographia.

55.4 **B.** The patient is suffering from dyskinesias from too much levodopa/carbidopa. Stopping levodopa/carbidopa is usually not an option for most patients; however, a reduction of the medication would be of the most benefit to her. Haloperidol would be a good choice if the patient was suffering from hallucinations. Donepezil is a medication used primarily for Alzheimer dementia and has no use in Lewy body dementia. Entacapone is a medication to enhance levodopa/carbidopa.

CLINICAL PEARLS

▶ Movement disorders have a profound impact on the quality of life of patients and their families. Family physicians should become adept at counseling patients about prognosis and the availability of support groups and community resources.

▶ The management of certain movement disorders including Parkinson disease is rapidly changing. It is important to find the latest information about emerging and alternative therapies, and to seek the help of a specialist when required.

REFERENCES

Crawford P, Zimmerman EE. Differentiation and diagnosis of tremor. *Am Fam Physician*. 2011;83(6): 697-702.

Gazewood JD, Richards DR, Clebak K. Parkinson disease: an update. *Am Fam Physician*. 2013;87(4): 267-273.

Kurlan R. Tourette's syndrome. *N Engl J Med*. 2010;363:24:2332-2338.

Novak MJ, Tabrizi SJ. Huntington's disease. *BMJ*. 2010;340:c3109.

Olanow C, Schapira AV, Obeso JA. Parkinson's disease and other movement disorders. In: Kasper D, Fauci A, Hauser S, et al., eds. *Harrison's Principles of Internal Medicine*. 19th ed. New York, NY: McGraw-Hill Education; 2015. Available at: http://accessmedicine.mhmedical.com. Accessed May 25, 2015.

A 25-year-old man presents to your office complaining of a 3-month history of rhinorrhea, itchy eyes, and exertional cough and wheezing. These symptoms have been progressively worsening over the past few months. His past medical history is significant for seasonal allergies to pollen and ragweed. His family history is significant only for hypertension in both parents. His siblings and children are in good health without allergies or respiratory illness. His social history is negative for smoking. He has worked as an animal laboratory technician for the last 6 months. On questioning, his symptoms were initially more severe toward the end of the work week but are now continuous. He has been taking over-the-counter antihistamines, which helped initially but have not relieved his allergic symptoms. On review of systems, he has noted hives that are less prominent now that he has been taking the antihistamines on a regular basis. On examination, his body mass index (BMI) is 23, blood pressure is 120/75 mm Hg, pulse is 72 beats/min, and respiratory rate is 18 breaths/min. His conjunctiva are injected, there is mild clear ocular discharge, and his nasal turbinates are boggy without visible polyps. His lung examination reveals prolonged inspiratory-to-expiratory ratio and end-expiratory wheezing at the bilateral bases. His heart examination is unremarkable and there is no peripheral edema.

▶ What is the most likely diagnosis?
▶ What further evaluation should be considered?
▶ What are the initial steps in therapy?

ANSWERS TO CASE 56:
Wheezing and Asthma

Summary: A 25-year-old man presents with classic signs and symptoms of asthma. The constellation of ocular, nasal, and pulmonary symptoms temporally related to work and environmental conditions to a common allergen is suspicious for occupational-related asthma. The physical examination also is consistent with this diagnosis.

- **Most likely diagnosis:** Occupation-related allergic asthma.

- **Further evaluation:** Peak flow measurements pre– and post–β-agonist treatment. Further workup should include a chest x-ray, pulmonary function testing with bronchodilator challenge, and consideration of allergen testing.

- **Initial therapy:** Initial treatment is with a short-acting inhaled β-agonist such as albuterol. A short course of oral steroids should be considered if the patient continues to have wheezing, decreased pulse oximetry, and decreased predicted peak flow measurements after β-agonist therapy. This patient should be removed from his current duties of working with laboratory animals.

ANALYSIS

Objectives

1. Recognize the presenting signs and symptoms of the common causes of wheezing.

2. Understand the etiologies and pathogenesis of asthma.

3. Understand the clinical evaluation, diagnosis, and staging of asthma.

4. Implement the treatment and management of asthma in children and adults.

APPROACH TO:
Wheezing

DEFINITIONS

ASTHMA: A chronic pulmonary disease characterized by inflammation and hyperreactivity of the airways.

REACTIVE AIRWAY DYSFUNCTION SYNDROME: Irritant-induced asthma usually associated with significant environmental exposures to chemical irritants and allergens.

INTERMITTENT ASTHMA: Symptoms of asthma occurring less than two times a week, nocturnal awakening less than two times a month, the need for oral corticosteroid treatment less than two times in a year, and *no* limitations in normal activities. Spirometry is normal in between exacerbations.

PERSISTENT ASTHMA: Signs and symptoms greater than the above. There are three classifications of persistent asthma: mild, moderate, and severe.

PEAK EXPIRATORY FLOW (PEF): An easily reproduced age- and gender-controlled measure of pulmonary function that is used as a measure of current levels of pulmonary obstruction that can be used to monitor and manage asthma.

CLINICAL APPROACH

Background

Asthma is one of the most common chronic diseases in the United States, and is accountable for a substantial number of emergency department evaluations and hospitalizations, many of which are preventable with appropriate management. It is diagnosed in approximately 10% of children and 5% of young adults with increasing prevalence in economically developed countries. Genetic and environmental factors play a significant role in the development of asthma. Work-related asthma is implicated in at least 10% of asthma cases in adults. Pathologic changes to the airways reflect inflammatory and remodeling changes including inflammatory cell infiltration, basement membrane thickening, shedding of epithelial cells, proliferation and engorgement of blood vessels, mucus plugging, smooth muscle hypertrophy, and fibrosis.

DIAGNOSIS

History

The characteristic history includes dyspnea, wheezing, productive or nonproductive cough, breathlessness, and chest tightness or discomfort. Depending on etiology and patient characteristics, the symptoms can be perennial or seasonal, episodic or continuous, and can have a diurnal pattern. Suggestive symptoms include episodic wheezing and cough with nocturnal, seasonal, or exertional characteristics in the absence of an acute upper respiratory tract illness. Frequent episodes of "bronchitis" are seen in young children who are likely to have asthma. Positive family histories for asthma and patient history of atopy when associated with symptoms are correlated with the diagnosis of asthma. It is important to realize that asthma can occur in all age groups and can present with a varied spectrum of signs and symptoms.

Physical Examination and Classification

The examination may be normal in between symptoms and exacerbations. The variable presentation and often normal examination can account for delays in diagnosis. The eyes and nose should be examined for signs of allergies, including conjunctivitis and nasal polyps. The neck should be evaluated for accessory muscle use in respiratory distress, or lymphadenopathy which may signify an infectious etiology. The chest should be examined for hyperexpansion and hunched shoulders.

Table 56–1 • DIFFERENTIAL DIAGNOSIS FOR WHEEZING
Allergic rhinitis and sinusitis
Foreign body in trachea or bronchus
Vocal cord dysfunction
Vascular rings or laryngeal webs
Laryngotracheomalacia, tracheal stenosis, or bronchostenosis
Enlarged lymph nodes or tumor (benign or malignant)
Bronchiectasis of various causes, including cystic fibrosis
Viral bronchiolitis or obliterative bronchiolitis
Cystic fibrosis
Bronchopulmonary dysplasia
Pulmonary infiltrates with eosinophilia
Chronic obstructive pulmonary disease (chronic bronchitis or emphysema)
Pulmonary embolism
Congestive heart failure
Cough secondary to drugs (angiotensin-converting enzyme [ACE] inhibitors)
Aspiration from swallowing mechanism dysfunction or gastroesophageal reflux
Recurrent cough not due to asthma

Adapted from Sveum R, Keating M, Lowe D, et al. Health Care Guideline: Diagnosis and Management of Asthma. *9th ed. Institute for Clinical Systems Improvement. June 2010.*

The skin should be examined for signs of atopy, eczema, or urticaria. The heart examination can reveal tachycardia and pulsus paradoxus during exacerbations. The lung examination may reveal wheezing heard predominantly on end expiration or forced end expiration with prolongation of expiration compared to inspiration. A differential diagnosis for wheezing is included in Table 56–1.

Classification of the severity of asthma is imperative in directing appropriate acute and maintenance care, and to minimize future exacerbations (Tables 56–2 and 56–3).

An acute asthma exacerbation presents with worsening of the classic symptoms and documented decrease from expected peak flow. Emergency treatment should be considered for the following:

- Peak flow less than 40% of predicted normal (based on age, gender, and height)

- Failure to respond to a β_2-agonist

- Severe wheezing or coughing

- Extreme anxiety due to breathlessness

- Gasping for air, sweaty, or cyanotic

- Rapid clinical deterioration over a few hours with hypoxia

- Severe retractions and nasal flaring

- Posture with shoulders hunched forward

Signs and symptoms for patients who are particularly at risk for poor control of the disease and outcomes including death are as follows:

Table 56-2 · CLASSIFYING ASTHMA SEVERITY IN CHILDREN 5-11 YEARS

Components of Severity		Classification of Asthma Severity (Children 5-11 y)			
		Intermittent	Persistent		
			Mild	Moderate	Severe
Impairment	Symptoms	≤2 d/wk	>2 d/wk but not daily	Daily	Throughout the day
	Nighttime awakenings	≤2 ×/mo	3-4 ×/mo	>1×/wk but not nightly	Often 7×/wk
	Short-acting β₂-agonist use for symptom control (not prevention of EIB)	≤2 d/wk	>2 d/wk but not daily	Daily	Several times per day
	Interference with normal activity	None	Minor limitation	Some limitation	Extremely limited
	Lung function	• Normal FEV₁ between exacerbation • FEV₁ >80% predicted • FEV₁/FVC >85%	• FEV₁ = >80% predicted • FEV₁/FVC >80%	• FEV₁ = 60%-80% predicted • FEV₁/FVC = 75%-80%	• FEV₁ <60% predicted • FEV₁/FVC <75%
Risk	Exacerbations requiring oral systemic corticosteroids	0-1/y	≥2 in 1 y		
		Consider severity and interval since last exacerbation, frequency and severity may fluctuate over time for patients in any severity category.			
		Relative annual risk of exacerbations may be related to FEV₁			

Abbreviations: EIB, exercise-induced bronchoconstriction; FEV₁, forced expiratory volume in 1 second; FVC, forced vital capacity.
Source: National Asthma Education and Prevention Program Expert Panel. Guidelines for the Diagnosis and Management of Asthma. Expert Report 3. *National Heart Lung and Blood Institute. NIH Publication number 08-5846. October 2007.*

Table 56–3 • CLASSIFYING ASTHMA SEVERITY IN YOUTHS AND ADULTS

Components of Severity		Classification of Asthma Severity (Youths >12 y and adults)			
		Intermittent	Persistent		
			Mild	Moderate	Severe
Impairment Normal FEV$_1$/FVC: 8-19 y 85% 20-39 y 80% 40-59 y 75% 60-80 y 70%	Symptoms	≤2 d/wk	>2 d/wk but not daily	Daily	Throughout the day
	Nighttime awakenings	≤2×/mo	3-4×/mo	>1×/wk but not nightly	Often 7×/wk
	Short-acting β$_2$-agonist use for symptom control (not prevention of EIB)	≤2 d/wk	>2 d/wk but not >1 ×/d	Daily	Several times per day
	Interference with normal activity	None	Minor limitation	Some limitation	Extremely limited
	Lung function	• Normal FEV$_1$ between exacerbation • FEV$_1$ >80% predicted • FEV$_1$/FVC normal	• FEV$_1$ ≥80% predicted • FEV$_1$/FVC normal	• FEV$_1$ >60% but <80% predicted • FEV$_1$/FVC reduced 5%	• FEV$_1$ <60% predicted • FEV$_1$/FVC reduced >5%
Risk	Exacerbations requiring oral systemic corticosteroids	0-1/y	≥2/y		
		Consider severity and interval since last exacerbation, frequency and severity may fluctuate over time for patients in any severity category.			
		Relative annual risk of exacerbations may be related to FEV$_1$			

Source: National Asthma Education and Prevention Program Expert Panel. Guidelines for the Diagnosis and Management of Asthma. Expert Report 3. National Heart Lung and Blood Institute. NIH Publication number 08-5846. October 2007.

At regular ambulatory visits:

- Previous admission for intensive care or intubations

- Three or more emergency department visits for asthma in the last year

- Two or more canisters of short-acting β-agonists in a month

- Failure to use controllers (inhaled corticosteroids) despite symptoms

- Current or recent cessation of oral corticosteroids

- Large fluctuations in peak flow

- Low socioeconomic status in an urban environment

- Mental disorders or substance abuse

At presentation with symptoms:

- A chest examination with minimal sounds on auscultation

- Distress and difficulty speaking on examination

- Tachycardia

- Extremely low peak flow (<50% of predicted)

- Elevated carbon dioxide on arterial blood gas with hypoxia. Typically, arterial carbon dioxide is low during an asthmatic attack due to increased respiratory rate. Normalization of carbon dioxide may be a sign of a severe exacerbation indicating CO_2 retention and impending respiratory failure.

Diagnostic Studies

Accurate spirometry is recommended in every patient 5 years or older at the time of diagnosis. Additional studies, tailored to the specific patient and symptoms, include the following:

- Bronchial provocation (eg, methacholine challenge) testing is the "gold standard" test for the diagnosis of asthma for patients with normal or near-normal spirometry

- Allergy testing (eg, skin testing, serum allergen radioallergosorbent test [RAST], in vitro–specific immunoglobulin E [IgE] antibody testing)

- Chest radiography, to exclude alternative diagnosis

- Arterial blood gas measurement

- Plain film radiographs or computed tomography (CT) scan of sinuses

- Evaluation for gastroesophageal reflux disease (GERD)

- Complete blood count (CBC) with eosinophils, total IgE, sputum culture

TREATMENT

Treatment for asthma always begins with education and counseling, environmental controls, and management of comorbid conditions. Proper use of inhalers is paramount to minimizing morbidity including hospitalization. Reduction in exposure to causative or aggravating environmental exposures including allergens, occupational exposures, smoking, and other irritants and allergens are paramount in limiting the long-term remodeling and damage associated with this chronic disease. **The chief cause of poor control in asthma is lack of adherence to environmental controls and prescribed medications.** Education in asthma self-management involving self-monitoring by peak expiratory flow or symptoms, along with regular monitoring and a written plan, improves outcomes for patients.

Pharmacologic measures to treat and manage asthma are instituted in a stepwise fashion based on staging of asthma (Table 56–4). Subcutaneous immunotherapy is an option for any patient with persistent allergic asthma in stages 2 to 4.

Medications—Fast-Acting Agents

Short-acting β₂-agonists (SABAs) are the most effective therapy for prompt relief of asthmatic symptoms. Albuterol, levalbuterol, and pirbuterol are the SABAs used in the United States and are generally considered equally effective in onset and duration of action. They have an onset of action of 5 minutes or less, peak in 30 to 60 minutes, and last 4 to 6 hours. They should be used only as needed for relief of symptoms or before anticipated exposure to known asthmatic triggers (eg, animals, exercise). Metered-dose inhaler (MDI) actuations can be taken in 10- to 15-second intervals, and nebulized treatment doses can be given continuously in severe cases. Increasing use or using them more than 2 days per week for symptom relief (not for prevention) generally indicates inadequate control of asthma or persistent asthma.

Dose-dependent side effects include tremor, anxiety, palpitations, and tachycardia (but not hypertension). B-Blockers may diminish the effectiveness of SABA, but are not contraindicated.

Metered-dose inhalers are the delivery mechanism of choice for all short-acting β₂-agonists, and the use of spacers is encouraged. **Nebulizer** treatments with SABAs are an alternative in those who cannot use an MDI, yet MDIs with spacers work as well as nebulizers when used correctly. If patients are not controlled with MDIs, the clinician should ensure that the medications are being used in the appropriate dosing intervals. In acute care settings, up to 10 puffs from an MDI given sequentially is equivalent to one nebulizer treatment.

Use of oral short-acting β-agonist is discouraged. They are less potent, take longer to act, and have more side effects compared to inhaled SABAs. **Anticholinergic bronchodilators,** such as ipratropium, combined with SABA are more beneficial in treating severe asthmatic attacks or those induced by β-blockers in the urgent care setting compared to treatment with a SABA alone.

Medications—Long-Acting Agents

The long-term daily use of control medications is indicated for persistent asthma to prevent symptoms, and eventually hospitalizations. These medications are **inhaled**

Table 56–4 • TREATMENT FOR ASTHMA BASED ON SEVERITY

Classification	Days With Symptoms	Nights With Symptoms	PEF or FEV₁ (PEF is % of personal best; FEV₁ is % of predicted)	Treatment[a] (for persons ≥12 y)
Severe persistent	Continual	Frequent	$\leq 60\%$	Preferred: high-dose inhaled steroid and long-acting β-agonist and consider omalizumab in patients with allergies If needed, high-dose inhaled steroid, long-acting β-agonist, and oral steroid and consider omalizumab in patients with allergies
Moderate persistent	Daily	>1 ×/wk but not nightly	>60%–<80%	Preferred: low-dose inhaled steroid and long-acting β-agonist or medium-dose inhaled steroid Alternative: low-dose inhaled steroid and leukotriene modifier, theophylline, or zileuton If needed (particularly in patients with recurring severe exacerbations): Preferred: increase inhaled steroid within medium-dose range and long-acting β-agonist Alternative: increase inhaled steroid within medium-dose range and add leukotriene modifier, theophylline, or zileuton
Mild persistent	>2 d/wk but not daily	3-4/mo	$\geq 80\%$	Preferred: low-dose inhaled steroid Alternative: cromolyn, nedocromil, leukotriene modifier, or theophylline
Intermittent	≤2/wk	≤2/mo	$\geq 80\%$	No daily medication needed; short-acting β-agonist as needed for symptoms Severe exacerbations may occur, separated by long periods of normal function and no symptoms, a course of systemic corticosteroids is recommended

[a]All patients: short-acting bronchodilator as needed for symptoms.

Data from National Asthma Education and Prevention Program (NAEPP) Expert Panel Report 3. Guidelines for the Diagnosis and Management of Asthma—Summary Report, 2007. *Washington, DC: National Institutes of Health, National Heart, Lung and Blood Institute; October 2007.*

corticosteroids (ICSs), leukotriene receptor antagonists (LRAs), and **long-acting β₂-agonists** (LABAs). Other long-acting agents that can be considered are cromolyn, methylxanthines, and immunomodulators, but are rarely used.

When ICSs are used consistently, they improve asthma symptoms more effectively than any other medications in both children and adults. There are no clinically meaningful differences among the various types of inhaled corticosteroids. The use of spacers improves the delivery of inhaled controllers. Except with long-term, high-dose use, systemic side effects of inhaled corticosteroids may occur but are not clinically important. Dysphonia, sore throat, and thrush can occur, but are generally managed well with the use of a spacer and rinsing with water after use.

Due to their delayed onset of action, inhaled steroids are insufficient for moderate-to-severe exacerbations. Instead, **oral steroid** treatment is recommended: 1 to 2 mg/kg/d for 3 to 10 days in children or 40 to 60 mg/d in one or two divided doses for 5 to 10 days in adults. Tapering steroid doses for short courses is typically not necessary.

The two most widely available LRAs are montelukast and zafirlukast. In patients who are unable or unwilling to use inhaled corticosteroids, montelukast and zafirlukast are appropriate alternative therapies for mild persistent asthma and have the advantages of ease of use. They also play a role in controlling many symptoms of allergic rhinitis. Combining LRAs and ICSs is a viable option for moderate persistent asthma. LRAs are indicated in exercise-induced asthma. They are the treatment of choice for **aspirin-sensitive asthma.**

The LABAs **salmeterol** and **formoterol** are β-agonists with duration of action of more than 12 hours. They have low rates of tremor and palpitations or tachycardia. However, the inhibition of exercise-induced asthma rapidly wanes with regular use. The effectiveness of SABAs is not impaired in regular users of LABAs. There appears to be an increase in severe exacerbations and deaths when LABAs are added to usual asthma therapy. It is recommended that **LABAs should never be used as monotherapy for long-term control of persistent asthma,** and should only be used in combination therapy. Use of LABAs has been associated with increased mortality. Increasing the dose of an ICS should be considered before adding a LABA if the initial dosage of the ICS is not effective.

Cromolyn sodium and nedocromil stabilize mast cells and interfere with chloride channel function. They are an alternative, but are not preferred, medication for the treatment of mild persistent asthma. They have few serious side effects including skin pruritis, irritability, and gastrointestinal upset, need to be dosed multiple times per day, and their use has markedly decreased due to the superiority of ICSs and LRAs.

Omalizumab is a monoclonal antibody that should be instituted only in collaboration or consultation with an asthma subspecialist for highest-risk patients 12 years or older, as additive therapy in patients with severe persistent asthma who have demonstrated immediate hypersensitivity to inhaled allergens. Anaphylaxis may occur in patients receiving this medication. It is administered subcutaneously every 2 to 4 weeks.

Sustained-release **theophylline** is a mild-to-moderate bronchodilator used as an alternative, adjunctive therapy with an ICS. Monitoring of serum theophylline levels is essential to minimize risk of toxicity and common side effects including tachycardia.

Stepped care can be increased or decreased seasonally and with good long-term management with the goal of minimizing medications as environmental and behavioral treatments decrease symptoms and improve PEF measurements. All medication changes should have a follow-up visit in 2 to 4 weeks with an asthma educator to assess effectiveness and frequency of symptoms.

Acute Management of Asthma

In the acute care setting, immediate treatment with a SABA with monitoring of vitals and PEF is indicated. If within 20 minutes, a patient has an **incomplete response** (PEF 40%-69% predicted), then three more SABA treatments within 1 hour (via MDI or nebulizer) should be given. If there is a **poor response** (PEF <40% or oxygen saturations <90%), then the addition of oral or intravenous corticosteroids is indicated. If the patient continues to have inadequate or poor response, then in-patient management with continuous oximetry and close monitoring should be considered.

Additional Measures

All asthmatics should have a yearly influenza vaccination, and remain up-to-date with age-appropriate pertussis and pneumococcal immunizations.

CASE CORRELATION

- See Cases 2 (Dyspnea), 19 (Upper Respiratory Infections), and 24 (Pneumonia).

COMPREHENSION QUESTIONS

56.1 A 25-year-old white woman who is in training for a competitive marathon complains of "hitting a wall" and "getting short of breath quicker than she should." She complains of coughing at the end of her training runs, and states that she may be expecting too much of herself. She does not smoke, has no significant family history, and no history of occupational or environmental exposures. Her physical findings including lung examination are unremarkable. Spirometry reveals normal values both pre- and post-albuterol treatment. What would be the most reasonable first step in treatment of this patient?

A. Trial of albuterol MDI before exercise

B. Chest radiograph

C. Chest CT

D. Counseling for athletic burnout or stress

E. An echocardiogram (ECG) to rule out pulmonary hypertension or cardiac disorder

56.2 A 34-year-old man with a past history of asthma presents to an acute care clinic with an asthma exacerbation. Treatment with nebulized albuterol and ipratropium does not offer significant improvement, and he is then admitted to the hospital. He is afebrile, has a respiratory rate of 24 breaths/min, pulse rate is 96 beats/min, and oxygen saturation is 93% on room air. On examination, he has diffuse bilateral inspiratory and expiratory wheezes, mild intercostal retractions, and a clear productive cough. Which one of the following should be the next step in the management of this patient?

A. Chest physical therapy

B. Inhaled corticosteroids

C. Azithromycin orally

D. Theophylline orally

E. Oral corticosteroids

56.3 A 13-year-old adolescent boy has a nonproductive cough and mild shortness of breath on a daily basis. He is awakened by the cough at least five nights per month. Which one of the following would be the most appropriate treatment for this patient?

A. A long-acting β-agonist daily

B. A short-acting β-agonist daily

C. Oral prednisone daily

D. An oral leukotriene inhibitor as needed

E. Inhaled corticosteroids daily

ANSWERS

56.1 **A.** Exercise-induced asthma or bronchoconstriction is a common, underdiagnosed condition in athletes. Many of the athletes are unaware of the problem. It is defined as a 10% lowering of forced expiratory volume in 1 second (FEV_1) when challenged with exercise. It is much more common in high-ventilation sports and in cold, dry air. The incidence among cross-country skiers is as high as 50%. A physical examination and spirometry at rest will be normal unless there is underlying asthma. Methacholine challenge testing can be ordered, but if it is not available, a trial with an albuterol inhaler is reasonable. Pulmonary or cardiac dysfunction not found during the physical examination is much less likely and, therefore, an ECG and chest x-ray would not be indicated until common etiologies have been ruled out. Psychological causes are also a less likely etiology.

56.2 **E.** Hospital management of acute exacerbations of asthma should include inhaled short-acting bronchodilators and systemic corticosteroids. The efficacy of oral versus intravenous corticosteroids has been shown to be equivalent. Antibiotics are not needed in the treatment of asthma exacerbations unless there are signs of infection. Inhaled ipratropium is recommended for treatment in the emergency department, but not in the hospital. Chest physical therapy and theophylline are not recommended for acute asthma exacerbations.

56.3 **E.** This patient has moderate persistent asthma. The most effective treatment is daily inhaled corticosteroids. A leukotriene inhibitor would be less effective and as a controller should be used daily. Oral prednisone daily is problematic due to the risk of adrenal insufficiency. Short- and long-acting β-agonists are not recommended as daily therapy because they are considered rescue medications rather than asthma controllers.

CLINICAL PEARLS

▶ Use the rule of twos to differentiate between intermittent and persistent asthma. Two or fewer symptoms or SABA use a week, two or less nocturnal awakenings a month, or two or less episodes needing for oral steroids in a year.

▶ The chief causes of inadequate control are poor adherence to medication plan, appropriate MDI utilization, and environmental control.

▶ As with any chronic disease, continuous education and follow-up is essential to optimal management.

▶ Persistent asthma should have controller therapy. Inhaled corticosteroids are the first-line controller.

▶ In adults with new-onset asthma, it is important to get a good occupational exposure history.

REFERENCES

Barnes PJ. Asthma. In: Kasper D, Fauci A, Hauser S, et al., eds. *Harrison's Principles of Internal Medicine.* 19th ed. New York, NY: McGraw-Hill Education; 2015. Available at: http://accessmedicine. mhmedical.com. Accessed May 25, 2015.

Cowl CT. Occupational asthma: review of assessment, treatment, and compensation. *Chest.* 2011;139 (3):674-681.

Elward KS, Pollart SM. Medical therapy for asthma: updates from the NAEPP guidelines. *Am Fam Physician.* 2010;82(10):1242-1251.

Pollart SM, Compton RM, Elward KS. Management of acute asthma exacerbations. *Am Fam Physician.* 2011;84(1):40-47.

Sveum R, Keating M, Lowe D, et al. *Health Care Guideline: Diagnosis and Management of Asthma.* 9th ed. Institute for Clinical Systems Improvement, Bloomington, MN. June 2010.

Tarlo SM, Lemiere C. Occupational asthma. *N Engl J Med.* 2014;370(7):640-649.

Tarlo SM, Liss GM. Prevention of occupational asthma. *Curr Allergy Asthma Rep.* 2010;10(4):278-286.

Weiler JM, Anderson SD, Randolph C, et al. Pathogenesis, prevalence, diagnosis, and management of exercise-induced bronchoconstriction: a practice parameter. *Ann Allergy Asthma Immunol.* 2010;105(suppl 6):S1-S47.

A 55-year-old white man presents to your office after an accident. He reports rear-ending another vehicle with his truck. He complains of some neck soreness, but no other injuries. Later, he admits to having fallen asleep at the wheel right before the accident occurred, and is somewhat amnestic of what happened prior to impact. He admits that he has frequently gotten sleepy while driving in the past, and even dozed off for a few seconds, but has never had a previous accident. He sleeps 7 to 8 hours per night but doesn't feel rested in the morning. His wife reports that he snores loudly and several times per night almost stops breathing. He smokes a pack of cigarettes daily and drinks a few beers on the weekends. On examination, he is an obese man with a short, wide neck. His body mass index (BMI) is 36 kg/m², blood pressure (BP) is 147/96 mm Hg, pulse rate is 88 beats/min, and respiratory rate is 16 breaths/min. On head, ears, eyes, nose, throat (HEENT) examination, you can only see his hard palate when he opens his mouth and says "ahhh." His cardiac and pulmonary examinations are unremarkable. On examination of his neck, he has mild paraspinal muscle tenderness, but no midline cervical tenderness and he has full range of motion.

▶ What condition is most likely to be responsible for his sleepiness?
▶ What should be the first step in his evaluation?
▶ What would be the most effective initial management?

ANSWERS TO CASE 57:

Obstructive Sleep Apnea

Summary: A 55-year-old man with snoring and excessive daytime sleepiness (EDS), resulting in a motor vehicle accident, presents to the office. On examination, he is an obese and hypertensive male with a short, wide neck.

- **Condition responsible for his sleepiness:** Obstructive sleep apnea (OSA)

- **Next step in his evaluation:** Comprehensive sleep evaluation including Epworth Sleepiness Scale and polysomnogram (PSG). If the PSG is positive, then continuous positive airway pressure (CPAP) titration is indicated.

- **Most effective initial therapy:** CPAP for nighttime use and lifestyle modifications including weight reduction, control of hypertension, and smoking cessation.

ANALYSIS

Objectives

1. Identify patients at risk for OSA, the common signs and symptoms of OSA, and indications for conducting a comprehensive sleep evaluation.

2. Understand the pathophysiology and differential diagnosis of OSA.

3. Understand the diagnosis and management of OSA and the importance of patient support and education.

4. Identify comorbid conditions associated with OSA.

Considerations

The patient in this case presents with a history and examination that suggest a diagnosis of OSA. The first step in his management is advising him not to drive, for the safety of himself and others, until further evaluation occurs and a treatment plan has been developed. A comprehensive sleep evaluation, including a sleep history, medical history, and physical examination, should be performed. Confirmation of the diagnosis of OSA is then obtained by overnight polysomnography. The initial treatment approach should include patient education, weight reduction, smoking cessation, and CPAP with close follow-up.

APPROACH TO:

Obstructive Sleep Apnea

DEFINITIONS

APNEA: Defined in adults as breathing pauses lasting at least 10 seconds accompanied by a 90% or more drop in airflow

HYPOPNEA: A 50% reduction in airflow lasting at least 10 seconds with a 3% drop in oxygen saturation, or a 30% reduction in airflow lasting at least 10 seconds with a 4% drop in oxygen saturation

APNEA HYPOPNEA INDEX (AHI): Number of apnea and hypopnea episodes per hour of sleep

RESPIRATORY DISTURBANCE INDEX (RDI): Number of apnea, hypopnea, and respiratory effort–related arousal (RERA) episodes per hour of sleep

RERA: Respiratory effort–related arousals

CLINICAL APPROACH

OSA is a chronic disease that affects 2% to 9% of adults and 2% to 5% of children. Its prevalence has increased dramatically in the last few decades with a direct correlation to obesity rates. It causes significant morbidity including EDS, cognitive impairment, increased risk of motor vehicle accidents, and impaired relationships, and has been associated with several metabolic and cardiovascular conditions (Table 57–1).

People with OSA experience repetitive collapse of the upper airway during sleep leading to hypopnea, apnea, and RERA episodes. The upper airway is comprised of flexible muscles, including the soft palate, that allow for the processes of speech, respiration, and eating. They lack rigid support and during normal sleep, this muscle tone decreases. In OSA, collapse of the flexible musculature of the upper airway during sleep leads to reduced or absent airflow despite continued respiratory effort. This phenomenon is demonstrated on the PSG by abdominal and chest wall movement during an obstructive event. In contrast, during a central apnea there is no respiratory effort, evidenced by absence of chest wall or abdominal wall movement on PSG. The collapse of the upper airway musculature results in occlusion and apnea (often preceded by snoring), which leads to hypoxia and hypercapnia. This results in arousal, wakefulness, and increased sympathetic activity in an attempt to restore airway patency, leading to fragmented sleep. Pathophysiologic factors associated with OSA are listed in Table 57–2.

Evaluation

The diagnosis of OSA is based on a comprehensive sleep evaluation, which includes a sleep-related history and physical examination. If OSA is suggested by the history

Table 57–1 • CONDITIONS ASSOCIATED WITH OSA
Obesity
Atrial fibrillation
Resistant hypertension
Acute coronary syndrome including acute myocardial infarction (MI)
Congestive heart failure
Type 2 diabetes
Stroke
Nocturnal dysrhythmias
Pulmonary hypertension

Table 57–2 • PATHOPHYSIOLOGIC FACTORS ASSOCIATED WITH OSA

• Anatomy that predisposes to narrow airway and obstructed airflow
  • Micrognathia—abnormally small mandible
  • Retrognathia—posteriorly displaced mandible
  • Enlarged tonsils or adenoids
  • Obesity causing increased adipose tissue
  • Nasal polyps
• Thyroid enlargement and acromegaly, both of which narrow the upper airway with increased tissue
• Decreased tone of upper airway dilating muscles
• Arousal threshold: arousal from sleep is a protective mechanism to restore airway patency; patients with OSA are less able to restore airflow without arousal

and physical, a PSG with CPAP titration must be performed to confirm the diagnosis and to determine the severity of OSA, which will help guide treatment. A differential diagnosis for OSA is included in Table 57–3.

A comprehensive sleep history includes asking the patient and their bed partner about snoring, daytime sleepiness not explained by other causes, witnessed apneas, choking or gasping during sleep, sleep amount, nocturia, decreased libido, morning headache, insomnia, frequent awakenings, concentration and memory, alertness, and history of falling asleep at the wheel. Often a patient's partner will be able to provide important information. It is important to ask about other medical conditions that could be related to OSA.

Several standardized scales are available to assess fatigue and sleepiness. The most widely used, the Epworth Sleepiness Scale, is a useful tool to help determine the extent of sleepiness, although a low score does not rule out sleep apnea. Other available tools include the Stanford Sleepiness Scale and the Fatigue Severity Scale.

The physical examination should include evaluation for features suggestive of the presence of OSA. They include BMI greater than 30 kg/m^2, hypertension, retrognathia, obesity, thick neck (likely correlated to a Mallampati class 3 or 4 score), macroglossia (large tongue), acromegaly, thyroid enlargement, large tonsils, enlarged uvula, enlarged nasal turbinates or polyps, and narrow or high-arched palate. The appearance of the oropharynx may be assessed using the Mallampati score (Table 57–4).

Diagnosis

According to the American Academy of Sleep Medicine (AASM), in-lab (PSG) and home testing with portable monitors are acceptable objective tests for OSA.

Table 57–3 • DIFFERENTIAL DIAGNOSIS FOR OSA
Snoring
Narcolepsy
Pulmonary disease
Periodic limb movements of sleep
Shift workers syndrome
Obesity hypoventilation syndrome (obesity and hypoventilation in the absence of other conditions that could account for hypoventilation; evidenced by a P_{CO_2} >45 mm Hg while awake; most people with this condition have concomitant OSA)

Table 57–4 • MALLAMPATI SCORE
1. Entire tonsil visible
2. Upper half of tonsil fossa visible
3. Soft palate and hard palate visible
4. Only hard palate visible
A score of 3 or 4 may be suggestive of OSA

PSG includes the following physiologic assessments: electroencephalogram (EEG), electrocardiogram (ECG) or heart rate, electrooculogram (EOG), chin electromyogram (EMG), airflow, and oxygen saturation. Additionally, anterior tibialis EMG can help assess for periodic limb movements which can coexist with sleep-related breathing disorders. According to the AASM, the diagnosis of OSA in adults is confirmed by the following:

- AHI or RDI greater than or equal to 15, defined by at least 15 obstructive events (apneas, hypopneas, RERAs) per hour on polysomnogram with or without symptoms

  Or

- AHI or RDI greater than or equal to 5, defined by five or more obstructive respiratory events per hour on polysomnogram in a patient who has symptoms of the following:

  - Daytime sleepiness

  - Unrefreshing sleep

  - Fatigue

  - Insomnia

  - Nighttime awakenings associated with gasping, choking, or breath holding, or witnessed loud snoring and/or breathing interruptions

Severe OSA is defined as having more than 30 RDI per hour; moderate OSA is defined as 15 and 30 RDI per hour; and mild OSA is defined as 5 to 15 RDI per hour.

TREATMENT

The medical, behavioral, and surgical therapies for OSA and treatment should involve a multidisciplinary approach. It is always important to include the patient in the decision-making process when deciding on treatment options. Positive airway pressure (PAP) is the treatment of choice for OSA of all severities, although alternative therapies may be indicated based on the patient's anatomy and severity of OSA.

All patients should be educated on behavioral changes. These include weight loss, smoking cessations, avoidance of alcohol and sedating medications, modifying risk factors, and driving precautions. There is a direct correlation between smoking and the development of sleep apnea, placing these patients at an increased risk of sudden cardiac death. Some individuals have elevated AHI or RDI in the supine, but not in other positions and may benefit from sleep-position measures to prevent sleeping in the supine position. One technique is to sew a tennis ball to the back of the sleepwear to prevent supine sleeping. After significant weight loss, the need for continued therapy or for PAP adjustment should be evaluated.

PAP acts as support to maintain patency of the upper airway and reduces the AHI. The level of PAP is determined by an in-lab attended overnight PSG and sometimes by a split-night diagnostic and titration study. A split-night study may occur if a patient has AHI greater than or equal to 40 during 2 hours of a diagnostic study; in this case, PAP may be applied and titrated in the same night.

Different modes of PAP delivery include continuous (CPAP), bilevel (BiPAP), and automatic titrating (APAP). PAP can be applied using a full face mask, oral mask, nasal mask, or nasal pillows. Heated humidification can assist in patient comfort. Adverse effects include nasal congestion and dryness, nosebleeds claustrophobia, inconvenience, air swallowing, skin rash, or minor trauma from the mask. Close follow-up with the health-care team is imperative, especially within the first few weeks after initiation.

Oral appliances work by enlarging the upper airway and preventing upper airway collapse. Examples include mandibular repositioning appliances (MRA) and tongue retaining devices (TRD). They are not as effective as PAP, but are indicated for people with mild-to-moderate OSA who have contraindications to the use of PAP, cannot tolerate PAP, or in whom PAP and behavioral therapy are ineffective. Patients should have a thorough dental examination prior to consideration of use. A repeat sleep study should be performed with the oral appliance in place in order to assess the treatment outcome. Regular follow-up with a dental specialist trained in sleep medicine should occur.

Surgical therapy may be considered as primary therapy if the OSA is mild, resistant to PAP, and when there is an anatomic cause of major airway obstruction that can be reversed. Surgery can be considered as secondary therapy after a trial of PAP or an oral appliance if treatment response is inadequate, or if the patient does not tolerate them. Surgery, specifically an uvulopalatopharyngoplasty (UPPP) may also be used as an adjunct to other therapies. Bariatric surgery may be a helpful adjunct to other OSA treatments in patients who have failed to lose weight through lifestyle modifications. Tracheostomy is curative and can be considered in extremely advanced cases refractory to treatment. There is no pharmacologic therapy for OSA aside from treating underlying diseases such as acromegaly or hypothyroidism that are causative etiologies. All patients with OSA require individualized care and regular follow-up to assess symptoms, treatment response, side effects, and to treat medical conditions associated with OSA.

CASE CORRELATION

- See Cases 2 (Dyspnea), 19 (Upper Respiratory Infection), 24 (Pneumonia), and 56 (Wheezing and Asthma).

COMPREHENSION QUESTIONS

57.1 A 47-year-old obese woman presents to your office complaining of excessive daytime sleepiness, snoring, and frequent awakenings from sleep. She is having difficulty concentrating and her sleepiness is affecting personal and professional relationships. She smokes three-fourths of a pack of cigarettes per day, averages two glasses of wine per night, and has hypertension and hyperlipidemia. You perform a comprehensive sleep history and physical examination and determine that she is at increased risk for OSA. Which of the following physical examination findings is most suggestive of OSA?

   A. Mallampati score of 2
   B. Obesity
   C. Acanthosis nigricans
   D. Peripheral edema
   E. Elevated blood pressure

57.2 You decide to perform an overnight PSG to confirm the diagnosis for the patient in question 57.1. The study is converted into a split-night study because her AHI was found to be over 40 in the first 2 hours of the study. What is the most likely diagnosis?

   A. Mild OSA
   B. Moderate OSA
   C. Severe OSA
   D. Positional OSA
   E. Central apnea

57.3 What is the next step in management of this patient?

   A. Dobutamine stress echocardiogram
   B. Treatment with PAP
   C. Referral for UPPP
   D. Pulmonary function testing
   E. Dental evaluation for oral appliance

57.4 A 54-year-old man comes to your clinic for a follow-up on OSA. He has been using PAP with a nasal mask for the last 3 years since he was diagnosed. He has recently purchased a CPAP machine and tells you he has been unable to use it because of facial discomfort. You check the machine and all the parts are in good condition. What is the next most appropriate step in management?

   A. Decrease the pressure
   B. Refer to surgery
   C. Refer for an oral appliance
   D. Change the mask
   E. Add heated humidification

ANSWERS

57.1 **B.** Obesity is the physical examination finding most suggestive of the presence of OSA. People who are obese are considered to be at high risk for OSA. A Mallampati score of 3 or more suggests increased risk for OSA. Acanthosis nigricans is suggestive of insulin resistance. Peripheral edema has a broad differential diagnosis and further evaluation is warranted. Elevated blood pressure, in contrast to resistant hypertension, is not a risk factor for OSA.

57.2 **C.** This patient has severe OSA based on a RDI over 30 per hour.

57.4 **B.** PAP is the treatment of choice for OSA and, as this patient had an AHI over 40 for 2 hours of the study, it was converted into a split-night study, meaning PAP was applied and titrated in the same night. Surgery and oral appliances are alternative treatment options, but for this patient the initial treatment should be PAP. Pulmonary function testing and cardiac stress testing are not indicated.

57.4 **E.** Heated humidification is indicated to improve patient comfort while using PAP. If the patient remains uncomfortable despite this addition, other measures should be taken such as a trial of a different type of mask (eg, nasal pillows), or pressure relief. If all modifications and patient comfort interventions fail, then an alternative treatment may be necessary.

CLINICAL PEARLS

▶ OSA is a chronic treatable disease that, if left untreated, is associated with increased risk of several cardiovascular disorders.

▶ A diagnosis of OSA should be considered in people with high-risk medical conditions, or features on history or physical examination that may suggest the presence of this disease.

▶ Polysomnography is required to confirm the diagnosis of OSA and determine the severity, which will help to guide treatment.

REFERENCES

Eckert DJ, Malhotra A. Pathophysiology of adult obstructive sleep apnea. *Proc Am Thorac Soc.* 2008;5(2):144-153.

Epstein LJ, Kristo D, Strollo PJ, et al. Clinical guideline for evaluation, management and long-term care of obstructive sleep apnea in adults. *J Clin Sleep Med.* 2009;5(3):263-276.

Greenstone M, Hack M. Obstructive sleep apnoea. *BMJ.* 2014;348:g3745.

Krishnan V, Dixon-Williams S, Thornton JD. Where there is smoke...there is sleep apnea: exploring the relationship between smoking and sleep apnea. *Chest.* 2014;146(6):1673-1680.

Myers KA, Mrkobrada M, Simel DL. Does this patient have obstructive sleep apnea? The Rational Clinical Examination systematic review. *JAMA.* 2013;310(7):731-741.

Ramar K, Olson EJ. Management of common sleep disorders. *Am Fam Physician.* 2013;88(4):231-238.

Wellman A, Redline S. Sleep apnea. In: Kasper D, Fauci A, Hauser S, et al., eds. *Harrison's Principles of Internal Medicine.* 19th ed. New York, NY: McGraw-Hill Education; 2015. Available at: http://accessmedicine.mhmedical.com. Accessed May 25, 2015.

A 62-year-old Asian woman who is new to your office presents complaining of moderate right-sided chest pain and difficulty breathing deeply after she accidentally stumbled and fell against a railing while walking home with her husband the previous day. She states that she has had no significant medical concerns or hospitalizations and is taking no medications or supplements. Her parents died of "old age" in their 90s, and her siblings and children are in excellent health. She does not drink or smoke, has lactose intolerance, is a vegetarian, and exercises occasionally by walking. She has been feeling well recently and has an unremarkable review of systems. On examination, her body mass index (BMI) is 19.5 kg/m^2, blood pressure is 108/75 mm Hg, pulse is 72 beats/min, and respiratory rate is 15 breaths/min. The general, head, ears, eyes, nose, throat (HEENT), neck, heart, abdominal, and extremity examinations are all unremarkable. The chest examination reveals normal lung sounds bilaterally but inspiration is limited secondary to pain. There is significant point tenderness and a moderate-sized bruise in the right anterior and lower ribs where she injured herself. Pulse oximetry is 97%. Electrocardiogram (ECG) reveals normal sinus rhythm without abnormality. Chest and rib radiographs reveal a nondisplaced fracture of the anterolateral right ninth rib at the site of injury.

► What additional diagnoses should be considered?
► What is the most likely underlying cause?
► What would be your next steps in evaluation and treatment?

ANSWERS TO CASE 58:

Osteoporosis

Summary: A 62-year-old woman presents with a fractured rib after a low-velocity trauma. She has a below-normal BMI and is of Asian ethnicity. She has no signs of cardiopulmonary compromise and appears clinically stable other than moderate pain.

- **Additional diagnoses that should be considered:** Underlying causes of pathologic fracture

- **Most likely underlying cause:** Osteoporosis

- **Next steps:** Incentive spirometry, pain management, and evaluation for pathologic fractures that include primary osteoporosis and secondary causes including chronic systemic diseases, endocrine disorders, metabolic disorders, malignancies, adverse drug effects (ADEs), and nutritional deficiencies

ANALYSIS

Objectives

1. Identify the risk factors and secondary causes of osteoporosis.

2. Understand the indications and recommendations for screening of osteoporosis in women and men.

3. Describe a rational evaluation for osteoporosis.

4. List the nonpharmacologic and pharmacologic options for prevention and management of osteoporosis.

Considerations

This 62-year-old female patient presents with a rib fracture from a low-impact trauma. Her age, ethnicity, weight, and dietary restrictions place her at an increased risk for developing osteoporosis. After preventing complications and treating pain for her rib fracture, assessment and management of the various causes of osteoporosis would significantly reduce this patient's risk for future fractures and disability associated with this disorder.

The evaluation of this patient should include a dual-energy x-ray absorptiometry (DEXA) scan. Considerations for laboratory testing to rule out secondary causes of osteoporosis should include serum alkaline phosphatase, calcium, and 25-hydroxy vitamin D. If there were other clinical symptoms or examination findings, additional testing of thyroid, liver, and kidney function tests to rule out hyperthyroidism, chronic liver disease, and renal insufficiency, respectively, should be considered. A complete blood count (CBC) could be considered if anemia, blood cell malignancy, or malabsorption syndromes are suspected.

APPROACH TO:
Osteoporosis

DEFINITIONS

OSTEOPOROSIS: A low-density, mass, and structural deterioration of bone that leads to an increased risk of fracture. The World Health Organization (WHO) defines osteoporosis as *"a hip or spinal mineral density (BMD) of 2.5 standard deviations or more below the T score (mean) for 'young normal' adult."* The **Z score** is the BMD compared with an average healthy individual of same gender and age. A Z score of less than or equal to −2.0 can be used with clinical signs in premenopausal women and men less than 50 years.

OSTEOPENIA: The WHO defines osteopenia as *"a hip or spinal mineral density (T score) of 1.0 to 2.5 standard deviations below the mean for 'young normal' adult."*

OSTEOMALACIA: A defect in bone mineralization that can lead to osteoporosis usually due to calcium or vitamin D deficiency.

CLINICAL APPROACH
PREVENTION

The National Osteoporosis Foundation (NOF) recommends that all men and women greater than 50 years should be counseled on risk of fractures from osteoporosis, be checked for possible secondary causes of osteoporosis, have adequate daily intake of calcium (1200 mg) and vitamin D (800-1000 IU), and perform regular weight-bearing exercises. Smoking cessation and alcohol reduction can further reduce risk. Additional pharmacologic options for preventive treatments that are Food and Drug Administration (FDA)-approved include hormone therapy, selective estrogen receptor blockers, and bisphosphonates. Due to cost and potential adverse drug effects, these medications are often reserved for those patients with high risk or DEXA scan evidence of significantly reduced bone density.

SCREENING

It is estimated that there are nearly 54 million people in the United States affected by osteoporosis and low bone mass, with 10.2 million diagnosed with osteoporosis (8.2 million women and 2 million men) and 43.4 million with osteopenia. If prevalence remains unchanged, it is estimated that 64.4 million people will be affected by 2020 and 71.2 million by 2030.

There are multiple recommendations for osteoporosis screening from medical societies and organizations across North America and Europe. **The United States Preventive Services Task Force (USPSTF) recommends that all women aged greater than or equal to 65 and those less than 65 years with risk factors that are equal to or greater than the risk of a healthy 65-year-old Caucasian woman should be screened for osteoporosis.** This 10-year risk is 9.3% based on the WHO's FRAX calculation tool (http://www.shef.ac.uk/FRAX/). **The USPSTF states that there is insufficient** evidence to assess the balance of benefits and harms of screening for osteoporosis in men. The NOF recommends that all men aged 70 and older and those aged 50 to 69 with risk factors undergo screening. The preferred screening modality is via DEXA scan of the femoral neck and lumbar spine. Quantitative ultrasound densitometry and peripheral DEXA can predict risk, but do not correlate adequately to be used diagnostically.

DIAGNOSIS

Osteoporosis can be diagnosed radiographically or clinically. A central DEXA T score of −2.5 or more of the femoral neck and lumbar spine is the standard radiographic diagnostic test. Quantitative computed tomography absorptiometry is limited by cost and radiation exposure. A clinical diagnosis of osteoporosis can present with low-impact fractures (eg, a fall below standing height) or by spontaneous fractures due to bone fragility. Patients who present with these fractures should undergo thorough evaluation to rule out secondary causes of fracture.

Evaluating for Secondary Causes of Osteoporosis

In postmenopausal women, secondary causes of osteoporosis are presumed unusual and, in the absence of other symptoms, additional testing may not be indicated. However, approximately 50% of pre- and perimenopausal women, and men of any age, with osteoporosis may have a secondary cause. Common secondary causes include hyperthyroidism, primary hyperparathyroidism, vitamin D deficiency, amenorrheic conditions (eg, female athlete triad, anorexia), and chronic use of corticosteroids. Tobacco use and alcohol use of greater than two drinks per day are also significant risks. Serologic testing, including a complete blood count, kidney and liver function tests, serum calcium, thyroid-stimulating hormone (TSH), and 25-hydroxy vitamin D levels should be considered standard components of the workup for the patient with suspected or diagnosed osteoporosis. When appropriate, estradiol levels in women and testosterone levels in men can screen for hypogonadism, as there is a direct correlation between osteoporosis and menopause and testosterone deficiency/late-onset hypogonadism.

TREATMENT

Recommendation for treatment varies between organizations. The NOF recommends treatment for postmenopausal women and men aged 50 and older presenting with the following symptoms:

• Hip or vertebral fracture

• T score less than or equal to −2.5 at femoral neck or spine after appropriate evaluation to exclude secondary causes

• BMD T score −1.0 to −2.5 at femoral neck or spine and greater than or equal to 3% 10-year risk of hip fracture and greater than or equal to 20% 10-year risk of major osteoporosis fracture based on the WHO FRAX algorithm (http://www.shef.ac.uk/FRAX/)

Treatment should be considered in patients with elevated risks or BMD above and below these recommendations, and based on patient preferences. Nonpharmacologic treatments include fall prevention along with treatments to mitigate risks from impaired vision, balance, gait, cognitive impairment, and dizziness/vertigo. Smoking cessation and avoidance of excessive alcohol consumption should be encouraged. Home safety evaluations for hazards and durable medical equipment (eg, grab bars, walkers, etc) needs should be undertaken. Hip protectors and lumbar braces have not been shown to be effective in prevention of falls in patients with osteoporosis.

A universal recommendation in postmenopausal women and patients with osteoporosis is calcium and vitamin D intake supplementation; although in recent years the latter has become controversial. It is recommended that patients with osteoporosis consume at least 1200 mg of calcium a day in divided doses (no more than 500 mg per dose). A dose of at least 800 to 1000 IU of vitamin D should be used in conjunction with the calcium. In proven vitamin D deficiency, loading doses of ergocalciferol (vitamin D_2) 50,000 IU weekly for 4-8 weeks is recommended, followed by maintenance dosing of 50,000 IU monthly or cholecalciferol (vitamin D_3) 1000 to 2000 IU daily. The treatment goal serum level of 25-hydroxy vitamin D is greater than 30 ng/mL. The Institute of Medicine recommends against routine screening of vitamin D levels in the general population.

FDA-Approved Pharmacologic Therapy

Bisphosphonates

Oral bisphosphonates are the first-line agent for treatment of osteoporosis. Alendronate, risedronate, and ibandronate inhibit osteoclastic activity and have antiresorptive properties. These medications have excellent evidence for reduction in fractures in the hip and spine. Depending on the agent, they can be dosed daily, weekly, or monthly. Intravenous bisphosphonates can be given four times a year (ibandronate) or yearly (zoledronic acid). Oral agents must be taken on an empty stomach with a full glass of water and the patient must stay in an upright or standing position for at least 30 minutes after dosing due to a risk of esophagitis. The optimal length of treatment continues to be debatable, as there are concerns about atypical bone fractures in patients taking bisphosphonates for 5 years or greater. There are also rare reported cases of osteonecrosis in the jaw (mostly with IV bisphosphonates in cancer patients) after dental procedures.

Hormone Replacement Therapy and SERMs

Estrogen replacement is FDA-approved for prevention of osteoporosis in women with significant menopausal vasomotor symptoms, yet this recommendation is fraught with controversy due to the increased risks of thrombosis and breast cancer. It should be used at the lowest effective dose and for the shortest possible duration. Women taking estrogen and who have not had a hysterectomy should also take progesterone to limit the risk of endometrial cancer. Raloxifene, a selective estrogen receptor modulator (SERM), is FDA-approved for prevention and treatment of osteoporosis, especially of the lumbar spine. Raloxifene has been shown to reduce the risk of breast cancer, yet increases vasomotor symptoms and risk of deep venous thrombosis. This medication may be best reserved for postmenopausal women who do not tolerate bisphosphonates, who do not have vasomotor symptoms, and who have a high risk for development of breast cancer.

Calcitonin

Calcitonin is an antiresorptive medication that is administered as a nasal spray. It has evidence for prevention of vertebral compression fracture reduction as well as a modest analgesic effect. It is considered as a second-line agent, as more effective medications are available.

Teriparatide

Teriparatide is a recombinant human parathyroid hormone that causes bone density growth through its effect on osteoblasts. It is administered as a daily subcutaneous injection for up to 2 years. Because of its osteoblastic activity, it is contraindicated in patients at risk for osteosarcoma, such as patients with Paget disease, a history of bone radiation, or unexplained elevated serum alkaline phosphatase levels (which can be fractionated via isoenzymes to discern origin of tissue). It is approved for patients with severe osteoporosis and in those who have not benefited from or cannot tolerate bisphosphonates.

Denosumab

Denosumab was approved by the FDA in June 2010 for women with severe risk of osteoporotic fracture who are intolerant of bisphosphonates. It is a monoclonal antibody that prevents osteoclast differentiation and limits bone turnover. It has evidence in prevention of all forms of osteoporotic fractures and has similar efficacy to bisphosphonates. Denosumab is given as a subcutaneous injection once every 6 months and has a warning of increased risk of serious infection due to its immunosuppressive properties.

Combination Therapy

Combining bisphosphonates with other agents has not been well studied, the cost may be prohibitive, and the potential for adverse drug effects is unknown.

Monitoring of Treatment Success

Little evidence is available to indicate how often and what kind of follow-up testing is needed for monitoring effectiveness of treatment for osteoporosis. The NOF recommends repeat BMD testing every 2 years. Biochemical markers of bone turnover can be used early on to assess effectiveness of treatment, but are of limited usefulness due to biological and laboratory variability. Reduced BMD after treatment usually indicates patient compliance issues, but could indicate inadequate calcium and vitamin D intake, an undiagnosed secondary cause of osteoporosis, or treatment failure.

COMPREHENSION QUESTIONS

58.1 According to USPSTF guidelines, which of the following patients should be routinely screened for osteoporosis via DEXA scan?

A. A 65-year-old African-American man who takes hydrochlorothiazide for hypertension

B. A 53-year-old postmenopausal Caucasian woman who takes hormone replacement therapy for hot flashes

C. A 67-year-old Caucasian woman who takes 1500 mg of calcium and 800 IU of vitamin D daily

D. A 45-year-old Asian woman who broke her hip by falling off of a ladder while cleaning her gutters

E. A 55-year-old African-American woman who used inhaled steroids for 10 years for the management of asthma, but who never took oral steroids

58.2 A 60-year-old woman presents for follow-up for a wrist fracture that she sustained when she tripped while walking her dog. Follow-up DEXA scanning revealed a T score of −2.9. She has been postmenopausal for 10 years and has not had a hysterectomy. Which of the following interventions is most appropriate for reducing her risk of subsequent osteoporosis-related fractures?

A. Daily exercise

B. Estrogen replacement therapy

C. Vitamin D and calcium supplementation with a follow-up DEXA in 2 years

D. Alendronate

E. Calcitonin

58.3 A 51-year-old newly menopausal, physically active woman of mixed Asian-European origin presents inquiring about bone density testing. Her BMI is 20.9 kg/m²; she has a history of lactose intolerance and a 15-year use of low-dose inhaled corticosteroids for allergy-induced asthma. She has no history of fracture, oral steroid use, heavy alcohol use, or smoking. Based on the USPSTF and NOF recommendations and FRAX calculations (http://www.shef.ac.uk/FRAX/), which of the following statements is true for this patient?

A. Her risk as an Asian is greater than her risk as a Caucasian.

B. DEXA scanning is recommended.

C. Inhaled steroids significantly increase her risk of osteoporosis.

D. Calcium and vitamin D supplementation is recommended.

E. Low-dose bisphosphonate therapy is recommended.

ANSWERS

58.1 **C.** The USPSTF recommends routine osteoporosis screening for women 65 years or older without previous known fractures or secondary causes of osteoporosis. They also recommend routine screening for women less than 65 years whose 10-year fracture risk is greater than or equal to that of a 65-year-old white woman with no additional risk factors. A hip fracture that occurred with a significant traumatic injury would not be an indication for bone density screening, but a hip fracture associated with a minor injury, such as falling from a standing position, would be. Inhaled steroids are not considered a risk factor for osteoporosis.

58.2 **D.** This patient meets the criteria for the diagnosis of osteoporosis. Supplementation with calcium and vitamin D along with weight-bearing exercise are appropriate but not likely, by themselves, to increase her bone density sufficiently to reduce her fracture risk. Bisphosphonates, such as alendronate, are the first-line treatment in this situation based on their effectiveness at reducing fracture risk. Estrogen therapy alone is not recommended in women with an intact uterus, as there is an increased risk of endometrial cancer. Calcitonin would be reserved for consideration in a patient who does not tolerate or has contraindications to the use of bisphosphonates.

58.3 **D.** Calcium of at least 1200 mg/d and vitamin D of at least 800 IU/d is a universal recommendation for menopausal women. The FRAX calculator shows that Caucasian and Asian women in the United States have a 10-year risk of 4.5% and 3.3%, respectively. DEXA scans for screening are recommended by USPSTF when women aged 50 to 64 have a 10-year risk of 9.7% or greater. Low-dose inhaled steroids are not associated with significantly increased risk of osteoporosis.

CLINICAL PEARLS

► Calcium supplementation is considered a universal recommendation for prevention and treatment of osteoporosis in postmenopausal women. The outcomes data on benefit for vitamin D supplementation remain controversial but the risk of harm is limited.

► The DEXA scan is considered as the diagnostic test of choice for both screening and diagnosis of osteoporosis and osteopenia.

► There is no universal agreement on screening for osteoporosis in men, but if a male patient has significant risk factors, screening should be conducted since approximately 20% of patients with osteoporosis are men.

► Vitamin D deficiency and heavy alcohol consumption are common secondary causes of decreased BMD and osteoporosis.

REFERENCES

Gourlay ML, Fine JP, Preisser JS, et al. Bone-density testing interval and transition to osteoporosis in older women. *N Engl J Med*. 2012;366:225-233.

Lindsay R, Cosman F. Osteoporosis. In: Kasper D, Fauci A, Hauser S, et al., eds. *Harrison's Principles of Internal Medicine*. 19th ed. New York, NY: McGraw-Hill Education; 2015. Available at: http://accessmedicine.mhmedical.com. Accessed May 25, 2015.

National Osteoporosis Foundation. *Clinician's Guide to Prevention and Treatment of Osteoporosis*. Washington, DC: National Osteoporosis Foundation; 2010.

Prockop DJ. New targets for osteoporosis. *N Engl J Med*. 2012;367:2353-2354.

Rao SS, Budhwar N, Ashfaque A. Osteoporosis in men. *Am Fam Physician*. 2010;82(5):503-508.

Sweet M, Sweet J, Jeremiah M, Galazka S. Diagnosis and treatment of osteoporosis. *Am Fam Physician*. 2009;79(3):193-200.

U.S. Preventive Services Task Force. Screening for osteoporosis: recommendation statement. *Am Fam Physician*. 2011;83(10):1197-1200.

A 58-year-old woman with known metastatic breast cancer presents for a follow-up visit. She was diagnosed with breast cancer 2 years ago, at which time she underwent a lumpectomy and local breast radiation therapy. Subsequently, she was found to have metastases to her thoracic spine and has started chemotherapy under the management of an oncologist. You have been trying to manage her pain with hydrocodone/acetaminophen, which provides temporary relief, but the pain returns a few hours after taking her pills. She has purposely been taking less than the recommended dosage in order to avoid addiction, and waits until the pain is severe before taking them. On average, she uses four to six hydrocodone/acetaminophen pills daily. The patient also complains of chronic constipation over the last few years. Her appetite is reduced by the chemotherapy, and the associated bloating and constipation make her not want to eat at all. Her last bowel movement was 4 days ago and she only has bowel movements when she uses enemas. On examination, she is wearing a bandana that covers her hair and does not appear cachectic. Her abdomen has hypoactive bowel sounds, and is mildly distended, firm, and tender to palpation without rebound or guarding.

► What is the likely cause of her constipation?
► What can you do to improve her pain control?
► How do you address her concerns about narcotic addiction?

ANSWERS TO CASE 59:
Chronic Pain Management

Summary: A 58-year-old woman with pain from bone metastases from breast cancer presents for follow-up of her pain management. She is using a short-acting narcotic/acetaminophen combination that modestly relieves her pain when she uses it, but she limits its use out of concern for addiction. She also has developed significant constipation.

- **Most likely cause of her constipation:** Side effect of her narcotic use.

- **Steps to improve her pain control:** Begin an extended-release opioid analgesic, such as extended-release morphine or fentanyl patches, with the addition of a short-acting opioid for breakthrough pain.

- **Steps to address her concerns about addiction:** Explain to her that addiction rarely occurs when pain medications are used as directed for the management of chronic pain.

ANALYSIS

Objectives

1. Be able to describe an appropriate evaluation of a patient presenting with chronic pain.

2. Be able to list treatment modalities for chronic malignant and nonmalignant pain syndromes.

3. Know common side effects of the pharmacologic agents used to treat chronic pain and list methods to overcome these side effects.

Considerations

This case represents a common primary care scenario of the management of a patient with chronic pain due to metastatic cancer. As treatment modalities for cancer improve, many people are living longer with cancer that would have been fatal in the past. Cancers can cause pain from direct invasion of organs or inflammation at the site of either the primary tumor or the metastases, with bony pain from metastatic disease being a common and especially painful complication. Some cancer treatments, such as surgery or radiation therapy, can be painful as well. Opioid analgesics are the mainstay of therapy for cancer pain, and there is little dispute or controversy regarding their use in this situation.

The management of chronic, nonmalignant pain syndromes can be much more challenging and controversial. Both physicians and patients may be concerned about the use of opioid therapy in these situations. The treatment of chronic, nonmalignant pain should be multidisciplinary and should utilize the biopsychosocial model of care to maximize outcomes. The use of pain medications is one option, with other modalities including exercise, physical rehabilitation, counseling, nonnarcotic medications, and complementary/alternative therapies as other viable options. The overall goals of chronic pain management should be to maximize function while minimizing pain and side effects of treatment.

APPROACH TO:
Chronic Pain Management

DEFINITIONS

NEUROPATHIC PAIN: Pain caused by damage or dysfunction of a nerve or of the nervous system

MUSCLE PAIN: Local or regional pain involving soft tissue of the musculoskeletal system

INFLAMMATORY PAIN: Pain due to the release of inflammatory agents, such as prostaglandins, in response to illness, injury, or inflammation-causing condition (eg, rheumatoid arthritis)

MECHANICAL/COMPRESSIVE PAIN: Most commonly musculoskeletal pain aggravated by activity and improved by rest and limitation of physical activity

CLINICAL APPROACH

Assessment

Acute pain is pain associated with an illness or injury that has a generally accepted time course and progression—the pain starts with the onset of the illness/injury, the pain may be constant or intermittent, and the pain improves as the illness/injury improves. In contrast, **chronic pain is persistent pain that negatively impacts the person's quality of life and functioning.** The pain can be constant, intermittent, or recurrent and may be associated with an illness or injury, but lasts longer than would be expected with the improvement of the condition.

Dealing with chronic pain can be frustrating for both the patient and the physician. Patients with chronic pain may have difficulties with personal and professional relationships due to their pain, may not be able to perform required or desired functions, and often do not get adequate pain relief. They can be accused of malingering, hypochondriasis, drug-seeking, and/or drug addiction. Physicians can become frustrated at the inability to diagnose the cause of the pain and may order numerous and repeated expensive tests or procedures out of concern for the patient or fear of malpractice suits. Physicians may also struggle with concerns about being tricked into prescribing narcotic medications and the legal ramifications for inappropriate and excessive prescribing of controlled substances.

Numerous guidelines and recommendations for the management of chronic, nonmalignant pain are available. The overall goal of chronic pain management is to create a comprehensive plan utilizing the biopsychosocial model with a specific emphasis on managing pain, minimizing dependence, and improving function while limiting disability and side effects.

Initially, an assessment should be made to identify the type and cause of the pain through a thorough history and physical examination. The history should focus on the location, duration, intensity, and type of pain (eg, neuropathic, musculoskeletal, etc). Time should be spent performing detailed psychological and social histories to evaluate for comorbid depression, other psychiatric conditions, or evidence of substance abuse. As it is legal for medicinal uses in many states, inquiring about marijuana use is paramount, as use of this drug may limit a clinician's ability to prescribe opioid-based therapy.

It is important to understand how the chronic pain condition has interfered with the patient's personal life, relationships, occupation, and other functioning. A detailed physical examination should be performed and documented at every visit. Functional assessment utilizing a standardized assessment tool should also be performed, as this allows for establishment of a baseline and provides for an objective assessment of improvement or deterioration over time. When available, previous medical records should be obtained and reviewed to avoid duplication of testing. If the history and examination suggest the presence of a treatable condition, and if the test has not previously been performed, then focused diagnostic testing should be performed. Some states have prescription audit registries that allow both state authorities and physicians to track and monitor controlled substance prescriptions that patients have been prescribed. Obtaining and reviewing such registries, where possible, should occur in all cases when a new patient presents to a practice for evaluation and treatment of chronic pain.

Nonpharmacologic Management

The comprehensive management of chronic pain should involve both pharmacologic and nonpharmacologic treatments. The patient, family, and physician should start by establishing realistic and achievable goals. The initial management should include nonpharmacologic therapies, including targeted exercise such as physical therapy or occupation-specific rehabilitation programs, psychological interventions such as counseling or cognitive behavioral therapy, and complementary or alternative modalities such as spinal and musculoskeletal manipulations, acupuncture, and meditation. Patient acceptance and participation are mandatory for success in reducing chronic pain. Unfortunately, third-party payers may not cover some of these treatment options and inability for patients to pay may limit access.

Pharmacologic Management

Initial pharmacologic management options should be based on the type, location, and severity of pain, the presence of comorbid conditions, and the need to minimize interactions with other medications that the patient may require. Nonnarcotic analgesics, such as acetaminophen or nonsteroidal anti-inflammatory drugs (NSAIDs), should be considered as first-line agents. However, these may not be viable options in the presence of significant liver (acetaminophen) or renal (NSAID) disease. Neuropathic pain may be relieved or reduced by the use of anticonvulsants (eg, gabapentin), and musculoskeletal pain may benefit from the judicious use of muscle relaxants. Antidepressant therapy (eg, selective serotonin reuptake inhibitors [SSRIs]) is also a beneficial adjunct to other therapies to help improve mood, sleep, and overall function. Benzodiazepines should be avoided in patients receiving chronic opioid analgesics to minimize the risk of oversedation and respiratory depression.

Opioid agonists (eg, hydrocodone, oxycodone, morphine, fentanyl) may be used for chronic, malignant, or nonmalignant pain when necessary in patients in whom pain cannot be controlled despite reasonable use of other modalities. In general, long-acting opioid agonists are preferred, as they provide greater duration of pain control and reduce the euphoria associated with short-acting opioid agonists, which may allow for improved patient function and less risk of abuse or addiction. The use of short-acting opioid agonists should be reserved for breakthrough pain. Common side effects of opioid agonists include sedation and constipation, a particularly bothersome issue for many patients. Follow-up of patients on chronic opioid therapy should include specific questioning about bowel movement frequency, and they should take daily stool softeners (eg, docusate) or stimulant/osmotic laxatives (eg, bisacodyl/polyethylene glycol 3350) to prevent chronic constipation.

Mixed opioid agonist-antagonists (eg, buprenorphine) act as partial agonists at one opioid receptor and antagonistic effects at another opioid receptor, and are becoming more viable options for patients with chronic pain. They provide a "ceiling effect" for analgesia, have the potential to induce acute abstinence in patients with physical dependency to agonist opioids, and are less preferred by patients who have opioid addiction. Tramadol, now considered a schedule 5 (V) drug by the Controlled Substances Act, is an opioid agonist with a mechanism of action that includes effects on monoamines including serotonin. It may be used as an adjunct for chronic pain, and carries a risk of lowering the seizure threshold.

Many physicians will encourage "controlled substance agreements" when their patients require long-term opioid analgesics. Such agreements provide guidelines for both physicians and patients regarding policies for use, follow-up visits, medication refills (eg, quantity of pills or patches, frequency of prescriptions, etc), and toxicology screening. These contracts may specify that the patient can only get controlled substance medications from one prescriber and one pharmacy. Typically, these agreements include the consent for urine toxicology screening as a mechanism to evaluate for drug diversion (eg, drug screen fails to show presence of the prescribed opioid in the urine) or unauthorized use of other drugs (eg, drug testing shows the presence of a nonprescribed or illicit drug). Agreements such as this, along with careful and thorough documentation in the medical record, can reduce physician concerns for legal issues regarding controlled substance prescriptions.

COMPREHENSION QUESTIONS

59.1 A 45-year-old diabetic patient presents for a routine follow-up. His diabetes has been uncontrolled although he is making good efforts to comply with his diet, exercise, and medication regimens. He has a long history of burning pain in his feet that has been uncontrolled by over-the-counter medications and is now worsening in severity such that he can no longer work. Your examination of his feet reveals no skin ulcerations, diminished but present and symmetrical pedal pulses, and reduced sensation on monofilament testing bilaterally. Along with aggressive management of his diabetes, which of the following interventions would be most appropriate at this time?

A. An NSAID

B. A long-acting opioid agonist

C. A short-acting opioid agonist

D. Gabapentin

E. Acupuncture

59.2 A 25-year-old patient who is a regular patient of the practice presents for an urgent evaluation. He has been receiving opioid analgesics from your practice for several months for back pain that was otherwise uncontrolled in spite of multidisciplinary treatments including physical therapy, chiropractic manipulation, and nonnarcotic medications. He has agreed to a controlled substance agreement that includes specification of the number of pills to be prescribed, frequency of refills, and urine toxicology screening. His last prescription was written by your practice partner last week.

The patient states that his prescription was stolen from his car this morning and he is very concerned that his pain will return if he doesn't get a new prescription right away. When you ask him to provide a urinalysis for a toxicology screen he states that he just urinated and can't wait until he urinates again, since he has to be somewhere in 15 minutes. Review of his chart indicates that he had one prescription rewritten earlier than agreed to in the recent past because he accidentally dropped his pills into the toilet. Which of the following is your best course of action at this time?

A. Refill his pain medication, with a warning that he needs to be more careful.

B. Refill his pain medication and refer him to an orthopedic surgeon for ongoing care.

C. Refuse to refill his pain medication, tell him it will be refilled on the appropriate date.

D. Refuse to refill his pain medication, refer him to Narcotics Anonymous.

E. Refuse to refill his pain medication, consider terminating him from your practice.

59.3 A 68-year-old man with prostate cancer metastatic to bone is going to be started on long-acting morphine for his pain. He denies depressed mood or insomnia. Which of the following adjunctive therapies should be considered along with long-term use of opioid agonists?

A. Bisacodyl

B. Trazodone

C. Tramadol

D. Gabapentin

E. Nortriptyline

ANSWERS

59.1 **D.** Diabetic neuropathy is the most common type of peripheral neuropathic pain. In many patients, it can be extremely painful and debilitating. Aggressive management of the patient's diabetes is extremely important, but improvement in neuropathic symptoms from diabetic control may take months and, in some patients, the neuropathy does not improve in spite of ideal diabetic control. An anticonvulsant, such as gabapentin, is often effective at alleviating or minimizing neuropathic pain. Antidepressants, especially tricyclic antidepressants, and NSAIDS, may also be effective. Physical therapy and acupuncture have no proven benefit in reducing symptoms of neuropathy. Opioid agonists are not indicated as first-line agents.

59.2 **E.** This patient is exhibiting several "red flags" for the misuse of narcotic medications. He is requesting refills more frequently than agreed and is refusing to provide urine for drug testing. Continuing to prescribe narcotic medications to the patient, even if waiting until an agreed upon date, would be inappropriate because of these concerns. While he may benefit from addiction counseling, he may not actually be using the medications himself—he could be giving them away or selling them to others. The most appropriate response provided would be to refuse this or any further, prescriptions and to terminate the patient from the practice.

59.3 **A.** Constipation is a common side effect of narcotic medication use. Establishing a bowel regimen for a patient who will be on a chronic narcotic program is an important adjunctive treatment. None of the other options are likely to be effective for chronic pain management due to metastatic disease to bone.

CLINICAL PEARLS

▶ The management of chronic pain is best performed by using a multidisciplinary approach that utilizes the biopsychosocial model of care. Medications are only one aspect of this model.

▶ Anticipate common side effects of your treatments, such as constipation associated with opioid agonists, and prophylactically provide your patient with the tools needed to address the problem.

▶ Perform urine toxicology screening often in patients whom you suspect may be using other drugs or illicit substances including medical marijuana.

REFERENCES

American Academy of Pain Medicine. Use of opioids for the treatment of chronic pain. Available at: http://www.painmed.org/files/use-of-opioids-for-the-treatment-of-chronic-pain.pdf. Accessed April 16, 2015.

Camilleri M. Opioid-induced constipation: challenges and therapeutic opportunities. *Am J Gastroenterol.* 2011;106:835-842.

Groninger H, Vijayan J. Pharmacologic management of pain at the end of life. *Am Fam Physician.* 2014;90(1):26-32.

Jackman RP, Purvis JM, Mallett BS. Chronic nonmalignant pain in primary care. *Am Fam Physician.* 2008;78(10):1155-1162.

Rockson SG. Current concepts and future directions in the diagnosis and management of lymphatic vascular disease. *Vasc Med.* 2010;15(3):223-231.

Schug SA, Goddard C. Recent advances in the pharmacological management of acute and chronic pain. *Ann Palliate Med.* 2014;3(4):263-275.

Smith H, Bruckenthal P. Implications of opioid analgesia for medically complicated patients. *Drugs Aging.* 2010;27(5):417-433.

Trayes KP, Studdiford JS, Pickle S, Tully AS. Edema: diagnosis and management. *Am Fam Physician.* 2013;88(2):102-110.

World Health Organization. WHO's pain relief ladder. Available at: http://www.who.int/cancer/palliative/painladder/en/. Accessed April 16, 2015.

A 52-year-old healthy man presents to your office complaining of a 2-year history of bilateral leg swelling and intermittent heaviness that has become more bothersome over the past 3 months. He works as a mailman and states that this heaviness is increasingly impairing his ability to complete his route. He tells you "The swelling in my legs is often worse in the evening, especially when I have been walking all day." By the end of the day, he has swelling up to his mid-calves and that the top of his socks leave deep indentations in his skin. He complains of brown spots and dryness and itching on his feet and ankles. He denies unusual shortness of breath, fatigue, sleep disturbance, but states that he has been using over-the-counter (OTC) ibuprofen for several months for knee pain. On examination, his body mass index (BMI) is 23 kg/m^2, blood pressure is 130/85 mm Hg, pulse is 72 beats/min, and respiratory rate is 16 breaths/min. His heart, lung, and abdominal examinations are unremarkable. On examination of his extremities, he has symmetrical bilateral edema to his mid-calves with pitting, prominent varicose veins, and brown 2-mm sized macules on his feet and ankles. His posterior tibialis and dorsalis pedis pulses are 2+ bilaterally and his feet are warm.

▶ What is the most likely diagnosis?
▶ What further evaluation should be considered?
▶ What is the initial step in therapy?

ANSWERS TO CASE 60:
Lower Extremity Edema

Summary: A 52-year-old man presents with classic signs and symptoms of peripheral venous insufficiency. It is bilateral, chronic, and dependent and without significant constitutional, cardiac, or pulmonary symptoms. Physical examination reveals varicosities and venous stasis dermatitis. The edema often interferes with and is aggravated by his work and is possibly worsened with the recent use of ibuprofen.

- **Most likely diagnosis:** Venous insufficiency and varicose veins, aggravated by use of nonsteroidal anti-inflammatory drugs (NSAIDs).

- **Further evaluation necessary:** Ensure that there are no comorbid conditions: sleep studies and echocardiography if obstructive sleep apnea (OSA) and pulmonary hypertension are considered; echocardiogram, chest radiograph (CXR), electrocardiogram (ECG), brain natriuretic peptide (BNP) if congestive heart failure (CHF) or other cardiac cause is considered; serum electrolytes, serum creatinine, and urinalysis if renal causes are considered; serum albumin if low-protein or malabsorption states are considered. Ankle brachial index (ABI) testing should be considered if potential treatments could aggravate peripheral arterial disease (PAD).

- **Beneficial treatment:** Leg elevation, compression stockings, low-sodium diet, and avoidance of medications that may cause edema. Consider oral horse chestnut seed extract for edema. Surgical options should be considered if comorbid PAD or venous stasis ulcers are present. Appropriate antibiotic and wound care therapy should be instituted when skin disruption is present to treat infection and maximize wound healing.

ANALYSIS

Objectives

1. Become familiar with the presenting signs and symptoms of common causes of lower extremity swelling.

2. Understand the clinical evaluation used to diagnose and identify low-risk lower extremity swelling from swelling indicative of severe comorbid conditions or those causes with significant risk.

3. Become familiar with the management of common causes of lower extremity swelling.

4. Define different types of lower extremity swelling and levels of lower extremity edema.

Considerations

In older people, chronic venous insufficiency is the most common cause of bilateral lower extremity swelling, affecting up to 2% of the general population, with increasing prevalence with age and obesity. Although venous insufficiency can often be diagnosed clinically without extensive testing, for persons older than 45 years there is an increased risk of **pulmonary hypertension** (most commonly secondary to obstructive sleep apnea) and **congestive heart failure** as the etiology of the lower extremity swelling. There are many **medications** also associated with fluid retention and should always be considered in the differential as a potential cause of or contributor to lower extremity swelling.

APPROACH TO:
Lower Extremity Edema

DEFINITIONS

VENOUS EDEMA: An excess of low viscosity, protein-poor interstitial fluid resulting in pitting in the affected area of the body.

LYMPHEDEMA: An excess of protein-rich interstitial fluid within the skin and subcutaneous tissue. Primary forms are rare and often genetically related. Secondary lymphedema is more common and often related to previous malignancies, surgery, radiation, and infections.

LIPIDEMA: A form of fat maldistribution that can appear to be leg swelling with foot sparing, and is not a true form of edema.

MYXEDEMA: A dermal edema secondary to an increased deposition of connective tissue components (mucopolysaccharides) seen in various forms of thyroid disease.

CLINICAL APPROACH

Edema is defined as a visible and palpable swelling comprised of interstitial fluid. The most common cause of leg edema in North American patients older than 50 years is venous insufficiency, as it affects up to 30% of the population. CHF affects around 1% of adults. The mostly likely cause of leg edema in women younger than 50 years is idiopathic edema, and may be confused with obesity. Most patients should be assumed to have one of these causes unless a history and physical indicate an underlying secondary cause. The two exceptions to this rule are in cases of pulmonary hypertension and undiagnosed CHF. These conditions may present with lower extremity edema prior to formal diagnosis.

DIAGNOSIS

History

The key elements of the history in evaluating the patient with lower extremity edema include the duration of edema (acute [≤72 hours], vs chronic), presence of pain, current medications, overnight improvement when sleeping (indicating dependent edema), signs or symptoms of OSA (eg, snoring, daytime somnolence), and history of chronic medical conditions including heart, liver, and kidney disease, or past history of pelvic or abdominal malignancies or radiation therapy. Family history of clotting disorders, varicosities, and lymphedema are also important to document.

Physical Examination

The key elements of the physical examination in the patient with lower extremity edema include signs of OSA including a body mass index (BMI) greater than 30 kg/m² and a thick neck circumference greater than 17 in (42 cm). Unilateral leg swelling is commonly seen with venous insufficiency, lymphedema, and deep vein thrombosis (DVT). Bilateral leg swelling is commonly seen with bilateral venous insufficiency, medication side effects, and idiopathic or systemic causes. Generalized edema is seen in advanced systemic diseases including CHF, renal failure, and liver failure. Tenderness of the swelling can be seen with DVTs and lipedema. Pitting is commonly encountered with venous edema, DVT, CHF, and early lymphedema; myxedema and chronic lymphedema do not cause pitting. Varicose veins are common in patients with chronic lymphedema, and a *Kaposi-Stemmer sign* (inability to pinch a fold of skin on dorsum of foot at base of second toe) is seen.

Common skin changes in lower extremity edema include hemosiderin deposition (brown pigmented spots), dry dermatitis, and skin ulceration (in cases of venous insufficiency), warm, tender, moist skin (as in complex regional pain syndrome), brawny induration, and warty texture with papillomatosis (lymphedema). Signs of underlying systemic disease include jaundice, ascites, and spider hemangioma (in liver disease and cirrhosis) and jugular venous distention, hepatojugular reflex, and rales on pulmonary examination (in congestive heart failure).

Diagnostic Studies

The majority of patients older than 50 years who present with leg swelling have venous insufficiency. Pulmonary hypertension (due to OSA or other causes) should always be in the differential of likely venous insufficiency. If the etiology is unclear, a complete blood count (CBC), comprehensive metabolic profile, urinalysis, and thyroid-stimulating hormone (TSH) can potentially rule out common systemic diseases associated with leg swelling. Proteinuria and serum albumin less than 2 g/dL are diagnostic for nephrotic syndrome. If the patient is found to have nephrotic syndrome, a fasting serum lipid profile should also be obtained.

If the clinical history and examination indicate a cardiac etiology, obtaining an electrocardiogram, echocardiogram, BNP, and chest radiograph should be obtained. A normal BNP can rule out CHF with a sensitivity of 90%.

In young women with idiopathic lower extremity edema who desire testing confirmation, or if the etiology is unclear, a morning to evening weight gain of greater than 0.7 kg may confirm the diagnosis. A water load test can be performed by drinking 20 cc/kg (max 1500 cc) in the morning and collecting all urine 1 hour prior to consumption until 4 hours after, then repeating. In the first trial, the patient must stand for the 4-hour time frame. In the second trial, the patient must remain recumbent. In cases of idiopathic edema, less than 55% of water consumed will be voided in the standing position and greater than 65% will be voided in recumbent position. Idiopathic edema is often associated with obesity and with depression.

Patients may complain of hand and face swelling in addition to leg swelling. On history, many patients may be taking diuretics to self-treat, or may be present asking for "water pills" to decrease the edema.

If a DVT is suspected (as in cases of acute edema), a D-dimer level should be obtained. Due to its high sensitivity yet low specificity, a normal D-dimer level essentially rules out a DVT, yet a positive D-dimer is not diagnostic of DVT. If the D-dimer is positive, then a venous Doppler ultrasonography of the lower extremities should be obtained. In patients with intermediate-to-high pretest probability of DVT, negative ultrasonography alone is insufficient to exclude the diagnosis of DVT. Further assessment is recommended, including repeating ultrasonography in 1 week if the D-dimer is elevated. An echocardiogram should be considered in patients greater than 45 years to rule out pulmonary hypertension or in any patient in whom OSA is suspected, and a polysomnogram should be obtained to evaluate this condition. If liver disease is suspected, then liver function tests and coagulation studies should be obtained. If a malignancy is suspected, then an abdominal and pelvic examination and computed tomography (CT) scan should be considered. Tumors commonly associated with lower extremity edema include prostate cancer, ovarian cancer, and lymphoma.

TREATMENT

Idiopathic Edema

Lifestyle modifications necessary to manage idiopathic edema include intermittent recumbency or leg elevation, avoidance of heat, low-sodium diet, decreased fluid intake, and weight loss. Patients with this disorder often have a secondary hyperaldosteronism due to this condition. Therefore, spironolactone dosed in the early evening has proven benefit in volume reduction. If not successful, a thiazide diuretic can be added as well. Loop diuretics should be avoided due to a higher risk of electrolyte abnormalities (eg, hypokalemia) and renal insufficiency. Compression stockings are less successful with this condition. Diuretic abuse is common among patients with idiopathic edema, and can lead to a mild hypovolemia that can stimulate renin-angiotensin-aldosterone secretion, which can lead to rebound edema when the diuretic is stopped. Diuretic-induced rebound edema can be minimized by weaning off the diuretic over a 3- to 4-week period. Patients need to be reassured that the initial worsening of edema is common with the withdrawal of diuretics but should normalize.

Venous Insufficiency

For patients with venous insufficiency, nonpharmacologic therapies include compression leg stockings and leg elevation. Often higher compressions of 30 to 40 mm Hg at the ankle are required to adequately control the swelling. If arterial insufficiency is a consideration, then venous and arterial Doppler ultrasonography should be performed prior to application of the stockings. Higher compression stockings can be difficult for some patients to put on, so patients should be instructed to put them on upon awakening before the leg swelling progresses. Advising the patient to roll the stockings off at the end of the day so that they can be rolled back on in the morning is also helpful. Stocking applicators can also be prescribed.

Horse chestnut seed extract inhibits elastin and hyaluronidase which in a 300-mg twice-daily dosing has been shown to modestly decrease symptoms associated with venous insufficiency. Loop diuretics in low doses can be used short term for patients who are severely affected. Surgical interventions are available for patients with severe disease who are unresponsive to less-invasive measures.

Lymphedema

Patients with lymphedema should be educated regarding the chronic nature of the condition. Reasonable expectations for treatment must be set and understood, as this condition is often difficult to manage. Treatments include exercise, elevation, intermittent pneumatic compression devices, manual lymph drainage massage, and surgical procedures. Diuretics are typically not helpful, but may be commonly used for comorbid conditions that contribute to volume overload including CHF and liver failure. Patients with chronic lymphedema are at a great risk of development of cellulitis. For patients with recurrent cellulitis, prophylactic antibiotics should be considered.

Deep Vein Thrombosis

Acute DVT requires prompt treatment with commencement of anticoagulation. Treatment options include low-molecular-weight heparin (eg, enoxaparin), warfarin, and direct Xa inhibitors (eg, rivaroxaban). The therapeutic goal for warfarin therapy should be a target international normalized ratio (INR) of 2.0 to 3.0. The duration of anticoagulation therapy varies based on cause and recurrence rate of the DVT. In initial cases of uncomplicated DVT, 3 months of anticoagulation is warranted. In cases of recurrent DVT and/or concomitant pulmonary embolism, then long-term anticoagulation is the standard of care. If anticoagulation therapy is contraindicated, then inferior vena cava (IVC) filter placement may be indicated to prevent life-threatening pulmonary embolism.

CASE CORRELATION

- See also Case 27 (Congestive Heart Failure).

COMPREHENSION QUESTIONS

60.1 A 60-year-old woman presents for follow-up of lymphedema that developed following a mastectomy and lymph node dissection for breast cancer. She finds the swelling to be very uncomfortable and limits the use of her right arm. Which of the following treatment options are recommended?

A. Intermittent pneumatic compression

B. Oral warfarin

C. Oral furosemide

D. Oral hydrochlorothiazide

E. Horse chestnut seed extract

60.2 Which patient would have the most benefit from a laboratory or diagnostic testing evaluation for systemic disease as a cause of lower extremity swelling?

A. A 35-year-old woman with cyclic bilateral ankle swelling without significant pain. She is taking OTC ibuprofen for her menstrual cramps. On examination, she has +1 pitting at the ankles.

B. A 44-year-old man with a 3-year history of left greater than right, pain-free, moderate swelling in his calves. He has a normal BMI, no daytime somnolence, and no constitutional symptoms. He is not taking any OTC or prescription medications. On examination, he has mild varicosities and hemosiderin skin deposits on both legs with nontender +1 pitting edema. Calf circumferences measure 17 cm on the left and 15.5 cm on the right.

C. A 50-year-old man with +2 bilateral lower extremity edema that has slowly been worsening over the last year. He has a history of hypertension and is taking hydrochlorothiazide, benazepril, and amlodipine. On review of systems, he complains of daily fatigue, and some increasing constipation.

D. A 25-year-old woman on oral contraceptives with bilateral +1 lower extremity pitting swelling over a 2-year period. On examination, she has a body mass index of 26 kg/m^2, no varicosities, no skin changes, and an otherwise negative review of symptoms. She does admit to using OTC weight-loss aids regularly.

60.3 A 65-year-old man with a history of prostate cancer and radiation therapy 3 years ago presents with chronic bilateral leg swelling. He denies dyspnea, chest pain, orthopnea, or wheezing. He denies daytime somnolence or snoring. On examination, he has nonpitting up to his calves with a "squaring" appearance of the foot. You are unable to pinch skin on dorsum of foot at second toe. What is the most likely diagnosis?

A. Deep vein thrombosis

B. Secondary lymphedema

C. Myxedema

D. Venous stasis

E. Hypoalbuminemia secondary to prostate cancer

ANSWERS

60.1 **A.** In lymphedema, diuretics unfortunately have little impact. Management options include support, pneumatic compression, manual lymph drainage, and surgery. In venous insufficiency, horse chestnut seed extract can be used to decrease signs and symptoms. Loop diuretics can be used short term to decrease edema burden.

60.2 **C.** Patients older than 45 with lower extremity edema and systemic signs such as fatigue, somnolence, and constipation could benefit from an evaluation for systemic disease as a cause for lower extremity swelling. A CBC, basic metabolic profile (BMP), urinalysis (UA), TSH, and serum albumin would be reasonable in this patient. Sleep studies and an echocardiogram would also be useful due to the increased risk for pulmonary hypertension as a cause of edema in patients older than 45 years. Liver function tests would be useful in patients who present with ascites. NSAIDs (5% risk of edema), calcium channel blockers (50% risk of edema), and oral contraceptives are medications that are associated with edema. The most common cause of unilateral edema without pain with onset more than 72 hours is venous insufficiency. Patients who cross their legs predominantly on one side can have greater disparity in leg swelling and varicosities.

60.3 **B.** The most common cause of lymphedema is secondary to malignancy (prostate, ovarian, lymphoma), surgery, and radiation therapy. The positive Kaposi-Stemmer is seen in lymphedema. Chronic bilateral lower extremity swelling is unlikely to represent a DVT. Myxedema is associated with thyroid disorders. Hypoalbuminemia is seen in advance malignancies, nephrotic syndrome, protein-losing enteropathies, and liver disease.

CLINICAL PEARLS

▶ Idiopathic edema and venous insufficiency are the most common causes of lower extremity swelling in patients without systemic disease and often can be diagnosed with history alone.

▶ Pulmonary hypertension secondary to sleep apnea should be considered in patients presenting with leg swelling who are older than 45 years, have a neck circumference greater than 17 in (42 cm), have daytime somnolence, and a history of snoring.

▶ If there is an unclear etiology of the lower extremity swelling, lipidema and lymphedema should be ruled out.

▶ Options for anticoagulation in the treatment of DVT include low-molecular-weight heparin, warfarin, and direct Xa inhibitors.

REFERENCES

Braunwald E, Loscalzo J. Edema. In: Kasper D, Fauci A, Hauser S, et al., eds. *Harrison's Principles of Internal Medicine.* 19th ed. New York, NY: McGraw-Hill Education; 2015. Available at: http://accessmedicine.mhmedical.com. Accessed May 25, 2015.

Buller HR, Prins MH, Lensin AW, et al. EINSTEIN-PE Investigators. Oral rivaroxaban for the treatment of symptomatic pulmonary embolism. *N Engl J Med.* 2012;366(14):1287-1297.

Eberhardt RT, Raffetto JD. Chronic venous insufficiency. *Circulation.* 2014;130:333-346.

Pittler MH, Ernst E. Horse chestnut seed extract for chronic venous insufficiency. *Cochrane Database Syst Rev.* Nov 14 2012;11:CD003230.

Raju S, Neglen P. Chronic venous insufficiency and varicose veins. *N Engl J Med.* 2009;360:2319-2327.

Review Questions

> The following are strategically designed review questions to assess whether the student is able to integrate the information presented in the cases. The explanations to the answer choices describe the rationale, including which cases are relevant.

R1. A 52-year-old obese man presents for follow-up of his hypertension. His blood pressure is well controlled on a daily dose of hydrochlorothiazide. You notice that he has thickened, velvety skin circumferentially around his neck. A finger-stick blood sugar test done an hour after he ate lunch was 130 mg/dL. Which of the following test results would be diagnostic for diabetes mellitus?

   A. The nonfasting, finger-stick sugar of 130 mg/dL is diagnostic. No further testing is needed.

   B. A hemoglobin A_{1c} level of greater than 6.0%.

   C. A fasting plasma glucose of 120 mg/dL.

   D. A random plasma glucose of 220 mg/dL and symptomatic polyuria.

   E. A plasma glucose of 130 mg/dL drawn 1 hour after a 50-g glucose challenge.

R2. For the patient in question R1, a diagnosis of type 2 diabetes mellitus is established. Along with diet and exercise, which of the following is the most appropriate initial management?

   A. Oral glyburide

   B. Oral metformin

   C. Oral pioglitazone (Actos)

   D. Mealtime injections of short-acting insulin

   E. Single daily injection of glargine insulin

R3. A 38-year-old African-American man is evaluated for the new diagnosis of hypertension. His workup has shown multiple elevated blood pressure readings in the past few months but no evidence of any other medical conditions. You plan to initiate an antihypertensive medication. Which of the following would be the best initial choice?

   A. Amlodipine (calcium channel blocker)

   B. Lisinopril (angiotensin-converting enzyme inhibitor)

   C. Losartan (angiotensin receptor blocker)

   D. Carvedilol (β-blocker)

   E. Doxazosin (α-blocker)

R4. A 45-year-old man presents for a routine physical examination. He has no known medical history and has not seen a doctor in several years. On a screening lipid panel he is found to have a total cholesterol of 330 mg/dL, high-density lipoprotein (HDL) cholesterol of 50 mg/dL, triglycerides of 100 mg/dL, and low-density lipoprotein (LDL) cholesterol of 220 mg/dL. These results are confirmed on repeat testing. According to the American Heart Association/American College of Cardiology guidelines, which of the following management options is most appropriate?

A. Therapeutic lifestyle changes (TLC) only

B. TLC and low-intensity statin

C. TLC and moderate-intensity statin

D. TLC and high-intensity statin

E. TLC and gemfibrozil

R5. A 50-year-old woman with hypertension presents for a routine well-woman examination. Review of her record shows that she had a Pap smear last year that was normal and included a negative test for human papillomavirus (HPV). She had a mammogram 6 months ago that was normal. She has no other chronic conditions besides hypertension, has not had any surgeries, has never smoked cigarettes, and is postmenopausal. For which of the following conditions would you routinely recommend screening at this encounter?

A. Cervical cancer

B. Ovarian cancer

C. Colon cancer

D. Osteoporosis

E. Lung cancer

R6. A 2-year-old girl is brought into the office by her mother for a routine well-child visit. This is the first time that you have seen her. Per her mom, the child has had no significant medical illnesses and is up-to-date on her vaccinations. Mom is concerned because she thinks that the child looks "cross-eyed" when she is showing her pictures in a book or watching TV. On examination, the child has appropriate growth and development for a 2-year-old. Careful examination of her eyes shows that the light reflex off of her corneas is not symmetric when you hold a pen light in front of her. When you cover and then uncover her right eye the light reflex on the left eye does not change. When you cover the left eye, the light reflex appears to move more central on the right cornea. When you uncover the left eye, the light reflex moves laterally on the right cornea and is central on the left. Which of the following should be your recommendation to the mother at this time?

A. We should refer to the child to a pediatric ophthalmologist at this time.

B. This is common in 2-year-olds and will get better as the child gets older.

C. She should hold her picture books to the child's right side to try to improve her rightward gaze.

D. The child will most likely require surgery to correct this problem.

E. No intervention is needed at this time but the child will likely need glasses when she starts school.

R7. A 24-year-old woman comes in for prenatal care at 10 weeks' gestation of her first pregnancy. Which of the following would be appropriate counseling to provide to her?

A. She should avoid sexual activity as it may precipitate early labor.

B. She should not have any x-rays during her pregnancy because of the risk to the fetus from ionizing radiation.

C. She should delay any vaccinations until the postpartum period.

D. She may use any over-the-counter medicine, if needed, as they are safe during pregnancy.

E. She should be screened for gestational diabetes at 24 to 28 weeks' gestation.

R8. A 40-year-old woman presents complaining of feeling a lump in her neck that has slowly enlarged over the past year. She has no pain in the area and no trouble swallowing. She denies palpitations, weight gain, weight loss, changes in her skin or hair. On examination you feel a nontender nodule in the left lobe of the thyroid. An ultrasound shows a 2.5-cm solid nodule in the thyroid and normal thyroid function tests. Which of the following is the next step in the evaluation?

A. Biopsy of the nodule

B. Nuclear medicine thyroid scan

C. Computed tomography (CT) scan on the neck

D. Referral for thyroidectomy

E. Careful observation with repeat blood tests and ultrasound in 6 months to assess for change

R9. A 62-year-old woman presents with 1 week of low back pain. She had no specific injury but stated that the pain started a day after she planted her vegetable garden, which she has done for many years without problem. She has no history of back problems in the past. The pain is mostly in the left lower back and gets worse when she bends forward. She has no neurologic symptoms, no fever, no weight loss, and otherwise feels well. Her general examination and vital signs are normal. She has left-sided paraspinal tenderness but no midline tenderness. She has limited forward flexion and rotation, but normal extension of her back. Straight leg raise test is negative, lower extremity reflexes are symmetric, and lower extremity strength testing is normal. Which of the following interventions would be appropriate at this time?

A. X-ray of the lumbar spine

B. Referral for physical therapy

C. Recommendation for 3 to 5 days of bed rest

D. Narcotic pain medication at bedtime to help her sleep

E. Recommendation to perform her normal daily activities

R10. A 2-year-old boy is brought in to your office as a new patient for the evaluation of a cough and fever. Your history and examination are consistent with a viral upper respiratory infection and you counsel the parent appropriately. However, you note that during the encounter, the child does not interact with you or his mother. He seems extremely focused on the toy motorcycle in his hands. On questioning, his mother notes that he is often sitting by himself with the motorcycle in his hands and doesn't interact much with other children. He has not yet started talking but she thinks that it is because he is "confused," as the family speaks both English and Spanish at home, so he doesn't know which words to use. Along with arranging for a hearing assessment, you also advise which of the following?

A. Comprehensive developmental screening

B. Reassurance that children from multilingual households often do develop speech at later ages, so this is likely normal

C. Assessment by child protective services for child abuse and neglect

D. Taking the toy motorcycle away to direct him to interact with others around him

E. Speaking only English or Spanish at home to reduce his language confusion

R11. A 7-month-old male infant is brought in for his first well-child examination. His mother says that she never brought him to the doctor because they didn't have insurance and he was doing fine at home. She said that he had a vaccine in the hospital on the day after he was born but otherwise has had no vaccines. Which of the following vaccines would be contraindicated in this child?

A. Hepatitis B

B. Influenza

C. Pneumococcal conjugate

D. Rotavirus

E. Inactivated polio virus

R12. A 24-year-old G_0P_0 woman presents for a pregnancy test. She has not had a menstrual period for 4 months. She has a history of chronically irregular menstrual cycles since menarche. She usually gets her period every 3 months and sometimes will go 6 months in between periods. On examination, she is a comfortable appearing obese woman. Her body mass index (BMI) is 41 kg/m² and her blood pressure is 138/90 mm Hg. She has some visible dark hair growth on her chin. The remainder of her general examination is normal and a urine pregnancy test is negative. Which of the following is required for you to make the diagnosis of polycystic ovarian syndrome (PCOS) in this case?

A. A pelvic ultrasound showing 12 or more follicular cysts.

B. Elevated serum estrogen level.

C. Elevated serum androgen level.

D. Menstrual bleeding induced after taking oral medroxyprogesterone for 10 days.

E. No further testing is needed for this diagnosis.

R13. An 80-year-old man is brought in by his daughter out of concern for problems with his hearing. He has worn hearing aids for several years in both ears but she says that his hearing has become acutely worse in his right ear in the past 3 weeks. She had the battery in the hearing aid replaced and it seems to be functioning normally. She is requesting a referral to an audiologist for repeat testing for her father. What is the most likely cause of this acute hearing reduction?

A. Presbycusis

B. Cerumen impaction

C. Hearing aid failure

D. Stroke

E. Brain tumor impinging on the eighth cranial nerve

R14. A 36-year-old G_2P_2 woman presents to discuss options for contraception. She isn't sure if she wants to have more children but wants to keep that as an option. She is generally healthy but smokes a pack of cigarettes per day and is not ready to stop. She says that, if possible, she wants something that would be very effective and that she wouldn't have to remember to use for it to be effective. Which of the following would be her best option?

A. Combined oral contraceptive pills (OCPs)

B. Progesterone-only "mini-pills"

C. Subdermal, etonogestrel-secreting implant

D. Tubal ligation with the option of reversal

E. Natural family planning

R15. A 48-year-old woman with chronic migraine headaches presents for an acute visit because she is having what she describes as the "worst migraine" she's ever had. She states that her migraines are usually very typical—one-sided throbbing pain, nausea, and photophobia that resolve after she uses her sumatriptan. She states that this headache feels different. It came on suddenly, is "15 out of 10" in intensity, involves her whole head, and even her neck hurts. On examination, she is lying very still on the examination table with the lights off. She can flex and extend her neck with some increase in her pain. She has no papilledema but doesn't like having the examination light shined in her eyes. Her neurologic examination is otherwise nonfocal. At this point you recommend which of the following?

A. Recommend giving herself another dose of sumatriptan, as she may be becoming resistant to the medication after being on it for many years.

B. Give her a shot of IM meperidine (Demerol) in the office to see if you can reduce the headache intensity.

C. Order an outpatient magnetic resonance imaging (MRI) of her head, with follow-up in 3 days.

D. Order an urgent outpatient CT scan of the head with follow-up in the clinic tomorrow.

E. Refer her immediately to the emergency room.

ANSWERS

R1. **D. A random plasma glucose of 220 mg/dL and symptomatic polyuria**

There are four diagnostic criteria for the diagnosis of diabetes:

- Fasting plasma glucose of 126 mg/dL or greater
- Hemoglobin A_{1c} of 6.5% or greater
- Plasma glucose of 200 mg/dL or greater 2 hours after a 75-g glucose challenge
- Random plasma glucose of 200 or greater and typical symptoms of hyperglycemia (polyuria, polyphagia, or polydipsia)

When possible, the result should be repeated to confirm the diagnosis (Case 51). In this question, only option D meets any of these criteria.

R2. **B.** In the absence of any contraindication, **metformin** should be the first-line treatment for type 2 diabetes in most cases. Studies have shown an improvement in outcomes, including mortality, in those taking metformin. It also does not induce hypoglycemia and is generally well tolerated. The safety, efficacy, and outcomes data generally make it the initial treatment of choice (Case 51).

R3.   **A. Amlodipine, a calcium channel blocker is the best choice.** According to the Eighth Joint National Committee (JNC 8) recommendations for treatment of hypertension, thiazide diuretics, angiotensin-converting enzyme inhibitors, angiotensin receptor blockers, and calcium channel blockers are the generally recommended initial medications for most patients with hypertension. The JNC 8 recommendations do state that **thiazide diuretics or calcium channel blockers are likely to be more effective than other medications in African Americans,** therefore amlodipine, a calcium channel blocker, would be the best choice out of the options provided (Case 30).

R4.   **D. TLC and high-intensity statin** should be initiated. The American College of Cardiology/American Heart Association guidelines for the management of hyperlipidemia recommend the use of β-hydroxy-β-methylglutaryl-coenzyme A (HMG-CoA) reductase inhibitors ("statins") as the appropriate treatment for hyperlipidemia in the following settings:

1. Anyone under the age of 75 with established atherosclerotic cardiovascular disease should be on high-intensity statin therapy.

2. Anyone with LDL cholesterol greater than 190 mg/dL should be on a high-intensity statin.

3. Anyone between the age of 40 and 75 with a 10-year atherosclerotic cardiovascular disease (ASCVD) risk of 7.5% or greater should be on a high-intensity statin.

4. All diabetics age 40 to 75 with an LDL of 70 mg/dL or greater should be on a statin. Moderate-intensity statins can be used if the calculated 10-year ASCVD risk is less than 7.5%; high-intensity statin should be used if the 10-year risk is 7.5% or greater.

See Case 35 for further discussion of hyperlipidemia as well as discussion of other guidelines and recommendations.

R5.   **C. Colon cancer screening.** The United States Preventive Services Task Force recommends colon cancer screening for all persons age 50 and above. This patient is up-to-date on her cervical cancer screening so she does not need that at this visit. Osteoporosis screening would routinely be recommended at the age of 65. Ovarian cancer screening in asymptomatic women is not recommended and lung cancer screening is only recommended in those with a history of smoking cigarettes (Cases 1 and 11)

R6.   **A. Referral to a pediatric ophthalmologist.** Examination of the eyes and vision screening is an important part of routine well-child care. Eye examinations should start in the newborn nursery. Children usually have a conjugate gaze by the time they are about 6 months old. This child is showing signs of strabismus, a misalignment of the eyes. Strabismus is the most common cause of amblyopia, an impairment of vision in one of the eyes. Children with suspected strabismus should be referred to a pediatric ophthalmologist as soon as the condition is suspected for evaluation and management. While surgery is sometimes necessary to correct the problem, this is not common. See Case 5 for further review of well-child care.

R7.   **E.** Counseling and anticipatory guidance are very important components of routine prenatal care. Case 4 discusses prenatal care in detail. The American College of Obstetricians and Gynecologists, along with the United States Preventive Services Task Force, recommend the routing screening of pregnant women for gestational diabetes at 24 to 28 weeks' gestation, as the identification and management of gestational diabetes can improve outcomes. There is no evidence that sexual activity may precipitate early labor in normal pregnancy, although there are some conditions in which counseling to avoid sexual activity may be warranted. X-rays during pregnancy may be done when the benefit of the x-ray outweighs the risk. Shielding of the pregnant abdomen would be recommended, when possible. While live virus vaccines should be delayed, other vaccines are not contraindicated during pregnancy. Influenza vaccine and tetanus, diphtheria, and acellular pertussis vaccines are recommended routinely. Finally, pregnant women should be advised to discuss the use of all medications, including over-the-counter, with their physician prior to use.

R8.   **A. Biopsy of the nodule.** About 5% to 6% of solitary thyroid nodules are malignant. The workup of a thyroid nodule should include an assessment of thyroid functioning by thyroid stimulating hormone (TSH) level and an ultrasound to assess the size of the nodule. A patient with a normal or reduced thyroid functioning (ie, normal or high TSH) and a thyroid nodule 1 cm in size or larger should have the nodule biopsied to assess for malignancy. Hyperfunctioning nodules (low TSH) are usually benign adenomas that are assessed with a radioactive iodine uptake study (Case 15).

R9.   **E. Normal activities.** This case is a very typical case of acute low back pain that is likely due to lumbosacral strain. This patient has no "red-flag" signs or symptoms that would warrant immediate imaging studies, such as numbness/tingling down the leg. The treatment of this common condition includes the use of anti-inflammatory medications, heat, and early mobility. Bed rest should be avoided and narcotic pain medications have shown no benefits in this setting. Physical therapy may have some short-term benefits but studies have not shown long-term benefit (Case 53).

R10.   **A. Developmental evaluation.** While not diagnostic, this child's behavior, lack of interaction with others, and speech delay are very concerning for autism spectrum disorders or other possible developmental conditions. While children in multilingual households may have some mild delays in speech at young ages, the lack of speaking any words at the age of 2 is a significant red flag that should lead to further testing. This testing should include both an assessment of hearing and a comprehensive developmental assessment (Case 54).

R11. **D. Rotavirus vaccine is contraindicated.** The evaluation and provision of vaccines is an important part of the scope of the family physician for patients of all ages. Key considerations include knowing both which vaccines are indicated and which, if any, are contraindicated for a specific patient. In this case, the rotavirus vaccine is contraindicated. Rotavirus should not be initiated after the age of 15 weeks per Centers for Disease Control and Prevention (CDC) schedule, because there is insufficient data about its safety in older infants. All other vaccines can be given and "catch-up" schedules provided by the CDC should be followed (Case 5).

R12. **E. No further diagnostic testing is needed.** This patient has evidence of PCOS clinically and meets the Rotterdam criteria for the diagnosis without further testing. The Rotterdam criteria are as follows:

- Hyperandrogenism, evidenced by hirsutism or elevated serum androgen levels (eg, testosterone, androstenedione, or dehydroepiandrosterone [DHEA])
- Oligomenorrhea with cycle length greater than or equal to 35 days
- Multifollicular ovaries on pelvic ultrasound, defined as 12 or greater small follicles in an ovary

Her evidence of hirsutism and oligomenorrhea are enough to meet the diagnostic criteria. Other causes of hyperandrogenism should be considered such as hypothyroidism and late-onset congenital adrenal hyperplasia. Management would include working with her to try to lose weight, consideration of the use of medroxyprogesterone or combined contraceptives to regularize her menses and consideration of the use of metformin or a thiazolidinedione agent to reduce insulin resistance (Cases 33 and 50).

R13. **B. Cerumen impaction is the most likely cause.** Presbycusis is the most common cause of hearing reduction in the elderly population. It is a progressive condition and is a diagnosis of exclusion. This patient has acute unilateral hearing reduction and is most likely caused by a cerumen impaction, an often overlooked condition. Examination of the external auditory canal may show near-complete, or complete, blockage with wax. Removal of the wax will often return the patient to his baseline level of hearing. See Case 18 for further review of common issues in the geriatric population.

R14. **C.** Of the options provided, the **subdermal implant** ("**Nexplanon**") would likely be her best option. Both combined and progestin-only OCPs require regular compliance to be effective. The combined OCPs are also relatively contraindicated in a woman over the age of 35 who smokes. A bilateral tubal ligation would be appropriate if she desired permanent contraception. While these can sometimes be reversed, if she has not yet made up her mind for permanent contraception, this would not be recommended. Natural family planning is less effective than other methods and does require effort on the part of the woman to be as effective as possible (Case 28).

R15.   **E. Direct referral to the emergency center, preferably by ambulance.** This patient has the acute onset of the worst headache of her life that is significantly different from her chronic migraine headaches. She is giving classic symptoms that are concerning for a **subarachnoid hemorrhage (SAH)**. Every minute of delay with SAH means the potential for brain tissue damage. Thus, this is a neurologic emergency! While she does have a history of migraines, it is important not to ascribe any headache that she has to migraines and it is important not to miss the red flags that should require urgent or emergent evaluation (Case 34).

INDEX

Page numbers followed by *f* or *t* indicate figures or tables, respectively.

adult male health maintenance
  analysis, 22
  case study, 21
  clinical approach, 23–24
  clinical pearls, 28
  comprehension questions, 27–28
  healthy lifestyle for, 26–27
  immunizations, 22, 26
  screening tests, 22, 24–25
Adult Treatment Panel (ATP), 354, 377
  on obesity, 354
advance directives, 200
advanced maternal age, 51, 52
adverse drug reactions and interactions
  adverse drug effects, 572
  analysis, 570–571
  Beers list, 571, 572
  case study, 569
  clinical approach, 572–574
  clinical pearls, 576
  comprehension questions, 575–576
  definitions, 571–572
  drug metabolism, 573–574
  etiologies, 572–573
  interventions to reduce risk of adverse drug
    effects, 574
  renal interactions, 573–574
  STOPP/START criteria, 572–573
  synergistic effects, 572
Advisory Committee on Immunization Practices
    (ACIP), 256, 318
age-related macular degeneration (AMD), 196
AHA. *See* American Heart Association
AHI. *See* apnea hypopnea index
AIDS. *See* HIV/AIDS
airway, breathing, circulation (ABCs), 475, 479
airway obstruction, 418–419
alanine aminotransferase (ALT), 507
alcohol abuse and misuse, 25, 444t, 447t, 507. *See
    also* substance abuse
  dementia and, 346–347
aldosterone antagonists, 294
alirocumab, 382t
allergic disorders
  allergic rhinitis, 77–81
  analysis, 76
  anaphylaxis, urticaria, and angioedema, 81
  background, 77
  case study, 75
  clinical approach, 77–79
  clinical pearls, 83
  comprehension questions, 82–83
  conjunctivitis, 82
  definitions, 77
  history, 77–78
  house dust mites and animals, 79–80
  large local allergic reactions, 467
  occupational rhinitis, 78
  pathophysiology, 77
  perennial rhinitis, 78, 79
  physical examination, 78–79

  pollens and, 79
  seasonal rhinitis, 78, 79
  symptoms, 78
allergic rhinitis
  causes, 79–80
  definition, 77
  pathophysiology, 77–78
  symptoms, 78
  treatment, 80–81
Alli. *See* orlistat
almotriptan, 369t
alosetron (Lotronex), 431
ALT. *See* alanine aminotransferase
Alzheimer disease
  antipsychotics and, 345
  criteria for probable, 344t
  dementia and, 344–346, 344t, 345t
  depression and, 344–345
  diagnosis, 344–345
  evaluation, 344
  medication used for, 345t
AMA. *See* American Medical Association
amantidine, 602
amblyopia, 63
ambulatory electrocardiographic rhythm monitor-
    ing, 458
AMD. *See* age-related macular degeneration
amelanotic melanoma, 142
amenorrhea, 280, 549
American Academy of Pediatrics (AAP), 63–64,
    68, 318
American Academy of Sleep Medicine (AASM),
    626–627
American Association of Clinical Endocrinologists
    (AACE), 558
American College of Rheumatology/European
    League Against Rheumatism (ACR/EULAR),
    43, 44t
American Heart Association (AHA), 68, 291,
    292–293
  guidelines for treating cholesterol, 380t
American Medical Association (AMA),
    318–319, 320
American Urological Association (AUA), 150
amiodarone, 459–460
Amitiza. *See* lubiprostone
amitriptyline (Elavil), 371t, 627t
amlodipine (Norvasc), 294
amniocentesis, 57
amoxapine (Asendin), 627t
amoxicillin, 519t
amphetamines, 442t, 444t
ampicillin, 116, 240t
anabolic steroids, 443t
Anafranil. *See* clomipramine
analogs, 440t, 441t
anaphylaxis, 77, 81
  insect stings and bites, 467–468
anemia
  in children, 66
  of chronic inflammation, 106–108

CHF. *See* congestive heart failure
chicken pox, 527–528
child abuse, 385–387, 389–391, 389*t*
child maltreatment, 387
childhood disintegrative disorder, 593*t*
childhood schizophrenia, 593*t*
children
abdominal pain and vomiting in, 334–339
accidents and injury and, 69
anemia in, 66
asthma classification in, 613*t*
BMI in, 63–64
car seats, 62, 69
dental health of, 68
developmental disorders, 590–596
fever and rash in, 526–534
foreign-body airway obstruction, 418–419
fractures, 399–400
gastrointestinal obstruction, 334–336, 337
high cholesterol/hyperlipidemia in, 68
hypertrophic pyloric stenosis, 335, 336
limping in, 396–404
malrotation with volvulus, 335, 336–337
poisoning, 337
well-child care, 62–72
wheezing and stridor in, 418–426
Chlamydia pneumoniae, 207, 238, 492
chlorpromazine, 370*t*
choking, 418–419
cholesterol, 377–378, 382*t*. *See also* hyperlipidemia
AAFP clinical practice guidelines for cholesterol
management, 381*t*
cholestyramine, 382*t*
chorea, 601
chorionic villus sampling (CVS), 57
chronic bronchitis, 31
chronic cough, 211
chronic daily headache (CHD), 366
chronic diarrhea, 113
chronic kidney disease (CKD)
analysis, 228–229
case study, 227
clinical approach, 229–232
clinical pearls, 234
Cockcroft-Gault equation, 230
comprehension questions, 232–234
definitions, 229
end-stage renal disease, 229
etiologies, 229
evaluation, 229–231
management, 231–232
MDRD, 230
chronic medical conditions, 372
chronic obstructive pulmonary disease (COPD)
analysis, 30–31
case study, 29
cigarette smoking and, 31, 32–33
classification, 33*t*
clinical approach, 31–35
clinical pearls, 37
comprehension questions, 35–36

evaluation, 31–32
management, of exacerbations of COPD,
34–35
management, of stable COPD, 32–34
chronic pain management
analysis, 644–645
assessment, 645–646
case study, 643
clinical approach, 645–647
clinical pearls, 650
comprehension questions, 648–649
definitions, 645
nonpharmacologic management, 646
pharmacologic management, 646–647
chronic renal failure, 380
chronic subdural hematoma, 347
cigarette smoking. *See* tobacco use
ciprofloxacin, 116
citalopram (Celexa), 627*t*
CKD. *See* chronic kidney disease
clarithromycin, 519*t*
clindamycin, 176–177, 240*t*
Clock Test, 343
clomipramine (Anafranil), 627*t*
clonidine, 372*t*, 603
cluster headache, 366, 370, 372
coagulopathies, 277, 550
cocaine, 442*t*, 444*t*
Cockcroft-Gault equation, 230
codeine, 441*t*
cognitive screening, 198
colesevelam, 382*t*
colestipol, 382*t*
colon cancer, 247
colon neoplasms, 247
colorectal cancer, 25
community-acquired pneumonia, 253–254, 255
complete blood counts (CBCs), 23, 475
compressive pain, 645
COMT inhibitors. *See* catechol-O-methyltransferase
inhibitors
condoms, 306
confidentiality
adolescent health maintenance and, 317–318
medical ethics and, 96
teenage pregnancy and, 97–98
congenital hypothyroidism, 64
congestive heart failure (CHF), 653
analysis, 286–287
case study, 285
chest x-rays, 290–291
classification of, 291, 291*t*
clinical approach, 287–292
clinical pearls, 297
comprehension questions, 295–297
definition, 287
diabetes and, 287
dyspnea and, 289
ECGs and, 290
echocardiography for, 291
electrolyte disorders and, 290